DISEASES TRANSMITTED
FROM
ANIMALS TO MAN

Fifth Edition

Diseases Transmitted
from
Animals *to* Man

Compiled and Edited by

Thomas G. Hull, Ph.D.

Contributors

CHARLES ARMSTRONG, M.D.
CARROLL L. BIRCH, M.D.
CHARLES H. BRIDGES, D.V.M., PH.D.
DORSEY W. BRUNER, B.S., D.V.M., PH.D.
CHARLES M. CARPENTER, D.V.M., M.D., PH.D.
DONALD L. COLLINS, PH.D., SC.D.
C. H. CUNNINGHAM, B.S., M.S., D.V.M., PH.D.
G. M. DACK, PH.D., M.D.
GORDON E. DAVIS, S.M., SC.D.
R. E. DYER, M.D.
CARL M. EKLUND, M.D.
ERNEST CARROLL FAUST, PH.D.
WILLIAM H. FELDMAN, D.V.M., M.S., D.SC.
J. H. S. GEAR, M.D.
ROBERT P. HANSON, PH.D.
W. T. HARDY, D.V.M.

WILLIAM T. HUBBERT, D.V.M., M.P.H.
THOMAS G. HULL, PH.D.
WILLIAM L. JELLISON, PH.D.
WILLIAM E. JENNINGS, D.V.M.
ALFRED G., KARLSON, D.V.M., PH.D.
KARL F. MEYER, D.V.M., M.D.,
  PH.D., SC.D., L.L.D.
ERSKINE V. MORSE, D.V.M., PH.D.
CORA RUST OWEN, PH.D.
RUDOLPH D. RADELEFF, D.V.M.
KARL R. REINHARD, D.V.M., PH.D.
HOWARD J. SHAUGHNESSY, PH.D.
CLARENCE D. STEIN, V.M.D.
ERNEST S. TIERKEL, V.M.D., M.P.H.
WARREN J. WARWICK, M.D.
TELFORD H. WORK, M.D.

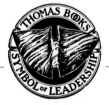

CHARLES C THOMAS · PUBLISHER
Springfield · Illinois · U.S.A.

Published and Distributed Throughout the World by

CHARLES C THOMAS • PUBLISHER

BANNERSTONE HOUSE

301-327 East Lawrence Avenue, Springfield, Illinois, U.S.A.

First Edition, January, 1930
Second Edition, February, 1941
Third Edition, March, 1947
Fourth Edition, January, 1955
Fifth Edition, October, 1963

Printed in the United States of America

U-6

LIST OF CONTRIBUTORS

ARMSTRONG, CHARLES, M.D.: *Medical Director Retired, United States Public Health Service.*

BIRCH, CARROLL L., M.D.: *Professor of Medicine, University of Illinois, College of Medicine, Chicago, Illinois.*

BRIDGES, CHARLES H., D.V.M., PhD.: *Head, Department of Veterinary Pathology, School of Veterinary Medicine, Agricultural and Mechanical College of Texas, College Station, Texas.*

BRUNER, DORSEY, W., B.S., D.V.M., PH.D.: *Professor of Veterinary Bacteriology, New York State Veterinary College, Cornell University, Ithaca, New York.*

CARPENTER, CHARLES M., D.V.M., M.D., PHD.: *Professor of Infectious Diseases, and Chairman of the Department of Infectious Diseases, School of Medicine, University of California, Los Angeles, California.*

COLLINS, DONALD L., PH.D., SC.D.: *Principal Scientist and State Entomologist, Biological Survey, New York State Museum and Science Service, University of the State of New York, Albany, New York.*

CUNNINGHAM, C. H., B.S., M.S., D.V.M., PH.D.: *Professor of Microbiology and Public Health, College of Veterinary Medicine, Michigan State University, East Lansing, Michigan.*

DACK, G. M., PH.D., M.D.: *Director, Food Research Institute and Professor of Microbiology, The University of Chicago, Chicago, Illinois.*

DAVIS, GORDON E., S.M., SC.D.: *Formerly, Principal Medical Bacteriologist, U. S. Department of Health, Education and Welfare, Public Health Service, National Institutes of Health, National Institute of Allergy and Infectious Diseases, Rocky Mountain Laboratory, Hamilton, Montana. Present address Campton, New Hampshire.*

DYER, R. E., M.D.: *Clinical Professor of Medicine, School of Medicine, Emory University, Atlanta, Georgia.*

EKLUND, CARL M., M.D.: *Medical Virologist, Rocky Mountain Laboratory, National Institute of Allergy and Infectious Diseases, Public Health Service, United States Department of Health, Education and Welfare, Hamilton, Montana.*

FAUST, ERNEST CARROLL, PH.D.: *Department of Tropical Medicine and Public Health, Tulane University, New Orleans, Louisiana.*

FELDMAN, WILLIAM H., D.V.M., M.S., D.SC.: *Chief, Laboratory Research in Pulmonary Diseases, Medical Service, Department of Mediicne and Surgery, Veterans Administration, Washington D. C. Emeritus Staff, Mayo Clinic and Mayo Foundation, Rochester, Minnesota.*

GEAR, J. H. S., M.D.: *Director, South African Institute for Medical Research, Johannesburg, South Africa.*

HANSON, ROBERT P., PH.D.: *Professor, Department of Veterinary Science and Department of Bacteriology, University of Wisconsin, Madison, Wisconsin.*

HARDY, W. T., D.V.M.: *Superintendent, Ranch Experiment Station, Texas Agricultural Experiment Station, Sonora, Texas*

HUBBERT, WILLIAM T., D.V.M., M.P.H.: *Department of Infectious Diseases, School of Medicine, University of California, Los Angeles, California.*

HULL, THOMAS G., PH.D.: *Associate Professor of Prevntive Medicine, Emeritus, University of Illinois, College of Medicine. Retired as Secretary, Council on Scientific Assembly, American Medical Association. Formerly, Chief, Division of Laboratories, Illinois Department of Public Health. Present Address, Yarmouth Port, Massachusetts.*

JELLISON, WILLIAM L., PH.D.: *Parsitologist, Rocky Mountain Laboratory, National Institute of Allergy and Infectious Diseases, National Institutes of Health, Public Health Service, United States Department of Health, Education and Welfare, Hamilton, Montana.*

JENNINGS, WILLIAM E., D.V.M.: *Colonel, Veterinary Corps, United States Army, Retired. Director, Meat Inspection Service, New York State Department of Agriculture and Markets, Albany, New York*

KARLSON, ALFRED G., D.V.M., PH.D.: *Consultant, Section of Microbiology, Mayo Clinic. Professor of Comparative Pathology, Mayo Foundation, Graduate School, University of Minnesota, Rochester, Minnesota.*

MEYER, KARL F., D.V.M., M.D., PH.D., SC.D., L.L.D.: *George Williams Hooper Foundation, University of California Medical Center, San Francisco, California.*

MORSE, ERSKINE V., D.V.M., PH.D.: *Profesor of Veterinary Microbiology and Dean of the School of Veterinary Science and Medicine, Purdue University, Lafayette, Indiana.*

OWEN, CORA RUST, PH.D.: *Bacteriologist, Rocky Mountain Laboratory, National Institute of Allergy and Infectious Diseases, National Institutes of Health, Public Health Service, United States Department of Health, Education and Welfare, Hamilton, Montana.*

RADELEFF, RUDOLPH D., D.V.M.: *Veterinarian in Charge, Animal Disease and Parasite Research Division, Agricultural Research Service, United States Department of Agriculture, Kerrville, Texas.*

REINHARD, KARL R., D.V.M., PH.D.: *Executive Secretary, General Medicine Study Section, National Institutes of Health, Public Health Service, United States Department of Health, Education and Welfare.*

SHAUGHNESSY, HOWARD J., PH.D.: *Chief, Division of Laboratories, Illinois Department of Public Health and Professor of Public Health, University of Illinois, College of Medicine, Chicago, Illinois.*

STEIN, CLARENCE D., V.M.D.: *Animal Diseases and Parasitic Research Branch, Agricultural Research Service, United States Department of Agriculture, Washington, D.C.*

TIERKEL, ERNEST S., V.M.D., M.P.H.: *Chief, Rabies Control Program, Veterinary Public Health Section, Communicable Diseases Center, Public Health Service, United States Department of Health, Education and Welfare, Atlanta, Georgia.*

WARWICK, WARREN J., M.D.: *Assistant Professor of Pediatrics, Department of Pediatrics, University of Minnesota Medical School, Minneapolis, Minnesota.*

WORK, TELFORD H., M.D.: *Chief, Virology Section, Communicable Disease Center, Public Health Service, United States Department of Health, Education and Welfare, Atlanta, Georgia.*

FOREWORD TO THE FIFTH EDITION

Since the first edition of this book was prepared some thirty-five years ago there has been a vast change in the zoonoses. At that time zoonosis was described as a "disease produced by animal parasites" (*The American Illustrated Medical Dictionary*, Dorland 1929). Since that time the field has broadened to include all animal diseases which might be transmitted to man. Zoonoses centers have sprung up in various parts of this country as well as elsewhere.

Thirty-two authors have each contributed one or more chapters to the fifth edition. Considerable freedom was given the different authors in the preparation of their respective subjects, and in the emphasis which they placed upon the various factors concerning the transmission of infection from animals to man. This was necessary in a work covering so many diverse fields.

It is hoped that the veterinarian, the physician, the health official and the research worker may find a common meeting ground in the work here presented. While each is engaged in a different phase of the problem and views the subject from a different angle, it will be through their concerted efforts that the number of infections which man contracts from animals will be reduced.

Appreciation is expressed to the various contributors to the fifth edition as well as to those who have contributed to previous editions and whose work may be carried over to some extent in the present edition. I also wish to thank the publisher and his assistants for their patience during a very grevious period. Especially I wish to thank Dr. William L. Jellison for his continued interest in the work and for his numerous suggestions. I wish also to express appreciation to my wife for her assistance in many ways.

THOMAS G. HULL

Yarmouth Port, Massachusetts

CONTENTS

SECTION ONE

DISEASES OF DOMESTIC ANIMALS AND BIRDS AND OCCASIONALLY OF WILD ANIMALS AND RODENTS

SECTION TWO

DISEASES OF RODENTS AND WILD ANIMALS AND OCCASIONALLY OF DOMESTIC ANIMALS

SECTION THREE

THE RELATION OF HUMAN AND ANIMAL DISEASES

LIST OF ILLUSTRATIONS

List of Illustrations

TABLES

DISEASES TRANSMITTED
FROM
ANIMALS TO MAN

SECTION ONE

**DISEASES OF DOMESTIC ANIMALS
AND BIRDS
AND OCCASIONALLY OF
WILD ANIMALS AND RODENTS**

Chapter 1

TUBERCULOSIS

WILLIAM H. FELDMAN, M.Sc., D.V.M., D.Sc. (HON.)

THE ABILITY of the respective pathogenic species of the genus *Mycobacterium* to infect one or more heterologous hosts makes tuberculosis in any species of animals a potential threat to the other species, including human beings. In fact, the transmissibility of tuberculous infections to other than natural hosts constitutes one of the most important problems in the control of this ubiquitous disease. That *Mycobacterium bovis,* the cause of bovine tuberculosis, is capable of infecting a diversity of species, such as swine, cats, dogs, canaries, parrots, and human beings, emphasizes the necessity of a comprehensive plan if tuberculosis is to be eradicated or even successfully controlled. Likewise, *Myco. tuberculosis,* the human type of the tubercle bacillus, is capable of inducing tuberculosis in cattle, swine, dogs, and parrots. The organism of avian tuberculosis *(Myco. avium),* in addition to being pathogenic for most birds, is capable of causing widespread destructive tuberculosis in swine and sheep. In addition, *Myco. avium* is capable of sensitizing cattle to diagnostic doses of mammalian tuberculin, thus frequently complicating the interpretation of a positive tuberculin test. These facts make it evident that to eliminate tuberculosis in one species and ignore the disease in others is not likely to solve the larger problem. The disease may exist in heterologous hosts in which the presence of tubercule bacilli constitutes a potential source of new infection, perhaps for natural hosts.

The natural occurrence of tuberculosis in most of the warm-blooded mammals and fowls and in such cold-blooded animals as alligators, iguanas, turtles, frogs, fish, fresh-water snails, and snakes, makes it evident that few, if any, species of animals have an absolute resistance to the disease.*

Those confronted with the multiplicity of problems which so uniquely characterize tuberculosis should be familiar with the different types of the causative agent, their natural, as well as their heterologous hosts, and the means of differentiating one type from the others.

ETIOLOGIC AGENT†

The causative agents responsible for tuberculosis belong to the genus *Mycobacterium* and are single-celled, rod-shaped micro-organisms that when properly stained have the distinctive characteristic of retaining the stain in the presence of acids diluted in alcohol. This acid-alcohol-fast property, although possessed by certain molds and actinomyces, constitutes the most distinguishing feature of the bacteria that are known generally as tubercle bacilli and are responsible for tuberculous disease in various species of animals, including human beings.

The genus *Mycobacterium* may be conveniently divided into three categories: 1) species that are pathogenic for warm-blooded animals, 2) species that are parasitic and pathogenic for cold-blooded animals, and 3) species that are saprophytic. The saprophytic species are widely distributed in nature, especially in soil, and are of importance to the student of tuberculosis, since they may be confused with pathogenic species of mycobacteria. Since we are concerned here primarily with tuberculosis as it affects warm-blooded animals, we may limit our consideration of the genus *Mycobacterium* to the following species: *Mycobacterium tuberculosis,* the natural host of which is human beings; *Mycobacterium*

---

*Those especially interested in the older literature of tuberculosis of animals should consult the comprehensive review by Eber (1917). This report lists a total of 1,677 papers published during the period of 1905 to 1914. The material in Chapter XX in Calmette's (1923) text is also of value. For a recent treatise on tuberculosis of animals, the admirable text by Francis (1958) is recommended. For a resumé, in the German language, of tuberculosis in domesticated and wild animals, the monograph of Pallaske provides a source of valuable information (1961).

†For those interested in detailed descriptions of the various species of the genus Mycobacterium that are pathogenic for warm-blooded animals, the following may be consulted: Smith (1905), Griffith and Munro (1944), Hagan and Bruner (1951), Rich (1951). Wilson and Miles (1955) and Middlebrook and Dubos (1958).

bovis, the natural host of which is cattle; and *Mycobacterium avium,* the natural host of which is gallinaceous birds.*

Although the three "types" of tubercle bacilli have certain biologic and morphologic features in common, there are other characteristics which distinguish each from the other two. These distinguishing characteristics are observed in the cultural behavior of the three types, by tests of pathogenicity, and to a lessor extent, by antigenic differences. Distinctions based on alleged morphologic characteristics of the three bacillary types of the tubercle bacillus observed microscopically do not constitute dependable criteria for identification of the respective types.

The essential physical characteristics of the three bacillary types of the tubercle bacillus, when initially cultured on solid mediums, may be summarized as follows:

HUMAN TYPE *(Myco. tuberculosis)*—This species is glycerophilic. Colonies are greyish ivory. The culture is dry, crumbly, and cauliflower-like. The growth is membranous, has a roughened surface, and may be luxuriant.

BOVINE TYPE *(Myco. bovis)*—Most strains on initial isolation are nonglycerophilic. They grow much more slowly than the human type; the culture is of a more delicate character, moist, glistening, and slimy. Growth is seldom luxuriant, and the organism is nonchromogenic on initial isolation.

AVIAN TYPE *(Myco. avium)*—The culture is moist, unctuous, and slimy. The growth is luxuriant. The rate of growth is relatively rapid when compared with the slow growth of the two mammalian types. This species grows well both with and without glycerin, and eventually the culture becomes ochroid.

The mycobacteria responsible for tuberculosis in man, cattle, and fowl are strictly aerobic. The organisms grow well in mediums con-

---

*In 1937, Wells of England reported a disease of wild voles *(Microtus agrestis),* which is due to a previously undescribed acid-fast bacillus. The disease produced by this organism resembles tuberculosis closely, and Brooke (1941) suggested *Mycobacterium tuberculosis* var. *muris* as a suitable name. The organism is avirulent for guinea pigs and rabbits in moderate doses, and so far as is known, it is of no significance in the production of tuberculosis in the higher mammals, including human beings. Additional information regarding the relationship of the vole bacillus to other pathogenic acid-fast bacilli has been contributed by Brooke. The presently accepted designation of this organism is *Myco. muris.*

taining egg yolk or potato. The optimal temperature for the growth of human and bovine types of tubercle bacilli is 37.5° C.; the avian type grows best at 40° C. An important distinguishing feature between *Myco. tuberculosis* and *Myco. bovis* is the ability of the former to produce an appreciable amount of niacin. A relatively simple test to demonstrate this substance was proposed by Konno (1956).

The physical appearance of the three types of tubercle bacilli, when grown on solid mediums, are illustrated in Figure 1. Other essential differences between the human, bovine, and avian species of tubercle bacilli are summarized in Table 1.

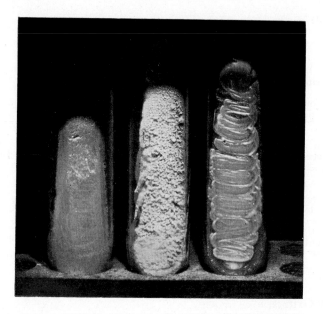

Fig. 1. Slant cultures representative of three types of *Mycobaterium tuberculosis*. From left to right the types are bovine, human and avian. (From Feldman, W. H.: *Avian tuberculosis infections*. (Baltimore, Willams & Wilkins Company, 1938.)

DETERMINATION OF TYPE

As mentioned previously, the physical characteristics of typical human, bovine, and avian strains of tubercle bacilli vary sufficiently under proper conditions of artificial cultivation to provide important criteria for at least preliminary classification. As has been

TABLE 1

SUMMARY OF IMPORTANT DIFFERENCES BETWEEN AVIAN, HUMAN, AND BOVINE TYPES
OF TUBERCLE BACILLI

Characteristic	Avian	Human	Bovine
Growth in liquid medium	Pellicle formation with crumbly granular growth at bottom	Pellicle formation with growth limited to surface	Pellicle formation with growth limited to surface
Miscibility with saline solution	Suspension easy. Organisms uniformly distributed	Suspension difficult. Organisms form clumps	Suspension difficult. Organisms form clumps
Tuberculin sensitivity	More intense for homologous than for heterologous tuberculin	More intense for mammalian than for avian tuberculin	More intense for mammalian than for avian tuberculin
Pathogenicity*	Virulent for chickens and rabbits. Slightly pathogenic for guinea pigs	Nonpathogenic for chickens. Markedly virulent for guinea pigs but only slightly so for rabbits	Nonpathogenic for chickens. Markedly virulent for guinea pigs and rabbits
In vitro sensitivity** to:			
(a) Streptomycin	Resistant†	Susceptible	Susceptible
(b) Isoniazide	Resistant†	Susceptible	Susceptible
(c) PAS	Resistant†	Variable	Susceptible
Test for:			
(a) Niacin	Negative	Positive	Negative
(b) Catalase	Positive	Positive‡	Positive‡
(c) Peroxidase	Variable	Positive‡	Positive‡

*When testing tubercle bacilli for pathogenicity, chickens and rabbits should be inoculated intravenously; guinea pigs, subcutaneously. Only tuberculin-negative chickens should be used.
**On initial isolation.
†Resistant to 10 mu or more.
‡Positive when INH susceptible, but this activity is lost at very low levels of resistance.

shown by Griffith and Munro (1944), by Stadnichenko, Sweany, and Kloeck (1945), and others, it is possible, by the use of glycerinated and nonglycerinated mediums, to differentiate with relative accuracy the bovine and human types of tubercle bacilli. Most bovine strains do not grow on initial isolation on mediums containing more than 0.75 per cent of glycerin, whereas the human type of the organism prospers on mediums containing 2 to 3 per cent of glycerin. This feature is of significance in distinguishing the two types by cultural methods. For this reason, all clinical materials suspected of containing bovine tubercle bacilli should be cultured on both glycerinated and nonglycerinated mediums.

Strains of tubercle bacilli, classified as avian, human, or bovine as a result of cultural differences and physical appearance, must be subjected to tests of virulence in suitable laboratory animals (guinea pigs, rabbits, chickens) if unequivocal proof of bacillary type is to be established. It must be recognized, however, that occasionally strains are encountered that do not possess the requisite characteristics to permit definitive classification. Such strains frequently have the physical appearance of one or the other of the recognized types of tubercle bacilli but fail to express the degree of virulence for rabbits, guinea pigs, or chickens that is necessary to establish their identity. These mycobacteria must be considered either as having reduced virulence or as representing unclassified members of the genus *Mycobacterium,* and their identity may be difficult to determine by present methods.*

The procedure for determining the type of tubercle bacilli by tests for virulence requires that young cultures be used, representing, if possible, the growth obtained on initial isolation. A weighed amount of the culture should be evenly suspended in sterile physiologic solution of sodium chloride.† For convenience in making subsequent dilutions, the volume should be adjusted so that 1 cc. of the suspension represents 1 mg. of bacteria. From the original suspension, dilutions containing 0.1 mg. and 0.01 mg. are prepared.

The standard test animals for typing tubercle bacilli are guinea pigs, rabbits, and chickens. It is essential that the animals used be free from naturally acquired tuberculosis. This is of the *utmost importance.* Although naturally acquired tuberculosis is of rare occurrence in guinea pigs and rabbits, the same is not true for chickens. In certain areas of the United States, tuberculosis of chickens is exceedingly prevalent, a fact which has not always been considered by some workers who have reported infection of human beings with *Myco. avium.* It should be the rule of every laboratory that *no chickens should be used for virulence tests of acid-fast bacilli unless the chickens have failed to react to an intracutaneous*

---

*The question of atypical strains of mycobacteria has been discussed by Price (1938 and 1939), Rich (1951), Stadnichenko, Sweany, and Kloeck (1945), Jensen (1950), Smith (1954 and 1958), and Runyon (1959).

†Miscibility of bovine and human strains of tubercle bacilli grown on solid medium may be enhanced by the addition of a few drops of sterile ox bile to the weighed cells just before they are ground.

*injection of avian tuberculin.** When possible, it is preferable to use young rather than old birds.

Each typing series of animals should consist of at least two guinea pigs, two rabbits, and two chickens. Each guinea pig should receive subcutaneously 0.1 mg. of the bacterial cells. The rabbits and chickens should be inoculated intravenously, each animal receiving 0.01 mg. of the bacteria. Guinea pigs should be killed for necropsy eight weeks after inoculation; rabbits and chickens, after ninety days. Animals which die before the stated intervals should be examined to determine cause of death and presence of tuberculous lesions.

The results of the test for virulence may be interpreted with confidence if one keeps in mind the susceptibility of the respective animals to the bovine, human, and avian species of the tubercle bacillus.

Briefly, the salient facts may be stated as follows: Guinea pigs are markedly susceptible to both *Myco. bovis* and *Myco. tuberculosis,* but have a high resistance to *Myco. avium.* Rabbits are highly susceptible to both *Myco. bovis* and *Myco. avium,* but have a very limited susceptibility to *Myco. tuberculosis.* Chickens are highly susceptible to *Myco. avium,* but have a formidable resistance to *Myco. bovis* and *Myco. tuberculosis.* Differences in the results of tests of virulence that distinguish the respective acid-fast bacilli responsible for tuberculosis in warm-blooded animals are summarized in Table 2.

TABLE 2

RELATIVE LABORATORY ANIMALS SUSCEPTIBILITY OF/TO THE FOUR SPECIES OF MYCOBACTERIA RESPONSIBLE FOR TUBERCULOSIS OF WARM-BLOODED ANIMALS*

Species	Animal			
	Guinea Pig	Rabbit	Chicken	Vole
Myco. tuberculosis	+	−	−	−
Myco. bovis	+	+	−	+
Myco. avium	−	+	+	−
Myco. muris	−	−	−	+

*Explanation of symbols
  − = Very resistant
  ± = Slightly susceptible
  + = Markedly susceptible

*The procedure for conducting a tuberculin test in chickens has been described by Feldman (1938).

Finally, in interpreting the results of tests of virulence, it must must be emphasized that typical strains of tubercle bacilli, when introduced into susceptible animals, produce progressive disease, usually with widespread dissemination to the organs of predilection. An alleged bovine strain that produces only localized lesions in guinea pigs and only minimal foci in the lungs of rabbits lacks the virulence necessary to qualify as a bovine type of the organism, regardless of its cultural characteristics. Likewise an alleged avian strain of tubercle bacilli that does not produce widely disseminated, progressive disease in rabbits and in previously tuberculin-negative chickens cannot be accepted as a representative of the avian species. Identification of types of tubercle bacilli, based on morphologic characteristics of the cells, physical characteristics of the culture, and tests for sensitivity to avian or to mammalian tuberculin, must be considered presumptive. Convincing evidence of the identification of a given strain obtained from clinical material can be established only by properly conducted tests of virulence.

TUBERCULOSIS OF CATTLE

From a consideration of economic loss, hazard to human health, and the ubiquitous character of the disease, tuberculosis continues to be one of the most important diseases of cattle. The insidious development of the infection, the tenacity of the causative agent, and its ability to infect heterologous hosts are factors that complicate the control and eradication of this disease.

Incidence*

Although precise information regarding the incidence of tuberculosis of cattle in the various countries is not available, accumulated data indicate that the disease occurs throughout the civilized world. The incidence in different countries varies greatly, depending on: 1) the type of animal husbandry practiced, 2) the commercial exchange of cattle from one country to another without proper regulatory supervision, and 3) the presence or absence of a militant and effective veterinary and medical program of detection, eradication, and control.

---

*Francis (1958) has provided much valuable data on the prevalence of tuberculosis of cattle in various parts of the world.

In the UNITED STATES, there are reasons to believe that tuberculosis in cattle will eventually become a rare disease. Although the incidence for the entire United States at the present time is impressively low, the disease still exists endemically. Fortunately, it is recognized that endemic areas constitute sources of new infection and that these foci must be reckoned with.

The incidence of bovine tuberculosis for the United States as a whole was never as high as in many other parts of the world. However, in some areas, the infection was formerly present to an alarming degree. According to Russell and Hastings in 1901,* the incidence of tuberculosis in cattle, as determined by the tuberculin test, varied in different areas from 4 to 50 per cent. The highest incidence occurred among the herds where dairying was practiced most intensively, while the range herds were practically free of the infection.

As a result of the concerted and militant plan of eradication set up co-operatively between the respective States and the Federal Government in 1917, the incidence of tuberculosis of cattle in the United States is at the present time as low, if not lower, than in any other country in the world. A graphic representation of the decline of the incidence of tuberculosis infection in cattle during a twenty-year period, as determined by the tuberculin test, is shown in Figure 2.

The figures presented in Table 3 reveal the continuous decline in the incidence of positive tuberculin reactors in the United States during the forty-five years since the eradication program has been in operation. Not shown in Table 3 are the percentage of reactors for 1952, 1953, and 1954. For each of these years, the percentage was 0.11, the lowest frequency recorded during the entire period that the eradication campaign has been in existence. (Tuberculin tests have been conducted annually since the eradication program was started in 1917. To conserve space in the table, figures during the first forty years are given at ten-year intervals.)

Further evidence of the low incidence of tuberculosis in cattle in the United States is contained in figures of the Meat Inspection Service of the United States Department of Agriculture for 1961. In a total of 19,861,262 cattle slaughtered, exclusive of reactors to

*Cited by Myers (1940).

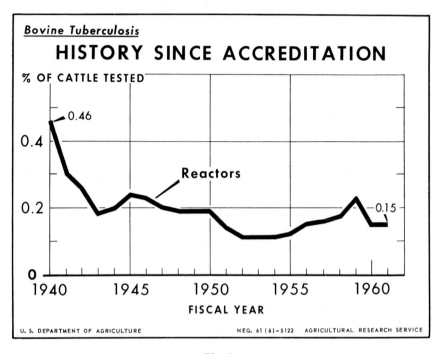

Fig. 2.

TABLE 3

Tuberculin Tests of Cattle in the United States at 10-Year Intervals From 1918
Through 1958, and the 3-Year Interval From 1958 Through 1961*

Year	Number Tested	Reactors	
		Number	Percentage
1918	134,143	6,544	4.9
1928	11,281,490	262,113	2.3
1938	14,180,871	89,359	0.6
1948	8,294,423	15,943	0.19
1958	8,883,813	15,361	0.17
1961	9,788,386	14,579	0.15

*Data from Animal Disease Eradication Division, United States Department of
Agriculture, Washington, D. C.

tuberculin, lesions considered tuberculous were found in 382
(0.0192 per cent). Among the 382, lesions were sufficiently severe
to require cooking or condemnation of only 87 carcasses (0.000438
per cent of the total number of cattle slaughtered, exclusive of

reactors to tuberculin, during 1961). The significance of this number is more apparent when compared with the number of carcasses cooked or condemned in the first fourteen years (1917-1930) that the eradication program was in effect. During that period, the average yearly number of carcasses cooked or condemned on account of tuberculosis (exclusive of reactors to tuberculin) varied from a high of 0.53 per cent to a low of 0.19 per cent. Expressed differently, the carcasses that were passed for cooking or were condemned, during the fourteen years referred to, represented a ratio of 1 to 353, while the ratio of carcasses in the same categories in 1961 was 1 to 228,290.

The remarkable diminution in the incidence of tuberculosis among cattle in the United States has been achieved by the ruthless application of what is, without doubt, the most effective method of eradicating tuberculosis among domesticated animals—the tuberculin test and the slaughter of the reactors.* According to official information, from 1917, when the tuberculosis eradication plan was initiated, until June 30, 1961, a total of 424,102,539 cattle had been tested with tuberculin. The number of animals that reacted to the tuberculin test was 4,125,637. During this period, the total amount of money expended to accomplish this stupendous and important task, including funds appropriated by the counties, States, and Federal Government, is probably more than one-half billion dollars. Considering the results achieved, the cost has not been excessive. That the task could be accomplished provides truly an amazing example of man's ability to integrate the efforts of the veterinary and the medical professions to free his environment of formidable and insidious factors that threaten his life and economic well-being.

The gains made in controlling bovine tuberculosis can be advanced or maintained only by sustained and militant action and by recognition of the fact that constant vigilance is imperative. As long as a single tuberculous animal exists, the possibility of the transmission of the infection to healthy animals and to human beings exists. The goal should be complete elimination of the disease. Those who would curtail the program of eradication on the assumption that

---

*For a detailed and interesting account of the attack against bovine tuberculosis, the reader should consult the book by Myers (1940).

tuberculosis is no longer a potential hazard, are guilty of serious disservice to human and to animal health.

In Canada, as in the United States, the eventual eradication of bovine tuberculosis was predicated on a well-formulated plan. The most important aspects of the procedure were the detection of infected animals by the use of tuberculin and the slaughter of the reactors. In 1952, approximately 80 per cent of the cattle in Canada were included in the official tuberculin testing programs, and the percentage of positive reactors reached a significant low of 0.34 per cent.* As the program has progressed, the incidence of the disease has diminished continuously. The present (1962) favorable situation is well reflected in the following information from the Health of Animals Division, Canada Department of Agriculture†:

"The eradication of bovine tuberculosis in Canada reached a milestone in 1961 with the completion of testing in the last area under the Restricted Area Plan. All areas in Canada have now been tested at least once. Completion of the testing program does not mean that tuberculosis has been eradicated from Canadian cattle. However, it has been reduced to such an extent that it will no longer be considered a serious threat to the Canadian cattle industry.

"This program, the Restricted Area Plan, commenced thirty-nine years ago. In the early stages of the program, the level of infection in some areas ranged as high as thirty per cent. In the fiscal year 1960-61, the level of infection had been reduced to 0.11 per cent. Eradication was begun systematically in 1919. The program has cost the Canadian Government more than $50,000,000 in compensation and administration costs. To date, it has involved over 49,000,000 tests, resulting in the discovery of 567,000 bovine cases of tuberculosis. Compensation paid to farmers for loss of infected cattle has been approximately $21,000,000.

"The contribution of the bovine tuberculosis testing program is reflected in the incidence of tuberculosis infection found on post-mortem at inspected establishments. This has been progressively reduced over the years, and today less than 0.01 per cent of swine and cattle carcasses are condemned on account of generalized tuberculosis."

---

*Personal communication in 1954 from Dr. Charles A. Mitchell, Quebec.
†Received in a personal communication in 1962 from Dr. K. F. Wells, Veterinary Director General, Ottawa.

Information concerning the prevalence of tuberculosis of cattle in Africa is meager. In 1940, Carmichael mentioned that in the District of Ankole, Uganda, the infection among cattle had reached serious proportions; as many as 70 per cent of the animals in different herds reacted to tuberculin.*

Reporting in 1943, Vaccarezza and Arena stated that the rate of tuberculous infection in cattle in Argentina was high. In 1941, more than 22,000,000 pounds (10,000,000 kg.) of meat were condemned on account of tuberculosis in national slaughtering establishments. In Buenos Aires, 25 to 40 per cent, in La Plata, 15 to 25 per cent, and in Cordoba, 12.2 per cent of the samples of raw milk contained tubercle bacilli. Fortunately, in these areas it is the general practice to boil milk intended for human consumption.

In Australia, the incidence of bovine tuberculosis has decreased markedly since the test-and-slaughter plan was put into effect in 1935. Between the years 1935 and 1949, cattle numbering 142,244 and representing herds in the five districts of Australia, were tested with tuberculin. The results revealed that in Queensland, New South Wales, Victoria, and South Australia, the average percentage of reactors was 6.4. For Western Australia, the occurrence of reactors was 40.5 per cent. The herds in the different geographic areas were tested again in 1951-52. The number of animals tested totaled 338,506, and the average percentage of reactors was 1.2[†] The Australian experience is an impressive example of what can be accomplished by detecting tuberculous animals and disposing of them with a finality that precludes the subsequent infection of healthy animals.

In Denmark, tuberculosis of cattle was exceedingly prevalent thirty years ago.[‡] Militant and effective methods of control and eradication were instituted in 1937, and the report for 1949 indicated that 99.8 per cent of the herds had been tuberculin tested and the percentage of positive tuberculin reactors had been reduced to 0.79 per cent (Bendixen, 1950).

---

*For additional information on the occurrence of tuberculosis among cattle indigenous to the tropics, see an earlier report by Carmicheal (1939).

†Seddou, cited by Francis, 1958.

‡For a concise history of bovine tuberculosis in Denmark and an account of the procedures used in successfully combatting the disease, the contribution by Bendixen (1950) may be consulted.

By 1950, Denmark was considered virtually free from bovine tuberculosis. In recognition of this singular triumph, according to Bendixen, the Joint Organization of the Danish Cooperative Dairies "proclaimed that from August 1, 1950, no milk producer with tuberculosis in his herd would be allowed to furnish milk to any dairy. . . ." This should provide the proper incentive to continue measures necessary to maintain the gains achieved.

In Eire, Dolan* in 1953 reported lesions of tuberculosis in 12 per cent of 65,774 carcasses slaughtered in Dublin.

According to Francis (1958), nearly 200,000 cattle are tuberculin tested annually in Finland. Although 3 per cent of the animals react positively, lesions of tuberculosis are found in only 0.001 per cent of slaughtered cattle. It is believed that the lesions represent infection with avian or human type tubercle bacilli, and that bovine tuberculosis has been entirely eliminated.

Indicative of the duration of the bovine tuberculosis problem in France is the report published in 1884 by Martin. Guinea pigs were inoculated with milk purchased in the city of Paris. It was established that virulent tubercle bacilli were present in nine of the thirteen samples. Martin recognized the hazard to human health and recommended that milk should always be boiled. Now—more than seventy-five years after Martin observations—tuberculosis of cattle in France continues to be prevalent. The highest incidence of infection occurs among dairy cattle maintained under conditions of permanent stabling. According to Van Es (1929), tuberculin tests, made between 1904 and 1921 of cattle supplying milk for Paris, revealed the presence of tuberculous infections in 21.2 to 41.75 per cent. The precise incidence of tuberculosis in cattle at the present time in France is not known. It is likely that the disease is still widespread; its control remains an important unsolved problem, and its existence continues to be a hazard to human health.†

Bovine tuberculosis is considered a serious problem in East Germany and in Czechoslovakia. The disease occurs frequently in

---

*Cited by Francis, 1958.

†In Paris in 1955, the author learned that tuberculosis was observed in approximately 3 per cent of the bovine carcasses at the time of slaughter. Furthermore, mammalian tubercle bacilli occurred in a significant percentage of specimens of milk marketed for human consumption.

Hungary. In Yugoslavia, the incidence is considered to be approximately 3 per cent (Steele, 1962).

According to Dalling and Gloyne (1942), about 40 per cent of the cows of Great Britain were infected with bovine tuberculosis. Furthermore, at that time, the annual loss from this disease due to replacements in the herd, condemnation of meat, and loss of productivity amounted to about £3,000,000 ($12,000,000). Of ominous significance to human health was the report in 1937 that in Great Britain five of every 1,000 dairy cows eliminated tubercle bacilli in the milk (Dalrymple-Champneys, 1937). In 1938, Griffith reported that the occurrence of tubercle bacilli in the milk of dairy cows in Great Britain, when determined by guinea pig inoculation tests, varied from 1 per cent to as high as 18 per cent.

Later information by Francis (1947) indicated that the incidence of tuberculosis of cattle in England was 20 per cent; in Wales, 7.4 per cent; and in Scotland, 14 per cent. For all of Great Britain, Francis believed the incidence of infection to be 17 to 18 per cent. The incidence of tuberculosis of dairy cows was much higher, probably between 30 and 35 per cent.

At the present time, there are many thousand officially recognized tuberculosis-free herds in Great Britain as a consequence of the Attested Herd Scheme, introduced in 1935. Francis (1958) stated that the incidence of tuberculosis of cattle in Great Britain "is rapidly decreasing."* Of a cattle population of approximately nine million, over four million dairy cattle were in attested herds. As of 1956, the attested areas embraced the western counties of Scotland and the Western Islands and most of Wales. If the currently successful program in Scotland, England, and Wales can be continued with uncompromsing vigor, the results within a decade will represent a noteworthy contribution to human and animal health.

In Holland, where a few years ago 80,000 of the cattle herds were considered to be tuberculous, the cattle population of 2.6 million was tested with tuberculin. Sixteen per cent of the animals reacted positively. A five-year plan of eradication was started in 1951. Attesting to the vigor of the attack on the problem is the fact that in

---

*For information concerning the operation of the Attested Herd Scheme, see Francis (1958, p. 75).

1952, 160,000 tuberculous cattle had been detected by the use of tuberculin, and were subsequently slaughtered (Francis, 1958).

Recently (1962), Ruys* provided the following additional information on the situation in Holland. By May 1956, all herds had been tuberculin tested, and the animals that reacted positively had been slaughtered. Continuing control of the disease is accomplished by means of annual or bi-annual testing, depending upon the previous incidence of the infection. It is assumed that to maintain the gains and accomplish the gradual elimination of the disease, it will be necessary to continue the control program for a period of years. An important aspect of the program is that every bovine animal that is tuberculin positive is slaughtered. Occasionally, a focus of tuberculosis infection originates from a human case due to Myco. bovis.

In Hong Kong, although bovine tuberculosis has been a problem of long dration, it is presently assumed to be under control. However, a considerable number of cattle are imported into Hong Kong from mainland China for slaughter. In these animals, tuberculosis is recognized frequently (Steele, 1962).

Tuberculosis of cattle in India was reported in 1942 by Mallick, Aggarwal, and Dua. In a survey of Amritsar, it was found that 25 per cent of 1,234 dairy cattle reacted to tuberculin.

Only meager information is available regarding the occurrence of bovine tuberculosis in Israel. According to Francis (1958), the incidence based on tuberculin tests and on meat inspection reports in 1946 was considered to be 13 per cent. Subsequent information, published in 1952, concerned the results of tuberculin tests of two groups of dairy cattle. In one, comprising 857 animals, the percentage of reactors was 7.5. The other group consisted of 169 animals, of which 51.4 per cent reacted positively. If the incidence of occurrence of tuberculosis in the cattle referred to reflects the present incidence of the disease in the cattle population of Israel, a formidable and difficult problem confronts those concerned officially with the protection of human and animal health.

Meager data concerning tuberculosis of cattle in northern Italy indicate that the disease is prevalent. De Gara (1942) reported

---

*Personal communication (1962) to author from Prof. Dr. A. Ch. Ruys, University of Amsterdam.

on the occurrence in Italy of the bovine type of infection in human beings. He emphasized the danger of drinking raw milk and mentioned that in one series, 37 (6.8 per cent) of 544 samples of market milk contained tubercle bacilli. The same author quoted Casco as having found bovine tubercle bacilli in seven of nine specimens of bovine feces and in two of nine specimens of saliva of bovine animals. The approximate incidence of bovine tuberculosis for all of Italy is not known. From the meager data, one may assume that the disease constitutes a serious burden on the cattle industry of that country. A more important factor is the hazard to human beings, particularly children, exposed to milk from tuberculous animals.

Japan, with a cattle population of about five million, has a relatively small amount of bovine tuberculosis. Data obtained by use of the tuberculin test and from the examination of slaughtered animals, indicate that the incidence of tuberculosis is 0.22 per cent (Steele, 1962).

In New Zealand, Holyoake[*] reported the results of tuberculin tests of 57,952 dairy cattle. Positive reactions were recorded in 6.6 per cent.

In the Philippines, dairy cattle are tuberculin tested annually. Positive reactions are seldom observed (Steele, 1962).

In Poland, the over-all incidence of tuberculosis of cattle is estimated to be 50 per cent (Steele, 1962). The disease constitutes an important problem in man and in animals. The cattle population is approximately eight and one-quarter million. The incidence of tuberculosis varies geographically from 5 per cent in the areas contiguous to or near the Russian border, to 50 per cent in the provinces along the East German border, to a high of 75 per cent in cattle on State farms. It is significant that in Poland, 15 to 25 per cent of tuberculosis in children is of bovine origin.

In Russia, but meager information is available concerning the occurrence of tuberculosis of cattle. However, it is the opinion of those with some knowledge of the situation that the incidence is between one and two per cent (Steele, 1962).

Magnusson[*] (1942), from necropsy statistics on 234,106 cattle in Sweden established the occurrence of tuberculosis in 19 per cent of the carcasses.

---

[*]Cited by Francis, 1958.

In Switzerland, bovine tuberculosis was prevalent for many decades. According to Fritschi (1960), 50 per cent of the cattle were tuberculous in regions where dairy husbandry was most intensive. In the Canton of Zurich, Hess (1960) mentioned that three years before bovine tuberculosis was considered eradicated from Switzerland, it was demonstrated by guinea pig inoculation tests, that 10 per cent of the milk specimens obtained at 237 dairy cooperatives, contained living tubercle bacilli (presumably *Myco. bovis*).* Effective measures for the eradication of bovine tuberculosis did not make significant progress until 1953. The program was essentially similar to that followed in the United States, the slaughter of tuberculin-positive animals and indemnification of the owners of animals slaughtered. During the period 1951-59, a total of 393,883 tuberculin-positive animals were removed from herds and subsequently sent to slaughter. By the end of 1959, the number of cattle considered to be noninfected was more than 1.6 million, representing more than 151,000 farms, and "the whole cattle population was declared tuberculosis-free" (Hess, 1960). Whether this statement is literally true may be questioned. However, the record shows that once an effective plan was activated, Switzerland was able to accomplish within a few years a noteworthy triumph over a major infectious disease of cattle. Constant vigilance will be required if the fruits of the victory are to be retained.

The Pathology of Tuberculosis in Cattle[†]

It is the consensus of those who have investigated the pathogenesis of tuberculosis of cattle that in adult animals the infection in the majority of instances is primarily in the lungs and that the tubercle bacilli reach the parenchyma of the lung by way of the respiratory tract. In suckling calves, according to Nieberle (1931), most of the primary infections occur in the gastro-intestinal tract (including the contiguous lymph nodes). In Nieberle's series of 100 suckling calves,

---

*Nabholz investigated a situation in the Canton of Zurich in which "one single milk spreader infected at least 108 head of cattle and 117 hogs through contaminated skimmed milk before being slaughtered" (Cited by Hess, 1960).

†Limitation of space does not permit a detailed account of the pathology of tuberculosis. For additional information see Van Es (1929). Hutyra, Marek and Manninger (1938), Medlar (1940), Stamp (1944), Stamp and Wilson (1946), Stamp (1948), and Francis (1958).

the primary focus occurred in the lung in 13 per cent of the animals.*

Being in most instances a chronic progressive disease, tuberculosis causes destruction of the tissues in the immediate vicinity of the original focus and may become caseous, fibrocaseous, cavitating, or calcareous (Figure 3). From the softening, destructive primary focus, the infection may spread to adjacent regions by continuity or to distant regions by way of the blood stream or the lymphatics. As a consequence, no tissue of the animal is immune to the formation of tuberculous lesions, although the sites of predilection are lungs, liver, spleen, serous membranes, and kidneys (Figure 4). Rarely is the musculature affected.†

In addition and of great importance to human health, the paren-

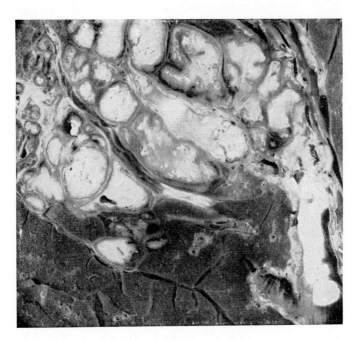

Fig. 3. Multiple caseocalcareous tuberculous nodules in the lung of a bovine. (Courtesy of Doctor Harry W. Schoening, Bureau of Animal Industry, United States Department of Agriculture.)

---

*The question of tuberculosis of the musculature of cattle is considered on p. 51.
†According to Stamp (1944), Nieberle expressed the opposite point of view, stating that pulmonary infection in the calf is much more frequent than alimentary infection.

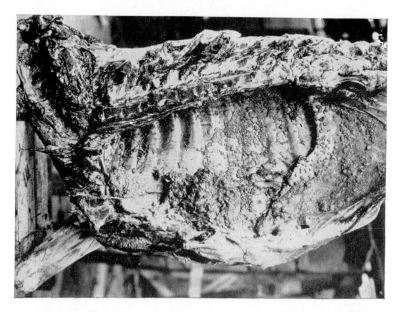

Fig. 4. Extensive pleural and peritoneal lesions of tuberculosis in carcass of a dairy cow. (From Van Es, L.: Bovine tuberculosis, Circular 23, University of Nebraska, College of Agriculture, Experiment Station, Lincoln, Nebraska. Revised 1929.)

chyma of the udder may be the site of tuberculous foci from which infectious material finds its way into the milk[†] (Figure 5). In the udder, the disease may affect all four quarters. The supramammary lymph nodes may or may not be involved.[‡] The disease in the udder may be chronic or acute and invariably leads to extensive tuberculous involvement of the duct system (Figure 6). As Stamp (1943) pointed out, in all cases of tuberculosis of the bovine udder, the lesions are "open" and enough functioning lactating lobules persist to provide for the secretion of at least some milk, which of course invariably contains tubercle bacilli. Although the disease is transmitted to the udder by the blood stream, local spread through the duct system probably occurs in all cases. In practically all instances,

---

[†]Detailed accounts of tuberculosis of the bovine udder have been supplied by Stamp (1943), and by Francis (1958).

[‡]According to Stamp (1943), the involvement of the supramammary lymph nodes does not indicate that the udder is tuberculous. Therefore, the condition of the supramammary lymph nodes is of no diagnostic value in detecting tuberculosis of the bovine udder.

the excretion of tubercle bacilli in the milk denotes demonstrable lesions in the udder. However, Wilson and Miles (1955) stated that tubercle bacilli may occur in the milk without demonstrable gross or microscopic lesions in the mammary gland. Whether tubercle bacilli can actually pass through the intact tissues of the parenchyma of the udder should be subjected to investigation. It seems more likely that when the organisms are present in milk as it is drawn from the udder, alterations of tissue are present, even though they may be exceedingly difficult to find.

The fact that bovine tuberculosis causes destruction of tissues, which may cause the morbid process to break into channels leading to the exterior of the body provides an important circumstance favorable to the transmission of the disease to other animals, including human beings. Lesions of the lungs may ulcerate into the bronchi. Tubercle bacilli may then be elimniated with the expired air during coughing, or the bacilli may be swallowed with mucous

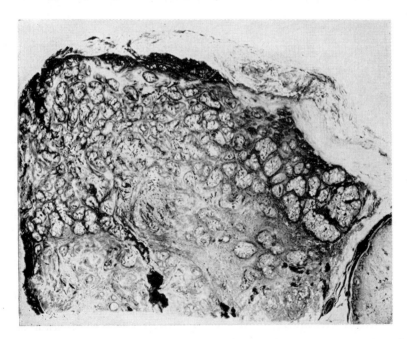

Fig. 5. Extensive and severe tuberculous involvement of the udder. There has been considerable destruction of the parenchymal tissues, which have been replaced largely by caseocalcareous lesions of tuberculosis. (Courtesy of Dr. Harry W. Schoening, United States Department of Agriculture.)

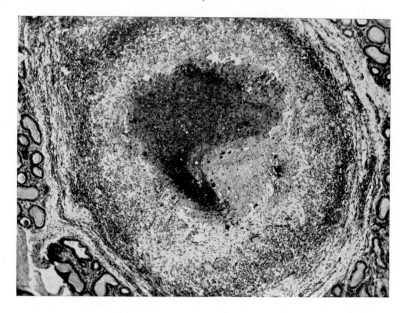

Fig. 6. Chronic nodular tuberculosis of the udder of a cow. Minimal calcification has occurred, and acid-fast bacillary forms were demonstrable among the cellular detritus (x55). (Courtesy of Dr. J. S. Bengston, United States Department of Agriculture.)

secretions and subsequently eliminated with the feces.* Feces may also contain tubercle bacilli if the disease is present in the intestinal mucosa or in the liver. Tuberculosis of the kidney may cause sufficient destruction to permit the infectious material to discharge into the renal pelvis and hence to egress with the urine. In tuberculosis of the testes, the semen may be infected, and if the disease affects the reproductive organs of the female, the vaginal discharges are likely to contain viable tubercle bacilli.

To recapitulate: Tuberculous cattle may excrete the infective bacteria in a variety of materials. These include discharges from the respiratory tract, milk, urine, semen, vaginal secretions, and feces. If infected, any and all of these may serve as a medium for the transmission of tuberculosis to previously noninfected hosts. *From every*

----

*In a study of feces from 391 apparently healthy cows in five counties in England, Williams and Hoy (1927) demonstrated tubercle bacilli in the feces of six (1.53 per cent).

*point of view, the tuberculous bovine is potentially a highly dangerous animal, not only for lower animals but also for man.**

Vaccination and Chemotherapy

That natural infection of cattle with tubercle bacilli might be prevented by vaccination or that the disease, when once established, would be amenable to specific chemotherapeutic substances, has been the hope of many. Unfortunately, the results have not justified the acceptance of either vaccination with BCG or specific chemotherapy as a practical means of effectively preventing or eradicating tuberculosis in cattle.†

Concerning the use of BCG and specific chemotherapy in controlling tuberculosis of cattle, the Joint WHO/FAO Expert Committee on Zoonoses stated in its second report (1959) "that generally speaking, vaccination has no place in the eradication of tuberculosis in cattle." Furthermore, the Committee concluded that chemotherapy in the treatment of tuberculous animals "is entirely impractical" and "should be discouraged."

TRANSMISSIBILITY OF *MYCO. BOVIS* TO OTHER SPECIES

As mentioned previously, one of the features of the organism responsible for tuberculosis of cattle is its ability to prosper in certain heterologous hosts, in which it may produce consequences as serious as those possible in the natural host.

Transmissibility: Cattle to Human Beings‡

The development of our knowledge concerning the virulence for human beings of the bacillus of bovine tuberculosis has been slow

---

*In a study of feces from 391 apparently healthy cows in five counties in England, Williams and Hoy (1927) demonstrated tubercle bacilli in the feces of six (1.53 per cent).

†Extensive experimental trials in the vaccination of cattle with BCG have been recorded by Haring *et al.* (1930). A more recent review and appraisal has been contributed by Rosenthal (1957).

‡A noteworthy review by Gervois of approximately 575 published reports concerning *Myco. bovis* as a causative agent of tuberculosis in human beings was made accessible in an English translation by Dr. Edward Kupka, with a foreword by Dr. Emil Bogen. The material was designated "W.P.A. Project #465-03-3-613," and was reproduced in 1939 at Olive View Hospital, California. The few copies were distributed to individuals and to a few medical libraries, including the National Library of Medicine, 8600 Wisconsin Avenue, Bethesda, Maryland.

and has frequently been interrupted by the temporary acceptance of opinions to the exclusion of facts. Fourteen years before Koch announced the discovery of the tubercle bacillus in 1882, Villemin (1868) proved by animal experimentation that tuberculosis is an infectious disease and is the effect of a specific causative agent. Twenty-five years after Koch's discovery, the danger to human beings of milk from tuberculous cattle was generally accepted. This point of view was influenced considerably by Koch's (1882) statement, made at the time he reported the discovery of the tubercle bacillus, that "bovine tuberculosis is identical with the disease in man and is thus a disease transmissible to man."

However, at the British Congress on Tuberculosis held in London in 1901, Koch (1902) reversed his former position and said, in effect, that human tuberculosis differs from that of cattle and cannot be transmitted to bovines.* Furthermore, Koch insisted that the susceptibility of human beings to bovine tubercle bacilli is uncertain and if infection of human beings with the bacillus of bovine tuberculosis occurs, it must be very rare. Finally he said, "I should estimate the extent of infection by the milk and flesh of tuberculous cattle, and the butter made of this milk, is hardly greater than that of hereditary transmission, and, therefore, do not deem it advisable to take any measures against it."

Koch's point of view as to the unimportance of the bovine tubercle bacillus as a hazard to human health was opposed by the officials of the Congress in London. This opposition was shared by many eminent scientists who attended the Congress, including Lord Lister. At a general meeting of the Congress, Ravenel (1901) reported that he had isolated from a human being a tubercle bacillus that was proved to be of the bovine variety. This was the first instance when the bacillus of bovine tuberculosis was definitely established as a human pathogen.[†]

---

*Smith, in 1898, reported the results of his studies that established distinct differences between human and bovine tubercle bacilli.

†As a matter of fact, Ravenel (1901) reported at the Congress five cases of probable bovine tuberculosis in human beings; one patient was Ravenel's laboratory assistant, three patients were veterinarians, and one was a cattle-car cleaner. The disease in all but one case was localized. Later, before the Pathological Society of Philadelphia, Ravenel (1902) reported a case of tuberculous meningitis in a child, seventeen months of age, from whom tubercle bacilli had been obtained and proved by cattle inoculation tests to be of the bovine variety. Smith (1905) also isolated bovine tubercle bacilli from a child.

The question of virulence of bovine tubercle bacilli for human beings became so pertinent after Koch's address at the London Congress that an official agency was formed to ascertain the facts. Thus, in 1901, there came into being the Royal Commission on Tuberculosis. In the several years of its existence, the Royal Commission made noteworthy contributions to the knowledge of tuberculosis. Exhaustive and careful studies were made of cultures of tubercle bacilli obtained from cases of human, bovine, and avian tuberculosis, and the results constitute a wealth of essential fundamental information that has served as an authoritative guide for subsequent workers. The final report of the Commission was issued in 1911.*

In an interim report, published by the Commission in 1907, the importance of the bacillus of bovine tuberculosis to human beings was emphasized by the following statement: "Cows' milk containing bovine tubercle bacilli is clearly a cause of tuberculosis and fatal tuberculosis in man. Our results clearly point to the necessity of measures more stringent than those at present enforced being taken to prevent the sale or the consumption of such milk."†

Several members of the British Royal Commission on Tuberculosis continued to explore the problem of the transmissibility of bovine tubercle bacilli for many years after the activities of the Commission had ceased. Among those was A. Stanley Griffith who by persistent and meticulous work and the conservative interpretation of his results was probably more responsible than any other individual for the final indictment of the bacillus of bovine tuberculosis as a menace to human health.

Koch, at the International Congress on Tuberculosis in Washington in 1908, did retreat somewhat from his previous dogmatic insistence that the danger of the bacilli of cattle tuberculosis for human beings is negligible. However, he continued to insist that satisfactory proof of chronic pulmonary tuberculosis in human beings due to bovine tubercle bacilli had not been established‡ Ac-

---

*An excellent account of the work of the British Royal Commission on Tuberculosis has been contributed by Francis (1958). His appraisal, more than a half century after the Commission was established, is timely. He discusses the factors that brought the Commission into being, what it accomplished, and the influence of its findings on the development of our knowledge of the pathogenesis of tuberculosis infections.

†Quoted from Griffith (1937).

‡From Munro and Walker (1935).

cording to Griffith and Munro, only two such cases could be quoted at the time of the meeting io Washington in 1908. In one of the cases, it appeared likely that human and bovine types of the tubercle bacillus were both present, and consequently unequivocal proof that the bovine tubercle bacillus contributed to the causation of the pulmonary disease was lacking. A few months later, in February 1909, Griffith (1937) in England obtained pure cultures of bovine tubercle bacilli from sputums of two men, twenty-one and thirty-one years of age, respectively. In 1913, Griffith isolated (in Edinburgh) bovine tubercle bacilli from a girl, sixteen years of age, who had pulmonary tuberculosis. In 1916, another instance of pulmonary tuberculosis due to the bovine tubercle bacillus was reported by Wang (1916) (also of Edinburgh), the patient being a man forty-one years of age.

Although Koch eventually modified his views regarding the danger of the bacilli of bovine tuberculosis to human beings, unfortunately the influence of his earlier belief was well entrenched. Koch's erroneous views must be held largely accountable for the tragic consequences that ensued from the denial that bovine tubercle bacilli are capable of producing in human beings a variety of tuberculous infections, including pulmonary forms of the disease.

The frequency of the bovine type of tuberculous infection in human beings is clearly dependent on the incidence of the disease in cattle and the quantity of raw milk and cream consumed. Regardless of the anatomic situation of the resultant disease, the most likely source of infection is one or a combination of the following: raw or improperly heated milk from tuberculous cows; the products of milk from tuberculous cows; and contaminated air expired from the lungs of tuberculous cattle or human beings infected with the bovine type of infection. In addition, it should be recognized that butchers and meat inspectors, whose duties require the exposure of the unprotected skin of the arms and hands to tuberculous carcasses, are in danger of cutaneous infection. Thus, the possibility of occupational tuberculosis must be recognized.* In fact, several cases of

---

*Hermansson (1939) inoculated guinea pigs with water in which a meat inspector had washed his hands after examining carcasses of tuberculous cattle, and demonstrated the presence of virulent tubercle bacilli. Similar tests showed the presence of tubercle bacilli in the water which had been used by butchers to wash their hands and in the water used to wash towels previously used by the meat inspector.

bovine tuberculous infection of butchers have been reported by Saenz (1939).

In presenting evidence involving the bacilli of bovine tuberculosis as a cause of infection of human beings, no attempt has been made to give a complete review of the literature. Price compiled and published in 1939 data on occurrence of the bovine type of infection in cases of tuberculosis in human beings in various countries of the world (Table 4). It must be recognized that her figures represent only approximations, but they provide sufficient evidence to leave no doubt that tuberculosis in cattle is a menace to human health. The figures given by Price for the United States (11.7 per cent) are largely based on studies made by Park and Krumweide during the period of 1910-1913. The true incidence of human infection with bovine tubercle bacilli in the United States at the present time (1962) is not known, but fragmentary evidence suggests that it is extremely low, especially among children, the age group in which the bovine type of infection is most prevalent.

The magnitude of the public health problem which tuberculosis in cattle previously created in the British Isles is evident from the information which Griffith compiled in 1937 from the reports of

TABLE 4

THE PERCENTAGE OF BOVINE TUBERCULOSIS AMONG CASES OF HUMAN AND BOVINE TUBERCULOSIS IN MAN IN DIFFERENT COUNTRIES OF THE WORLD
(DATA COMPILED BY PRICE AND PUBLISHED IN 1939)

Country	Total	Human	Bovine	
			Number	Per Cent
France	1,083	1,055	28	2.6
Germany	1,165	1,007	158	13.6
Netherlands	767	701	66	8.6
Switzerland	218	201	17	7.8
Sweden	14	14	0	0
Norway	107	101	6	5.6
Poland	160	149	11	6.9
Italy*	871	846	25	2.9
Spain	95	90	5	5.3
Hungary	334	328	6	1.8
Greece	327	327	0	0
Australia	280	246	34	12.1
Japan	272	264	8	2.9
United States	1,362	1,202	160	11.7
Canada	901	847	54	6.0

*In Italy there were sixty-four atypical strains.

several investigators. The data pertaining to England are presented in Table 5, while data for Scotland are shown in Table 6.

Table 5 and Table 6 pertain only to extrapulmonary infection due to the bacillus of bovine tuberculosis. The data concern cases of cervical adenitis, lupus, peritonitis, meningitis, and infections of the bones and joints. These statistics do not disclose the total number of cases of the bovine type of infection among patients fifteen

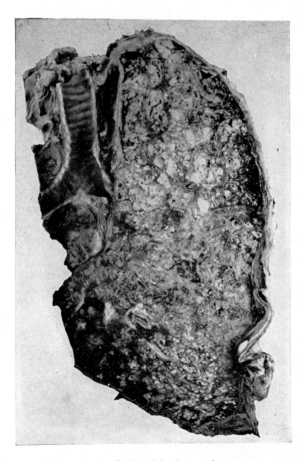

Fig. 7. Pulmonary tuberculosis of the right lung of a young woman due to the bovine variety of the tubercle bacillus. The patient had worked for several years as a dairy maid, starting at the age of fourteen years. Both lungs were extensively affected. (From Myers, J. A.: *Man's Greatest Victory Over Tuberculosis.* Springfield, Thomas, 1940.)

years of age or less, but experience has shown that the organism affects children more frequently than it affects adults.*

Although it was recognized that infection with the bovine type tubercle bacillus might affect almost any tissue of the body, pulmonary disease due to this organism was considered infrequent until the important investigations of several workers, especially Griffith and his colleagues in Britain, and Jensen in Denmark, proved the situation to be otherwise (Figure 7). According to Griffith (1937),

TABLE 5

PERCENTAGE IN ENGLAND OF THE BOVINE TYPE OF INFECTION AMONG 1,428 CASES OF EXTRAPULMONARY HUMAN TUBERCULOSIS (GRIFFITH)

Variety of Tuberculosis or Source of Material	Cases	Percentage of Cases in Different Age Groups in Which the Bovine Type of Bacillus Was Found		
		Less than 5 Years	5 to 15 Years	All Ages
Adenitis (cervical)	126	90.9	53.4	50.0
Lupus	191	58.4	44.4	48.7
Scrofuloderma	60	53.3	43.3	36.6
Bone and joint	553	29.5	19.1	19.5
Genito-urinary	23	—	—	17.4
Meningeal	265	28.1	24.5	24.6
Necropsies	187	28.6	15.5	22.5
Miscellaneous	23	33.3	9.1	8.7

TABLE 6

PERCENTAGE IN SCOTLAND OF THE BOVINE TYPE OF INFECTION AMONG 873 CASES OF EXTRAPULMONARY HUMAN TUBERCULOSIS (GRIFFITH)

Variety of Tuberculosis or Source of Material	Cases	Percentage of Cases in Different Age Groups in Which the Bovine Type of Bacillus Was Found		
		Less than 5 Years	5 to 15 Years	All Ages
Adenitis (cervical)	93	65.0	62.3	51.6
Lupus	13	100.0	71.4	69.2
Bone and joint	218	46.2	28.9	29.8
Genito-urinary	42	—	—	31.0
Meningeal	203	34.4	14.0	29.6
Necropsies	290	33.6	38.5	32.4
Miscellaneous	14	—	—	71.4

*Rich (1951) pointed out that 2,000 children died annually in Great Britain from infection with bovine tubercle bacilli because of the lack of social responsibility on the part of powerful dairy interests, which had frustrated all attempts to enact legislation making pasteurization of milk sold to the public compulsory. Since the time referred to, much has been accomplished in protecting the consumers of milk in Britain from infection by bovine tubercle bacilli. The number of tuberculous cows in dairy herds has been significantly reduced, and effectively pasteurized milk has become generally available.

up to 1922, only four cases of human pulmonary tuberculosis due to *Myco. bovis* had been established. In 1922, Munro* found two additional cases among 100 cases of pulmonary tuberculosis studied. The latter finding, according to Griffith, provided an impetus for numerous, prolonged, and extensive investigations. These studies showed that in countries where bovine tuberculosis is prevalent and milk is consumed in a raw state, pulmonary tuberculosis due to the bovine tubercle bacillus may be expected to occur.

The evidence presented by Griffith and Munro in 1944 was most impressive and belatedly provided an unequivocal answer to Koch's skepticism regarding the ability of this type of the tubercle bacillus to produce pulmonary disease in human beings. The report was based on a study of 6,963 cases of pulmonary tuberculosis in Great Britain. In every instance, tubercle bacilli were isolated from the sputum, and the bacillary type of each strain was determined by appropriate laboratory procedures. Some of the more important findings follow: 1) In Scotland, among 2,769 cases, the percentage of pulmonary infections due to the bovine tubercle bacillus was 5.8, the highest percentage being in the Orkney Islands (25.8) and the lowest (4.4) in the city of Aberdeen, where it was believed that many of the infections had originated in rural areas. 2) Among 3,671 strains of tubercle bacilli obtained from patients in England, 79 (2.15 per cent) were bovine in origin. 3) In Wales, the bovine type of infection was found in two of 203 cases. 4) In Eire, an examination of 320 cases of pulmonary tuberculosis did not disclose any instance of bovine infection. 5) In the entire series of 6,963 cases of pulmonary tuberculosis affecting human beings a total of 241 cases (3.5 per cent) were due to infection with the bacillus of bovine tuberculosis. 6) The strains from 232 of the 241 cases were fully virulent by animal tests of pathogenicity, while nine strains showed varying degrees of attenuation. 7) Previous cervical and abdominal tuberculous adenitis and involvement of bones and joints in a considerable proportion of the cases suggested the alimentary canal as the portal of entry of the infection. 8) There was no doubt that the great majority of the patients from whom bovine tubercle bacilli were obtained had been infected through the agency of cow's milk. 9) In five instances, both human and bovine species of mycobacteria

---

*Cited by Griffith, 1937.

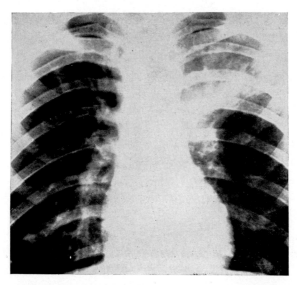

Fig. 8. Thorax of a man, nineteen years of age, who worked on a farm near Lund, Sweden. There was no tuberculosis in the man's family but the disease was present among the swine and the cattle of the farm where he worked. Sputum from this man yielded tubercle bacilli of the bovine type. (From Myers, J. A.: *Man's Greatest Victory Over Tuberculosis.* Springfield, Illinois, Charles C Thomas, 1940.)

were obtained from a single patient. 10) The possibility of infection from one human being to another was presumptive in a few instances, but not proved. 11) *Pulmonary tuberculosis in human beings caused by bovine tubercle bacilli was indistinguishable clinically, radiologically, and by post mortem examination from pulmonary tuberculosis due to tubercle bacilli of the human type* (Figure 8). These observations are of much significance. They emphasize the importance of proper laboratory procedures if the diagnosis of pulmonary tuberculosis of man due to *Myco. bovis* is to be established unequivocally.

Little precise information is available concerning the role of *Myco. bovis* as the infective agent in tuberculosis of human beings in Eire. In 1940, Mushatt published the results of an investigation of a relatively small series of extra-pulmonary cases of tuberculosis of children (one to 14 years of age). Of the fifty cases studied, twenty-five were from the city of Dublin, two from rural areas of County Dublin, and the remainder from twelve counties other than Dublin.

The cultures of tubercle bacilli obtained from the respective cases were studied bacteriologically and by tests for virulence. Seventeen (34 per cent) of the strains were typed as bovine. The strains of bovine tubercle bacilli were obtained from ten of fourteen cases of tuberculous cervical adenitis, four of twenty-two cases of bone and joint tuberculosis, and three of twelve cases of tuberculous meningitis. Only two cases of primary abdominal tuberculosis were studied, and in both instances human-type tubercle bacilli were isolated.

During the period of 1945 to 1948, Kerr, Lamont, and McGirr (1949) found, by testing with tuberculin, an incidence of 33 per cent tuberculous infection among 600 dairy cows in North Ireland. In addition, tubercle bacilli were found in 7.5 per cent of "churned samples of milk." In contrast, a study reported by Reilly* in 1950, indicated that in North Ireland the bovine type of infection in pulmonary tuberculosis of man was infrequent. Among 1,060 cases, *Myco. bovis* was established in only one instance. Whether or not the findings of Reilly are a true reflection of the situation at the present time is uncertain.

The National Tuberculosis Survey of the Republic of Ireland (1954) recounts the typing of 903 strains of tubercle bacilli from human beings. Of 860 strains from pulmonary sources, nine (1 per cent) were *Myco. bovis;* of forty-three strains from nonpulmonary sources, five (10.4 per cent) were *Myco. bovis.*†

That the bovine type of tubercle bacilli at one time constituted a major problem in the epidemiology of tuberculosis of human beings in Denmark is evident from the data presented in Table 7. Additional data of historical value on the prevalence in Denmark of bovine tuberculosis infections of human beings during the period when the disease in cattle was rampant are revealed in the report by Jensen, Lester, and Tolderlung (1940). These workers, during the years 1930-1935, studied cultures of tubercle bacilli from 5,476 cases of various forms of clinical tuberculosis and found *Myco. bovis* in 644 (11.8 per cent). Great strides have been made during the past decade in suppressing bovine tuberculosis in Denmark, and the incidence of human infection by *Myco. bovis* has undoubtedly dimin-

---

*Cited by Francis, 1958.

†For additionl information regarding the relationship of *Myco. bovic* to tuberculosis in Ireland, the report of the National Tuberculosis Survey (1954) may be consulted.

TABLE 7

Incidence in Denmark of the Bovine Type of Infection Among 2,946 Cases of Human Tuberculosis (Jensen and Frimodt-Moller. Quoted by Price)

Variety of Tuberculosis	All Ages			Less Than 15 Years			15 to 29 Years			30 Years and More		
	Total	Bo-vine	Per Cent	Total	Bo-vine	Per Cent	Total	Bo-vine	Per Cent	Total	Bo-vine	Per Cent
Respiratory	1,824	88	4.8	432	29	6.7	1,007	50	5.0	385	9	2.3
Bone and joint	567	105	18.5	98	24	24.5	255	57	22.4	214	24	11.2
Lymph nodes	251	123	49.0	80	66	82.5	97	47	48.5	74	10	13.5
Meningeal	304	75	24.7	176	58	33.0	92	13	14.1	36	4	11.1
Total	2,946	391	13.3	786	177	22.5	1,451	167	11.5	709	47	6.6

ished proportionately. However, due to the relatively long period of residual infection in some persons, instances of human infection with *Myco. bovis* will probably be found long after the disease in cattle has been eradicated.

Data obtained from extensive studies of the problem in other North European countries disclose that infection of human beings, especially children, by bovine tubercle bacilli is of common occurrence. Ruys (1939), for example, working among Dutch children (under 15 years of age) from large towns and rural districts, found that 9 per cent of the cases of pulmonary tuberculosis were due to *Myco. bovis*. In large towns, among adults who had pulmonary tuberculosis, the incidence of bovine type of infection was 1 per cent, whereas among adults from rural areas, the incidence was 6 per cent. In cases of extrapulmonary tuberculosis, *Myco. bovis* was the infective agent in 20 per cent of both rural and urban patients.*

During a period of three years, Hedvall (1940) investigated the occurrence of pulmonary tuberculosis due to the bovine type of the tubercle bacillus among patients in southern Sweden. About 3,300 specimens were examined, and 746 separate cultures of acid-fast bacilli were obtained. Sixty-five strains were *Myco. bovis*. The age

---

*In another report, Ruys (1937) mentioned that about 35 per cent of all cattle slaughtered in Amsterdam in 1933 and 1934 were tuberculous and that 40 per cent of 11,000 cattle in the provinces tested with tuberculin reacted positively. In a later report, Ruys (1950) stated that as a consequence of efforts to control and eradicate tuberculosis among cattle, the prevalence of the disease in Holland was reduced considerably. As evidence of the success of the eradication program, there were several areas in Holland in 1950 where the disease had practically disappeared.

of the patients who had the bovine type of infection varied from
seven months to sixty-eight years, and the majority lived in rural
areas.

Lange (1937), working at the Robert Koch Institute, Berlin, determined the type of tubercle bacilli present in the sputum of certain tuberculous patients—milkers, veterinarians, and butchers—
who, as a consequence of their occupations, were especially liable
to exposure to tuberculous cattle. During the years 1927 to 1937,
sputums from 171 patients were studied, and cultures of acid-fast
bacilli were obtained from 148. When finally classified by appropriate studies, 136 strains of tubercle bacilli of human type and nine
strains of bovine type were recognized. In three of the cases, mixed
cultures of human and bovine tubercle bacilli were recorded. The
ages of the patients ranged from seventeen to fifty-one years.

That there was an occupational factor in Lange's series may be
inferred from the following: Among sixty-nine patients who were
milkers, human type tubercle bacilli occurred in sixty; bovine type
tubercle bacilli occurred in eight; and in one, both human and
bovine types of the bacillus occurred. Among forty patients comprising butchers and veterinarians, thirty-seven were infected with
tubercle bacilli of the human type, one with bacilli of bovine type,
and two with a mixture of both human and bovine types. In a third
group totalling thirty-nine patients, composed of masons, carpenters,
and others, all infections were found to be due to the human type
of organism. Lange quoted the report of Goeters in Leipzig, who
obtained material at necropsy from 118 cases of pulmonary tuberculosis and identified the bovine type of infection in six. In four
of the six cases of bovine type of infection, the subjects were adults.

In Table 4, the incidence in Germany of infection by *Myco. bovis*
among 1,165 cases of tuberculosis in man is given as 13.6 per cent.
More recently (1955), Lebek and Steinert contributed information
on the incidence of nonpulmonary tuberculosis due to *Myco. bovis*
in children in Bavaria. By bacteriologic procedures, including the
inoculation of guinea pigs, they typed 109 strains of tubercle bacilli
from children sixteen years of age. The organisms were identified
as *Myco. bovis* in 34 per cent, as *Myco. tuberculosis* in 63.3 per cent,
and as "mixed" in 2.7 per cent. Obviously at the time this study was
under way, effective means were not employed for safeguarding consumers in Bavaria from milk containing virulent bovine tubercle

bacilli, and tuberculosis of cattle remained a major threat to human beings.

In France, although numerous reports leave no doubt of the prevalence of tuberculosis in the bovine population, the incidence of the bovine type of infection in human beings is much lower than one might expect. This is undoubtedly because in France, cow's milk is seldom consumed without previously being heated. In 1939, Saenz reported on the role of the bovine tubercle bacillus in human tuberculosis in France. Among 903 strains of tubercle bacilli isolated from patients with various forms of tuberculosis, of whom more than half were children, only 22 (2.4 per cent) were of bovine origin.* In seven of the cases of bovine infection, the patients were butchers, who presumably were occupationally exposed to the infection. In the other fifteen cases of bovine infection, most of the patients were children. Saenz also reported on twenty-four cases of lupus, in only two of which were the lesions due to bacilli of bovine origin. He mentioned that in other countries, bovine tubercle bacilli accounted for 50 per cent or more of the cases of lupus. Recently (1962), the results of a nine-year study of the incidence of occurrence of *Myco. bovis* infection in human beings were reported by Bernheim, Viallier, and Cayré. The material studied was from persons residing in Lyons or vicinity. From a total of 722 specimens, mostly from children, 36 (or approximately 5 per cent) yielded *Myco. bovis*. Thirty-two of the 36 cultures were extrapulmonary in origin, 3 were from sputum, and 1 from a gastric lavage. That the source of the *Myco. bovis* infections in this series was tuberculous cattle is a reasonable assumption.

The occurrence in Italy of infection of human beings by *Myco. bovis* was described in 1942 by de Gara. In addition to summarizing the findings of previous investigators, de Gara included in his report an account of cases that he had studied† (Table 8). The data shown in Table 8 indicate that in Italy, during the period when the information was obtained, the bovine type of infection did not constitute any large part of the problem of human tuberculosis. However, the fact that the disease slowly smolders in its natural host makes it a

---

*Not all of the twenty-two strains of tubercle bacilli designated as of the bovine type by Saenz were identified by animal inoculation tests, which fact provokes certain reservations regarding the true bacillary type of some of the strains.

†Work done at the Hygienic Institute, University of Milan.

TABLE 8

PERCENTAGE OF BOVINE TUBERCULOSIS IN ITALY (DE GARA)

Variety of Tuberculosis	Total Number Examined	Bovine Type	
		Number	Per Cent
Bone and joint	8	1 (?)	12.5 (?)
Cervical lymph node	27	1	3.7
Other extrapulmonary	217	14	6.5
Pulmonary	657	20	3.0
Total	909	36	4.0

constant menace to those of the rural population who live or work in close contact with tuberculous animals. In addition, those who presumably drink only cooked or adequately heated milk, may sometimes forget or disregard this important safeguard. Evidently in Italy, at the time of de Gara's observations, pasteurization was not practiced except in the larger communities, and as a consequence, milk was rendered safe by the household practice of boiling it to prevent souring. Indicative of the hazard are de Gara's data, showing that tubercle bacilli were found in 6.8 per cent of 544 samples of market milk. De Gara stated that more than 1,000 strains of tubercle bacilli, obtained throughout Italy, had been typed, and the incidence of the bovine type was 4.8 per cent.

DuToit and Buchanan stated in 1942 that tuberculosis of cattle was of common occurrence in South Africa, but infection of human beings with the bacilli of bovine tuberculosis had rarely been demonstrated. They studied the published data for South Africa and found that of 242 strains of tubercle bacilli, obtained largely from tuberculosis of bones and joints, lymph nodes, and meningeal lesions, only one strain—that obtained from a case of tuberculous meningitis —proved to be bovine in origin.

Carmichael (1940) studied pulmonary tuberculosis in the natives of Uganda. He reported a survey by Wilcocks in 1939 in Tanganyika, in which sputums of sixty-seven natives affected with pulmonary tuberculosis were studied, and all strains were of the human type. Carmichael's own observations include the fact that the cattle of the district of Ankole were severely infected with tuberculosis, as many as 70 per cent of the animals reacting positively to the tuberculin test. Using cultural methods and the inoculation of rabbits, Carmichael determined the type of 283 strains of tubercle bacilli isolated in cases of pulmonary tuberculosis; only four were of the bovine type.

Webster, reporting in 1941 on the incidence of human and bovine types of tuberculosis among the people of Victoria, Australia, stated that among 183 adults affected with a variety of clinical forms of tuberculosis, no instance of bovine type of infection occurred. Among 123 children, eleven (8.9 per cent) were infected with the bovine type of the tubercle bacillus. The lesions occurred in the tonsils and cervical and mesenteric lymph nodes. According to Webster, in Victoria, the bacillus of bovine tuberculosis had little or no part in the causation of tuberculosis of the bones and joints.

Chapple and Abrahams (1956) reported from Queensland, Australia, six cases of pulmonary tuberculosis in man in which *Myco. bovis,* by pathogenicity tests, was established as the causative agent. All of the patients were males. The average age of five of the patients was fifty-three years; the sixth was twenty-seven years old. An occupational factor seemed to be of significance in explaining the disease, which the authors believed had been acquired by inhalation. The occupations of the respective patients were as follows: abattoir employee, two; dairy farmer, two; stockman, one; and bullock driver, one. The findings indicated potential hazard to those whose daily work brought them in intimate contact with aerosols from morbid tissues containing *Myco. bovis.**

According to Kimura and Kondo (1939), Kitasato was the first in Japan to investigate the role of *Myco. bovis* in human infections. A total of 152 cases were studied, but in none was the bacillus of bovine tuberculosis recognized. Kimura and Kondo summarized the reports of various Japanese workers and found, as of February 1939, that a total of 1,323 cases of tuberculosis (in all of which the patients were Japanese) had been studied bacteriologically and that the human type of infecting agent had been present in 1,310 cases, whereas in only thirteen cases (0.98 per cent) were bovine tubercle bacilli recognized. The thirteen strains were obtained from the following anatomic sites: lung and pleura, one strain; bone and joint, two strains; cervical lymph nodes, two strains; genito-urinary tract, one strain; skin, seven strains. The authors attributed the low rate

---

*The report of Chapple and Abrahams (1956) contains a useful listing of many published accounts of the occurrence of infections by *Myco. bovis* in human beings.

of infection with the bovine type of the tubercle bacillus largely to the fact that the amount of raw milk consumed by the Japanese is minimal.

Although reports indicate that tuberculosis is prevalent among the cattle in Argentina, relatively few instances have been reported in which *Myco. bovis* has been obtained from human beings. The first report, according to Vaccarezza and Arena (1943) was made by Ligniers in 1904. The same authors quoted Poire and Arseno-Carranza as having studied 150 strains of tubercle bacilli obtained from sputums of patients with pulmonary tuberculosis; none was bovine in type. Vaccarezza and Arena mentioned that in a few instances, the bacilli of bovine tuberculosis had been identified in cases of pulmonary and extrapulmonary tuberculous disease in human beings in Argentina. The fact that boiling of milk is generally practiced probably accounts for this apparently low rate of infection.

Delgado and Ilukevich (1957) investigated the incidence of infection with *Myco. bovis* in patients with various forms of tuberculosis in Venezuela. Among 164 patients, mycobacteria of bovine tuberculosis were obtained from eight (4.88 per cent). The authors concluded in part "that the infection of bovine origin plays a very important role in the human tuberculosis epidemiology of our environment."

Indicative of the part that milk from tuberculous cows may have in incapacitating children are the results of a study by Price (1938) in Toronto, Canada. Price had accumulated data during thirteen years on 500 tuberculous children and found that 9.6 per cent of the extrapulmonary tuberculosis was due to the bovine type of infection. The youngest child in Price's series was six and one-half months of age, and without exception, the children came from an environment that did not provide for pasteurization of milk.

In 1942, Beattie and Nicewonger reported an investigation in the United States on the occurrence of *Myco. bovis* in human pulmonary tuberculosis. A total of 366 strains of tubercle bacilli from the sputums of persons in sanatoriums and hospitals in various parts of California were studied. The strains were "screened" by cultural methods, and those that were dysgonic or not typically eugonic were subjected to tests for virulence in rabbits. No strains considered to be bovine in type were found.

Earlier reports on the incidence of infection with bovine tubercle bacilli in human beings in the United States vary as follows: Of the 564 cases of tuberculosis reported by Park and Krumwiede in 1910, the bovine type of infectious agent was present in 7.6 per cent. In Aronson and Whitney's (1930) series and in the report by Van Es and Martin (1930), the incidence of the bovine type of infection was 3.8 and 3.9 per cent, respectively. In 1933, Chang reported the results of a study he had made at a sanatorium in Massachusetts. In approximately one-fourth of the 200 cases studied, the infective organisms were of the bovine type. The figures of Chang are unusual and probably did not represent a true indication of the extent of infection of human beings with the bacilli of bovine tuberculosis generally throughout the United States at the time of his studies.

At the present time (1962) in the United States, the occurrence of bovine tubercle bacilli in milk must be extremely rare. Human beings who are now infected with *Myco. bovis* are probably elderly persons—those in the fifth to seventh decades—who were infected before the tuberculin testing of cattle and the pasteurization of milk were generally practiced. Exceptions are, of course, possible. In rural areas, where the family obtains its milk from the so-called "family" cow, an occasional animal in this category that has not been tuberculin tested may harbor tubercle bacilli. Such an animal could be a source of tuberculosis in man.

From the foregoing incomplete review of reports and investigations that have yielded information on the infectivity of *Myco. bovis* for human beings, several pertinent facts become apparent:

1) *Myco. bovis* is an important pathogen for human beings.

2) A review of the literature by Price in 1939, revealed that among approximately 18,000 cases of human tuberculosis in which the type of the infectious agent was determined, *Myco. bovis* was responsible in 10 per cent of the cases.

3) The marked decrease in the incidence of tuberculosis in cattle has been paralleled by striking reduction in the incidence of infection with *Myco. bovis* in human beings. The detection of the disease by testing cattle with tuberculin, and the further safeguard provided by the proper pasteurization of milk, give impressive assurance that milk can be produced that will not expose the consumer to the danger of bovine tuberculosis.

4) Cases of bovine tuberculous infections of human beings have had widespread geographic distribution, although it must be em-

phasized that, excepting in the countries of Western Europe, the problem has been insufficiently explored.

5) The organism of bovine tuberculosis is capable of producing in human beings every form of tuberculosis of which the human type of organism is capable.

6) Children are much more commonly infected with the bovine type of the tubercle bacillus than are adults. The incidence is highest among children less than five years of age.*

7) The usual portal of entry of bovine tubercle bacilli in human beings is by way of the alimentary canal through the medium of contaminated milk and other dairy products. This probably accounts for the extrapulmonary situation of the vast majority of infections with bovine tubercle bacilli in man.

8) Although the extrapulmonary forms of tuberculosis predominate in the statistics, several hundred cases of pulmonary tuberculosis in man, caused by *Myco. bovis,* have now been established.

9) According to Price (1939), lesions of extrapulmonary tuberculosis in a child in the absence of demonstrable tuberculosis in the parenchyma of the lungs or in the tracheobronchial lymph nodes, should be regarded as due to the bovine type of infectious agent unless proved otherwise.

10) According to Griffith (1938), the latent period of human pulmonary tuberculosis of alimentary origin from *Myco. bovis* may vary from less than one year to twenty-six years or more.

11) The tuberculous dairy cow is a serious menace to human health and should not be tolerated by an informed society.

Transmissibility: Man to Bovine

Since tuberculosis is a contagious disease, it would be remarkable indeed if *Myco. bovis* could be transmitted only from the natural host—the cow—to other cattle and to human beings. Griffith and Munro (1944) gave a brief account of a herd that had been tested repeatedly with tuberculin and the reactors eliminated. Every new test revealed that some previously negative animal had become a reactor. Although initially the source of the continuing infection

---

*It is Rich's (1951) opinion that the difference in the frequency of infection in adults and in children due to the bovine tubercle bacillus can be explained on the basis of greater exposure of children to the infectious agent, since milk constitutes a large part of the diet of children, and the greater degree of natural resistance to tuberculosis possessed by adults.

was not suspected, the herdsman was known to have been affected with pulmonary tuberculosis due to the bovine type of the organism, and it is likely that the contagion in this case was from man to animal.

Another example of the role of human beings in the transmission of bovine tuberculosis to previously noninfected cattle was reported by Tice (1944) of New York State. In this instance, in spite of repeated tuberculin tests, the removal of all reactors, and strict measures of sanitation, infection continued to occur in new additions to the herd. It was not until three complete herds had been slaughtered on account of positive tuberculin reactions that the owner was suspected as the possible source of the infection. Investigation revealed that he had been a patient at a tuberculosis sanatorium for a few weeks just prior to the first tuberculin test of the dairy herd. Subsequent study of sputum from the owner of the dairy and of infected lymph nodes from the cattle that had reacted to tuberculin revealed tubercle bacilli of the bovine type. The evidence in Tice's report indicates definitely that the owner had contracted pulmonary tuberculosis from his original herd and had subsequently infected three new replacement herds within a period of two and one-half years. Tice's observation emphasizes the importance of medical examination of human beings who may have access to the premises of a dairy in which repeated tuberculin tests of the herd reveal the presence of tuberculosis of obscure origin.

An analysis of the source of new infections which occurred among 915 previously tuberculosis-free herds in Jutland (1950) showed that in 10.4 per cent of the herds, the disease was apparently re-introduced by tuberculous human beings presumably infected with bovine tubercle bacilli (Bendixen, 1950). Several additional instances of infection of previously tuberculosis-free cattle by human beings infected with bovine tubercle bacilli have been reported by Plum* of Copenhagen.

A few cases have been reported in which human tubercle bacilli were demonstrated in naturally infected, tuberculous cattle. Feldman and Moses (1941) reviewed the literature up to 1941, and reported a case of their own. In several of the 10 cases reviewed, it was known that exposure to human beings with pulmonary tuber-

---

*Cited by Jensen *et al.,* 1940.

culosis had occurred. In most of the cases, the infective process had remained localized in one or more lymph nodes of the bovine recipient, although in one instance, lesions occurred in the lung, bronchial lymph nodes, and one of the mesenteric lymph nodes.

It is obvious that persons who have active pulmonary tuberculosis should be excluded from premises frequented by cattle. Exposure to tubercle bacilli of the human type seldom produces demonstrable lesions in cattle. However, such exposure may result in the development of tuberculin hypersensitivity.

Transmissibility: Man to Man

Griffith and Munro (1944) also discussed the possibility of pulmonary tuberculosis of the bovine type being disseminated from one person to another. The evidence in support of this happening if circumstances are propitious is impressive. Certainly the sputum of a patient who has pulmonary tuberculosis of the human type plays an important role in the spread of the disease from person to person, and there is no reason for believing that sputum containing the bovine form of the tubercle bacillus would be less contagious. It is generally agreed by those who have had experience with the subject that the bovine type of the tubercle bacillus is not less virulent for human beings than the human type. To quote Griffith and Munro, "It would be very surprising if these bacilli are not sometimes transmitted to healthy persons through the inspired air." They recounted instances in which strong presumptive evidence existed for the "man-to-man" transmission of the bovine type of infection. Cumming (1933) presented evidence suggesting that air-borne infection with the bovine type of tubercle bacilli does occur in dairy workers.

In 1939, Munro reported a case in which it appeared likely that there had been transmission of the disease from father to child. The child, two and one-half years of age, had received no other than pasteurized milk. Bovine tubercle bacilli had been cultured from the sputum of the father, who was exceedingly careless in his personal habits and practiced no safeguards to avoid infecting others. Clinically, the child gave evidence of tuberculosis of an ankle joint, and roentgenographically there were signs of minimal tuberculosis in the lungs. Bovine tubercle bacilli were cultured from gastric contents obtained by lavage and from the urine of the child.

Ruys (1939) reported a case in which pulmonary tuberculosis in a human being was due to the bovine variety of the tubercle bacillus. It appeared that the infection had its source from a friend who had open pulmonary infection also due to *Myco. bovis.*

Another tragic example of the transmission of the bovine type of tuberculosis infection from an infected human being to others was reported by Van der Hoeden and de Raadt of the Medical University Clinic of Utrecht (1940). A girl, sixteen years of age, with severe productive pulmonary tuberculosis due to bovine tubercle bacilli, infected two younger sisters and a younger brother. The oldest girl, one sister, age fifteen years, and the brother, age ten years, all died with rapidly progressing tuberculosis, and tubercle bacilli of the bovine type were demonstrated from each. The other sister, twelve years of age, was also infected, but at the time of the report was not clinically ill. A significant circumstance that perhaps explains the transmission of the infection is the fact that each of the younger children had occupied for one night the same bed as the oldest sister during the period when she was seriously ill and was expectorating much infective material.

DETECTION OF BOVINE TYPE OF INFECTION IN HUMAN BEINGS

Since there are no recognizable clinical, roentgenographic, or pathologic features that provide reliable means whereby one can definitely distinguish human from bovine forms of tuberculous infection in man, laboratory procedures are necessary for the precise diagnosis. As was mentioned previously (p.), most mammalian strains of tubercle bacilli can be "typed" as bovine or human on the basis of certain cultural features. Most strains of the human type will grow in a medium containing glycerin, but bovine strains on initial isolation prefer a nonglycerinated medium, or one in which the glycerine content does not exceed 0.75 per cent. Furthermore, most strains of *Myco. tuberculosis* are eugonic; conversely, strains of *Myco. bovis* are usually dysgonic.* It must be kept in mind that the distinguishing characteristics mentioned constitute presumptive,

---

*Atypical strains of tubercle bacilli and instances of "mixed" infections with human and bovine types of tubercle bacilli are considered in the review articles by Price (1939) and by Griffith and Munro (1944).

rather than unequivocal, proof of the type of tubercle bacillus under consideration. To obtain convincing proof of the type of the organism, it is necessary to inoculate guinea pigs and rabbits, and sometimes chickens, following the procedures mentioned previously (p. 10). With the results of a properly conducted animal test available, it should be possible to type or classify definitely nearly all strains of acid-fast bacilli responsible for mammalian tuberculosis.

CONTROL OF INFECTION FROM CATTLE TO MAN

As was mentioned previously, milk from tuberculous cows is frequently contaminated with tubercle bacilli. Butter, cream, and cheese made from such milk may likewise contain the organisms. Even if the milk from tuberculous cows does not contain *Myco. bovis* before it is excreted from the udder, there is always the possibility that contamination with tubercle bacilli may occur from extraneous sources, of which manure in the dairy barn or in the barnyard is hazardous. Data assembled by Williams and Hoy (1927) established that dung from tuberculous cattle, and even from cattle that were apparently healthy, contained tubercle bacilli virulent for guinea pigs. The contamination of milk by barnyard filth occurs fairly commonly, and should fecal material containing tubercle bacilli fall into the milk from the soiled surface of the udder and sides of the cow, the milk at once becomes dangerous to human health.*

A sound and well-proved method of safeguarding the public from the tuberculous dairy cow is the periodic tuberculin testing of all cattle and the slaughter of those animals that react positively to the test. As a further safeguard, the proper pasteurization of milk intended for human consumption should be compulsory. (An exception would be "certified" milk.)

Tonney, White, and Danforth (1927) compiled data from European cities and found that of 16,700 samples of market milk examined, 8.66 per cent contained tubercle bacilli. The specimens were collected from several large centers of population, and the studies were made by a large number of investigators during the period from 1893 to 1925. The occurrence of contaminated milk varied

---

*Maddock (1933) showed that in some instances virulent bovine tubercle bacilli can survive six months' exposure in soil, in soil and dung mixture, and in dung.

from 2.7 per cent of specimens to 61.5 per cent. It should be pointed out that these data were compiled at a time when the danger of the bovine type of tubercle bacilli to human health was not generally recognized, and as a consequence, little had been done to exclude tuberculous cows from dairy herds.

In a recent (1959) report by Maglione and Cavallero of Italy, information was presented that established the presence of *Myco. bovis* in the washings of the skin of the mammary gland of naturally infected cattle. It is evident that where a high percentage of a dairy herd is infected, the environmental factors are of much significance in the transmission of the disease to other animals and to human beings.

The data concerning transmission of tuberculosis from cattle to man provide formidable evidence that milk, unless produced under the strictest sanitary and regulatory control, may not be a safe food for human consumption.

The literature contains many reports of the efficacy of pasteurization in killing tubercle bacilli in cow's milk. The reports of Price (1938, 1939) after her long experience with the situation in Toronto and the surrounding province of Ontario, Canada, provide unequivocal evidence of the effectiveness of proper pasteurization in eliminating tubercle bacilli from the milk supply of a large city. Relative to the situation to Toronto, Price wrote as follows in 1939: "Since 1916, when pasteurization was made compulsory, there has not been a single proven case of bovine infection in the generation of children using city milk." This statement was based on the careful study of the etiologic factor in a series of 500 tuberculous children whom Price had investigated during a period of thirteen years. She found that tubercle bacilli of the bovine type were responsible for 9.64 per cent of the extrapulmonary tuberculous infection. It was of much significance that without exception children infected with *Myco. bovis* had their residence elsewhere than in the city of Toronto. Price also established the fact that the children infected with *Myco. bovis* had consumed raw milk for some time.

Confirmatory of the effectiveness of pasteurization in rendering milk containing tubercle bacilli safe for human consumption are the observations of Ruys of Amsterdam. Before, during, and after World War II, Ruys (1946, 1950) investigated by precise bacteriological methods the types of tubercle bacilli obtained from patients with various forms of clinical tuberculosis in Amsterdam. The figures show that before the war, infections with bovine tubercle bacilli, especially in children, were common. During and after the war, the incidence of the infection in children declined strikingly. Furthermore, among children not in contact with persons known to have active tuberculosis, the percentage of positive tuberculin reactors gradually diminished during the years of the war and thereafter. Although infection with bovine tubercle bacilli had markedly diminished, infection with human-type tubercle bacilli during this period had shown an increase of serious magnitude.

In explanation of the reduction of new infections due to bovine tubercle bacilli, Ruys (1950) mentioned that since 1940 there had been in Amsterdam compulsory pasteurization of all milk sold for human consumption. This practice was instituted during the war by the Germans and has continued ever since.

Further evidence of the ability of the pasteurization process to render bovine tubercle bacilli nonviable was obtained by Price (1938). She subjected to tests in guinea pigs, 200 samples of pooled raw milk which were obtained from the pasteurization tanks prior to heating. In 26 per cent of the samples, virulent tubercle bacilli were demonstrated by animal inoculation tests. After heating the milk, from which the samples had been obtained, at 145°F. for thirty minutes and cooling it quickly, 100 additional samples were removed and used to inoculate guinea pigs. None of the samples in the second series produced tuberculosis in the inoculated animals.*

With modern equipment, pasteurization of milk is an economical and efficient procedure for rendering milk safe without impairing to any measurable degree its value as a highly important and nutritious food. Pasteurization plants should be operated under some public health authority and in strict conformity with regulations designed to provide maximal efficiency.

Improper pasteurization of milk may be harmful in that the designation "pasteurized milk" implies a factor of safety that may not be

---

*The most reliable method for detecting tubercle bacilli in milk is by the inoculation of guinea pigs. A 50 to 100 cc. sample of the suspected milk is centrifuged for thirty minutes at 3,000 r.p.m. The cream and the sediment are mixed, the intervening fluid is discarded, and the resultant material is divided into two equal portions and used to inoculate two healthy guinea pigs subcutaneously. The animals are killed for necropsy eight weeks after inoculation and examined for lesions of tuberculosis.

present.* Modern equipment, proper supervision, and frequent inspections are the essential factors for obtaining pasteurized milk that is safe for human consumption.

Another factor to be considered in the possible transmissibility of tuberculosis of animals to human beings is the infectivity of the musculature and other edible tissue of meat-producing animals. Tuberculosis in animals is ordinarily not a self-limiting disease. The infective agents are conveyed from an initial lesion to other situations of predilection by continuity, by the lymphatics, and by the blood stream. If the disease is severe and of widespread distribution, it is likely that at some phase of its progression, the tubercle bacilli had a hematogenous spread, and, as a consequence, all tissues are likely to have received a deposition of few-to-many tubercle bacilli. It is true that certain tissues, such as the smooth and striated muscles, have considerable intrinsic resistance to tuberculous infection, and it is exceptional that a focus of the disease will develop and prosper in the musculature. For this reason, lesions of tuberculosis are found most frequently in the lymph nodes and parenchymal organs, such as the lungs, liver, spleen, mammary glands, and testes.

In 1932, Day reported the incidence of tuberculosis of the musculature of cattle slaughtered in Federally supervised abattoirs. During a period of twenty-three years, a total of twenty-five cases involving the voluntary muscles were recorded. Five of the animals were bulls, two-to-six years of age; three were steers, two-to-three years of age; two were heifers, two years of age; and fifteen were cows, four-to-ten years of age. In all cases, lesions of tuberculosis were also found elsewhere in the respective carcasses; and in fourteen of the twenty-five cases, the disease was generalized throughout the internal organs. In view of the millions of carcasses of cattle examined during the period when Day's material was obtained, the few cases of tuberculosis involving the voluntary musculature demonstrate the rarity of this form of the disease.

The meat inspection service, administered by the United States Department of Agriculture, is highly efficient. However, Federally-supervised meat inspection is required only for meat prepared for food by concerns engaged in interstate commerce. According to data

---

*According to Ruys (1939), Boer found that inadequately pasteurized milk may contain living tubercle bacilli and hence provide a false sense of security.

from the Agricultural Research Service, USDA, the foregoing represents about 80 per cent of the meat and poultry prepared for human consumption in the United States. The remainder of the meat and poultry products in the United States amounts to 6.3 billion pounds annually and may be sold under city, county, or State inspection or without the benefit of any inspection whatever.* Local inspection may be inadequate owing to lack of trained personnel and the failure of public health authorities to insist on adequate examination by qualified inspectors.

In inspecting meat of tuberculous animals to determine wholesomeness for human consumption, the Federal inspector is guided by regulations which are based on the principle that no meat shall be passed for food if it contains tubercle bacilli or if there is a reasonable possibility that it contains tubercle bacilli or if it is impregnated with the toxic substances of tuberculosis or associated septic infections.† To be effective, meat inspection should include both antemortem and postmortem examinations.

TUBERCULOSIS IN MAMMALS OTHER THAN CATTLE

Dogs

Dogs are apparently equally susceptible to *Myco. bovis* and *Myco. tuberculosis*. They have a high resistance to *Myco. avium* and are difficult to infect with this species even experimentally.‡ Tuberculosis in dogs produces few symptoms that are characteristic, and as a consequence the disease is seldom recognized while the animal is living. The disease frequently affects the lungs, where the lesions commonly undergo necrosis with extension of the bacilli-laden cellu-

---

*From item pertaining to the need for additional meat inspection legislation by Dr. M. R. Clarkson: *J.A.V.M.A., 140:*424-425, Mar. 1, 1962.

†For data pertaining to the presence of virulent tubercle bacilli in voluntary striated muscle, heart, blood, spleen, liver, and lymph nodes of a variety of food animals affected with tuberculosis, see report by Müller and Ishiwara (1914).

‡Plum (1936) reported an instance of presumably naturally acquired avian tuberculosis in a dog. Miliary lesions occurred in the lungs, kidneys, and spleen. A culture of mycobacteria was obtained from the kidney, with the characteristics of *Myco. avium.* The bacteria were tested for virulence in a rabbit, a chicken, and guinea pigs. From the results, it was concluded that the organisms were avian tubercule bacilli. The resistance of dogs to experimental infection with *Myco. avium* invokes reservations as to the validity of this case. Plum also suggested that some of the circumstances of the case were inexplicable.

lar detritus into the larger respiratory channels. Tuberculous tracheitis may occur. Consequently, the tuberculous dog is a potential danger to human beings and especially to children, who frequently fondle and play with their canine pets in an intimate manner.*

The exact incidence of tuberculosis in dogs is unknown. In the United States only an occasional case has been reported. Most of the data are derived from the observations of investigators in Europe, including Great Britian. A compilation of 182 cases in which the bacillary type of the infecting agent was determined is shown in Table 9.

TABLE 9

TYPES OF TUBERCLE BACILLI IN 182 CASES OF NATURALLY ACQUIRED
TUBERCULOSIS IN DOGS (FELDMAN AND CODE)

Geographic Area	Bacillary Type		
	Human	Bovine	Avian
England and Scotland	29	11	0
Continental Europe	103	32	1
Dutch East Indies	2	0	0
United States	3	1	0
Total	137	44	1

From the data presented in Table 9, it is evident that the frequency of infection of dogs with the human type of tubercle bacillus is about three times as great as the frequency of infection with the bovine type. However, this does not indicate that dogs are more resistant to *Myco. bovis* than to *Myco. tuberculosis*. The disparity in the incidence of the two types of infection can best be explained on the basis that there was a greater opportunity for exposure to infectious material containing tubercle bacilli of the human type.

Scott (1930) investigated the probable source of exposure of 100 tuberculous dogs and found that fifty-one had lived in restaurants or cafes where human sputum was at all times present on the floors, and twenty-eight had lived in intimate contact with sick persons.

Urwitz (1949) mentioned that at the Veterinary College in Stockholm, during the ten-year period beginning 1938, necropsy was per-

---

*For additional information on tuberculosis in dogs, the following may be conculted: Scott (1930), Feldman and Code (1942), Lovell and White (1940), Hjarre (1939), Hawthorne *et al.* (1957), and Francis (1958).

formed on 3,673 dogs. Instances of tuberculosis in the dogs were observed every year, with a total of fifty-two for the period.

In 1955, during a four-months' period, 175 consecutive dogs were examined at necropsy at the University of Glasgow Veterinary Hospital. Generalized tuberculosis was observed in eight, approximately 4.5 per cent (Hawthorne *et al.*, 1957).

In 1956, Berg reported 8 cases of tuberculosis among 1,750 dogs examined at the Norwegian Veterinary College (Oslo) during 1949-53. In 7 of the dogs, the etiologic agent was found to be *Myco. tuberculosis;* in the 8th dog, although mycobacteria were

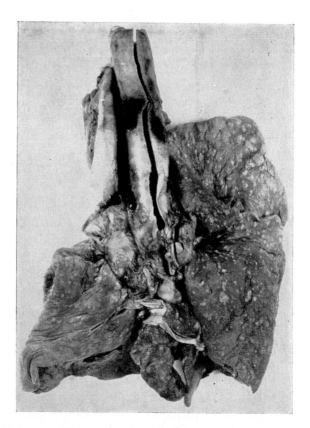

Fig. 9. Multiple nodular lesions of tuberculosis of the lungs of an adult dog. An enlarged tracheobronchial lymph node occupies the left central area between the lung and the trachea. There was present also a large tuberculous mass in the wall of the terminal portion of the ileum. Infection was due to the human type of the tubercle bacillus.

observed in smear from a peritoneal exudate, no culture was obtained.

In the above-mentioned series it may be assumed that few, if any, of the dogs were diagnosed as tuberculous during life. The potential hazard for human beings of such seedbeds of infection is obvious.

Some of the characteristics of tuberculosis in dogs may be summarized briefly as follows: 1) The disease occurs most frequently in animals from one to five years of age. 2) Symptoms, while not pathognomonic, may include loss of weight, cough, and enlargement of the lymph nodes of the head and neck. 3) The lungs and tracheobronchial lymph nodes are affected in about 60 per cent of the cases (Figures 9 and 10). Other organs of predilection include the liver and the kidneys. Less frequently, the pleura, pericardium, and peritoneum are involved. 4) The morbid anatomic manifestations may be caseous granulomatous nodules, exudative tuberculous pneumonitis, or circumscribed neoplastic-like masses; the last occur especially in the liver and kidneys. Microscopically, giant cells of the Langhans type, frequently associated with tuberculosis in many other mammals, do not occur. 5) Acid-fast bacillary forms are often

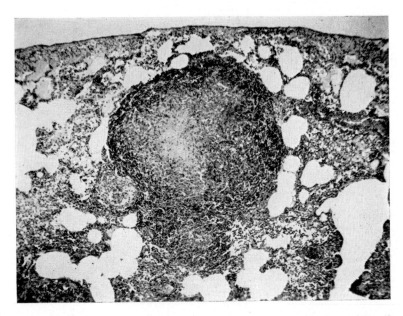

Fig. 10. Tuberculous nodule near the periphery of a lung of a dog (x70). (Same case as shown in Fig. 9.)

numerous in preparations made from the caseous portions of the lesions.

In the diagnosis of tuberculosis in dogs, consideration should be given to: 1) possibilities for infection as a consequence of contact with a human being who has active pulmonary tuberculosis or by the ingestion of contaminated cow's milk or tissue containing bovine tubercle bacilli; 2) suggestive symptoms such as loss of weight and cough of variable duration; and 3) the results of the tuberculin test.

In conducting a tuberculin test on dogs, 0.1 cc. of a 1:100 dilution of tuberculin (OT or PPD) should be injected intracutaneously. The results of the test should be recorded after 48 hours (Colwell and Mills, 1940). The degree of induration, not erythema, is significant in interpreting the reaction. In animals in the terminal stages of the disease, or those in poor general health due to mange or distemper, the sensitivity to tuberculin may be suppressed.

The public health aspect of tuberculosis in dogs is worthy of consideration. The possibility of transmission of the infection from a tuberculous dog to man certainly exists, although few such instances have been reported.

Urwitz (1949) of Stockholm reported that a dog infected with *Myco. tuberculosis* was the probable source of infection in five cases of pulmonary tuberculosis in human beings. The dog had presumably become infected as a consequence of frequent association with a man who had active cavitary pulmonary tuberculosis, proved bacteriologically. Two of the patients were ten to twelve years of age; the third was an infant. The fourth patient, mother of the infant, was in her early twenties. These four patients were members of two families that shared a two-story cottage. The fifth patient was a playmate of the other children, all of whom frolicked frequently with the infected dog.

Urwitz also briefly mentioned a case, observed by Bjure, of miliary tuberculosis in an infant due to *Myco. bovis*. The child had contact with an Alsatian wolfhound that was affected with bilateral pulmonary tuberculosis in which the causative organism was also *Myco. bovis*.

De Kock and le Roux (1956) reported a case in which a tuberculous lesion developed on a finger of a veterinarian after he performed necropsies on two dogs with generalized tuberculosis. The organisms obtained from the patient's finger and from the dogs all were shown by subsequent studies to be *Myco. tuberculosis.* The patient was successfully treated by excision of the morbid tissue, followed by specific chemotherapy.

In tuberculous dogs having pulmonary lesions in which there is bronchogenic spread or exudative tuberculous pneumonitis, countless numbers of tubercle bacilli find egress with the respiratory excretions mixed with the saliva. Many of the organisms are undoubtedly swallowed and eliminated with the feces. In severe destructive tuberculosis of the kidneys, tuberculous bacilluria is probably common. These facts, in addition to the inference that may be drawn from the instances of human infections recounted, constitute sufficient reasons for considering tuberculosis in the differential diagnosis of sick dogs. Obviously, a tuberculous dog should be destroyed, and for public health reasons, the type of infection should be determined by appropriate laboratory procedures.*

Cats

Tuberculosis of cats is an uncommon disease in the United States. In Europe, the incidence of the disease varies from 2 per cent to 13 per cent of cats examined.[†]

Cats have a formidable resistance to infection with *Myco. tuberculosis* and *Myco. avium,* but they are susceptible to *Myco. bovis.*[‡] Available evidence indicates that in most instances, the infection in cats is by way of the digestive tract. This coincides with the fact that in districts where bovine tubercle bacilli occur in the milk and the milk is not boiled or pasteurized, tuberculosis of cats is likely to occur.

Despite the many failures to induce experimentally in cats tuberculous infections with *Myco. tuberculosis,* a few instances have been reported in which naturally acquired infections with this type of the tubercle bacillus have occurred. Hjarre (1939) reported one of seven

---

*A report of an epidemiologic study if the inter-relationship between tuberculosis of human beings, dogs, and cats in Glasgow, Scotland, has been contributed by Hawthorne and Lauder (1962).

†A brief account of tuberculosis in cats, due in most instances to *Myco. bovis,* has been given by Karlson (1960).

‡Kuwabara (1938) attempted to infect a series of cats with *Myco. tuberculosis* by inoculation, by feeding, or by exposing them for two-to-three years in the homes of tuberculous patients. In none of the animals did tuberculosis develop. Progressive tuberculosis developed among all cats inoculated with *Myco. bovis.*

cases of tuberculosis in cats to be due to the human type of the tubercle bacillus.

A most unusual tuberculous infection in a cat was described recently by Hix, Jones, and Karlson (1961). At necropsy of a four-
year-old spayed female Siamese cat, a culture of mycobacteria was
obtained from the lungs. By appropriate laboratory procedures, including animal inoculation tests, the organism was proved to be
Myco. avium. The animal had been ill for some months. Symptoms
included a persistent cough, intermittent dyspnea, and loss of weight.
Aside from a general lymphadenopathy, evidence of the infection
was confined to the lungs. The morbid changes in the lung produced
areas of consolidation by the proliferation of epithelioid cells, which
obliterated alveolar spaces. Sections of the morbid tissue—lymph
nodes and lungs— when appropriately stained, revealed myriads of
mycobacteria.

Another unusual instance of mycobacterial infection in a cat was
reported by Huitema and van Vloten (1960) of Rotterdam. Lesions
from the lungs and mesenteric lymph nodes failed to yield cultures,
but from the spleen and lymph nodes of guinea pigs inoculated with
the morbid material, cultures were obtained that were considered
to be the murine (vole) type of mycobacteria.

Transmission of tuberculous infection of cats to human beings
appears to be of rare occurrence. One such case, with fatal termination, was reported from Sweden by Lewis-Jonsson (1946). The patient was a previously healthy boy, approximately three and one-half
years of age. About three weeks before being seen by a physician, the
child had been bitten on the right forearm by "a diseased cat." The
wounds of the dermis were pinprick-like. These healed initially in
twenty-three days, but infiltration then ensued, followed by ulceration. The child became febrile, and tenderness developed in the
right axilla. The patient's condition showed a slow but continuous
worsening, and he died 110 days after being bitten. The salient features of the necropsy findings were ulcerous tuberculosis of the
skin in the area of the cat bite, miliary lesions in the lungs, spleen,
liver, and kidneys, and tuberculous meningitis. Morbid tissue, obtained at necropsy, was used to inoculate a guinea pig and a rabbit.
Lesions developed in each animal, and *Myco. bovis* was obtained by
culture from lesions in the guinea pig. It is unfortunate that circumstances precluded a necropsy of the cat that bit the child. How-

ever, the evidence relating the bite of the sick cat to the infection of the child is convincing.

Information regarding the pathologic characteristics of natural tuberculous infections among cats was contributed by Dobson (1930), working at Edinburgh, Scotland. Dobson observed the disease in eleven of a total of 505 cats examined. In every instance, the bovine type of the organism was the etiologic agent. Among the infected cats, the sexes were about equally represented. Emaciation was the most commonly observed symptom. The lesions occurred most frequently in the mesenteric lymph nodes, lungs, spleen, kidneys, and liver. In three cases, open cutaneous lesions were present. Tuberculous lymphadenitis also occurred. In one instance there was pleural effusion; in two, tuberculous peritonitis; and in one, a tuberculous nodule in the small intestine. Dobson was unable to demonstrate acid-fast bacilli in the saliva or in the urine of the infected cats.

The pathologic character of tuberculosis in cats is that of a disseminated miliary or nodular process that is commonly characterized by liquefaction (Figure 11). Although the route of entry of the infective agent is through the mucosa of the intestine, the intestine may be without demonstrable lesions. In some instances severe tuberculous enteritis may occur, but this would appear to be due to autoreinfection from tubercle bacilli in the ingesta when an animal that has "open" pulmonary tuberculosis swallows its own infective respiratory secretions. It is likely that in the lungs the primary focus occurs subpleurally. Extension of the process into the pleura and beyond may produce a purulent or fibrinous pleural reaction. The pleura becomes greatly thickened and may eventually consist of a dense structure of fibrous connective tissue without distinguishing signs of tuberculosis.

As the disease progresses in the lungs, diffuse and striking pneumonitis may ensue. As a consequence large regions of the lungs become solidified. These eventually caseate or liquefy, with the destruction of pulmonary tissue and the formation of cavities. Entrance of tuberculous debris into the bronchioles may occur. As a result bronchogenic spread of the infection is probably fairly common.

Except in the early miliary form, the tuberculous character of the lesions may not at once be recognized microscopically. Giant

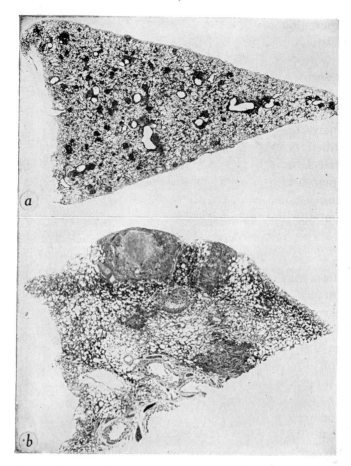

Fig. 11. Pulmonary tuberculosis of the cat. *a*. Miliary type showing a moderate number of small dark colored discrete tuberculous foci (x4). *b*. Nodular type showing large tuberculous nodules near the periphery. The center of one nodule has undergone considerable caseation necrosis (x8). (Prepared from material kindly supplied by Dr. J. T. Stamp, Royal [Dick] Veterinary College, University of Edinburgh.)

cells of the Langhans type do not occur. When caseation is present, calcification may occur, but this is uncommon. Appropriately stained tissue may contain acid-fast bacilli in sufficient numbers to be seen microscopically.

The disease seems to have special predilection for the lungs, judging from the severity of the reaction in these organs. In instances in

which tuberculous pneumonitis is present, large regions of the parenchymal tissue are distorted and destroyed beyond recognition.

In many respects, the pathologic anatomy of naturally acquired
tuberculosis in cats is similar to inoculation tuberculosis in the
highly susceptible guinea pig. The disease in both species is widely
disseminated and highly destructive, and there are many similarities
in the microscopic appearance of the lesions in the various organs.

The tuberculous cat, like the tuberculous dog, must be considered
a potential source of tuberculous infection to other mammals including man and particularly children. Especially likely as a source
of infection to man are open cutaneous lesions, the discharge from
which contains numerous tubercle bacilli.*

Swine

The susceptibility of swine to infection with mycobacteria is
unique in that this animal may be infected by either of the three
common species of tubercle bacilli responsible for tuberculosis in
warm-blooded animals. Because of this fact, the incidence of tuberculosis in this common domestic animal provides an index to the
amount of tuberculosis in cattle, man, and chickens in a given community. It must be recognized, however, that the preceding statement
is subject at least to one reservation in that the possibility for exposure constitutes an important factor in the incidence of infection
by the respective species of the genus.

A fairly satisfactory concept of the incidence of tuberculosis in
swine in the United States during the past 44 years may be obtained
by referring to Table 10.† The incidence of infections due to each
of the respective bacillary types of the tubercle bacilli among the
tuberculous animals represented in Table 10 is not known. Thirty-
seven years ago, observations by Van Es and Martin (1925) showed
that in tuberculous swine from Nebraska, the avian tubercle bacillus
was responsible for more than 88 per cent of the infections. Since
1925, the incidence of tuberculosis in swine has steadily lessened in
the United States, probably as a consequence of the lowered inci-

---

*Additional information regarding tuberculosis in cats will be found in the report
by Lovell and White (1941), and in the text by Francis (1958).

†A brief review of the occurrence of tuberculosis in swine in certain other areas of
the world has been prepared by Karlson (1960).

dence of the disease in poultry (Figure 12). For many years, infection of swine by *Myco. bovis* has been at a relatively low level. At the present time in the United States, tuberculosis of swine is, in

TABLE 10

Swine Slaughtered under Supervision of Federal Meat Inspection Service. Shown Are the Total Number Slaughtered for Different Years and the Percentages of the Total Number That Were Sterilized or Condemned for Tuberculosis. (Data Compiled from Statistical Material Supplied by the Animal Disease Eradication Division, U. S. Department of Agriculture.)

Year	Number Slaughtered	Percentage Retained Tuberculosis Suspected*	Percentage Sterilized or Condemned
1917	40,210,847	9.89	0.41
1927	42,650,443	13.5	0.31
1937	36,226,309	9.5	0.08
1947	45,073,370	8.5	0.04
1957	62,238,519	2.9	0.0167
1961	64,210,887	2.47	0.01244

*The vast majority of tuberculous lesions found in carcasses of swine retained during inspection at the time of slaughter are of small size and limited in extent. The lesions are confined, in most instances, to lymph nodes of the head and neck and of the mesentery, with no demonstrable involvement of the parenchymal organs. Severe and extensive lesions that require the diseased carcass be sterilized or condemned, are relatively infrequent.

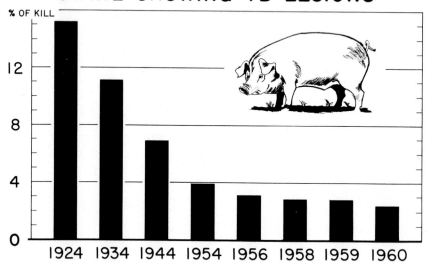

SWINE SHOWING TB LESIONS

FROM FEDERAL MEAT INSPECTION RECORDS OF CARCASSES RETAINED

U. S. DEPARTMENT OF AGRICULTURE   NEG. 60(9)-5002   AGRICULTURAL RESEARCH SERVICE

Fig. 12.

the vast majority of instances, still due to the organism of avian tuberculosis.[†]

Tuberculous chickens, which are permitted the freedom of the farm premises, deposit fecal material containing tubercle bacilli throughout the barnyard and hog lots. As improved methods of poultry husbandry are practiced and the incidence of tuberculosis of chickens continues to decline, tuberculosis in swine will likewise continue to become more infrequent.

Another source of tuberculous infections in swine is uncooked garbage. Garbage may contain uncooked viscera of tuberculous chickens which constitute potent sources of infection for susceptible hosts, such as swine.

Tuberculosis of swine due to *Myco. tuberculosis* probably occurs rather infrequently, although precise information regarding this is not available. In a study of the type of tubercle bacilli responsible for tuberculous lesions in hogs fed uncooked garbage, it was shown that among 264 animals examined after slaughter, 28.4 per cent had tuberculosis. Subsequent studies to determine the type of the infecting organisms in each of the diseased carcasses showed that 74.5 per cent of the bacterial strains were of the avian type, and 25.5 per cent were of the human type (Feldman, 1939).

Generally speaking, the bovine type of the tubercle bacillus is capable of producing in swine a more severe and more widely disseminated tuberculosis than either of the other two species of the organism. However, it has been shown that although avian tuberculosis in swine is predominantly a localized disease of the lymph nodes, the disease may become widely distributed with involvement of the liver, spleen, lungs, and kidneys (Feldman, 1938a) (Figure 13). When infected perorally, swine seem to be more resistant to *Myco. tuberculosis* than to *Myco. bovis* or *Myco. avium*. Infection of swine with *Myco. tuberculosis* (human type tubercle bacilli) seldom causes more than localized tuberculous adenitis. The lymph nodes of predilection are the mesenteric, the submaxillary, and the cervical.

One should recognize that lesions of tuberculosis in swine constitute a possible occupational hazard for slaughterhouse employees and meat inspectors. Meat inspectors especially are likely to come

---

*A detailed account of avian tuberculosis in swine has been prepared by Feldman (1938) and by Karlson (1958).

in contact with infectious material, since handling of diseased viscera and lymph nodes with the bare hands is a routine procedure. Manipulation of diseased tissues cannot be avoided, and the possibility for cutaneous infection with virulent tubercle bacilli exists.

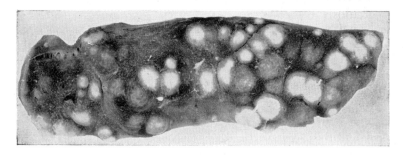

Fig. 13. Numerous nodular lesions of tuberculosis of the spleen of a swine. Infection in this instance was due to the avian type of the tubercle baccillus.

When, in a community, infection of swine by human tubercle bacilli can be demonstrated, the fact should be of concern to those responsible for the public health. If the dissemination of human tubercle bacilli is occurring in sufficient numbers to produce tuberculous lesions in swine, it is reasonable to believe that the source of such pathogens is a potential danger to human beings.

The public health aspect of the avian type of tuberculous infection in swine is probably negligible, since human beings appear to have a marked resistance to this type of the tubercle bacillus (see p. 70).

Horses*

Horses have a low-to-moderate susceptibility to *Myco. bovis,* but are relatively resistant to *Myco. tuberculosis* and *Myco. avium.* Although only a few cases have been reported of horses being infected naturally with the avian type of tubercle bacilli, severe and fatal infection can be accomplished experimentally by the intravenous injection of fully virulent cultures of this organism (Feldman, 1938).

In the United States, tuberculosis of horses has been observed rarely. In 1961, no instance of tuberculosis infection was seen among

*A useful compilation of information pertaining to tuberculosis in horses, mules, and asses has been provided by Francis (1958).

49,394 carcasses of horses slaughtered in abattoirs supervised by the Federal meat inspection service*

Most of the reported cases of tuberculosis of horses have been of European origin, but even in Europe, it is not of common occurrence. In Germany, for example, from 1904 to 1924, the incidence of tuberculosis in cattle was 18.98 per cent; in swine, 2.10 per cent; in goats, 0.85 per cent; in sheep, 0.16 per cent; and in horses, 0.14 per cent (Feldman, 1938).

Myco. bovis is responsible for most instances of tuberculosis in horses. In a series of fifty-five cases reported by Griffith (1937a) from England, bovine type tubercle bacilli were obtained in all except two. In one of the latter cases, human type tubercle bacilli were identified, and in the other, avian.

Since *Myco. bovis* is the organism usually responsible for tuberculosis in horses, it is evident that the occurrence of the disease in the horse is largely dependent on the occurrence of tuberculosis in cattle. The extremely low incidence of tuberculosis in cattle in the United States provides adequate explanation for the paucity of the disease in horses in this country. The transmissibility of the bovine type of infection in the horse to previously noninfected cattle maintained on the same premises should be considered in situations where the source of infection in cattle cannot be explained.

A horse affected with the bovine type of tuberculosis, with involvement of the lungs and kidneys, could become a hazard to human beings. However, the likelihood of this type of infection in horses in the United States is so slight that equine tuberculosis is of no significance to public health.

Monkeys†

Monkeys, probably the most agile, mischievous, fascinating, and perennially popular mammals exhibited at zoological gardens, are, unfortunately, extremely susceptible to tuberculosis.‡ In addition to

---

*Information kindly supplied by Dr. H. H. Pas, Meat Inspection Service, U. S. Department of Agriculture.

†For those especially interested in tuberculosis in monkeys, apes, marmosets, lemurs, and other captive wild mammals and fowl, the review by Francs (1958) may be consulted.

‡Mencken (1960) quotes Thomas Fuller as saying, " 'What pretty things man will make for money,' quoth the old woman when she saw a monkey."

their popularity with those who enjoy their antics in zoos and circuses, monkeys, as well as other primates, have become exceedingly important in some aspects of experimental medicine. For many reasons, monkeys are the animals of choice in certain research projects pertaining to infectious diseases. Complicating the care and maintenance of a colony of monkeys in captivity, is tuberculosis, which may become a virtual scourge.*

It is generally believed that monkeys living in their natural or wild environment do not contract tuberculosis. However, when they are in captivity and subjected to exposure from infected human beings or other infected primates, their susceptibility to tuberculosis becomes impressively evident. If overcrowding and unsanitary conditions prevail, once the disease is established in the colony, most of the animals are likely to die of tuberculosis within a period of four to six months. According to information compiled by Schroeder (1938), the average annual mortality rate of monkeys in captivity is approximately 10 per cent, and 80 per cent of all deaths are due to tuberculosis.

Monkeys, chimpanzees, baboons, and lemurs appear to be susceptible to *Myco. tuberculosis* and *Myco. bovis* equally. A large dosage of *Myco. avium,* given intravenously, induces an infection that may be rapidly fatal.

It appears that monkeys captured in their wild state are most likely to contact tuberculosis from persons with the disease with whom they are in close proximity during transportation from their native haunts to quarters maintained by dealers. Additional sources of contagion are individuals with active tuberculosis, employed by dealers, who frequent the premises where the monkeys are maintained.

In naturally acquired tuberculosis of monkeys due to either *Myco. bovis* or *Myco. tuberculosis,* the lung is the organ of predilection. The focus of infection is usually found in either an apical lobe or a diaphramatic lobe. Generalization frequently occurs, and bronchogenic spread may result in extensive pulmonary involvement (Fig. 14). Lesions may also occur in the pleura, intestines, mesenteric

---

*For an account of means used in controlling tuberculosis in a monkey colony maintained for medical research, one may consult the report by Benson, Fremming, and Young (1955).

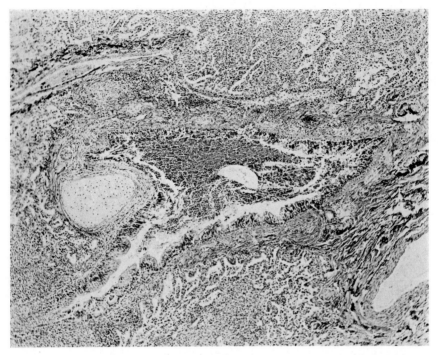

Fig. 14.

lymph nodes, liver, kidney, spleen, and peritoneum. Infection in most instances seems to be by inhalation of aerosols containing tubercle bacilli exuded from active tuberculous pulmonary or upper respiratory lesions.

For the control of tuberculosis in monkeys, it is necessary to: 1) isolate all new acquisitions, 2) administer two tests with tuberculin, one month apart,* and 3) remove from the colony monkeys that react positively and dispose of them immediately. *This is of the utmost importance!* Even though a monkey may be without recognizable symptoms of illness, experience indicates that if it is positive to

---

*Monkeys may be tested with tuberculin as follows: With sterile physiologic sodium chloride solution, make a 1:10 dilution of Koch's old tuberculin. Inject 0.1 cc. of the diluted solution intracutaneously into an upper eyelid. Record results after forty-eight hours. If no reaction occurs after seventy-two hours, the test should be recorded as negative. A positive reaction is characterized by edema of the upper eyelid, with thickening and narrowing of the palpebral opening. Erythema in the area of injection is of no significance.

tuberculin, it will probably die of tuberculosis within six months after it became hypersensitive.

Animal caretakers, assigned to monkey colonies, should have pre-employment physical examinations, including a roentgenogram of the chest, to detect those with active pulmonary tuberculosis. Personnel in contact regularly with colonies of primates should have a Mantoux test every six months. If the test is positive, roentgenograms of the chest should be taken and examined for possible signs of tuberculosis.

Sheep and Goats*

Tuberculosis is extremely rare in sheep. According to Feldman (1938), among 147,000,000 sheep slaughtered in abattoirs in the United States under Federal supervision from 1928 to 1936, tuberculosis was recognized in less than fifty. In 1937, of approximately seventeen and one-half million sheep slaughtered under Federal supervision, only twenty-two were condemned for tuberculosis. Further evidence of the continued rarity of tuberculosis in sheep in the United States is found in the figures of the U. S. Meat Inspection Service for 1961, when nearly fifteen million sheep were slaughtered and tuberculosis was not detected in a single carcass.[†] In European countries, the disease is likewise seldom encountered.

Sheep are known to be susceptible to both *Myco. bovis* and *Myco. avium*.[‡] An instance of generalized tuberculosis in an old ewe due to *Myco. bovis* was reported by Stubbs and Live (1939). The lesions were from a carcass examined in a Federally supervised abattoir, hence no antemortem information regarding the animal was available. Grayish-white nodular lesions of variable sizes occurred throughout the lungs, spleen, liver, and kidneys. Lesions were also present in the diaphragm. Calcification of some of the lesions was noted. An emulsion, prepared from an affected lymph node and the spleen, was used to inoculate rabbits, guinea pigs, and a chicken.

---

*For a more detailed account of tuberculosis in sheep and goats, the treatise by Francis (1958) may be consulted.

†For a consideration of naturally acquired and experimentally induced *Myco. avium* infection in sheep, the monograph by Feldman (1939) may be consulted.

‡Information kindly supplied by Dr. H. H. Pas, Meat Inspection Service, U. S. Department of Agriculture.

The results of these tests of pathogenicity identified the mycobacteria as tubercle bacilli of the bovine type. Although a few instances of natural infection of sheep due to the human type of the tubercle bacillus have been reported, it is generally believed that sheep are fairly resistant to this organism.

On the basis of limited statistics, tuberculosis in goats appears to be extremely infrequent. During 1961, among 85,540 goats slaughtered and examined by the Federal Meat Inspection Service of the United States Department of Agriculture, in no instance was the presence of tuberculosis established.* However, the fact that goats are highly susceptible to *Myco. bovis* is sufficient reason for not considering too lightly the part that goats might play in the transmission of the infection to man. If associated with tuberculous cattle, goats are likely to contract tuberculosis. Golden is quoted by Myers (1940) as having found six tuberculous goats in a herd of forty-two. The bacillary type of the infectious agent was not mentioned, but it is reasonable to assume that it was bovine. It is obvious that goats that provide milk for human use should be subjected to the tuberculin test. As a further safeguard, Myers recommended that "goats' milk should always be pasteurized if it is to be used for human consumption."

TUBERCULOSIS OF CHICKENS[†]

Tuberculosis of chickens is widely distributed throughout most of the northern hemisphere and is one of the most common and, in some areas, one of the most serious diseases affecting the domestic chicken. The highest incidence of the disease in the United States occurs in those states of the North Central area (Figure 15). The incidence is variable, depending upon the type of poultry husbandry practiced. In some areas, tuberculosis of fowl is practically non-existent; in others, the incidence of the disease in farm flocks may exceed 10 per cent.

When infected naturally, chickens are susceptible only to the avian type of the tubercle bacillus. However, *Myco. avium* is viru-

---

*Information kindly supplied by Dr. H. H. Pas, Meat Inspection Service, U. S. Department of Agriculture.

†For a comprehensive account of tuberculosis in chickens, see the monograph by Feldman (1938).

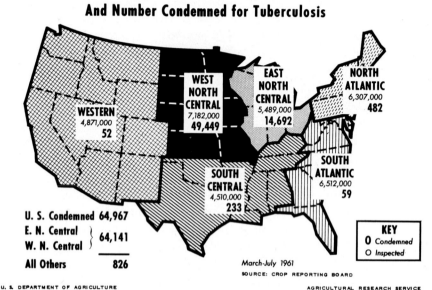

Fig. 15.

lent in varying degrees for several heterologous hosts, including
swine, sheep, and to a lesser degree, cattle (Table 11).*

Tuberculosis in chickens is characterized by its insidious course,
its chronicity, the presence within the lesions of exceedingly large
numbers of *Myco. avium,* and ulcerative lesions of the intestine

TABLE 11

COMPARATIVE PATHOGENICITY OF MYCOBACTERIUM AVIUM FOR CERTAIN MAMMALS

Animal	Susceptibility	Animal	Susceptibility
Cat	Highly resistant	Marsupials	Infection reported
Cattle	Infection occurs; usually localized	Mink	Readily infected
Deer	Infection reported	Monkey	Highly resistant
Dog	Highly resistant	Mouse	Relatively resistant
Goat	Assumed to be relatively resistant	Rabbit	Readily infected
Guinea pig	Slightly susceptible	Rat	Relatively resistant
Horse	Assumed to be highly resistant	Sheep	Moderately susceptible
Man	Highly resistant	Swine	Readily infected

*Pertinent information regarding the pathogenicity of *Myco. avium* for cattle may
be found in the publication by Minett (1932) and by Feldman (1938). For an account
of tuberculosis of wild crows due to avian tubercle bacilli, the report by Mitchell and
Duthie (1950) is of value.

which provide for a gross dissemination of the infectious agent mixed with fecal material.

The disease is acquired in most instances by ingestion. The *Myco. avium* enters the digestive tract with food or water. Infection by way of the respiratory tract has been reported. Lesions occur most frequently in the intestines, spleen, liver, lungs, and bone marrow. Occasionally, cutaneous lesions have been observed.

In chickens the infection is characterized by the production of firm, discrete, granulomatous nodules of variable sizes. A few-to-many nodules may occur along the intestines, and firm, yellowish, elevated foci are present usually in the spleen and liver (Figure 16). In some cases, the progression of the infection in the spleen or liver is so great and so rapid that rupture of the organ takes place as a consequence of the hypertrophy. When this happens, fatal hemorrhage usually ensues.

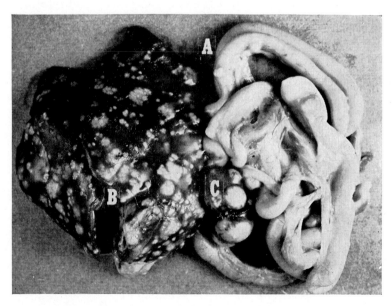

Fig. 16. Naturally acquired tuberculosis of the abdominal viscera of an adult chicken. Nodular lesions are present in the intestines (A), the liver (B), and the spleen (C).

Tuberculous chickens are likely to be thin or even emaciated. The disease can be detected best in the living bird by testing with avian tuberculin. However, chickens in the later stages of the disease may fail to react to tuberculin.

Spread of the disease can be controlled by denying the birds the freedom of the farm premises and by the application of hygienic measures in poultry husbandry. A tuberculosis-free flock of young chickens, confined to clean and noncontaminated enclosures, will probably remain free from tuberculosis. The yearly addition of young, though noninfected, chickens to a previously established flock where tuberculosis exists and where the birds range unrestricted throughout the barnyard will insure the perpeutation of the disease.

Where tuberculous chickens exist, there is abundant opportunity for the infection to spread to other chickens and to susceptible heterologous hosts. As mentioned previously, the fecal material abounds in viable tubercle bacilli, which can remain viable outside the body of the host for a long time. In the litter and soil of an infected barnyard, the organisms have been known to remain viable and pathogenic for several years after the premises had become contaminated.

The question whether eggs laid by tuberculous birds contain avian tubercle bacilli has been the subject of considerable investigation.* The accumulated evidence indicates that this occurs infrequently—probably in less than 1 per cent of the eggs laid by infected chickens. Because most of the eggs from chickens are consumed by human beings, it is important to know the temperature necessary to render the bacilli nonviable. The temperature necessary to prepare an egg that is "soft-boiled" is not sufficient to kill the bacteria; some survive in the zone between the soft and firm portions of the egg. Time and temperature sufficient to prepare eggs that are "hard-boiled" are ordinarily sufficient to kill avian tubercle bacilli that may be present. However, there is some evidence to indicate that the time of boiling must be extended to ten minutes to insure the desired results.

INFECTION OF MAN BY *MYCO. AVIUM*[†]

One of the most important, yet most confusing, questions concerning tuberculosis in chickens is whether or not the infection is

---

*For a detailed consideration of the question of eggs containing avian tubercle bacilli, see the review by Feldman (1938).

†The role of *Myco. avium* in tuberculosis of man has been the subject of critical reviews by Fontana (1935), Feldman (1938), and Rich (1951).

communicable to human beings. The question has been the subject of much speculation, and a careful review of the literature reveals that many of the cases of alleged infections with *Myco. avium* in man have been either described inadequately or studied incompletely or incorrectly. As a consequence, the reviewer, if he is critical, must come to the conclusion that in most of the reported instances, infection of human beings with *Myco. avium* has not been established by acceptable evidence. Feldman (1938) reviewed the cases reported up to 1938 and concluded that "in the majority a diagnosis of avian tubercle bacillus infection was questionable or erroneous." Rich (1951) analyzed the data presented up to 1944 and concluded that "if progressive tuberculosis is ever produced in the human being by the avian bacillus it must be only very rarely. . . ."

In spite of the skepticism that logically follows a critical examination of the evidence presented to support most of the reported cases of alleged avian tubercle bacilli infections in man, it must be accepted that at least in a few cases, *Myco. avium* has been demonstrated in morbid materials from human beings.

The reader particularly interested in infection of human beings with *Myco. avium* may review the cases described by the following: Jensen, Lester, and Tolderlund (1940); Bradbury and Young (1946); Finlayson (1948); Dragsted (1949); Karlson (1959); Furniss *et al.* (1960); and Furniss *et al.* (1961). The cases reported by these workers were studied carefully. Impressive evidence was obtained in each instance to justify the conclusion that acid-fast bacilli with the bacteriologic and pathogenic characteristics of *Myco. avium* were associated with and probably responsible for the tuberculous processes in the respective patients.*

Although the possibility of infection of man by the organism which causes tuberculosis of chickens must be recognized, it is also true

---

*Through the kindness and generosity of Prof. Dr. Med. Gertrud Meissner, Tuberkulose-Forschungsinstitut, Borstel, über Bad Oldesloe, Deutschland, it is possible to mention briefly three unpublished instances of pulmonary infections of human beings with *Myco. avium*. Each of the patients was an adult white male with chronic pulmonary disease. The mycobacteria obtained in the respective cases were identified by animal pathogenicity tests as avian tubercle bacilli. Doctor Meisner's studies of the mycobacteria obtained from these patients have been comprehensive. The conclusion that the mycobacteria in each case were *Myco. avium* is based on sound experimental evidence. It is hoped that Doctor Meissner will prepare and publish a detailed account of her important observations.

that the pathogenicity of this type of tubercle bacillus for the vast majority of human beings is practically nil. The possible relation of *Myco. avium* to Hodgkin's disease has been discussed by Feldman (1938) and Rich (1951).

The extreme rarity of proved infections of human beings with avian tubercle bacilli, and the skepticism of many who doubt that such infections ever occur, make it exceedingly important that every reported case be firmly established by convincing data. To establish the bacillary type of some strains of the genus *Mycobaterium* is not a simple matter, and extensive studies frequently are necessary. The most convincing evidence is obtained from properly conducted tests of pathogenicity. (Procedures for the determination of type of tubercle bacilli are given on page 8.)

ITEMS OF NOTE

1) It is generally recognized that *Myco. tuberculosis, Myco. bovis,* and *Myco. avium* produce tuberculosis in man, cattle, and fowl, respectively. However, the ability of each of the three species to produce progressive tuberculosis in heterologous hosts is not universally appreciated. If this fact is fully understood and its importance completely realized, the necessity of a comprehensive plan of control and eradication of tuberculosis becomes evident. Ideally, the goal should be the elimination of tuberculous infections from all species.

2) From a public health point of view, tuberculous cattle constitute the most important animal source of tubercle bacilli that are virulent for man. In the United States, bovine tuberculosis has been reduced to an impressive level; yet so long as a single focus of infection remains, there exist the essentials necessary for the dissemination of the infection. The attack against the tubercle bacillus must be intensified and pursued without compromise. An attitude of complacency, or one in which satisfaction with past achievements minimizes the importance of the task yet to be done, will defeat any plan of approach, no matter how adequate it may appear to be.

3) If tuberculosis occurs in animal groups which had previously been free of the infection, it is imperative that the source of the infection be determined. An investigation, guided by the principles of modern epidemiology should be initiated immediately. The species of the infective *Mycobacterium* must be established, and if the

organism is *Myco. bovis* or *Myco. tuberculosis*, public health officials should be notified.

4) Finally, the remarkable achievement of the veterinary profession in practically eliminating tuberculosis from cattle in the United States constitutes a notable example for the guidance of physicians who are concerned with eliminating tuberculosis of human beings. *The problem must be attacked nationally and with vigor, and with the thought ever in mind that tuberculosis is a highly contagious disease. Those who have the disease in the contagious phase must be segregated from those who are not infected.*

ACKNOWLEDGEMENT

The author expresses his thanks and appreciation to the following friends and colleagues who rendered valuable assistance in the preparation or certain portions of the chapter on Tuberculosis: Mr. Frank P. Dunbar, Dr. A. G. Karlson, and Dr. Roy E. Ritts.

REFERENCES

ARONSON, J. D., and WHITNEY, CAROLINE E. (1930): The types of tubercle bacilli found in tuberculous lesions and in nontuberculous tissue in man. *J. Infect. Dis., 47:*30-55.

BEATTIE, MARGARET, and NICEWONGER, ROBERT (1942): Bovine tubercle bacilli in sputum. *Am. Rev. Tuberc., 45:*586-588.

BENDIXEN, H. C. (1950): Bovine tuberculosis. In: *The Fight Against Tuberculosis in Denmark.* Copenhagen, NYT Nordisk Forlag Arnold Busck, pp. 75-90.

BENSON, R. E., FREMMING, B. D., and YOUNG, R. J. (1955): A tuberculosis outbreak in a Macaca Mulatta colony. *Am. Rev. Tuberc. & Pul. Dis., 72:*204-209.

BERG, OLAV A. (1956): Tuberculosis in Dogs. *Acta Tuber. Scand., 32* (3/4):351-361.

BERNHEIM, M., VIALLIER, J., and CAYRÉ, R. -M. (1962): La tuberculose humaine a bacilli bovin. Sa relative fréquence, ses caracteres distinctifs *La Presse Medicale, 70* (5):197-199 (Jan 27).

BRADBURY, F. C. S., and YOUNG, J. A. (1946): Human pulmonary tuberculosis due to avian tubercle bacilli; report of a case. *Lancet, 1:*89-91.

BROOKE, W. S. (1941): The vole acid-fast bacillus: 1. Experimental studies on a new type of Mycobacterium tuberculosis. *Am. Rev. Tuberc., 43:*806-816.

CALMETTE, ALBERT (1923): *Tubercle Bacillus Infection and Tuberculosis in Man and Animals.* English translation by Willard B. Soper and George H. Smith. Baltimore, Williams and Wilkins Co., pp. 689.

CARMICHAEL, J. (1939): Bovine tuberculosis in the tropics, with special reference to Uganda. Part I. *J. Comp. Path. & Therap., 52:*322-333.

CARMICHAEL, J. (1940): Pulmonary tuberculosis in Uganda natives; a bacteriological survey. *Tr. Roy. Soc. Trop. Med. & Hyg., 33:*453-459.

CHANG, C. S. (1933): Human and bovine infection in extrapulmonary tuberculosis. *New England J. Med., 209:*690-692.

CHAPPLE, I. L., and ABRAHAMS, E. W. (1956): Bovine phthisis in Queensland, *M. J. of Australia,* pp. 995-997.

COLWELL, CHARLOTTE A., and MILLS, MOORE A. (1940): Experimental tuberculosis in the dog—I. Cutaneous sensitivity to tuberculin in the dog, *Am. Rev. Tuberc., 42:*259-270.

CUMMING, W. M. (1933): Pulmonary tuberculosis in dairy-farm workers and others coming much in contact with cattle; type of causal organism in 14 cases. *Tubercle, 14:*205-207.

DALLING, T., and GLOYNE, S. R. (1942): Discussion on the control of diseases of cattle inimical to man; tuberculosis. *Proc. Roy. Soc. Med., 35:*469-478.

DALRYMPLE-CHAMPNEYS, W. (1937): L'incidence de la tuberculose humaine d'origine bovine en Grande-Bretagne. *Bull. Office Internat. Hyg. Pub., 29:*329-336.

DAY, L. E. (1932): Tuberculosis of the voluntary muscles. *Bureau Vet., 8:*1-2.

DE GARA, P. F. (1942): Bovine tuberculosis: Its incidence in bone, joint, and cervical lymph node lesions in Italy. *Am. Rev. Tuberc., 45:*576-585.

DE KOCK, G. and LE ROUX, J. (1956): Studies on Tuberculosis in Dogs, and on a Case of Human Tuberculosis Contracted from a Dog. *Onderstepoort Journal of Veterinary Research, 27* (2): 227-238, Oct.

DELGADO, BLANCO, J., and ILUKEVICH, A. (1957): Contribucion al estudio de la variedad bovine del mycobacterium tuberculosis en el hombre en Venezuela. *Revista de la Policlinica Cararas, 25* (143):145-164, Oct./Dec.

DOBSON, N. (1930): Tuberculosis of cat. *J. Comp. Path. & Therap., 43:*310-316.

DRAGSTED, INGER (1949): Avian tuberculosis in man. *Lancet, 2:*103-105.

DU TOIT, C. J., and BUCHANAN, G. (1942): Tuberculous meningitis of bovine origin; report of case. *South African M. J., 16:*10-11.

EBER, A. (1917): Die Tuberkulose der Tiere Bericht über die Jahre 1905-1914. *Ergebn. d. All. Path. u. Path. Anat., 18:*1-371, Abb. 2.

FELDMAN, W. H. (1947): Animal tuberculosis and its relationship to the disease in man. In: The relations of disease in the lower animals to human welfare. *Ann. New York Acad. Sc., 48:*469-505, Art. 6.

FELDMAN, W. H. (1938): *Avian Tuberculosis Infections.* Baltimore, Williams and Wilkins Company, 483 pp.

FELDMAN, W. H. (1938a): Generalized tuberculosis of swine due to avian tubercle bacilli. *J. Am. Vet M. A., 92:*681-685.

FELDMAN, W. H. (1939): Types of tubercle bacilli in lesions of garbage-fed swine. *Am. J. Pub. Health, 29:*1231-1238.

FELDMAN, W. H., and MOSES, HAROLD (1941): Human tuberculosis in a bovine; case report of a spontaneous infection in an adult bovine. *Am. Rev. Tuberc., 43:*418-424.

FELDMAN, W. H., and CODE, C. F. (1942): Tuberculosis in dogs, with a report of a case in which surgical procedures may have influenced the pathogenesis. *J. Tech. Methods, 22:*49-56.

FINLAYSON, MARGARET K. (1948): A case of human tuberculosis due to avian tubercle bacilli. *New Zealand M. J., 47:*362-367.

FONTANA, ALFRED (1935): *La Tuberculosi Aviaria.* Milan, Dottor Francesco Vallardi, 179 pp.

FRANCIS, JOHN (1958): *Tuberculosis in Animals and Man: A Study in Comparative Pathology.* London, Cassell and Company, Ltd., 357 pp.

FRITSCHI, E. (1960): Organization and carrying out of the official campaign against bovine tuberculosis in Switzerland. *Zooprofilassi, 15:* (11):832-842.

FURNISS, A. L., COLLINS, C. H., and MARKS, J. (1960): A Case of Infection with Avian Type Tubercle Bacilli. Great Britain Ministry of Health, *Monthly Bulletin, Public Health Laboratory 20:*126-128, July.

GRIFFITH, A. S. (1937): Bovine tuberculosis in man. *Tubercle, 18:*529-543.

GRIFFITH, A. S. (1937a): Types of tubercle bacilli in equine tuberculosis. *J. Comp. Path. & Therap.*, *50*:159-172.

GRIFFITH, A. S. (1938): Bovine tuberculosis in the human subject. *Proc. Roy. Soc. Med.*, *31*:1208-1212.

GRIFFITH, A. S., and MUNRO, W. T. (1944): Human pulmonary tuberculosis of bovine origin in Great Britain. *J. Hyg.*, *43*:229-240.

HAGAN, W. A., and BRUNER, D. W. (1951): *The Infectious Diseases of Domestic Animals with Special Reference to Etiology, Diagnosis and Biologic Therapy* (2nd Ed.). Ithaca, New York, Comstock Publishing Co., Inc., Chapter 24, pp. 299-363.

HARING, C. M., TRAUM, J., HAYES, F. M., and HENRY, B. S. (1930): Vaccination of calves against tuberculosis with Calmette-Guerin culture, BCG. *Hilgardia, 4*, 307.

HAWTHORNE, V. M., JARRETT, W. F. H., LAUDER, I., MARTIN, W. B., and ROBERTS, G. B. S. (1957): Tuberculosis in man, dog, and cat. *Brit. M. J.*, *2*:675-678.

HAWTHORNE, V. M., and LAUDER, I. M. (1962): Tuberculosis in Man, Dog, and Cat. *The American Review of Respiratory Diseases, 85* (6):858-869.

HEDVALL, ERIK (1940): An investigation into the occurrence of bovine pulmonary tuberculosis in man in the South of Sweden. *Lancet, 60*:151-155.

HERMANSSON, K. A. (1939): Föreligger risk för besiktningsveterinär att under sitt på offenligt slakthus eller kontrollslakteri bliva infekterad med tuberkelbakterier? *Scandinav. VetTidskr., 29*:926-933; (abstr.) *Vet. Bull., 10*:491-492, July, 1940.

HESS, E. (1960): Tuberculosis—eradication—programme in Switzerland. *Zooprofilassi, 15* (11):843-846.

HIX, JERROLD W., JONES, T. C., and KARLSON, ALFRED G. (1961): Avian tubercle bacillus infection in the cat. *J. Am. Vet. M. A.*, *138*, No. 12: 641-647.

HJÄRRE, A. (1939): Ansteckungsquelle für den menschen über tuberkulose bei hunden und katzen. *Acta Tuberc. Scandinav., 13*:103-124.

HUITEMA, H., and VAN VLOTEN, J. (1960): Murine tuberculosis in a cat. *Vet. Bull., 31*, No. 2:53-106.

HUTYRA, FRANZ, MAREK, JOSEF, and MANNINGER, RUDOLPH (1938): *Special Pathology and Therapeutics of the Diseases of Domestic Animals*. Chicago, A. Eger, *1*:355-660.

JENSEN, K. A. (1950): Cooperation of the bacteriological laboratory. In: *The Fight Against Tuberculosis in Denmark*. Copenhagen, NYT Nordisk Forlag Arnold Busck, pp. 54-74.

JENSEN, K. A., LESTER, V., and TOLDERLUND, K. (1940): The frequency of bovine infection among tuberculous patients in Denmark. *Acta Tuberc. Scandinav., 14*:125-127.

Joint WHO/FAO Expert Committee on Zoonoses, Second Report (1959): *World Health Org. Tech. Report*, Series No. *169*, Geneva.

KARLSON, A. G. (1958): Tuberculosis. In Dunn, H. W.: *Diseases of Swine*. Ames, Iowa, Iowa State College Press, pp. 277-391.

KARLSON, A. G. (1959): Avian tuberculosis. *Minn. Med., 42*:1399-1402.

KARLSON, A. G. (1960): Tuberculosis caused by human, bovine, and avian tubercle bacilli in various animals. *64th Ann. Proc., U.S. Livestock Sanitary Association*.

KARLSON, A. G. (1963): From Tuberculosis, Ch. 26, *Diseases of Swine*, 2nd Ed. Iowa State Univ. Press, Ames, Iowa.

KERR, W. R., LAMONT, H. G., and McGIRR, J. L. (1949): Further Studies on Tuberculin Sensitivity in the Bovine, *Vet. Rec. 61* (32):466-475.

KOCH, ROBERT (1882): Die aetiologie der tuberculose. *Klin. Wchnschr., 19*:221-230.

KOCH, R. (1902): Address before the second general meeting. *Tr. Brit. Cong. Tuberc., 1*:23-35.

KIMURA, REN, and KONDO, HISASHI (1939): Ueber das Seltene Vorkommen des bovinen typus von Tuberkelbazillen bei Japanern. *Zentralbl. Bakt., 144:*365-369.

KONNO, K. (1956): New Chemical Method to Differentiate Human Type Tubercle Bacilli from Other Mycobacteria. *Science 124:*985.

KUWABARA, T. (1938): Susceptibilty of cats to tubercle bacilli. *Kitasato Arch. Exper. Med., 15:*318-329.

LANGE, BRUNO (1937): Perlsuchbazillen als erreger der Lungenschwindsucht. *Deutsche med. Wchnschr., 63:*1465-1469, Sept. 24; 1506-1508, Oct. 1.

LEBEK, G., and STEINERT, C. (1955): The incidence of bovine nonpulmonary tuberculosis in children in Bavaria. *Ztschr. f. Hyg. u. Infektionskr., 141:*218-234.

LEWIS-JONSSON, JOHANNES (1946): The transmission of tuberculosis from cats to human beings (Report of a case). *Acta. Tuberc. Scandinav., 20:*102-105.

LOVELL, R., and WHITE, E. G. (1940): Naturally occurring tuberculosis in dogs and some other species of animals. I. Tuberculosis in dogs. *Brit. J. Tuberc., 34:*117-133.

LOVELL, R., and WHITE, E. G. (1941): Naturally occurring tuberculosis in dogs and some other species of animals. II. Animals other than dogs. *Brit. J. Tuberc., 35:*28-40.

MADDOCK, E. C. G. (1933): Studies on the survival time of the bovine tubercle bacillus in soil, soil and dung, in dung and on grass, with experiments on the preliminary treatment of infected organic matter and the cultivation of the organism. *J. Hyg., 33:*103-117.

MAGLIONE, ENRICO, and CAVALLERO, GIUSEPPE (1959): Sulla Presenza Del Micobatterio Tubercolare Nell'acqua di Lavaggio Della Cute Mammaria di Bovine Tubercolino-positive. *Atti Della Societa Italiana Delle Scienze Veterinarie, 13:*607.

MALLICK, S. M., AGGARWAL, H. R., and DUA, R. L. (1942): An investigation into the incidence and type of tuberculous infection in cattle at Amritsar with special reference to human infections. *Indian M. Gaz., 77:*668-672.

MARTIN, M. HIPPOLYTE (1884): Recherches ayant pour but de démontrer la fréquence de la tuberculose consécutive a l'inoculation du lait vendu, à Paris sous les portes cochères. *Rev. Med., Paris, 4:*150-161.

MEDLAR, E. M. (1940): Pulmonary tuberculosis in cattle; the location and type of lesions in naturally acquired tuberculosis. *Am. Rev. Tuberc., 41:*283-306.

MEISSNER, GERTRUD (1961): Vorkommen und Eigenschaften (bakteriologisch und tierexperimentell) von atypischen Mycobakterien, *Jahresbericht Borstel,* Funfter Band, pp. 408-480.

MENCKEN, H. L. (1960): *A New Dictionary of Quotations.* New York, Alfred A. Knopf, p. 806.

MIDDLEBROOK, GARDNER, and DUBOS, RENÉ J. (1958): The mycobacteria. In: *Bacterial and Mycotic Infections of Man,* 3rd Ed., Edited by René J. Dubos. Lippincott, Philadelphia, pp. 277-309.

MINETT, F. C. (1932): Avian tuberculosis in cattle in Great Britain. *J. Comp. Path & Therap. 45:*317-330.

MITCHELL, C. A., and DUTHIE, R. C. (1950): Tuberculosis of the common crow. *Canad. J. Comp. Med., 14:*109-117.

MÜLLER, M., and ISHIWARA, T. (1914): Ueber den tuberkelbacillengehalt der muskulatur, des blutes, der lymphe und der fleischbeschaulich nicht infiziert erscheinenden organe tuberkulöser schlachttiere. *Zentralbl. Bakt., 74:*393-455.

MUNRO, W. T., and WALKER, GILBERT (1935): Pulmonary tuberculosis due to the bovine type tubercle bacillus; a case report with autopsy findings. *Lancet, 1:*252-254.

MUNRO, W. T. (1939): Epidemiological aspects of pulmonary tuberculosis due to bovine type tubercle bacilli. *Edinburgh M. J., 46:*165-179.

MUSHATT, C. (1940): Nonpulmonary tuberculosis caused by the bovine type of tubercle bacillus in children in Eire. *J. Hyg., 40:*396-405.

MYERS, J. A. (1940): *Man's Greatest Victory over Tuberculosis.* Springfield, Thomas, p. 380.

National Tuberculosis Survey (1954): *Report of Tuberculosis in Ireland,* Dublin, Hely's, Ltd., pp. 301.

NIEBERLE, K. (1931): In: Tuberculose der Tiere. B. Pathologische Anatomie und Pathogenese. *Ergebn. d. allg. Path. u. path. Anat., 25:*631-812.

PALLASKE, G. (1961): *Pathologische Anatomie und Pathogenese der spontanen Tuberkulose der Tiere.* Stuttgart, Gustav Fischer Verlag, 152 pp.

PARK, W. H., and KRUMWIEDE, CHARLES, JR. (1910): The relative importance of the bovine and human types of tubercle bacilli in the different forms of human tuberculosis. *J. M. Res., 23:*205-364.

PLUM, N. (1936): Tre tilfaelde af tuberkulose hos hunden. *Maanedsskrift for Dyrlaeger, 48:*193-202.

PRICE, R. M. (1938): Bovine tuberculosis in children. *Canad. J. Pub. Health, 39:*251-254.

PRICE, R. M. (1939): The bovine tubercle bacillus in human tuberculosis. *Am. J. M. Sc., 197:*411-427.

RAVENEL, M. P. (1901): The comparative virulence of the tubercle bacillus from human and bovine sources. *Lancet, 2:*349;443.

RAVENEL, M. P. (1902): The intercommunicability of human and bovine tuberculosis. *Proc. Path. Soc., 23:*181.

REILLY, L. V. (1950): Human tuberculosis of bovine origin in Northern Ireland. *J. Hyg. 48:*464-471.

RICH, A. R. (1951): *The Pathogenesis of Tuberculosis,* 2nd Ed. Springfield, Thomas, pp. 28-101.

ROSENTHAL, SOL ROY (1957): *BCG Vaccination Against Tuberculosis.* Boston, Little, Brown & Co., pp. 389.

RUNYON, E. H. (1959): Anonymous mycobacteria in pulmonary disease. *M. Clin. North America, 43:*273.

RUYS, A. CHARLOTTE (1950): Bovine tuberculosis in man in Amsterdam before, during, and after the War. *Acta Tuberc. Scandinav., 24:*177-181.

RUYS, A. C. (1939): On tuberculosis in man due to bovine type of tubercle bacillus in the Netherlands. *Tubercle, 20:*556-560.

RUYS, A. CHARLOTTE (1946): The influence of war conditions on bovine tuberculosis in man in Amsterdam. *Monthly Bull. Ministry of Health and the Emergency Public Health Laboratory Service.* Med. Res. Council, London, 67-71, March.

RUYS, A. C. (1937): Frequence de la tuberculose du type bovin chez l'homme dans les Pays-Bas. *Bull. Office internat. hyg. pub., 29:*342-347.

SAENZ, A. (1939): Progrès récents réalisés dans les méthodes de culture du bacille de Koch; rôle du bacille bovin dans l'infection tuberculeuse de l'homme en France. *Paris Méd., 1:*536-543.

SCHROEDER, C. R. (1938): Acquired tuberculosis in the primate in laboratories and zoological gardens. *Am. J. Pub. Health, 28:*469.

SCOTT, H. H. (1930): Tuberculosis in man and lower animals. *Med. res. Council. Special Report Series, 149:*1-270.

SMITH, H. WILLIAMS (1954): The isolation of mycobacteria from the mesenteric lymph nodes of domestic animals. *J. Path. & Bact., 68:*367.

SMITH, H. WILLIAMS (1958): The isolation of Mycobacterium johnei and other acid-fast bacilli from the retropharyngeal and ileocaecal lymph glands and spleen of apparently normal cattle. *J. Path. & Bact.,* 76:201.

SMITH, THEOBALD (1898): A comparative study of bovine tubercle bacilli and of human bacilli from sputum. *J. Exper. Med., 3:*451-511.

SMITH, THEOBALD (1905): Studies in mammalian tubercle bacilli. III. Description of a bovine bacillus from the human body. A culture test for distinguishing the human from the bovine type of bacilli. *J. M. Res., 13:*253-300.

STADNICHENKO, A. M. S., SWEANY, H. C., and KLOECK, J. M. (1945): Types of tubercle bacilli in birds and mammals: Their incidence, isolation, and identification. *Am. Rev. Tuberc., 51:*276-293.

STAMP, J. T. (1943): Tuberculosis of the bovine udder. *J. Comp. Path. & Therap., 53:*220-230.

STAMP, J. T. (1944): A review of the pathogenesis and pathology of bovine tuberculosis with special reference to practical problems. *Vet. Rec.,* 56:443-446.

STAMP, J. T. (1948): Bovine pulmonary tuberculosis. *J. Comp. Path. & Therap.,* 58:1-23.

STAMP, J. T., and WILSON, A. (1946): Some aspects of the pathogenesis of bovine tuberculosis, based on abattoir returns. *Vet. Rec.,* No. 2:11-15.

STEELE, JAMES H. (1962): Veterinary Public Health, U. S. Department of Health, Education, and Welfare. Personal communication to author.

STUBBS, E. L., and LIVE, I. (1939): A case of sheep tuberculosis due to the bovine type. *J. Am. Vet. M. A.* 95:173-176.

TICE, F. J. (1944): Man, a source of bovine tuberculosis in cattle. *Cornell Vet., 34:*363-365.

TONNEY, F. O., WHITE, J. L., and DANFORTH, T. F. (1927): Tubercle bacilli in the raw milk of the Chicago dairy district. *Am. J. Pub. Health, 17:*491-493.

URWITZ, S. (1949): Tuberculous Infection From Dogs. *Acta Tuberc. Scandinav, 23:* 211-219.

VACCAREZZA, R. F., and ARENA, A. R. (1943): Tuberculosis de origen bovino. *Rev. Assoc. med. argent, 57:*10-22; (abstr.) *Am. Rev. Tuberc., Abstr. Section,* 48:57.

VAN DER HOEDEN, J., and DE RAADT, M. F. (1940): Interhumane lesmetting met. het. bovine type van den tuberkelbacil. *Nederl. Tijdschr. Geneesk., 84:*45, 4390-4397.

VAN ES, L. (1929): *Bovine Tuberculosis.* Circular 23, Univ. Nebraska, Coll. Agric. Exper. Sta., Lincoln (Revised), 77 pp.

VAN ES, L., and MARTIN, H. M. (1925): An inquiry into the cause of the increase of tuberculosis of swine. Res. Bull. *30,* Univ. Nebraska, Coll. Agric. Exper. Sta., Lincoln, 78 pp.

VAN ES, L., and MARTIN, H. M. (1930): The incidence of avian tuberculosis in mammals other than swine. Res. Bull. *49,* Univ. Nebraska, Coll. Agric. Exper. Sta., Lincoln, 132 pp.

VILLEMIN, J. A. (1868): *Études sur la Tuberculose; Preuves Rationnelles et Expérimentales de sa Spécificité et de son Inoculabilité.* Paris, Baillière, pp. 640.

WANG, C. Y. (1916): Isolation of tubercle bacilli from sputum and determination of their type. *J. Path. & Bact.,* 21:14-21.

WEBSTER, REGINALD (1941): Studies in tuberculosis: II. The relative incidence of human and bovine types of Mycobacterium tuberculosis in human disease in Victoria. *M. J. Australia,* 2:49-55.

WELLS, A. Q. (1937): Tuberculosis in wild voles. *Lancet, 1:*1221.

WILLIAMS, R. S., and HOY, W. A. (1927): Tubercle bacilli in the faeces of apparently healthy cows. *J. Hyg.,* 27:37-39.

WILLIAMS, STENHOUSE, and HOY, W. A. (1928): Tubercle bacilli in bovine faeces. *Lancet,*
   *1:*245.
WILSON, G. S., and MILES, A. A. (1955): *Topley and Wilson's Principles of Bacteriology
   and Immunity,* 4th Ed., Baltimore, Williams and Wilkins, pp. 1482-1542.

Chapter 2

ANTHRAX

Clarence D. Stein, V.M.D.

Anthrax is primarily a disease of animals; secondarily, man is infected from an animal, either by direct or indirect means. Other designations for the disease which have been used are malignant pustule, splenic fever, charbon, murrain, and wool sorters' disease.

HISTORY

The origin of anthrax is lost in antiquity. About 1491 B.C. Moses is quoted as threatening Pharoah with an epizootic among his horses, cattle, and sheep as follows:

"The hand of the Lord will fall on your livestock in the fields, on horses, asses, camels, herds and flocks, with a very severe pest."[88]

The disease is considered by many authors to have been anthrax. The severity of the outbreak is indicated by the statement that all the cattle of Egypt died.

Classical writers in the centuries that followed alluded to outbreaks among animals that in all probability were anthrax. Homer mentions it; Virgil describes it quite accurately in epizootic form in animals; Hippocrates, Galen, and Pliny describe carbuncles which are considered to be anthrax by modern authorities. Numerous writers during the medieval ages mention devastating epizootics of the disease in animals. Not until near the end of the sixteenth century, however, was it suspected that the disease was transmissible to man. In 1613, in the south of Europe, it developed into a scourge which carried off 60,000 people. In ancient Anglo-Saxon records there appear accounts of recipes, charms, and incantations for the cure or prevention of "black bain" as anthrax was then called.

The beginning of scientific literature on anthrax is marked by the publication of *Charbon Malin* by Fournier in Dijon, France, in

1769. The Academy of Dijon offered a prize essay on the subject which resulted in some remarkably accurate descriptions of the disease in man and animals. Chabert[15] in 1780 distinguished different forms of anthrax in man from other septic conditions of the skin, and Barthelemy in 1823 proved the contagious nature of the disease in animals.

The cause of anthrax at this time was a moot point, theories being bound up in all the hazy and illogical notions of the pre-Pasteur period. Delafond, a French veterinarian, held that anthrax in sheep was caused by an "excess of blood circulating in the vessels due to too copious and substantial feeding." Heusinger was of the opinion that anthrax in man was due to a malarial neurosis dependent on various conditions of the soil and climate. Other ideas included the influence of soil, summer heat, storms, insanitary conditions of the stables, and the like.

Among such a confusion of ideas, with anthrax killing off from 25 to 50 per cent of the flocks of sheep and so prevalent in France and other European countries that farming was almost at a standstill,[112] a period of observation and investigation began about 1850 which culminated in the identification of the anthrax bacillus by Koch in 1876[52] and the production of a preventive vaccine by Pasteur in 1880.[71]

Historically anthrax has a triple signficance. It was the first disease of man and animals shown to be caused by a micro-organism, the first disease against which a bacterial vaccine was found to be effective, and it constituted the principal subject for study by the early investigators who laid the groundwork for the modern science of bacteriology.

THE ETIOLOGIC AGENT

Anthrax bacilli in the blood were first seen by Pollender[75] in 1849. His description was not published until 1855, however, and meanwhile Davaine and also Rayer[78] had called attention to these peculiar bodies "about twice the size of a red blood corpuscle" which were present in the blood of infected animals. Brauell[11] in 1857 and Delafond in 1860[20] both observed the same organisms but none of the investigators up to this time realized their full significance. The researchers of Pasteur into the field of what was destined to become the science of bacteriology stimulated Davaine[17] again to take up the study of these organisms. In 1863 he demonstrated that only the blood of animals sick with the disease contained the organism,[17a] and in 1873 he showed that when this blood was passed through a clay filter it was harmless for other animals.[17b] In 1876 Robert Koch[52] cleared up the whole matter by cultivating the organisms outside the body in pure culture and again producing the disease.

Bacillus anthracis is one of the largest organisms among the pathogenic bacteria, measuring from 1 to 1.25 microns in thickness and 5 to 10 microns in length. It is a non-motile, Gram-positive, spore-bearing rod and has the further distinction of being one of the most resistant of organisms among the pathogens. In its spore stage it is very resistant to heat, low temperatures, chemical disinfectants, and prolonged drying and can survive for many years in contaminated soil and animal products such as hides, hair, wool, bone meal, and dried blood. The remarkable tenacity of anthrax spores and their great resistance to such environmental influences as heat, freezing, and drying have been demonstrated by a number of investigators.

Murray[66] reported evidence, based on extensive and well-controlled experiments, that a temperature of 135° C. for five to ten minutes was necessary to kill dry anthrax spores in the absence of moisture, whereas under moist conditions spores suspended in normal (0.8 per cent) saline solution were killed in five to ten minutes at a temperature of 100° to 105° C.

Stein[99] showed that moist spores resisted successive rapid freezings at −72° to −78° C. and thawing at 37° C. for forty-five consecutive times and that dry spores contained in dried blood swabs from field cases were both viable and virulent after storage at 25° to 30° C. for thirteen years.

Graham Smith[37] showed that dry anthrax spores kept at room temperature in the presence of diffuse sunlight were capable of germinating after ten years, and in progressively smaller numbers up to twenty-two years, but not after twenty-two and one half years.

On the other hand, McCullough[59] reported that dry spores can still germinate after being kept at room temperature for forty years, and Umeno and Nobata[110] reported that dry spores on cotton threads kept at room temperature in the absence of light for more than forty years were viable and pathogenic for mice. Chemical disinfectants are not very effective against the spores except in strong solu-

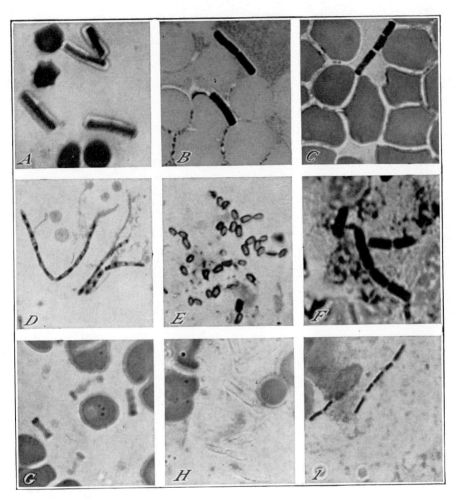

Fig. 17. Stained anthrax bacilli and spores. *A,* bacilli in sheep blood (methylene blue), x1,700. *B,* bacilli in guinea pig blood (Giemsa's stain), x1,600. *C,* bacilli in guinea pig blood (Hasting's stain), x1,600. *D,* sporulating organisms from spleen (from case of anthrax in cattle), x1,400. *E,* anthrax spores from culture, x1,900. *F,* bacilli in blood, stained with methylene blue (photograph taken with polarized light), x2,000. *G* and *H,* so-called shadow or ghost forms, x1,500. *I,* bacilli from spleen of guinea pig (note long chains), x1,400. (From Stein, C. D.: *Vet. Med.,* 1943, 38, 130-139.)

tions or over long periods of time—5 per cent liquor cresolis compositus for seven hours, 5 per cent carbolic acid for two days, 10 per cent mercury bichloride for twenty minutes, and 10 to 20 per cent

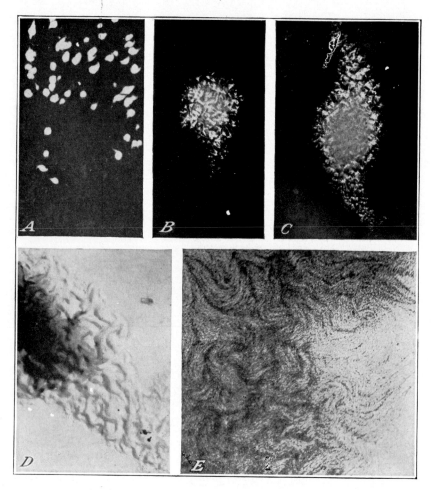

Fig. 18. Anthrax colonies on surface of plain agar plates, eighteen-hour growth, made direct from suspension in saline solution of spleen swab from case of anthrax in cattle. *A*, small and medium irregular shaped colonies, natural size. *B*, small colony (note ground glass appearance), x10. *C*, large comet-shaped colony (note ground glass appearance), x10. *D*, portion of colony *C* showing border, x30. *E*, border of colony *C*, x100. (From Stein, C. D.: *Vet. Med.*, 1943, 38, 130-139.)

formaline for 10 minutes. In dry air the organisms are destroyed at 200° F. in twenty-four hours. (Smyth)[89] Lye in 5 per cent solution is one of the most effective disinfectants against anthrax infection. To disinfect contaminated objects or premises, they should be thoroughly saturated with the disinfectant, which should not be washed off for at least twenty-four hours. The vegetative forms, free from spores, are easily destroyed by the usual methods of disinfection, and likewise show little resistance to heat and drying.

In culturing, other less resistant types of bacteria will overgrow *Bacillus anthracis,* but when the former have been destroyed by the proper degree of heat, the latter is easily cultivated on all ordinary nutrient media, forming characteristic colonies which are not difficult to identify. These colonies have a ground-glass or medusahead appearance, curled, with marginal filaments always returning to the

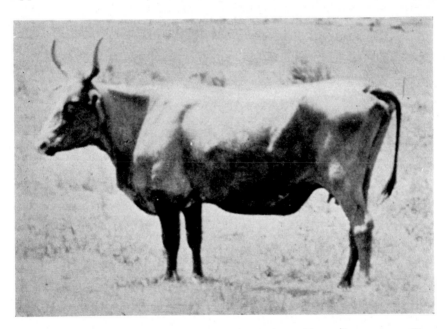

Fig. 19. A subacute case of bovine cutaneous anthrax. Note edematous swelling in the region of shoulder, brisket and ventral portion of abdomen. (Courtesy of Dr. I. P. Coulter, Florida Livestock Sanitary Board.)

colony and not showing free ends. In filaments of a twenty-four hour culture, cell divisions are not easily seen when examined under the oil immersion lens through a cover-glass. Spores do not develop until after twenty-four hours on standard agar. As with several other pathogens, two types of colonies have been noted—rough and smooth, the rough or "R" type being the more virulent. After the use of some antiseptics, "R" colonies may disappear and only the "S" type remain, coincident with loss of virulence.

It has been shown that there is a definite antagonism between the anthrax organism and the colon bacillus.[36] When allowed to grow in mixed culture the anthrax organisms not only decrease in relative number but also in virulence. A similar antagonism has been shown between the *anthrax bacilli* and *Pseudomonas aerugenosa* and also one of the "mycoides" group of organisms.

While generally referred to as an aerobic organism, the anthrax bacillus can be grown anaerobically under which condition it has a somewhat altered morphology, produces no spores, and is less virulent.[70] This behavior corresponds somewhat with that in man as it is a non-spore-former in the body, forming spores only in the presence of an abundant supply of oxygen. This fact is the basis for the regulation regarding the disposal of anthrax-infected carcasses mentioned later.

GEOGRAPHIC PREVALENCE

Anthrax occurs in all parts of the world. In certain European countries where restrictive measures, together with preventive vaccination, as in England, France, and Germany have been enforced, the disease in animals is now rather infrequent. In other parts of the world, especially the Asiatic countries of Siberia, Iran, Tibet, China, India, and Arabia, where sanitary science has not been developed, anthrax in animals is very prevalent. It occurs in many parts of South America, Africa, and Australia. Legg[55] lists the following countries as most likely to supply infected materials such as wool, hair, hides and skins: China, India, Central Asia, Straits Settlements, Persia (Iran), Mesopotamia, Asia Minor, Japan, Russia, Egypt, and Africa. American experience would add South America and Mexico to this list.

Glassman[31] in his report on the world incidence of anthrax in man during the thirty year period (1924-1953) states that outside North America human cases were prevalent in the following areas: Africa (French West Africa, Kenya, Ruanda Urundi, Tanganyika); South America (Argentine, Chile, Uruguay, Venezuela); Europe (Bulgaria, Italy, Portugal, Rumania, Spain, Yugoslavia); The Near and Middle East (Iran, Iraq, Turkey and Eurasia) and U.S.S.R.

According to Glassman countries providing statistics on incidence of human anthrax to the World Health Organization report a total of approximately 9,000 cases per annum. In recent years he also estimated that 20,000 to 100,000 cases of human anthrax occurs per annum throughout the world.

Kaplan[50] of The World Health Organization in 1953 reported that anthrax is found in practically all parts of the world with the heaviest areas of infection in the Mediterranean region, Africa and Asia.

The outlook for a gradual reduction in the incidence of animal anthrax, however, is more hopeful for the future, since vaccination of livestock against anthrax and better methods of control are being carried out in many of the world's endemic areas. Prophylactic vaccination is being used extensively in the United States, but as yet this country continues to have many outbreaks in animal anthrax, and human anthrax arising from the handling of domestic materials is not uncommon.

Anthrax occurred in North America early in colonial days.

Fleming[29] in his book on *Animal Plagues* states that anthrax in epizootic proportions occurred in 1769, 1783, and 1795 in the West Indies taking a heavy toll of livestock and human life.

Hanson[38] has pointed out, that probably the first published account of anthrax in animals and man in North America was the report made in 1824 by J. Kercheval, a physician from Bardstown, Kentucky.

Kercheval described an outbreak of an acute fatal disease of livestock transmissable to man that occurred during the summer of 1819 in the vicinity of Bardstown, Kentucky. The symptoms and lesions he described were characteristic of anthrax. Carpenter[13] traced the infection in Louisiana back to the time of its settlement by the French. The disease was believed to have been prevalent among the deer of that region. The cattle were likewise attacked annually so that by 1835 it existed in all parts of the state. Carpenter states, however, that it "seems not to have been even noticed in the medical annals of America." In 1835 he reported a large number of human cases. Later references in that state as well as in other lower Mississippi and Gulf States in the years that followed indicate that anthrax was more or less endemic in that region.[2] The first human case in the state of Pennsylvania of which there is record occurred in Philadelphia in 1834.[73] "Murrain," or anthrax, was at that time prevalent among cattle fed on the common. Several person who skinned such animals developed lesions on the hands.

In New England, Osborn[69] could find no mention of anthrax in

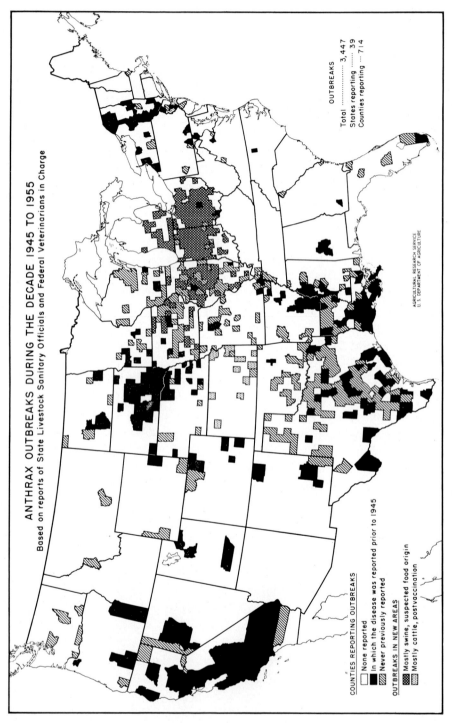

Fig. 20.

the colonial records of Massachusetts. In 1852, a report appeared by a physician in Salem who had seen six different cases in previous years. From 1853 to 1869 at Walpole, Massachusetts, twenty-six cases occurred, traceable to a hair factory.

Outbreaks in livestock are reported to have occurred in Mississippi in 1865, in Texas in 1860, in New York in 1881, in Vermont and Massachusetts in 1887, and in California in 1888. Infected areas still exist in most of these states.[97]

Numerous references in medical literature have appeared since that time indicating that anthrax has existed especially in the northern states of the Atlantic seaboard, in California, and in the Central Gulf States. In Louisiana in 1924, 20,000 head of cattle perished from the disease in forty-three of sixty-four parishes.[68]

Animal anthrax tends to appear in river valleys. Stein[94] states that recognized areas of infection exist in the San Joaquin and Sacramento Valleys of California, southeastern South Dakota, northeastern Nebraska, the Texas Gulf coast, the delta region of the lower Mississippi, and in the Mississippi valley in Arkansas, Mississippi, and Louisiana, in all of which areas widespread outbreaks occur from time to time. Streams are often contaminated with surface drainage from anthrax soil and may carry the infection to distant points, especially during floods and overflows. The outbreaks usually occur when livestock are on pasture, and tend to follow hot, dry summers in which normally swampy areas are dried up and the regular growth of herbage becomes scanty, necessitating grazing close to the soil.

Smyth[90,91] as Chairman of the Committee on Anthrax of the Industrial Hygiene Section of the American Public Health Association, reported anthrax incidence in the United States from 1919 to 1944. In the first five year period (1919-23) covered by his investigations, only fifteen states reported human cases, while twenty-three additional states and the District of Columbia reported cases in man during the twenty year period (1924-1943). At some time during the twenty-five year period 1919-1943 every state except Idaho and South Carolina reported one or more human cases.

From Table 12, which shows the geographic distribution of animal and human anthrax in the United States, it may be seen that with the possible exception of Idaho, there is not a state in which either animal or human anthrax has not been recognized in the twenty-five period preceding 1944. In each succeeding five-year period new states

TABLE 12
Geographical Distribution of Anthrax in the United States 1919-1943

State	Animal Anthrax Occurring		Human Anthrax Occurring		Comments
	Before 1939	1939-1943	Before 1939	1939-1943	
Alabama	+	+	−	+	
Arizona	−	−	+	+	
Arkansas	+	+	+	+	
California	+	+	+	+	
Colorado	+	+	+	+	
Connecticut	+	−	+	−	
Delaware	+	?	+	+	"No animal anthrax in 1942 or 1943." Human cases chiefly industrial.
D. C.	−	−	−	+	Probable source: hairbrush.
Florida	+	−	+	−	
Georgia	+	+	+	+	
Idaho	−	−	−	?	Diagnosis disputed.
Illinois	+	+	+	+	
Indiana	+	−	+	−	
Iowa	+	+	+	+	
Kansas	+	−	+	−	
Kentucky	?	?	+	−	No reports received re animal cases.
Louisiana	+	+	+	+	
Maine	+	−	+	+	
Maryland	+	+	+	−	
Massachusetts	+	+	+	+	Human cases chiefly industrial.
Michigan	−	−	+	−	
Minnesota	+	+	+	−	
Mississippi	+	+	+	+	
Missouri	+	+	+	+	
Montana	+	+	+	?	Diagnosis disputed.
Nebraska	+	+	+	?	Doubt completeness of reporting human cases; animal anthrax prevalent.
Nevada	+	+	+	−	
New Hampshire	+	−	+	+	Human cases chiefly industrial.
New Jersey	+	+	+	+	Human cases chiefly industrial.
New Mexico	?	?	+	+	No reports received re animal cases.
New York	+	+	+	+	Human cases chiefly industrial.
N. Carolina	+	+	+	+	
N. Dakota	+	+	+	+	
Ohio	+	−	+	+	
Oklahoma	+	−	+	+	
Oregon	+	+	+	+	
Pennsylvania	+	+	+	+	Human cases chiefly industrial.
Rhode Island	?	?	+	−	No reports received re animal cases.
S. Carolina	+	−	−	−	
S. Dakota	+	+	+	+	
Tennessee	?	?	+	?	Human case diagnosis disputed. No animal cases '41-'43; previous records destroyed.
Texas	+	+	+	+	
Utah	+	+	+	+	
Vermont	+	−	+	+	
Virginia	?	?	+	−	No reports received re animal cases.
Washington	+	−	+	−	
West Virginia	+	−	+	+	
Wisconsin	+	+	+	+	
Wyoming	+	−	+	−	

which had not previously reported human cases of agricultural orgin, have so reported, until now at least three quarters of the states have so reported. Although the larger number of human cases are of industrial origin, they are concentrated in a few states and are quickly recognized and promptly treated. The more serious problem lies in the widely scattered cases of agricultural origin.

Schrack[82] reported that during the eighteen year period 1934-1951 1229 cases of anthrax in man occurred in the United States. Seventy percent of these occurred in the New England and Middle Atlantic States and 326 or more than one quarter of the cases occurred in Pennsylvania.

Data compiled from the U. S. Public Health Reports for the sixteen year period (1945-1960)[64] reveals that 640 anthrax cases in man were reported from the United States. Although anthrax in man showed a decrease in incidence during the period from 1954 to 1960, it still is a problem among workers in industries handling imported hair, wool and hides (Table 13).

TABLE 13

REPORTED CASES OF ANTHRAX IN MAN, UNITED STATES 1945-1960**

Year	Number of Cases	Year	Number of Cases
1945	40	1953	45
1946	40	1954	22
1947	69	1955	39
1948	60	1956	38
1949	54	1957	26
1950	49	1958	16
1951	60	1959	12
1952	47	1960	23

**From reports of U. S. Public Health Service, National Office of Vital Statistics.

Epidemiological studies of anthrax in animals in the United States made by Stein and his associates[97,98,99,100,101,102,103,104,105] revealed that during the thirty year period (1915-1945) outbreaks had been reported from 438 counties in forty-three states and the infection appeared to be spreading slowly into new areas. During the eleven year period (1945-1956) 3569 outbreaks of anthrax were reported from forty states with losses of 17,868 head of livestock. Two outbreaks occurred in zoo animals with a loss of 27 animals and 10 outbreaks occurred in mink with a loss of 460 animals. Thirty-seven cases of agricultural anthrax in man, nine of which occurred in veterinarians were also reported. A marked increase in incidence occurred in 1951 when 483 anthrax outbreaks were reported from twenty-five states. The greatest losses were reported from southeastern Missouri and adjoining areas along the Mississippi River in Kentucky and Tennessee where 302 outbreaks with losses of 1,152 head of livestock occurred. For the first time in more than twenty years anthrax also appeared in Florida when twenty-one outbreaks were reported from three counties with a loss of 206 cattle. In 1952, 1,644 outbreaks were reported from thirty-two States with a total loss of 1,578 cattle, 1,614 swine, twenty horses, six mules, and 233 sheep. This was the greatest number of outbreaks ever to be recorded for any single year. This tremendous increase in incidence was due chiefly to widespread outbreaks of food origin that occurred in swine herds in the Midwest during the first two quarters of the year, and to postvaccination outbreaks that occurred principally in cattle herds in Kansas and New Jersey (Table 14). The Animal Morbidity Reports of the Agricultural Research Service, United States Department of Agriculture for the five year period (1956-1960) show that anthrax outbreaks in animals were reported from twenty-seven different states. Outbreaks occurred in 1879 herds of cattle and 153 herds of swine.

This five years period was highlighted by a major epizootic of anthrax that occurred in Oklahoma and Kansas in 1957 with loss of 1,627 farm animals on 741 premises.

TABLE 14

SUMMARIZED DATA ON THE YEARLY INCIDENCE OF ANTHRAX IN LIVESTOCK FROM 1945 TO 1955, INCLUSIVE

Year	No. States Reporting	No. Counties Involved	No. Outbreaks	Livestock Losses*
1945	14	52	97	583
1946	18	82	163	4,019**
1947	19	65	124	880
1948	14	63	120	1,654**
1949	16	57	93	773
1950	12	55	61	595
1951	25	113	483	2,753
1952	32	432	1,644***	3,451
1953	26	121	233	597
1954	23	74	429	2,299**
1955	20	61	122	264

*In some states losses were estimated. **Heavy losses were reported during severe epizootics of the disease in Louisiana. ***Greatest number of outbreaks in swine herds in the Midwest and postvaccination outbreaks in cattle in Kansas and New Jersey.

An unusual outbreak of anthrax occurred in 1956 among cattle and moose in the Wyoming Mountains. The epizootic occurred in animals on summer ranges in three National forests at an elevation of 8,000 to 10,000 feet and resulted in the loss of fifty-eight cattle and eighteen moose.

A study of annual reports on the incidence of animal anthrax from 1945 to 1960 indicates a gradual extension of the disease in some areas and its restriction in others.

THE DISEASE IN ANIMALS

Practically all animals are in some degree susceptible to anthrax. Cattle, horses, mules, sheep, goats, and the wild herbivores are most commonly affected. Omnivora (man and swine) possess the greatest natural resistance to the disease. Under certain conditions, carnivora (dogs, cats, and wild animals of prey), birds, frogs, and toads may become infected. Mice, guinea pigs, and rabbits, which are commonly used in the laboratory diagnosis of anthrax, are very susceptible, while rats show considerable resistance. Although insects may transmit the disease in a purely mechanical manner, they appear to be immune.

Fowls are highly resistant to the disease, but they can be infected experimentally. Outbreaks in ostriches have been reported by Henning,[40] Robertson,[79] and Theiler;[107] outbreaks in ducks, by Gerlach,[30] outbreaks in geese, by Ubertini;[109] and a case in an eagle, by Almeyew.[1]

Outbreaks in wild animals in captivity and cases in farm dogs and cats occasionally occur from eating infected meat. Stein[100] refers to outbreaks in mink, deer, and buffalo in the United States, and to an outbreak in a zoological garden in which deaths from anthrax were reported in three mountain lions, three honey bears, and one each of the following: badger, leopard, tiger, fox, jaguar, civet cat, bobcat, and an owl. Somers[93] mentions an outbreak in a traveling menagerie in England in which polar bears, lions, pumas, racoons, leopards, a badger, an anteater, a coypu, and a vulture were affected with anthrax.

The disease occurs in elephants in India, Siam, and Burma[27,28] and in antelopes in Africa.[40]

Spontaneous outbreaks in wild animals under natural conditions have been reported in wild pigs, wild dogs and dingoes in Australia;[5] and in wolves, hares and elk in Russia.[53]

Although anthrax in livestock in the United States is principally confined to cattle, outbreaks in horses, mules, sheep, and swine are also encountered. Infection in livestock usually is the result of grazing on infected pasture land rather than by contact. Infection may also be caused by contaminated fodder or artificial feed-stuffs, such as bonemeal, fish meal, oil cake, and tankage; by drinking from contaminated pools; or by the bites of contaminated flies. Dogs, cats, and other carnivores, as well as swine, usually acquire the infection from consuming infected meat.

In the United States, anthrax in livestock occurs in epizootic form in regions in which the soil is known to be seriously contaminated with anthrax spores. However, it may occur, sporadically, anywhere at any time and thus may appear where previously not identified or where it has been quiescent for a long period.

Since anthrax organisms may persist for long periods of time in certain types of soil, it is more or less confined to areas commonly designated as "anthrax districts." In such districts, it constitutes a perennial problem, making its appearance during a definite period known as the anthrax season, usually late in the summer and early in the fall when grazing is close, due to scanty pasturage, and when flies are very numerous. In such areas, the disease can be kept in check by preseasonal vaccination with appropriate types of immunizing agents.

Pastures in which infected cattle have roamed may remain contaminated for years and prove fatal to any stock turned thereon to graze. Pastures contaminated by tannery wastes have been described by Eichhorn[22] and by others as a menace to cattle, as are streams into which tannery wastes are discharged and from which cattle or other animals may drink. Anthrax organisms may be carried from place to place by birds and small animals. They have been found on the beaks and feet of buzzards which have fed on animals dead of the disease. Dogs, cats, rats, opossums, and chickens all may harbor live spores in the feces after eating infected flesh and thus serve as dangerous carriers in spreading the contagion to new territory. Infection by ingestion may occur from eating hay, forage, or other crops which have been grown on infected pasture land or are otherwise contaminated with anthrax spores. The use of artificial feedstuffs appears with great frequency in association with outbreaks, bone meal seemingly being the source of infection in several instances.

Outbreaks in South Africa[19] and the United States[102] were traced directly to imported contaminated bone meal. Since 1951 numerous outbreaks of anthrax in livestock due to contaminated feeding stuffs have been reported from England[12] and Sweden.[4]

To prevent the introduction of anthrax infection into the United States, Federal regulations governing the importation of bones, or bonemeal for use in animal feeds or fertilizer are enforced by the Department of Agriculture. These regulations require that such material be subjected to heat at sufficiently high temperatures to destroy the spores of *Bacillus anthracis*.

Biting flies may be a factor in the spread of anthrax not only from animal to animal, but also from animal to man. Non-biting flies, after feeding on infected meat, may also carry anthrax organisms on their proboscises and feet, infecting wounds in animals and contaminating feedstuffs and other material on which they settle. Anthrax spores have remained alive in flies for twenty days, being found in the feces. Infection through abrasions, cuts, and scratches, can likewise spread the disease, but such factors, compared with ingestion, are of small importance in animals.

The disease in animals may occur in a peracute (apoplectic), acute, subacute, or chronic form.[99]

The peracute form is most common in cattle, sheep, and goats, and occurs at the beginning of an outbreak. It is characterized by a sudden onset and rapidly fatal course. Victims are frequently found dead without showing any previous evidence of disease.

In the acute and subacute forms the disease develops more slowly, but after the first symptoms are noticed becomes well established in twelve to twenty-four hours. There is, first, excitement, followed by depression, spasms, respiratory or cardiac distress, trembling, restlessness, staggering, convulsions, and death. During the course of the disease, pregnant animals may abort, rumination ceases, and the milk secretion is reduced. Bloody discharges may emanate from the natural body openings, and edematous swellings may appear on different parts of the body. The acute form usually terminates in death in a day or two. The subacute form may result in death in three to five days or longer, or in complete recovery after several days. These types of the disease are common in cattle, horses, and sheep (Figure 19).

Chronic anthrax occurs mostly in swine, affects the mesenteric and submaxillary lymph glands, and is usually recognized only on post-mortem examination. When infection in hogs follows feeding on an anthrax-infected carcass, some of the animals may be found dead without having shown any previous signs of illness. Others of the group may show symptoms of illness, with rapidly progressing swellings about the throat which, in some cases, cause death by suffocation. A relatively large percentage of the group may become visibly sick for a few days, with or without moderate swellings about the throat, and recover.

In horses and mules, the first indication of the disease may be severe colicky symptoms, accompanied by high temperature, chills, loss of appetite, extreme depression, muscular weakness, and the passage of blood-stained feces. Hot, painful, and rapidly progressing swellings frequently develop over the body, especially about the neck and lower abdomen.

Dogs are affected chiefly with pharyngeal anthrax or anthrax of the tongue, in which swelling may occur about the head and the throat. Anthrax of the intestines also occurs in dogs, manifested as a severe gastroenteritis.

Isolated or sporadic cases are usually of the subacute form, and are sometimes limited to the formation of a tumor or carbuncle at the point where the organisms gain entrance to the body.

ANTHRAX IN MAN

The number of human cases of anthrax in the United States is not large.

Epidemiological reports of the United States Public Health Service on the yearly incidence of anthrax in man for the sixteen year period (1945-1960)[64] indicate there were less than seventy cases annually. In areas where anthrax in man and animals rarely occurs many physicians and veterinarians may practice a lifetime without encountering a case (Table 12).

In the first decade of this century British authorities placed anthrax mortality in Europe at about 25 per cent.[7] Holtzmann[43] showed that in the tannery industry in Germany in 1927-32 fatalities averaged 9.3 per cent as compared with 12 per cent in the same industry in the United States during the same period.[90] Anthrax fatalities in the United States have decreased from approximately 20 per cent in 1910-20, to about 8 per cent in 1939-43.

This improvement occurred principally in the tannery and woolen mill cases and was undoubtedly due to earlier diagnosis and more prompt and efficient treatment. Since 1945, the death percentage rate in the United States has been further reduced by treatment with penicillin and other antibiotics. During the five years prior to 1960 the mortality rate for cutaneous anthrax was about one percent.

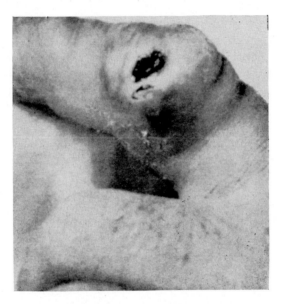

Fig. 21. Anthrax lesion on the finger, five days following autopsy and skinning of an anthrax carcass. Typical black center is surrounded by edematous tissue, beefy-red in color. (Courtesy of the *Wisconsin Medical Journal*. From Wyatt, E. T. and Epstein, S.: Anthrax in Wisconsin, 1941.)

Human anthrax infection is usually through a skin lesion, generally a slight abrasion, scratch, or small wound on an exposed surface, producing primarily the local lesion of malignant pustule, carbuncle, or charbon. Less frequently infection may enter the upper respiratory tract in the form of dried spores in dust from wool sorting or from storage lofts for dried skins or hair, and produce the massive pneumonia of "woolsorters' disease." Less often still in man, internal anthrax may take the form of an intestinal infection, resulting from eating improperly cooked meat. Milk is rarely responsible for human anthrax infection, as infected cattle are usually too ill to be secreting milk.

Solowieff,[92] reporting autopsies on twenty-two cases of intestinal anthrax, states that the lesions are usually limited to a comparatively small section of the bowel, most frequently the cecum and adjacent part of the small intestine. Jean[48] reports one case of renal anthrax with multiple kidney abscesses, unsuccessfully treated by excision.

Occasionally no portal of entry is recognizable and infection may localize or at least predominate as a meningitis. Cernaianu[14] states that the brain is much more receptive to anthrax bacilli than the skin. McCowen and Parker[60] report a fatal case of anthrax meningitis with no evident external lesion. Several similar cases have been noted in the United States.

Internal anthrax of any type is usually fatal, although prompt energetic treatment may occasionally be successful. One case has been reported[61] of pulmonary anthrax in a two and one-half year old child, diagnosed by finding anthrax organisms in the sputum. The child recovered under serum therapy, but with damaged vision, the eyes apparently being affected at the start. Another case of pulmonary and intestinal anthrax developing after a primary ankle lesion recovered after treatment with serum and arsenicals.[90]

An Epidemic of Pulmonary Anthrax

While very few cases of inhalation anthrax in the United States have been reported prior to 1957, Brachman and his associates of the U.S. Public Health Service[10] in 1958, reported an epidemic of nine cases of anthrax that occurred among the employees of a goat hair processing mill in Manchester, New Hampshire between August 27 and November 5, 1957. Four of the nine cases were non-fatal cutaneous anthrax. The five remaining cases were inhalation anthrax, four of which were fatal.

The clinical picture of inhalation anthrax in these five cases was characterized by an onset of symptoms of a mild upper respiratory tract infection, followed in about three and one-half days by symptoms of acute respiratory distress and shock. Four of the patients died from seven to twenty-five hours after the acute symptoms developed and two of these patients revealed clinical and pathological evidence of meningitis.

All of the nine cases were associated with handling one particular shipment of black goat hair imported from India. During the sixteen and one-half years prior to this epidemic 136 cases of cutaneous anthrax with one fatality have been reported from among employees of this mill.

The external form of anthrax presents a very typical clinical picture. In two or three days after contact with infected material, a small reddish blister appears, surrounded by an area of erythema. At this stage diagnosis is not always easy unless the serous fluid is examined bacteriologically. This should be done at once, since early diagnosis is of the greatest importance. Clinical diagnosis becomes almost certain, however, within twenty-four to twenty-eight hours, with the very characteristic further development of the lesion. The center becomes infiltrated and dark red, increases rapidly in size, and soon becomes black. In fact, the name *anthrax* is derived from this characteristic black center. The lesion may become nearly two inches in diameter, surrounded by a wide area of edema, which later becomes hard but not particularly painful unless touched. Systemic manifestations, fever and prostration, often occur out of proportion to the size of the lesion. If adequate treatment is not instituted early, infection tends to spread rapidly through the lymphatics to the circulation, resulting in an almost always fatal bacteriemia. Square-ended rods may be cultured from the local lesion if discharging, from serum from the edematous area, and later, on post-mortem, from the blood and internal organs, as liver, spleen, and kidney. If the carbuncle has a sloughing, necrosed center, the rods will contain central spores, but otherwise organisms from body tissues do not show spores when freshly stained.

The most usual sites for local lesions are the head, neck, and upper extremities, as these are the most exposed areas. Legge's *Industrial Maladies*[55] gives the distribution of primary lesions in 937 cases reported in England (Table 15). Osborn's Massachusetts figures[69] correspond to these, except that lesions of the neck were more frequent than those of the head and face. These give more detailed distribution areas. Smyth reports on the location of primary lesion in 640 cases (Table 16).

Human anthrax may be derived from direct contact with animal secretions, excretions, or infected tissues, or by contact with animal products, as hides, skins, or hair, or may be transmitted by biting flies from animals to man.

TABLE 15

ANATOMIC DISTRIBUTION OF PRIMARY ANTHRAX LESION IN 937 CASES (LEGGE)

Site	*Percentage Distribution*
Head and face	44.6
Neck	31.2
Upper extremity	20.4
Lower extremity	1.9
Trunk	1.9

TABLE 16

LOCATION OF PRIMARY ANTHRAX LESION IN 640 CASES (SMYTH)

Total internal anthrax		11	1.7% of total
Pulmonary	4		
Pulmonary and intestinal	2		
Intestinal	2		
Meningeal	3		
Total external anthrax		629	98.3% of total
Face, head and neck	309		49.1% of external cases
Upper extremity	264		42.0
Lower extremity	23		3.65
Chest, abdomen and back	23		3.65
Multiple lesions	9		1.4
Not stated	1		0.1

During the years (1919-43) covered by the Smyth reports,[90] few human cases in the United States have been attributed to infection from animals other than sheep, cattle, horses, and mules, and none from animal products other than hides and skins of cattle, goats, horses, and mules, horse-hair, imported wool, blood meal, and fertilizer. Many cases due to skinning or autopsying cows, shearing sheep, butchering, and milking, were reported. Other cases occurred in rendering plants and from the use of fertilizers, the material in one instance being wool waste. Cases were reported as resulting from cattle feed, in one instance a blood meal; one case developed in a cordage factory from handling sisal fiber from Mexico, probably infected from animals. One girl in Louisiana apparently developed a fatal case while carving statuettes from horse bones. One man became infected while caring for a dog that had fed on a dead sheep; another while caring for a sick mule. Cases contracted from minks have also been reported.

Seidman and Wheeler in 1947[86] reported a fatal case in a worker in the piano key industry attributed to infection from imported elephant tusks. Washings from elephant tusk scarpings, when injected into guinea pigs, produced the disease.

Dried bones and bone meal from the Far East have been incriminated in a number of cutaneous anthrax cases in man, thirteen cases were reported from Wales in 1953,[18] six cases from England in 1955[47] and nine cases from Scotland in 1958.[3]

There are a few cases on record in which anthrax has passed from one person to another, but they are comparatively rare. One case was reported of a three-year-old child contracting ocular anthrax while sleeping with her father who had an anthrax lesion.[91] There have been several reports of familial anthrax.[91] In Pennsylvania in 1930-31, in a family on a small farm, seven cases developed. The first case was reported as small-pox, with multiple skin lesions, rather unusual, but died of meningitis, anthrax organisms being isolated from the cerebrospinal fluid; the second case, overlapping the first, and also fatal, was first diagnosed as erysipelas; a third case with multiple skin lesions and anthrax bacteriemia recovered after serum treatment, as did four other subsequent cases. All seven cases occurred in two months, with a return case in the next year in one of the four. Recurrences have been reported by three other writers.[67,87,111]

Bites of bloodsucking insects may at times be a factor, but such cases often can be traced to an infected animal rather than to an infected person on whom the insect has previously fed. According to Heeren[39] biting flies have been frequently mentioned as agents of transmission in early reports on anthrax in Louisiana, and insect transmission has been accepted in that state as one of the important modes of dissemination. Stein[101] mentions four cases in man in widely separated areas that developed following insect bites.

Bites from pets which have recently fed on the carcasses of animals dead of anthrax have been known to cause anthrax infection. This again is of animal origin.

Contact with the animal may be direct, as a farmer caring for a sick animal or skinning one which has died from the disease. As an illustration of the manner in which anthrax may spread from animals to man the following incident is cited. During a severe outbreak in cattle in the southern part of Florida in 1951 the disease was acquired by five persons as follows: a cowboy who had skinned a cow that had died of anthrax, two veterinarians who had vaccinated exposed cattle in the area, a laboratory technician who had handled suspected specimens from the area, and a child of the nurse who waited on the two infected veterinarians[25] Contact may be more remote, as handling hides which have been shipped long distances. Cases are recorded of workmen in tanneries carrying the infection home to members of their families, though escaping themselves. Such a happening may be due to a housewife mending or washing her husband's work clothes, and the fact that this has occurred is a strong argument for having work clothes autoclaved and laundered at the work place. The contact may be very remote, such as a man living in a hotel in a large city and rarely even seeing an animal, becoming infected by a shaving brush made from hair of an infected animal in China.

RELATION OF ANTHRAX TO FOOD HYGIENE

The importance of preventing the transmission of anthrax to man through the consumption of meat and other products from animals affected with the disease has been emphasized by public health officials.

Although the intestinal form of anthrax in man has been reported from countries where the flesh of animals dead of disease is consumed, there is little likelihood of infection being acquired from meat in civilized countries, where stringent meat inspection regulations are enforced. Some element of danger, however, may exist from the consumption of uncooked meat of animals slaughtered in uninspected abattoirs, or from the use of meat as animal food from local rendering plants.

The danger of infection from milk containing bacilli, as previously mentioned, is remote, as the milk secretion usually diminishes greatly, and the bacilli, as a rule, are present in the blood in great numbers only just before death and rarely occur in the milk secretion.

When an outbreak of anthrax occurs in a dairy herd, the dairy should be placed under strict quarantine, and all milk should be withheld from distribution until the public health officials and state livestock sanitary officials consider circumstances satisfactory for issuing a clean bill of health. Precautions should be taken to prevent the contamination of milking cans, mechanical milkers, buckets, and other dairy equipment by direct or indirect contact with diseased animals and their excreta. The question may also arise as to whether the meat and milk from vaccinated animals are dangerous. No instance has been reported to indicate that milk from vaccinated animals contains the organisms. However, milk from cows showing a marked reaction following vaccination should not be used until the animals return to normal.

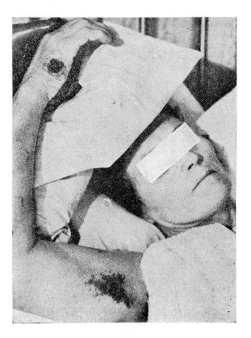

Fig. 22. A case of human anthrax, acquired from handling fat trimmings from a hog suspected of dying from choke. Two cats, fed on meat from the hog, died suddenly of anthrax. Diagnosis confirmed by laboratory examination. (Courtesy of *The Norden News*. Human case of anthrax, April-May, 1934 issue.)

Due to the fact that viable anthrax spores may persist at the site of inoculation for a considerable time after vaccination, the Federal meat inspection regulations require that carcasses of food-producing animals treated with spore vaccines be condemned, if the animals are slaughtered *less than six weeks* after vaccination, or if evidences of the reaction to the injection remain, such as inflammation, tumefaction, or edema, regardless of the period of time elapsing between treatment and inspection.

ANTHRAX AN INDUSTRIAL HAZARD

Human anthrax in the United States is primarily an industrial hazard. The number of cases among workers in the hide, skin, leather, hair, and wool industries is greater than among those in other occupations, followed by transportation workers, farmers, and veterinarians.

Statistics collected by Smyth[90] from 1919 to 1943 showed that in the first five-year period the majority of cases were in tanneries, nearly all of which are located in Delaware, Massachusetts, New Jersey, New York, and Pennsylvania. Although the percentage of tannery cases dropped from fifty-three in the first five-year period to nineteen in the last five-year period, the percentage of cases due to contact with wool and hair increased from fifteen to fifty-eight. Nearly all these cases occurred in woolen mills in Massachusetts, New Hampshire, New Jersey, New York, and Pennsylvania, with over half of such cases in the last period occurring in Pennsylvania. Agricultural anthrax, or anthrax due to direct contact with infected animals, has also appeared to increase over the years and to be recognized in an increasing number of states, although much of this apparent increase may be due to better diagnosis and reporting. In 1951 Wolff and Heimann[114] showed that 80 per cent of the human cases reported from 1939 to 1949 were of industrial origin and occurred in New England and the Middle Atlantic States, whereas 14.5 per cent of the cases for the same period were of agricultural origin and occurred in Arkansas, California, Louisiana, Mississippi, Missouri, Nebraska, and South Dakota. Goat hair and wool were the sources of 82 per cent of cases of industrial origin, and hides and skins were responsible for only 18 per cent. They further pointed out that of the cases due to hair and wool, 76 per cent were of wool origin and that of the cases due to hides and skins, 90 per cent were caused by infected goat and kid skins. The infected wool, goat hair, and goat skins originated principally in areas having a high incidence of anthrax in sheep and goats, such as India, Pakistan, Western Asia, China, North Africa, and southern Europe.

While there has been an apparent decrease in tannery anthrax, since 1939 there has been a marked increase in anthrax cases in workers in the woolen and hair industries.

Goat hair and wool from countries where anthrax is prevalent are the greatest sources of human infection.

In this connection, it is noteworthy that sixteen of the twenty-three cases of anthrax in man reported during 1960 by the U.S. Public Health Service occurred in South Carolina and were related to the processing of *imported goat hair*. These were the first cases of human anthrax ever to be reported from that State.

"Pulled" wools obtained from the skin of dead animals are more likely to be contaminated than grease wools obtained by clipping live animals. Virtually all cases of anthrax from handling hair and coarse wool occur during procedures prior to the making of yarn, and to the weaving and finishing operations. It is generally believed that the anthrax organism in wool does not survive the usual dyeing process, but some cases resulting from handling finished wool products have been reported.

One case was attributed to carrying finished rugs, although no organisms could be isolated from the rugs. Another was attributed to rags imported from Europe for use in paper-making. Various cases were attributed to scoured and so-called sterilized wool, the "sterilizing" process used being inadequate. The outbreak of seven cases with one death in a small primitive industrial village of Pennsylvania among wool-carpet-yarn-mill employees[90] was reported in 1934. Cases have also been attributed to the use of wool wastes as fertilizers.

Hoffmann,[42] in Germany, reports finding, in the textile industry, anthrax bacilli on goat hair, on textile machinery, and on finished yarn. One cannot help wondering if, with the decided increase in anthrax in the woolen industry in this country, some of the untraced cases here may not have been infected from clothing.

Industrial anthrax infection may occur in those workers not directly handling infected skins, hides, wool, or hair. Smyth, in his 1934 report, lists four cases in mechanics infected while doing repair work, a machinist and carpenter in Massachusetts, a paint cleaner in New York, and a stockyard worker in Kansas. One case is also given of a New York laborer cleaning out a sewer, one of an insurance inspector in Massachusetts, two of laboratory workers, and one of a man presumably infected from handling a fertilizer in Maine.

ANTHRAX FROM SHAVING BRUSHES

The nearest approach to a human epidemic of anthrax during the Twentieth century occurred during World War I and in the years that followed, when there was much excitement over anthrax from shaving brushes, both in this country and in England. The source of nearly all the hair for shaving brushes was horsehair from Siberia and China, where anthrax was prevalent.[45] During the course of shipment in normal times the material was cleaned and disinfected, usually in France or Germany. With the advent of World War I, shipments were made directly to the United States across the Pacific. Faulty or careless processes for insuring protection against the disease were responsible for a considerable number of cases.

The first recorded case of anthrax from a shaving brush was on July 9, 1915, in a British soldier.[24] From that time on similar cases occurred not infrequently in both the British and American forces as well as in the civil population. In the United States troops there occurred during the war 149 cases of anthrax with twenty-two deaths, due to infected shaving brushes. In New York City from 1919 to 1923, there were thirty-two cases reported from this source. In Illinois Hull examined one lot of three dozen brushes, every one of which was contaminated with virulent anthrax spores.

This hazard, formerly so widespread and justly feared and guarded against, had, until 1938, very materially lessened, due to stringent regulations as to the sterilization of hair for brushes. Another outbreak, however, occurred in 1938-39, traced to importation of 35,000 allegedly sterilized brushes from Japan. An investigation by the North Dakota Health Department and by the United States Public Health Service, showed that a considerable proportion of these brushes were contaminated by anthrax spores. Many of the brushes in this shipment were traced and withdrawn from sale. In 1939-1943, no cases were reported from this source, although two cases were attributed to a hair brush and a toothbrush.

As an illustration of the way in which such shaving brush infection may remain a latent danger for years, the London Letter of the *Journal of the American Medical Association* for August 10, 1935, notes that three years previously a consignment of twelve shaving brushes came into Lambeth and was found infected. Eleven were seized, but the twelfth had been sold and could not be traced. Every one of the eleven contained anthrax. Eventually the twelfth brush was found, but unfortunately not until after causing a fatality. A boot repairer had used this infected brush daily for two years, at last becoming infected only after cutting himself. One other case was also reported in 1935 (Pawan).[72]

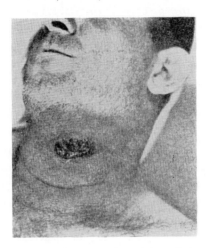

Fig. 23. Anthrax in man, acquired by use of an infected shaving brush. (Courtesy of North Dakota Livestock Sanitary Board.)

PREVENTION AND CONTROL

The prevention and control of anthrax in man depend on three factors: eradication of the disease in animals, elimination of industrial infections, and finally, earlier diagnosis and more prompt and energetic treatment of infected cases.

The control of anthrax in animals is difficult, but is being accomplished by vaccination and strict sanitary police measures. Vaccination of livestock in infected areas well in advance of the anthrax season is the most effective measure known for preventing the disease. Such vaccinations do not afford protection for more than a year and must be repeated annually and irrespective of whether the disease has already appeared on the premises or not.

Vaccination against anthrax dates from Pasteur's epoch-making demonstration in 1881 at Poully le Fort, France. The results of that experiment are well known: all the vaccinated animals resisted exposure to anthrax whereas all the non-vaccinated animals (controls) died.

The vaccine prepared by Pasteur was composed of cultures of live anthrax organisms of reduced virulence attenuated by growing at high temperatures. The Pasteur vaccine was widely used for a number of years and did much to control the disease, but was found to have definite limitations because of its rapid deterioration, long period required to produce immunity, and its failure to impart a full measure of protection in badly infected areas.

The deficiencies of the Pasteur vaccine were recognized by many investigators who devised other methods of immunization. In 1902, Sobernheim advocated simultaneous injection of virulent anthrax bacilli and anti-anthrax serum for immunization; while a decade later the successful vaccination with attenuated spore vaccines was demonstrated in Russia by Zenkowsky, in Hungary by Detri, and in Japan by Nitta. In 1916 Eichhorn[21] in the United States demonstrated that a high degree of immunity could be produced by simultaneous vaccination with a potent anti-anthrax serum and an attenuated spore vaccine.

Besredka, in 1921, introduced a new method for production of immunity by the intradermic injection of attenuated spore vaccines which conferred a solid immunity of long duration five days subsequent to vaccination. This method of vaccination is widely used in badly infected areas in the United States with excellent results. Anthrax bacterin was first used for prophylactic vaccination in the United States about 1930.

In 1939, Sterne[106] developed a non-virulent living spore vaccine made from an avirulent, non-capsulated, variant strain of *Bacillus anthracis*. This vaccine, which consist of a heavy suspension of avirulent spores in a glycerine-saline solution containing saponin, has been used with considerable success in Africa, England, India and a number of other countries. Since 1957 the Sterne Vaccine has been steadily gaining in favor for vaccination of livestock in endemic areas in the United States.

According to Stein:

"The recognized immunizing agents now being used in the United States for vaccination of animals against anthrax are of two types:

Anthrax bacterin, a sterile product, and two kinds of living spore vaccines; A. the Sterne type avirulent vaccine and B. the Pasteur type attenuated vaccine.

Anthrax bacterin which produces an immunity of low degree without danger of infecting non-exposed animals is used on premises where there is a minimum exposure.

Experience, however, has shown that living-spore vaccines, which are widely used in known infected areas, produce a higher degree of immunity than do bacterins.

"The selection of the anthrax biologic to be used in a given lot of animals should be left to the local veterinarian or state livestock sanitary officials who, because of their experience and knowledge of the local conditions, are in a position to know which products are best suited to the needs of the herd. Each of the immunizing agents mentioned has a particular field of usefulness and also definite limitations."

In outbreaks of anthrax in livestock, the following control measures, if properly carried out, will materially assist in checking the disease and preventing its spread to other areas: prompt disposal of dead animals by complete cremation; isolation of sick animals and immediate treatment with anti-anthrax serum, terramycin or penicillin; vaccination of apparently well but exposed animals; destruction of manure, bedding, and other contaminated material by burning; disinfection of contaminated stables; fly control with effective repellents; and a strict quarantine of the infected premises, rigidly enforced to prevent the movement of livestock from or into the infected area. Fields once infected with anthrax bacilli are difficult to cleanse. These should be turned to purposes other than grazing wherever possible. Animals dead of the disease should not be carried to new localities, but should be disposed of on the premises. They should either be burned or buried deeply with quick-lime, without opening the carcasses or removing the skins. In the absence of oxygen, spores are not easily formed and the vegetative forms of the organism are easily destroyed. When the skin is opened, spores form with the access to oxygen, and the problem of destruction is greatly increased.

If anthrax is suspected consult your veterinarian or state livestock sanitary officials but never open a carcass to determine the cause of death. More than one cattleman or other animal owner has become infected from autopsying an animal for the purpose of making a diagnosis.

For the recognition of anthrax in suspected materials, as animal tissues, hides, skins, and hair, the use of culture methods for isolation in pure culture is recommended. The following procedure is suggested.

Make broth culture of suspected material, incubate twenty-four hours, heat and hold in water bath at 80° C. for ten minutes to kill nonspore-formers.

Inject 0.5 to 1.0 cc. subcutaneously in the abdomen of a guinea-pig. The animal may die in twenty-four hours to seven days. Hold the inoculated animal under observation eight days before regarding it as negative. If the test animal dies, immerse completely in 10 per cent formaldehyde for a half hour before autopsy, and autoclave cage before cleaning.

Autopsy, if positive, should show gelatinous edema at site of inoculation, increase of serous fluids, dark uncoagulated blood and congestion of internal organs, especially large, dark friable spleen. Gram-positive, irregularly stained, square-ended rods, single or in short chains without spores, should be found in smears from edematous area, cut surfaces of liver, kidney, and spleen, and from heart blood. Smears stained with Geimsa or McFadden Methylene blue method should reveal encapsulated bacilli. Confirm by characteristic colonies on agar, no hemolysis on blood agar plates and by growth in bouillon, gelatin, and litmus milk.

Always confirm diagnosis by inoculation of a second guinea-pig with pure culture isolated from heart blood or from the liver, spleen, or kidney. The second animal should die in one to four days with the same findings as the first. (For further details of laboratory diagnosis, see Stein.[95,96]) In Europe, however, especially for diagnosis of anthrax in hides, much dependence seems to be placed on the Ascoli precipitin reaction[6] rather than on animal inoculation. The former reaction depends on the use of a heat-stable antigen obtained from organ extracts of animals dead from anthrax, and requires a potent precipitating serum and careful technique for successful use of the test. These extracts give a precipitate with antianthrax serum.[117]

The elimination of industrial infections depends chiefly on the proper disinfection of all raw materials likely to be infective, the disinfection of the workplace, and the education of employers and employees as to the need of prompt care of all skin wounds among workers liable to infection.

The primary consideration should be the prevention of infective materials from reaching the workplace, which, of course, concerns chiefly the disinfection of wool, hair, skins, hides, etc. Many devices have been suggested for the sterilization of hides, none of which have been entirely satisfactory. Two considerations are of prime importance: economy of cost which will make the process come within the possibility of commercial use, and lack of injury to the hides and skins. Horsehair and wool can be sterilized satisfactorily, as is done at the central disinfecting station in England.

The government disinfecting station at Liverpool[77] is planned to receive all wool and hair imported from countries where anthrax is prevalent. Material is washed in hot, alkaline suds in a wool-washing machine, followed by a hot 2 per cent formaldehyde solution and storage for several days in a holding room. The British feel that such a central cooperative government plant is the only safe and sure means of disinfecting raw wool and undressed hair, as the small dressers and spinners will not, and cannot, carry out proper methods. (For detailed information on the English method of wool disinfection see Wolff and Heimann.[114])

In the United States, government regulations[49] originally required the disinfection of horsehair and wool from suspected sources by subjection to dry heat at 165° F. for fifteen minutes, but inspectors now require a twenty-four hour holding period preceded by washing in hot, nearly boiling, alkaline suds. Autoclaving with steam under pressure is much more certain than this but may be objected to by some manufacturers using horsehair for brushes, for fear of setting a curl in the hair. The English formaldehyde method is much more satisfactory.

The problem of disinfection in tanneries is a more difficult one because of the possibility of injuring the hides in the process. No thoroughly satisfactory method has as yet come into general use in the United States. The English Seymour-Jones method[76] of soaking for twenty-four hours in a 1/5000 bichloride of mercury solution with 1.0 per cent formic acid requires a two-week holding period after treatment to insure success. The Austrain Schattenfroh method[83] of soaking in a 2 per cent hydrochloric acid and 10 per cent sodium chloride solution for forty-eight hours at room temperature can be depended on to kill anthrax spores but it leaves a harsh skin which is hard to tan satisfactorily.

Robertson,[80] in 1932, reported excellent results in the disinfection of dry hides with hydrogen sulphide gas, but long exposures were necessary to insure results (seven to 16 days, depending on temperature). No statements are given as to gas concentration and no tests on a commercial scale are reported.

Provided a generally satisfactory method for disinfecting skins and hides can be developed for the greatest protection of all handlers, it should be carried out in central government stations at ports of entry or, even better, at disinfecting stations under international management, at the shipping ports of countries of origin.

Since no successful method of preventing infective material from reaching the workplace has been devised, second consideration must be to prevent the worker from becoming infected.

Prevention, therefore, is primarily a problem of immunity. Since the sterile anthrax antigen recently developed by Wright and others[116] is now available for immunization of man, the vaccination of employees in plants where industrial exposure is a constant hazard should materially reduce the incidence of anthrax in such establishments.

In tanneries, soak vats are likely to hold infection, once acquired, for some time. These should be periodically completely drained, scrubbed, thoroughly whitewashed, and allowed to be idle for one or two days. At the same time the platform around them and under the milling drums should be whitewashed, and the drums rinsed with strong milk-of-lime. Lime is suggested because, though not killing all spores, it will greatly reduce their number, and residual lime will not harm skins that go into liming vats later.

As a protection to the consumer, MacDonald,[57] on the basis of experimental work, recommends the sterilization of carpets in the factory on the sizing machine with the use of hot formalin solution. This again offers no protection to the factory worker making the carpet.

Clothing worn by workers in wet processes and by handlers of untanned skins, especially in goat-skin tanneries, should not be taken out of the tannery unless first disinfected. The best method of disinfection is by steam under pressure in an autoclave at fifteen pounds pressure for thirty minutes.

Tannery workers and workers in hair and uncombed wool should be required to wash their hands thoroughly with soap and hot water before lunching, and they should take showers before changing to street clothes. Adequate washing facilities should be provided. A Philadelphia tannery has a washroom and shower room located between the locker room for street clothes and the room where work clothes are put on and taken off. When not in use, work clothes hang on pegs in the open room in order to dry. Workers should not be permitted to take lunches into the work rooms, but should be provided with lunch tables and chairs or benches in a room separated from the working area.

Employees should be instructed to pay attention to every skin wound, even the most trivial, and to apply to the plant dispensary or a near-by physician to have such skin breaks disinfected at once and covered with a protective dressing. These should be kept under observation by physician or nurse until completely healed. No one should work with unprotected open wounds of any kind. If the wound cannot be properly covered by an impervious dressing, rubber finger stall, or glove, the employee should quit work until it is healed. Skin infections cannot occur through unbroken skin. Cuts after shaving should be properly protected and workers should be instructed to keep their hands away from their faces while at work, especially if they have cuts or open pimples on the face.

The successful control and cure of those cases developing where adequate protection has not been afforded, depend upon early diagnosis and prompt efficient treatment. Although in the well-established anthrax pustule diagnosis can be made by inspection, wherever possible diagnosis should be confirmed bacteriologically by the finding of irregularly stained Gram-positive rods in the secretion from the wound or in serum obtained from a small puncture into a forming lesion; or when bacteriemia has developed, in a blood smear. When in doubt surely, and always if possible, morphologic diagnosis should be confirmed by isolation of the organism in pure culture and by animal inoculation. Freshly isolated virulent anthrax should kill a guinea-pig in one to seven days, usually in four days. After the death of the animal, the organism may be isolated from all body tissues and fluids.

When anthrax is suspected, however, treatment should be begun at once and not delayed pending positive diagnosis.

As to the most effective means of treatment, developments in new methods are progressing so rapidly that any recommendation made here might well be outmoded before this material is published.

In the early days of anthrax the recommended treatment was the removal or destruction of the lesion by excision, cauterization, or injection of 50 per cent phenol about the lesion. This was, however, soon found to be ineffective, especially when not properly carried out or carried out too late. Often the infection was spread to other tissues through such manipulation.

After Koch's discovery of the anthrax bacillus in 1876,[52] Pasteur[71] successfully vaccinated sheep against the disease in 1880, and about the same time Toussaint[108] discovered that blood from animals dead of the disease, when heated and injected into other animals, would protect them against infection. Vaccination of animals has been successfully carried out since that time, but as this is accomplished by the use of attenuated cultures (killed cultures not being very effective), humans are not vaccinated against this disease with such vaccines because of the danger of occasional increase in virulence of the culture.

A STERILE ANTHRAX IMMUNIZING AGENT
DEVELOPED FOR USE IN MAN

In 1954, Wright and his associates (Wright, Schlingmann et et.)[116-81] at Camp Detrick, Frederick, Maryland reported the development of a sterile alum-precipitated protective anthrax antigen for the immunization of man against anthrax. The antigen produced immunity in rabbits for more than three months and in monkeys for more than fourteen months.

Immunity against anthrax for short periods was also demonstrated in sheep[8] and cattle[46] injected with the antigen.

In preliminary tests the antigen was injected subcutaneously into 660 persons each receiving three subcutaneous injections of 0.5 cc. at intervals of two weeks followed by a similar booster injection after six months. The antigen injections in man were well tolerated, producing no serious systemic reactions and moderate local reactions in only a few of the persons injected.[115]

Dr. Brachman[9] of the U. S. Public Health Service, who has been closely associated with evaluation of this vaccine in tests conducted among employees of four goat hair processing mills over a period of four years advised the author, that the statistical analysis of the data collected indicates the antigen is highly effective. The U. S. Public Health Service is currently advocating the immunization of all employees in goat hair mills and are providing vaccine for this purpose.

In 1895 Sclavo[84] in Italy produced a serum that has been widely used for the cure of anthrax in man. His original serum, however, has been modified by the use of ass serum instead of horse serum. In this country, we use an anti-anthrax serum produced by inoculating horses with virulent organisms. With the advent of this specific serum, the fatality rate for anthrax was cut sharply. Sclavo[85] in 1903 published statistics showing a fatality of 6 per cent in 164 patients treated with serum as compared with 24 per cent for Italy as a whole. In 1911, the British Ministry of Health,[63] in a report on 800 cases of anthrax, gave the fatality rate for serum-treated cases as 4 per cent as compared with 48 per cent for those not so treated. For thirty or forty years serum remained the most effective treatment known and was emphatically recommended as the treatment of choice.

The early practice of combining excision or cauterization with the use of serum, is to be condemned. Another practice usually carried out until a decade or so ago was the injection of serum about the lesion, as well as its administration intravenously, but the generally accepted policy today is one of "hands off the local lesion." Immobilization of the patient during the infective stage, to avoid possibility of blood-stream infection, has always been considered important by practically all physicians who have treated any number of cases.

The recommended treatment with anti-anthrax serum is 10 to 20 cc. intravenously as a desensitizing dose, followed by 50 to 100 cc. in two hours. If indicated, the larger dose may be repeated in twenty-four, forty-eight and seventy-two hours, depending on the spread of the vesicles and the swelling of surrounding tissues.

Severe serum reactions frequently result, either immediately after administration of the first dose, or from five to ten days, later, and for this reason, many physicians now prefer chemotherapy to serum.

Since there is now little or no demand for anti-anthrax serum many biological institutions in the United States have discontinued its production.

In 1926 and 1933 two British writers reported on the use of neo-

arsphenamine. Pijper[74] obtained excellent results with neoarsphenamine alone, and Eurich[27] treated over 200 cases with combined
serum and neoarsphenamine with a fatality rate of 5 per cent. Meshtschaninoff[62] treated twenty-one patients successfully with neoarsphenamine. Hodgson[41] reviewed 107 cases of anthrax treated med-
ically—six of fifty-two patients received large doses of anti-anthrax
serum died, whereas fifty-five patients who, in addition to serum,
were given full doses of neoarsphenamine, recovered. In this country arsenicals were not used before 1932, and then in only a few
cases. Since then, however, they have been used more extensively
with apparently excellent results. In a few cases mapharsen and
neosalversan were used, but the most satisfactory and most widely
used arsenical is neoarsphenamine, given intravenously, 0.6 gm.
initially, and 0.9 gm. the following day, repeated in twenty-four
hours if indicated. No reactions have resulted from this treatment
as with serum, and recovery has been more prompt.[56]

In some instances it has been considered advisable in very severe
cases to combine the use of serum with neoarsphenamine, and in
such cases smaller doses of each are given than when either is used
alone.

Sulfonamides have also been successfully used for treatment. In
1939 two papers, one by Cruickshank[16] and one by May and Buch[58]
on experimental work with mice, showed sulfanilamide and sulfapyridine to be effective in treating these animals. Neoprontosil, sulfanilamide, sulfapyridine, sulfadiazine, and sulfathiazole have all been
used, but the most widely recomemnded is sulfathiazole, 3 to 4 gms.
by mouth initially, with 1 to 1.5 gm. every three to four hours up to
seven days is indicated. In 1942 Gold[32] published his results on the
treatment of forty cases with various sulfa-drugs. He feels that recovery is more prompt with sulfathiazole than with any other treatment,
and that this is the treatment of choice.

The results obtained in the treatment of a large number of cases
with anti-anthrax serum, arsenicals, or sulfadrugs, are shown in
Table 17 compiled by Smyth.

Except for those cases treated by serum alone, the figures shown
in Table 17 may be considered only suggestive, since no rates should
be based on fewer than 200 cases for any degree of accuracy, but they
do give some idea of results obtained by various treatments, from
case records sent in to Smyth.

TABLE 17

Results from Various Methods of Treatment of Anthrax Cases (Smyth)

Treatment	No. of Cases	Fatality Rate Per Cent
None; wrong diagnosis	25	88
Non-specific local treatment; incision; excision, cautery	60	28.3
Serum only	519	8.6
Arsenicals only	62	0
Sulfa-drugs only	64	4.7
Serum and arsenicals	72	8.3
Serum and sulfa-drugs	32	9.4

The successful use of penicillin in the treatment of human patients was first reported in 1944 by Murphy, LaBoccetta and Lockwood.[65] Prompt recovery occurred in three women wool workers affected with an uncomplicated cutaneous form of the disease. In August 1945, the American Medical Association[51] approved the use of penicillin in the treatment of anthrax.

In 1946 Ellingson, Kadull, Bookwalter, and Howe[23] successfully treated twenty-five cases of cutaneous anthrax with 60,000 units of penicillin intramuscularly in each of five doses followed by 30,000 units every three hours, the total dosage being between 1 and 4 million units.

LaBoccetta[54] in 1948 reported thirty-six cases of cutaneous anthrax that were successfully treated with sodium penicillin in doses of 100,000 to 200,000 units daily, administered intramuscularly at three-hour intervals. The treatment was continued until smears and cultures became negative on two successive days.

In 1950 Gold[33] reported the successful treatment of two cases of cutaneous anthrax by oral administration of aureomycin, 500 to 750 mg. every four hours until 11.25 to 19.75 gm. were injected.

Gold and Boger[34] later reported eight cases which were successfully treated with the newer antibiotics—two with aureomycin, four with chloromycetin, and two with terramycin. Organisms disappeared from lesions somewhat more slowly with the use of these three antibiotics than with penicillin. Ingestion of aureomycin produced intense nausea and vomiting in some patients, but chloromycetin and terramycin produced no untoward reaction.

The obvious advantages of oral medication, namely, ease of administration, comparative lack of sensitizing reactions, and ambulatory management, make the newer antibiotics, aureomycin, chloromycetin, and terramycin ideal agents for the treatment of anthrax infection.

In 1955, Gold[35] made a report summarzing his wide experience in treating 117 cases (116 cutaneous and 1 pulmonary) of human anthrax with different types of curative agents between 1933 and 1955. The pulmonary case and the first cutaneous case treated were fatal. The first twenty-one patients were treated with anti-anthrax serum and next fifty-six with sulfonamide compounds. Both were effective but caused reactions.

The remaining forty patients were successfully treated with antibiotics as follows: five with penicillin, seven with chloramphenicol, six with chlortetracycline (aureomycin) fourteen with oxytetracycline (Terramycin) six with tetracycline (achromycin) and two with erythromycin. Gold states that because reactions that occurred with penicillin and chloramphenicol, the last four antibiotics mentioned are the drugs of choice in the treatment of anthrax providing adequate dosage is used. He further pointed out that the control of the spreading edema, with subsidence of systemic toxicity, is the only reliable method with which to measure adequate dosage.

White[113] in 1956 reported 502 cases of cutaneous anthrax in Magadi, Kenya, Africa treated with penicillin with a mortality rate of less than 0.5 per cent. The disease occurred in African natives over a seven year period (1950 to 1956). Treatment of adults consisted of intramuscular procaine penicillin in oil in doses of *300,000* units daily until twenty-four hours after they become afebrile (usually three or four days). Children required heavier dosage.

Lucchesi gives the following criteria for the ideal treatment:
1. It should not harm the patient.
2. It should produce the lowest mortality.
3. It should cause the shortest absence from employment.
4. It should be the least expensive.
5. It should be easily given.

And to this we would add that it should be readily available.

It would seem from the information at present that to meet these requirements, penicillin, the broad-spectrum antibiotics, and neo-arsphenamine would be the agents of choice. Serum is not always readily available, and promptness of treatment is extremely important. It is also costly, and produces more or less severe reactions.

Although sulfathiazole is easily administered by mouth and meets the requirements, it must be administered every three or four hours for perhaps a week.

In recent years specific anti-serum, arsenicals and the sulfonamides have been largely supplanted by penicillin and other antibiotics for human treatment, which also have been found to be highly effective in the treatment of anthrax in livestock.

While treatment with penicillin has been highly successful, some of the newer antibiotics, such as aureomycin, chloromycetin, and terramycin, may prove extremely effective, but too few cases have been reported to permit any definite evaluation at this time.

Regardless of the type of treatment administered the importance of early treatment cannot be overemphasized.

ITEMS OF NOTE

1) Anthrax is primarily a disease of animals.

2) Practically all human infections arise from contact with animals, either direct or remote.

3) Anthrax in man in the United States is primarily an industrial hazard at the present time, but agricultural anthrax is also apparently of increasing importance.

4) The anthrax bacillus in its spore stage is among the most resistant of pathogenic bacteria.

5) The control of anthrax in man depends on the promulgation of educational measures among industrial workers exposed to infection, and the immunization of such workers together with better devices for sterilization of infected hair, hides, and wool; and also upon the control of the disease among domestic animals.

6) For treatment, immune serum, arsenicals, sulfa-drugs, and antibiotics such as penicillin, aureomycin, chloromycetin, and terramycin are now being used, the treatment of choice probably being penicillin.

7) Penicillin and the broad spectrum antibiotics have simplified the once prolonged treatments for cutaneous anthrax and reduced the mortality rate of this serious and often fatal disease to less than one per cent.

8) Promptness of diagnosis and treatment are of even greater importance than type of treatment.

REFERENCES

1. ALMEYEW, H. S.: *Deutsch. Tierärztl., Wchnschr., 44:*375, 1936.
2. ANDREWS, J. B.: United States Department of Labor, Bureau of Labor Statistics Bulletin, *267:*58-98, 1920.
3. ANON: Anthrax and Bone Meal. *J.A.M.A., 314:*Sept. 20, 1958.
4. ANON: Anthrax in Sweden. *Nord. Vet. Med., 641:*Sept. 1957.
5. AUSTRALIA: Diseases of Domestic Animals in Australia. Part 5, Vol. 1 Bacterial Diseases, Dept. of Health, Commonwealth of Australia 1933.
6. BAECKMANN, K.: *Muench. med. Wchnschr., 83:*134-137, 1936.
7. BELL and LEGGE: Cited from ALLBUTT and ROLLESTON's System of Medicine, p. 252, 1906, by ANDREWS, in United States Department of Labor, *Bureau of Labor Statistics Bulletin, 267:*100.
8. BOOR, ALDEN K. and TRESSELT, HUGH B.: *Am. J. Vet. Res., 16:*425-428, July, 1955.
9. BRACHMAN, PHILIP S.: Personal communication May 8, 1960.
10. BRACHMAN, PHILIP S., PLOTKIN, STANLEY A., BUMFORD, FORREST H., ATCHINSON, MARY M., *Am. J. Hyg., 72-*1—July 1960—pp. 6-23.
11. BRAUELL: *Virchows Arch. Path. Anat.,* 132-144, 1857.
12. BRENNAN, A. D. J.: *Vet. Rec., 17:*65 Apr. 25, 1953.
13. CARPENTER, W. M.: *South. M. J.,* 257-274, Feb., 1839.
14. CERNAIANU, C.: *Compt. rend. Soc. biol., 109:*1385-1386, 1932.
15. CHABERT, P.: *Description and Treatment of Charbon in Animals.* Paris, 1780.
16. CRUICKSHANK, J. C.: *Lancet, 2:*681-682, 1939. Quoted by WYATT and EPSTEIN, *Wisconsin Medical Journal,* Feb., 1941.
17a. DAVAINE, C.: *Compt. rend. Acad. sc., 57:*386-387, 1863.
17b. DAVAINE, C.: *Rev. Phot. hop. rend. Acad. sc. Paris, 5:*221-222, 1873.
18. DAVIES, D. G. and HARVEY, R. W. S.: *The Lancet, 11:*880-881, Oct. 24, 1953.
19. DEKOCH, G. W., STERNE, MAX and ROBINSON, E. M.: *J. South African Vet. Med. A., 11:*4, December, 1940.
20. DELAFOND: Cited by ANDREWS, J. B. *United States Bureau of Labor Statistics Bull., 267:*9, 1920.
21. EICHHORN: *U. S. Dept. Agri., Bur. of Animal Ind., Bull., 340:*1916.
22. EICHORN, A. and EDMUNDS, A. L.: *J. Am. Vet. M. A., 58:*278-288, 1920.
23. ELLINGSON, H. V., KADULL, P. J., BOOKWALTER, H. L. and HOWE, C.: *J.A.M.A., 131:*1105-1108, 1946.
24. ELWORTHY, R. R.: *Lancet, 1:*20-23, 1916.
25. *Epedemiological Reports:* Weekly Morbidity Report, Federal Security Agency, Public Health Service; National Office of Vital Statistics, *2:*45, Nov. 12, 1951.
26. EURICH, F. W. and HEWLETT, R. T.: Bacillus anthracis—A system of bacteriology. *Med. Res. Coun. Great Britain, 5:* 1930.
27. EURICH, F. W.: *Brit. M. J., 21:*50-53, 1933. Quoted by Lucchesi et al.
28. EVANS, G. H.: *Elephants and Their Diseases, Rangoon, Burma,* 1910.
29. FLEMING, GEORGE: *Animal Plagues,* Vol. 1. London, Chapman and Hall, 1871 pp 439-522.
30. GERLACH, F.: *Wien. Tierärztl. Monatschr., 10:*481, 1923.
31. GLASSMAN, H. N.: *Pub. Health. Rep.,* 73-1—1958, pp 22-24.
32. GOLD, H.: *Arch. Int. Med., 70:*785, 1942.
33. GOLD, H.: *Am. J. Med., 8:*31-33, 1950.
34. GOLD, H. and BOGER, W. P.: *New England J. Med., 244:*391-394, 1951.
35. GOLD, HERMAN: A. M. A. *Arch. Int. Med., 96:*387-396, Sept. 1955.

36. GOLDMANN, W.: *Zentralbl. Bakt., 136:*345-352 (abt. 1), 1936.

37. GRAHAM-SMITH, G. S.: *J. Hyg., 41:*5, 6, 1941.

38. HANSON, ROBERT P.: *J. Am. Vet. M. A., 135*-9: 463-466, Nov. 1, 1959.

39. HEEREN, RALPH H.: *New Orleans M. & S. J., 99:*545-551, 1947.

40. HENNING, H. W.: *Animal Diseases in South Africa* (2nd edition), 1949.

41. HODGSON, A. E.: *Lancet, 11:*5, July, 1944.

42. HOFFMANN, R.: *Centralbl. Bakt., 113:*541-543 (abt. 1), 1929.

43. HOLTZMANN, F.: *Med. Welt., 9:*671-674, 1935.

44. HEUSINGER, C. F.: *Anthrax: The Disease in Animals and Men.* Erlangen, Enke, 1850.

45. Investigation of the Shaving Brush Industry, with Special Reference to Anthrax. *United States Public Health Report, 34:*994-995, 1919.

46. JACKSON, F. C., WRIGHT, GEORGE G. and ARMSTRONG, JAMES: *Am. J. Vet. Res., 18:*771-777, Oct. 1957.

47. JAMIESON, W. M. and GREEN, D. M.: *The Lancet, XI:*560, 1955: No. 6863 Vol. CCLXVII 521-574.

48. JEAN, G.: *J. urol., Paris, 28:*101-103, 1929.

49. Joint Order No. 2, U. S. Dept. Treas. and Dept. Agri., Jan., 1918.

50. KAPLAN, MARTIN M.: Proceedings of the Symposium on Anthrax in Man. Philadelphia, Pennsylvania, October 8, 1954, pp. 4-12.

51. KEEFER, CHESTER S. *et al.: J.A.M.A.,* 1162, Aug. 18, 1945.

52. KOCH, ROBERT: *Beitr. Morphol. Biol. Pflanzen, 2:*303, 1876.

53. KRYUCHKOV, I. I.: *Vet. Moscow, 30:* No. 6, 1953.

54. LaBOCCETTA, A. C.: *A.J.M. Sc., 216:*407-410, 1948.

55. LEGGE, SIR T. M.: *Industrial Maladies.* London, Oxford, 1934, p. 234.

56. LUCCHESI, P. F. *et al.: The Treatment of Anthrax.* Symposium on Anthrax. Bur. of Industr. Hyg., Pa. Dept. of Health, Apr. 1, 1941, pp. 29-33.

57. MacDONALD, I. G.: *J. Indust. Hyg. & Toxicol., 18:*357-362, 1936.

58. MAY, H. B. and BUCH, S. C.: *Lancet, 2:*685-686, 1939. Quoted by WYATT and EPSTEIN, *Wisconsin M. J.,* Feb., 1941.

59. McCULLOUGH, E. C.: *Disinfection and Sterilization.* Effect of Temperature upon Microbial Life. Philadelphia, Lea, 1936, p. 121.

60. McCOWEN, G. R. and PARKER, H. B.: *J. Roy. Nav. M. Serv., 18:*278-280, 1932.

61. McKITTERICK, J. C. and PEARSON, G. J.: *Am. J. Dis. Child., 38:*1250-1255, 1929.

62. MESHTSCHANINOFF: Cited by GAY "Agents of Disease and Host Resistance," Springfield, Thomas, 1935. Quoted in.[56]

63. MITCHELL, WM.: Anthrax and fatalism. *Brit. M. J.,* 751-752, 1911.

64. Morbidity and Mortality Reports U. S. Dept. of Health Education and Welfare— Supplement 193-1945; Supplement 206-1948; Reprint 2943—June 24, 1949; Reprint 3020, May 12, 1950; Reprint 3087, May 25, 1951; Supplement 1-54 Oct. 1953; Supplement 2-52 Jan. 1954; Supplement 2-53 Sept. 1954; Supplement 3-52 Jan. 1955; Supplement 8-53 Sept. 16, 1960; Report 9-52 Jan. 6, 1961; 2.

65. MURPHY, T. D., LaBOCCETTA, A. C. and LOCKWOOD, J. S.: *J.A.M.A., 126:*948-950, 1944.

66. MURRAY, T. J.: *J. Infect. Dis., 48:*457-467, 1931.

67. NATIN, I.: *Semana méd., 1:*1332; *2:*314, 1931.

68. NEWS NOTE: *J.A.M.A., 83:*538, 1924.

69. OSBORN, S. H.: *Am. J. Pub. Health, 10:*657-665, 1920.

70. PAGNINI, U.: *Gior. batteriol. e immunol., 16:*876-885, 1936.

71. PASTEUR, L.: *Compt. rend, Acad. sc., 91:*86, 455 & 677, 1880.

72. PAWAN, J. L.: *J. Trop. Med., 38:*170, 1935. Abstr. in *Arch. Dermat. & Syph., 33:*890, 1936.
73. PENNOCK, C. W.: *Am. J. M. Sc., 19:*13-25, 1836.
74. PIJPER, ADRIANUS: *Lancet, 210:*88, 1926. Quoted by Lucchesi.
75. POLLENDER: *Vierteljschr. f. gerichtl. Med., 8:*103-114, 1855.
76. PONDER, C. W.: *Wien. klin. Wchnschr., 24:*735-736, 1911.
77. *Prevention of Anthrax Among Industrial Workers.* Memorandum on the Disinfecting Station Established in Great Britain for Disinfection of Wool and Hair, 1921. H. M. Stationery Office, London.
78. RAYER, M.: *Compt. rend. Soc. biol.,* 141-143, 1850.
79. ROBERTSON, W.: *J. Comp. Path. & Therap., 21:*361, 1908.
80. ROBERTSON, M. E.: *J. Hyg., 32:*367-374, 1932.
81. SCHLINGMAN, A. S., DEVLIN, H. B., WRIGHT, G. G., MAINE, R. J., and MANNENY, MARY C.: *Am. J. Vet. Res., 17:*256-261, April 1956.
82. SCHRACK, W. D.: Proceedings of the Symposium on Anthrax in Man. Philadelphia, Pennsylvania, Oct. 8, 1954, pp 20-24.
83. SCHATTENFROH: *Wien. klin. Wchnschr., 24:*735-736, 1911.
84. SCLAVO, A.: *Centralbl. Bakt., 18:*744-745 (abt. 1), 1895.
85. SCLAVO, A.: *Riv. Igiene Sanit., 14:*519, 1903.
86. SEIDEMAN, R. M. and WHEELER, K. M.: *J.A.M.A., 135:*837-838, 1947.
87. SINDERSON, H. C.: *Brit. M. J., 1:*612, 1933.
88. SMITH, J. M. P. and GOODSPEED, E. J.: *The Complete Bible.* Chicago, Univ. Chicago Press, *Exodus, 9:*3.
89. SMYTH, HENRY FIELD: *Am. J. Hyg., 1:*541-555, 1921.
90. SMYTH, HENRY FIELD: A 20-year survey of anthrax in the United States: Sixth report of the Committee on Anthrax, Industrial Hygiene Section, American Public Health Association, 1939.
91. SMYTH, HENRY FIELD: *Am. J. Pub. Health,* Aug., 1945.
92. SOLOWIEFF, N.: *Arch. Hyg., 104:*132-143, Abst. in *J.A.M.A., 95:*1950, 1930.
93. SOMERS, F.: *Vet. Rec., 1181:*543, 1911.
94. STEIN, C. D.: Anthrax. *Yearbook of Agriculture,* 250-262, 1942.
95. STEIN, C. D.: *Vet. Med., 38:*4, 1943.
96. STEIN, C. D.: *J. Vet. Res., 14:*38-54, 1944.
97. STEIN, C. D.: *Vet. Med., 40:*10, 340-349, 1945.
98. STEIN, C. D.: Anthrax in animals and its relationship to the disease in man. *Annals. New York Acad. Sc., 48:*507-534, April 10, 1947.
99. STEIN, C. D.: *Vet. Med., 42:* January, 1947.
100. STEIN, C. D.: *Vet. Med., 43:*463, 1948.
101. STEIN, C. D.: *Vet. Med., 45:*5, May, 1950.
102. STEIN, C. D. and STONER, M. G.: *Vet. Med., 47:*8, 1952.
103. STEIN, C. D. and STONER, M. G.: *Vet. Med., 48:*7, 1953.
104. STEIN, C. D. and VAN NESS, G. B.: *Vet. Med., 50:*11, 1955.
105. STEIN, C. D. and VAN NESS, G. B.: *Vet. Med., 51:*11, 1956.
106. STERNE, M.: Avirulent Anthrax Vaccine Onderstepoort, *J. Vet. Sc. & Animal Ind., 21:*1, March, 1946.
107. THEILER, A.: *Agr. Jour. of Union of So. Africa, 4:*370, 1912.
108. TOUSSAINT, H.: Quoted by M. BOULEY in "Anti-anthrax Vaccination," *Bull. Acad. Med., Paris, 45:*792, 1880.
109. UBERTINI, B.: *La Clinica Veterinaria, 62:*72, 1939.
110. UMENO, S. and NOBATA, R.: *Soc. Vet. Sci. J., 17:*221-223, 1938. (In Japanese. English abstract p. 87.)

111. VACCAREZZA, R. F.: *Semana méd., 1:*1481-1483, 1931.
112. VALLERY-RADOT, R.: *The Life of Pasteur.* New York, Doubleday Page, 1916.
113. WHITE, T. H.: *British M. J.,* No. 5004, Dec. 1, 1956 (correspondence) 1300.
114. WOLFF, A. H. and HEIMANN, H.: *Am. J. Hyg., 53:*1, 1951.
115. WRIGHT, G. G., HEEDBURG, M. A., and SLEIN, J. B.: *J. Immunol., 72:*263, 1954.
116. WRIGHT, GEORGE G. and WEDUM, A. G.: Proceedings of the Symposium on Anthrax in Man. Philadelphia, Pennsylvania, October 8, 1954, pp. 136-144.
117. ZINSSER and BAYNE-JONES: *Textbook of Bacteriology.* New York, Appleton, 137, 1934, p. 689.

Chapter 3

BRUCELLOSIS

CHARLES M. CARPENTER, D.V.M., PH.D., M.D.
WILLIAM T. HUBBERT, D.V.M., M.P.H.

BRUCELLOSIS is primarily a disease of domestic animals which, under special circumstances, may be readily transmitted to man. The disease is named in honor of Sir David Bruce, discoverer of *Brucella melitensis,* one of the three species of *Brucella.* Brucellosis is a worldwide disease but is most prevalent in areas in which extensive cattle, swine, and goat herding is practiced. It causes serious economic loss to the animal industry and extensive morbidity in man, thus constituting an important public health problem.

Brucellosis is manifested in many forms in animals and in man. It cattle, abortion is the most frequently observed symptom and accounts for the designation of the disease as infectious abortion. In swine, in addition to abortion, arthritis is a frequent sequella. Man, on the other hand, usually experiences a febrile illness, long known as undulant fever.

Three species of the genus *Brucella* are recognized: *Brucella abortus,* of bovine origin: *Brucella suis,* of swine; and *Brucella melitensis,* of caprine sources. Two additional organisms which have been tentatively classified as members of the genus *Brucella: Brucella ovis,* a cause of genital disease among sheep;[1] and *Brucella neotomae,* recovered from the desert wood rat, *Neotoma lepida.*[2]

The relationship of the disease in animals to human infection was not well understood until comparatively recently. Although Zammit, a member of the British Mediterranean Fever Commission, discovered in 1905 that man acquired Malta fever from drinking infected goat's milk, human infection from other domestic animals was not demonstrated until after Evans in 1918[3] pointed out that *"Micrococcus melitensis"* described by Bruce and *"Bacillus abortus"* isolated by Bang were morphologically and antigenically similar and should be classified in a single genus now designated *Brucella*. The summation of the present knowledge of brucellosis is an outstanding example of the cooperative effort of the veterinarian, the physician, and the public health worker, which was required to unravel the intricate epidemiology of the disease.

Prior to the use of the all inclusive term "brucellosis," the various syndromes in animals and in man were known by many names. In cattle, infectious abortion is referred to as "Bang's disease," "contagious abortion" and "slinking of the calf." In man, Malta fever, Mediterranean fever, intermittent fever and goat fever are often used synonomously for undulant fever.

HISTORY

Bang's Disease and Undulant Fever. Abortion in animals, particularly in cattle, swine, sheep, and goats, has long been a scourge of husbandmen. Before the era of scientific medicine, a variety of noninfectious causes were held responsible for the premature expulsion of fetuses. In the great cattle raising areas of Central Europe, however, where abortion was rampant, the disease was considered to be infectious even in the 16th century. In 1876, Franck[4] demonstrated that the disease could be reproduced in normal pregnant cows by introducing into the genital canal of normal pregnant cows, uterine discharges and fetal membranes from diseased animals. The specific cause, however, remained for Bang[5] to discover twenty years later. He isolated *Bacillus abortus* from the placenta of aborting cattle and reproduced the disease with pure cultures for the first time, thereby proving that the disease was caused by an infectious agent.

Undoubtedly, Bang's disease was introduced into the Eastern United States with the early importation of cattle from Europe. McNeal and Kerr first described the disease in this country in 1910.[6] In the following two years, 1911 and 1912, Schroeder and Cotton,[7] and Smith and Fabyan,[8] respectively, reported the isolation of Bang's bacillus from cow's milk. As happens so often in science their findings were fortuitous. In searching for the tubercle bacillus in cow's milk the inoculation of guinea pigs revealed a tuberculosis-like disease from which no acid-fast bacilli could be demonstrated. The causative agent was finally identified as *Br. abortus*.

Although farmers throughout the world were suffering serious losses from abortion in cattle and swine little thought had been given to its possible public health significance. The isolation of *Br. abortus* from cow's milk suggested a possible relationship to human disease. Mohler and Traum[9] in 1911 searched for human infections. They tested the blood of forty-two individuals for specific agglutinins for *Br. abortus* and inoculated guinea pigs with suspensions of tissues prepared from adenoids and tonsils of fifty-six children. All of the guinea pigs were normal at autopsy, with the exception of one inoculated with tonsil tissue from which *Br. abortus* was isolated. Thus, this was the first instance in which the organism was isolated from a human source. Although Mohler and Traum failed to find agglutinins for *Br. abortus* in human blood, two years later, 1913, Larson and Sedgwick[10] demonstrated specific agglutinins and complement-fixing bodies in the blood of seventy-three of 425 children. In 1915, they further reported that the blood tests on the children who drank milk from a herd of cattle free from Bang's disease were negative, whereas the children with agglutinins for *Br. abortus* had been drinking mixed market milk. In 1916, Cooledge[11] detected agglutinins in the blood of three of six adults who had drunk raw milk, and in one of four persons who had consumed only pasteurized milk but failed to find them in the blood of four other individuals who said they were not milk drinkers. Another significant discovery in this same period was that of Traum[12] who, in 1914, detected a third species of *Brucella* in fetuses from aborting swine. Thus, *Br. suis* was isolated and destined to become an important human pathogen.

Malta Fever—Man and Goats. In the Mediterranean littoral and particularly on the Island of Malta in the Mediterranean Sea, an investigation was being carried out to determine the circumstances under which man acquired Malta fever from drinking goat's milk. The disease had become a serious disability among the Royal Military and Naval Forces in the area. In 1887, approximately ten years prior to Bang and Stribolt's discovery of *Br. abortus,* Sir David Bruce[13] had isolated *Micrococcus melitensis* from the spleen of a patient who had died from the prevailing febrile illness designated Malta fever. In 1904, the British Mediterranean Fever Commission, with Sir David Bruce as Chairman, was appointed to inquire into the disease. The investigation led to Zammit's, a member of the Commission, fruitful discovery that the source of Malta fever was goat's milk. The observation was outstanding and one of the most significant advances in the epidemiology of brucellosis.. Zammit also demonstrated specific agglutinins for the organism in goat's milk and first used the agglutination test to detect animals discharging Brucella in milk.

In the same year of Zammit's discovery, an interesting incident took place in the United States. The Bureau of Animal Industry of the United States Department of Agriculture commissioned one of its employees, Mr. Thompson, to purchase milch goats in Malta. On August 19, 1905, sixty-one female and four male goats were shipped on the SS Joshua Nicholson to Antwerp, Belgium, and from there aboard the SS St. Andrew to the United States. Eight of twelve crewmen who drank the unboiled goat's milk while on the Joshua Nicholson developed Malta fever. On arrival in the United States, the goats were condemned and quarantined in Athenia, New Jersey. Prior to their slaughter, a woman who drank some of the raw milk likewise acquired the disease.

Another unrelated focus of goat infection was detected in Southwestern United States in 1911 at about the same time Bang's disease was discovered in the Eastern United States. Gentry and Ferenbaugh[14] observed cases of Malta fever in Texas and traced them to goat's milk. Evidently, the disease had prevailed along the Mexican border for many years and Mexican goat herders were already boiling the milk because they believed that goat fever or Rio Grande fever—their designation for Malta fever, was acquired from drinking raw goat's milk.

Recognition of Relationship of Infectious Agents to Disease Entities. The next striking observation in the disease complex was that of Evans[3] in 1918, approximately two decades after the discovery of *Br. abortus*. By special bacteriologic and serologic studies she demonstrated that *"M. melitensis"* and *"B. abortus"* were very closely related morphologically and antigenically, and proposed that the two species be classified in the genus *Bacterium*. Her studies set the stage which led to the clarification of the host-range and host-parasite relationships of the heretofore supposedly two unrelated bacterial species. Because the cocco-bacillary forms of certain strains of *Br. melitensis* resemble cocci, present day bacteriologists who are students of the *Brucella* readily understand why Bruce originally described the organism as a "micrococcus." The circumstances which led to the comparative study of the two organisms is interesting. Evans in 1917 was engaged in a study of the bacterial flora of cow's milk in the Dairy Division of the U. S. Department of Agriculture. In discussing the presence of *Br. abortus* in milk with Dr. Adolph Eichhorn, then Chief of the Pathology Division of the Bureau of Animal Industry, he suggested that a comparative study be made of "*B. abortus*" and "*M. melitensis*" because of their occurrence in the mammary gland. Evans carried out her classic work which bridged another important gap between veterinary and human medicine. Her work renewed interest in the possibility that *Br. abortus,* the cause of infectious abortion in cattle, might be pathogenic for man as was the presence of *Br. melitensis* in goat's milk.

Not until 1924, was another strain of the "abortus" type isolated from man. Keefer[15] recovered the organism from the blood of a patient with undulant fever, which later was determined to be *Br. suis.* The patient was a technician who on occasions had collected porcine fetuses from an abattoir in Baltimore, which explained the source of infection.

In the following year, 1925, Carpenter[16] made blood cultures from a group of students at Cornell University, Ithaca, New York, who were suffering from fevers of undetermined origin. The symptoms varied somewhat in character but a persistent or recurrent fever was the chief complaint. The symptoms in a few were suggestive of mild typhoid fever but no corroborative laboratory evidence could be adduced, and therefore, the illnesses were often referred to as paratyphoid fever. A series of blood cultures from two of the patients finally revealed *Br. abortus.* Subsequently, seventeen cases of undulant fever were detected. Intravenous inoculation of several of the cultures into pregnant heifers produced abortion.

An epidemiologic study by Carpenter and Baker[17] indicated the source of the infection to be an infected supply of raw milk from a herd of pure bred cattle owned by one of the distinguished professors in the New York State College of Agriculture. Guinea-pigs inoculated daily for thirty days with mixed milk from the herd showed extensive infection with the Bang's bacillus. Thus. *Br. abortus* was isolated from the blood of patients known to have drunk raw milk proven to be contaminated with the organism. Furthermore, proof was adduced by producing abortion in cattle with cultures isolated from the blood of patients with undulant fever, and subsequently recovering the organism from the placentas and fetuses of the experimental animals. Thus, the evidence was complete that *Br. abortus* in cow's milk produced undulant fever in man.

With definite proof that undulant fever could result from drinking unpasteurized milk containing *Br. abortus,* physicians throughout the United States and in foreign countries searched for and reported cases of undulant fever. Early reports were made by Huddleson,[18] Moore and Carpenter,[19] Evans,[20] Gage and Gregory,[21] Knowlton,[22] and by Hull and Black.[23] It was soon evident that sources of infection other than milk and dairy products were responsible for human infection. Man may acquire the disease from contact with infected animals or with meat from diseased animals, especially swine.

In addition to infection resulting from direct contact with or ingestion of infected animal tissues, recent investigation has firmly established the importance of aerosols in the transmission of *Brucella* to man in an abbatoir. In an Iowa swine abattoir outbreak involving 128 cases, *Br. suis* was isolated from the air.[24] Variations in the attack rate among employees further supported the airborne hypothesis.

Extensive investigations on laboratory methods of diagnosis, prevention, and treatment in man and animals have been made. The relevant reports will be reviewed under those sections. The above historical survey points out that brucellosis is not only one of the most serious diseases of animals but is as yet an important disease of man.

ETIOLOGIC AGENTS

Three closely related species of the genus *Brucella* are recognized as causing brucellosis; *Br. abortus, Br. melitensis,* and *Br. suis.* No known human cases have been reported due to either *Br. ovis* or *Br. neotomae.* The generic name was proposed by Meyer and Shaw in 1920 and has been accepted by the Society of American Microbiologists. The changing and confusing nomenclature of the former two species since their discovery is set forth in Table 18.

The difficulties encountered by the bacteriologist in studying *Brucella* have been concerned with isolation, varying morphology, differentiation and classification of strains isolated from human and animal sources. The changing morphology of the *Brucella,* however, is better understood as a result of extensive studies of bacterial dissociation. Variation among bacteria is now expected when formerly it was only suspected. Outstanding work on colonial dissociation of *Brucella* was carried out by Henry,[25] in 1933 who observed several factors which brought it about. Smooth ("S") and rough ("R") types are rather well defined, but as in the case of many bacterial species intermediate colonial types appear during dissociation.

TABLE 18

NOMENCLATURE OF *Brucella* ORGANISMS

Brucella Abortus	*Brucella Melitensis*
Bacillus abortus, 1897—Bang	*Micrococcus melitensis*, 1887—Bruce
Corynebacterium abortus, 1903—Preisz	*Bacillus melitensis*, 1912—Jordan
Bacterium abortus, 1918—Society of American Bacteriologists	*Bacterium melitensis*, 1918—Society of American Bacteriologists
Alcaligenes abortus, 1919—Castellani and Chalmers	*Alcaligenes melitensis*, 1919—Castellani and Chalmers
Brucella abortus, 1920—Meyer and Shaw	*Brucella melitenesis*, 1920—Meyer and Shaw

The typical virulent smooth strain is a Gram-negative, nonmotile, short rod or coccobacillus varying from 0.3 to 0.6μ in width and from 0.5 to 1.0μ in length. Most stock cultures of *Brucella* can be maintained on standard laboratory media. Isolation, however, is not always easily accomplished. *Br. suis* and *Br. melitensis* are more readily cultivated than *Br. abortus,* many strains of which require an atmosphere of from 10 to 20-per cent CO_2. Inasmuch as the species of *Brucella* to be isolated cannot be predicted, an enriched medium and an increased carbon dioxide tension should always be employed. Better results are obtained when several suitable media, such as chocolate or blood agar, trypticase soy agar and Albimi's *Brucella* agar are inoculated. In the case of blood cultures or clots embryonated eggs or an enriched broth may be used. Castaneda[26] recommends the combined use of agar and broth in a small bottle or flask in which a few milliliters of broth are layered over the lower segment of the agar slant. Cultures should be incubated at from 35 to 36° C. and not discarded as negative until after at least two weeks' incubation.

Identification of *Brucella* may be made tentatively on the appearance of the smooth type of colony which is usually small, convex, moist, and glistening. It has a grayish-blue opal-like appearance, is not sticky and does not adhere firmly to the medium. The colony gradually becomes larger and after a week or ten days is more opaque and acquires a light brown color, particularly the center which is elevated. Confirmation is dependent upon agglutination of the organism by a specific *Brucella* antiserum.[2]

TABLE 19

BIOCHEMICAL REACTIONS DIFFERENTIATING THE SPECIES OF *Brucella*

Species	Type#	Dye Concentration (μg)			H_2S Production	Urease Production
		Basic Fuchsin (10)	Thionin (10)	(50)		
Br. abortus	I	+	−	−	++	(+, ++)
	II	−	−	−	++	
	III	+	+	−	−, +, ++	
Br. melitensis	I	+	+	−	−	(+, to ++++)
Br. suis	I	−	+	+	++++	(++++)
	II	−	+	+	−	
	III	+	+	+	−	

10μg/ml $= 1:100,000; +$, or $−$ denotes presence or absence of growth in dye medium, degree of blackening from H_2S, or rapidity of urease reaction. #Meyer and Cameron described the following types within the three species based on dye inhibition and H_2S production.[27] (Type I is considered to be typical of the species.)

The World Health Organization Expert Committee on Brucellosis (1953) recommends the following procedures for identification of *Brucella* species:[28]

1. Use of mono-specific *Brucella* antisera, if available.
2. Addition of CO_2 for initial isolation of *Br. abortus*.
3. Observe hydrogen sulfide (H_2S) production.
4. Dye inhibition tests, particularly basic fuchsin and thionin.
5. Determine urease production.

Brucella ovis and *Br. neotomae* have the following characteristics:

Br. ovis[29]

Antigenically distinct from other *Brucella* species, requires 10% CO_2 for initial isolation, uninhibited by basic fuchsin (10 μg.) or thionin (10 μg.) inhibited by methyl violet (10 μg.), H_2S production − or +, and urease negative.

Br. neotomae[2,40]

Antigenically indistinguishable from *Br. abortus,* inhibited by both basic fuchsin (10 μg.) and thionin (10 μg.), H_2S production ++++, young S colonies examined by the method of Henry (1933) produce bright orange color, and does not require CO_2 on initial isolation.

Rough and mucoid types may be differentiated from smooth types by the acriflavine test of Braun and Bonestell[30] and by the 2, 3, 5,-triphenyl tetrazolium chloride test of Huddleson and Baltzer.[31] Examination of colonies under obliquely-transmitted light affords a dependable method for distinguishing smooth from non-smooth cultures.[25] Stinebring and Braun, working with an anti-*Br. abortus* bacteriophage prepared in a Russian laboratory at Rostov on the Don, reported the phage showed specific lytic activity against smooth and intermediate strains of *Br. abortus* including strain 19.[32]

Meyer and Cameron[27] determined a pattern of oxidative reactions employing standard manometric techniques for a number of strains representing the *Brucella* species when grown in either a variety of amino acid or carbohydrate substrates. The method is useful in the classification of members of the genus *Brucella*. Utilizing this finding they consider *Br. neotomae* to be transitional between the three recognized species of *Brucella*, it resembles *Br. suis* in carbohydrate utilization, CO_2 requirements, and H_2S production, and *Br. abortus* and *Br. melitensis* in amino acid utilization.[27] They believe *Br. ovis* should not be included in the genus *Brucella* because of differences observed in oxidative metabolism and in serologic reactions.[33]

Antigenic studies indicate that *Brucella* have two antigenic factors; namely "melitensis" and "abortus-suis." Many antigenically-related subtypes have been reported among the smooth types in addition to several recognized variants. Their differentiation requires the use of specially adsorbed antisera. Although variants have been primarily of academic interest, their role in the epidemiology of brucellosis and in the pathogenesis of the disease is currently being investigated with renewed interest. Studies by Olitzki and Sulitzeanu[34] utilizing "agar gel" precipitation indicate the presence of a number of common precipitin antigens among the *Brucellae,* and in addition they were able to demonstrate a precipitin arc distinct for *Br. abortus* strain 19. Their work indicated no correlation between the soluble precipitin antigens and the insoluble agglutinating antigens, the latter apparently being contained within the cell wall. Carrere, Roux, and Serre[35] prepared gluco-lipido-polypeptide (GLP) antigens from the three species and observed two antigenic types based on formation of precipitin arcs, "abortus" *(Br. abortus* and *Br. melitensis)* and "suis" *(Br. suis* only). Phillips, Braun, and Plescia[36] prepared material rich in DNA from *Br. abor-*

tus which produced five diffusion arcs. One arc produced a strong positive Feulgen reaction indicating DNA in the precipitate.

EPIDEMIOLOGY

The epidemiology of brucellosis presents one of the most fascinating chapters in medical annals. The *Brucella* enjoy an extensive host range including man, cattle, horses, mules, swine, goats, sheep, cats, dogs and chickens. Brucella have also been recovered from a number of wildlife species, including deer, buffalo, European hares, jack rabbits, and the desert wood rat. Thus, a vast animal reservoir of infection is available to infect man. Experimentally, the disease may be transmitted to monkeys, rabbits, guinea pigs, rats, hamsters, mice, and chickens.

Brucellosis in man and animals may be caused by any one of the three species of *Brucella*. In general, however, *Br. abortus* is predominant in cattle, *Br. suis* in swine, and *Br. melitensis* in goats and sheep. Bovine brucellosis is most prevalent in the dairy industry in which large herds of cows are in close contact. The disease occurs among beef cattle, but the nature of the industry, namely, grazing over wide areas, castration of males, and annual slaughtering of large numbers of animals tend to control natural spread of the infection. Cows may become infected with *Br. suis* or *Br. melitensis* from contact with hogs and goats, respectively. Horses are more susceptible to infection with either *Br. melitenis* or *Br. abortus*. Although swine may become infected with all three species they are most susceptible to *Br. suis*. Chickens likewise are susceptible to each species.

There is emerging evidence that wildlife play a significant role in the epidemiology of brucellosis. Bendtsen, Christiansen, and Thomsen[37,38] have incriminated the hare as an important reservoir of *Br. suis* infection for swine in Denmark. A strain of *Br. suis* similar to that isolated from Danish hares was recovered in blood cultures from an Alaskan Eskimo girl who apparently was infected from ingesting raw caribou bone marrow.[39] In addition a strain of *Br. suis* has been isolated from a tissue pool prepared from jack rabbits *(Lepus californicus)* in Utah.[40] *Br. neotomae,* isolated from the desert wood rat, has been shown experimentally to produce an inapparent infection in young swine, with no gross lesions evident at autopsy.[41] Further ecologic investigation of the disease in wildlife will elucidate their role both in transmission of *Brucella* infection to man and as reservoirs of infection for domestic animals which may complicate eradication.

Geographic Prevalence. Brucellosis is practically worldwide and prevails wherever domestic animals and man cohabit. The United States, British Isles, Central Europe, South Africa, Mexico, Canada, and Northern Japan are the areas of greatest bovine infection with *Br. abortus.*

Brucellosis due to *Br. melitensis* is confined chiefly to the countries in which goat raising is extensively practiced. The caprine type of the disease thrives in a subtropical climate usually where the standards of living are low and poor sanitation exists. The infection is endemic in Southern Europe south of the 46° latitude, particularly in the Mediterranean littoral. It prevails in certain parts of Russia, South America, North Africa, Persia, Central America, Mexico, and in the Southwestern United States. *Br. melitensis* has been reported in several other areas in the United States. Carpenter and Boak[42] reported it in New York State in 1934. It was isolated from milk from a dairy in contact with goats. In 1945, Stiles[43] reported goat milk cheese as a source of human infection in Colorado, and in 1946 Jordan and Borts[44] reported human cases resulting from melitensis infection in swine in Iowa. Sheep and horses in contact with infected goats acquire infection with *Br. melitensis.*

Brucellosis in swine has been recognized in Central Europe. In the United States it is endemic in the great Midwestern swine-raising states and on the West Coast. Human infection is widespread, and its epidemicity depends upon the prevalence of the disease in animals and the customs of the people in those areas. The pattern of human infection is set by that of the animal reservoir in a particular environment.

Seasonal Prevalence. The seasonal prevalence of abortion in cattle occurs at that time of the year when the majority of cows are pregnant. The husbandman is impressed with the slinking of the calf which, in many areas, is predominant in the spring and early summer months. Undoubtedly, the same is true in porcine brucellosis. Many infections are acquired as the result of cows grazing in pastures contaminated with infected exudates from abortion. The same is true of hogs in feeding lots. Observers often fail to recognize that most animals remain infected for many, many months. Thus, the chronicity and latency of the disease, in addition to the lack of dependable methods for detecting the infection, make epidemiologic studies difficult.

More human cases of brucellosis are reported in the summer months than at any other season of the year, which indicates that the typical acute form of the disease is recognized most often during this season. This may be due to vacationers consuming unpasteurized milk in rural areas. Malta fever, however, is four times more prevalent in summer than in winter.

Incidence. The incidence of brucellosis in man and animals is not accurately known. Not all states require physicians to report cases of undulant fever, and veterinarians do not report cases of infectious abortion to public health authorities. Many farmers make every effort to conceal abortion in their animals. Thus, the reported cases of the disease fail to provide accurate information concerning the prevalence of brucellosis.

Most surveys for the incidence of the disease in man and animals have been carried out by means of the agglutination test which is the simplest and most economic procedure, particularly among animals. Such data provide only a general index to the incidence of the infection in our animal and human populations. Many cases are not detected because of vagaries in the agglutination test and because of absence of agglutinins or detection of only a few agglutinins—"low titres"—in an infected host. Skin tests for dermal sensitivity, particularly in man, are more specific than serologic tests. Early in the course of the disease neither test is positive, however.

From 1935 to 1961, inclusive, data on the prevalence of Bang's disease among 230,618,972 cattle in the United States have been obtained by the Agricultural Research Service of the U.S. Department of Agriculture. In 1935, the agglutination test detected a total of 381,010 reactors, or 11.5 per cent of 3,317,760 cattle. In 1961, however, only 139,894 cattle, or 1.0 per cent of 13,418,657 animals tested reacted positively to the test, showing a marked decrease in the incidence of bovine brucellosis during the past twenty-seven years (Table 20).

In Western New York State, data obtained from agglutination tests in both man and cattle for a period of seven years, 1935-1941, indicated that as an average the ratio of human to bovine reactors

TABLE 20

RESULTS OF AGGLUTINATION TESTS FOR BRUCELLOSIS IN CATTLE IN THE UNITED STATES, 1935-1961

(U. S. DEPARTMENT OF AGRICULTURE FIGURES)

Year (Ending June 30)	Cattle Tested	Reactors Number	%
1935	3,317,760	381,010	11.5
1936	6,674,709	457,104	6.8
1937	8,021,167	397,864	5.0
1938	7,837,443	324,532	4.1
1939	7,591,398	219,165	2.9
1940	6,937,428	171,953	2.5
1941	7,465,254	182,075	2.4
1942	6,891,219	209,238	3.0
1943	5,185,228	196,329	3.8
1944	5,235,912	226,079	4.3
1945	5,213,458	243,050	4.7
1946	4,876,866	245,786	5.0
1947	5,133,814	232,293	4.5
1948	5,434,792	232,199	4.3
1949	5,671,347	226,691	4.0
1950	5,974,721	208,298	3.5
1951	5,640,836	172,322	3.1
1952	7,491,327	314,260	4.2
1953	7,860,870	268,348	3.4
1954	9,002,109	235,660	2.6
1955	14,186,241	365,247	2.6
1956	16,754,195	366,524	2.2
1957	15,913,396	280,253	1.8
1958	16,251,440	260,322	1.6
1959	14,168,909	214,331	1.5
1960	12,468,476	147,805	1.2
1961	13,418,657	139,894	1.0
TOTALS	230,618,972	6,919,638	3.0

approximated 1:25. The data on man were obtained in the Health Bureau Laboratory of the City of Rochester, New York, in which agglutination tests were carried out routinely on all samples of blood submitted for serologic tests for syphilis. Thus, the specimens do not represent an unselected sampling of the population. In 1935, 127, or 0.32 per cent, of 39,374 human blood tests were positive. In 1941, only 33, or 0.13 per cent, reactions were discovered among 25,204 patients. A similar decline in reactors was noted in blood tests on cattle in New York State. In 1935, 4,777, or 9.1 per cent, of 52,490 were positive and in 1941, only 4,245, or 2.6 per cent, of 163,279 cows tested reacted to the agglutination test (Table 21).

The incidence of the disease in man is difficult to determine because of the lack of agreement concerning an agglutinin titre diagnostic of brucellosis and the marked variation in results of serologic

TABLE 21

COMPARISON OF RESULTS OF AGGLUTINATION TESTS FOR BRUCELLOSIS ON
HUMAN AND BOVINE SERA IN NEW YORK STATE

Year	Human*		Bovine	
	Tests No.	Positive Per Cent	Tests No.	Positive Per Cent
1934	35,484	0.48		
1935	39,374	0.32	52,490	9.1
1936	45,381	0.21	83,714	5.9
1937	51,510	0.09	105,267	7.2
1938	47,883	0.26	107,579	6.7
1939	62,712	0.14	144,121	3.6
1940	58,620	0.12	172,232	3.0
1941	25,204	0.13	163,279	2.6
Total	366,168	0.218	828,628	5.44

*Data obtained from individuals in Western New York on whom blood was obtained for a serologic test for syphilis.

TABLE 22

RESULTS OF AGGLUTINATION TESTS FOR BRUCELLOSIS IN SWINE IN THE UNITED STATES, 1953-1961

Year	Swine Tested	Reactors Numbers	%
1953	47,792	1,068	2.2
1954	71,974	3,264	4.5
1955	116,416	3,544	3.0
1956	123,657	3,850	3.1
1957	124,737	3,813	3.1
1958	137,805	2,320	1.7
1959	171,503	2,612	1.5
1960	170,406	2,302	1.4
1961	177,379	1,902	1.1
TOTALS	1,141,669	24,675	2.2

tests obtained in different laboratories. Carpenter, Boak and Chapman,[45] McAlpine and Mickle,[46] Hardy,[47] and Hardenbergh[48] have, by means of the agglutination test, reported positive results that range from 0.6 to 7.0 per cent. The total annual number of reported cases of brucellosis in the United States increased steadily from twenty-four in 1925 to a peak of 6,321 in 1947. Since 1947, there has been a rapid decline with only 742 cases reported in 1960. Unreported cases occur, however. The disease is more prevalent among males than females, the ratio being approximately 3:1. Males are undoubtedly exposed to the infection more frequently than females. More cases of undulant fever occur among young, adult males from twenty to forty years than from any other age group. Veterinarians and dairy husbandmen who come in contact with infected animals experience the infection most frequently. Many cases are detected among employees in abattoirs and in the meat packing industry who handle uncooked meat. Laboratory personnel who work with cultures of *Brucella,* with infected experimental animals and other animal tissues often acquire the disease. Another large percentage of the cases of brucellosis are observed among individuals who drink unpasteurized milk or consume dairy products prepared from unpasteurized milk. Undulant fever has been reported following blood tranfusion from an infected person. Several veterinarians who have accidentally inoculated themselves with *Br. abortus* vaccine, Strain 19, employed for the vaccination of cattle, have developed acute brucellosis. Gilman[49] describes a case of undulant fever in a man who, while using a defective syringe, accidentally sprayed some of the vaccine into his eyes.

TABLE 23

RESULTS OF AGGLUTINATION TESTS FOR BRUCELLOSIS IN GOATS IN THE UNITED STATES, 1953-1961

Year	Goats Tested	Reactors Numbers	%
1953	17,256	17	0.1
1954	15,360	32	0.2
1955	16,911	66	0.4
1956	13,368	49	0.4
1957	14,974	58	0.4
1958	12,185	30	0.3
1959	11,414	19	0.2
1960	11,533	14	0.1
1961	12,142	10	0.1
TOTALS	125,143	295	0.2

DIAGNOSIS

Clinical Diagnosis. Abortion in cattle and hogs suggests brucellosis. Numerous other infectious agents may interrupt pregnancy, however. Retention of the placenta or sterility may be the only clinical evidence of the disease in some herds. Although abortion may herald the disease in sheep and goats, most often they show no evidence of infection except occasional lameness and mastitis.

Frequently the disease is not suspected in goats until human infection results from contact with the animals or from ingestion of goat milk or cheese. In horses, the most common symptoms are those occasioned by fistulous withers or poll evil.

The diagnosis of acute human brucellosis may be suspected among patients presenting symptoms of headache, malaise, weakness, chills, fever, and night sweats. Often the first symptoms resemble those of a respiratory infection. In chronic brucellosis, the chief complaints may be only continuous or intermittent malaise and a low grade fever extending over a period of weeks, months, or even several years. In others, the predominant symptoms may stem from a localized infection in joints, the genital tract, gall bladder and reticulo-endothelial system. An accurate diagnosis cannot be made without the aid of the laboratory, however.

Laboratory Diagnosis. Laboratory procedures for the diagnosis of brucellosis include: 1) bacteriologic examination; 2) immunologic tests; and 3) animal inoculation.

Bacteriologic Examination. Demonstration of *Brucella* in cultures constitutes the most dependable diagnosis, but it is a prolonged, difficult procedure. A negative culture does not necessarily exclude brucellosis because often cultures are negative from patients and animals with brucellosis. In man, blood cultures are made most often. Other sources of *Brucella* are bone marrow, biopsied lymph nodes or liver, bile, joint and spinal fluids, uterine discharges, purulent exudate from abscesses, urine, stools, and surgical specimens such as pulmonary granulomas. Similar specimens from animals may be cultured, but milk, fetuses, placentas, vaginal and uterine exudates are more suitable. Semen from infected bulls may contain the organism. Careful collection of the specimen is very essential because the result is directly dependent upon the selection of the material and the precautions observed during transportation to prevent drying or overgrowth with bacterial contaminants. A cool temperature or refrigeration to delay bacterial growth is preferable. The specimen should not be obtained during chemical or antibiotic therapy, because minimal concentrations of those agents are bacteriostatic for *Brucella*. From seven to ten days should elapse between termination of therapy and collection of the specimen. In the case of long acting penicillin, however, collection should be made at least a month after last administration of the drug.

Details of the growth requirements and identification of *Brucella* are described in many standard textbooks. Specially enriched media, such as blood agar and liver infusion agar, are necessary for isolation. Commercially-prepared media, such as Albimi's *Brucella* agar, Bacto-tryptose agar, and trypticase soy agar are likewise suitable. For blood cultures, a broth medium may be employed. Huddleson suggests that a 0.1-per cent aqueous solution of crystal violet be incorporated into the medium to yield a final concentration of 1:1,000,000. The dye inhibits the growth of Gram-positive bacteria, but does not affect the *Brucella*. Such a medium is useful when attempts are being made to recover *Brucella* from contaminated specimens. Weed[50] described the use of a modified W medium (Kuzdas and Morse) for the isolation of *Brucella* from contaminated clinical specimens. Castaneda[26] has described a combined agar and broth medium contained in a small bottle in which the lower half of the agar surface is immersed in the broth. Pickett and Nelson[51] reported that the cultures made from the sediment of blood cells lysed with sterile distilled water will detect more cases of brucellosis than standard methods for making blood cultures. Certain strains of *Brucella,* especially *Br. abortus,* are microaerophilic and require for isolation a reduced oxygen tension which can be supplied by use of a candle jar or by obtaining CO_2 directly from a tank. Most strains are aerobic, however, and require an atmosphere with increased carbon dioxide. A concentration of from 8 to 10 per cent is recommended. Incubation should be carried out at 36° C. An experienced bacteriologist is essential to secure successful results.

Immunologic Tests

a. **Agglutination Test.** Specific agglutinins for *Brucella* may be detected in milk serum—whey—and in blood serum from infected animals, and in the blood serum, spinal, joint, and pleural fluids of man. Agglutinins appear in from ten to fourteen days after onset of symptoms. They may be detected in the blood serum for months and even years after subsidence of symptoms. Either the "plate" or "tube" test may be employed to demonstrate agglutinins. A dependable *Brucella* antigen prepared from smooth cultures is essential. Multiple dilutions of human serum from 1:10 to 1:1280 are employed in the tube test. They may be incubated either in a water-bath at 56° C. for eighteen hours and read immediately or at 50° C. for two hours and then read after remaining overnight in a refrigerator at 4° C. A procedure known to be reliable is that recommended by the Agricultural Research Service, U.S. Department of Agriculture. Incubation is carried out for forty-eight hours at 37° C. The plate test provides a rapid method of agglutination in which the results are read in from five to eight minutes after mixing the serum with a specially-concentrated antigen stained with gentian violet and brilliant green. Certain investigators prefer to use the plate test as a screening procedure and support it with the tube test. Agglutination tests on bovine serum are usually carried out in dilutions of 1:50, 1:100, and 1:200. The generally accepted interpretation of the agglutination test in cattle is as follows:

(1) Non-vaccinated over six months of age or adult vaccinated.
Negative—no agglutination or incomplete agglutination at 1:50
Suspect — agglutination at 1:50 or incomplete agglutination at 1:100
Positive— agglutination at 1:100 or in greater dilution

(2) Calfhood vaccinated (strain 19 at 4-8 months of age) over 30 months of age.
Negative—incomplete or complete agglutination at 1:50
Suspect — agglutination at 1:100 or incomplete agglutination at 1:200
Positive— agglutination at 1:200 or greater dilution

Cows with "suspect" reactions should be retested at intervals of from one to two months.

Interpretation of the agglutination test on certain human sera is occasionally difficult because of a "prozone reaction" in the lower serum dilutions in which agglutination is not observed. In such specimens typical agglutination occurs at 1:80 or at 1:160 and in succeeding higher dilutions. The phenomenon is explained by the presence of "blocking antibodies" which are eliminated by dilution. The arbitrary requirement of a titre of 1:80 or of 1:160 as a criterion to establish the diagnosis of human brucellosis is not tenable. Higher agglutinin titres may be more significant. On the other hand, titres as low as 1:20 and 1:40 may be diagnostic if associated with dermal sensitivity and with clinical symptoms of brucellosis. Other causative factors must be ruled out, however. The same principle is true in interpreting blood tests on cattle and hogs. Non-specific agglutination is frequently observed in both animal and human sera, particularly in the former. The sera from patients with tularemia, and from individuals vaccinated against cholera often agglutinate a *Brucella* antigen.[52,53]

Goats infected with *Br. melitensis* may develop only a few agglutinins. Therefore, multiple dilutions of goat serum should be made from 1:10 to 1:320. Agglutination in such low dilutions as 1:10, 1:20, and 1:40 should be considered as evidence of infection. The agglutination test for brucellosis in hogs is not a dependable procedure for controlling the disease in a herd because many infected animals fail to react. On the other hand, the test is a useful aid in detecting herd infection.

A modification of the agglutination test to detect *Brucella* agglutinins in milk was developed by Fleischauer[54] in 1937. It has been designated the "ring test," "BRT," or "ABR" (Abortus-Bang-Ring) test. It is a useful and relatively inexpensive procedure for testing pooled samples of milk from a herd for agglutinins, thereby serving as a screening measure for Bang's disease. It may be used on milk samples from individual cows, but is not as accurate as the blood test. On the other hand, the ring test is more sensitive than the standard agglutination test on whey because it is less affected by the dilution factor. The success of the test is dependent upon a suitable antigen prepared from a heavy suspension of *Brucella* stained with hematoxylin. The test is carried out by adding one drop of antigen to each milliliter of milk. After incubation at 37° C. for one hour or at room temperature, 22° C., for two hours the sample is centrifuged. If agglutinins are present the agglutinated, stained organisms adhere to the fat globules and rise to the surface with the fat forming a purple layer of cream. The milk beneath is pale blue. In the absence of agglutinins, the layer of cream remains unstained and the color of milk beneath is distinctly blue. The test is used extensively in Scandinavian countries. In Denmark, where the test is employed to accredit herds officially for absence of Bang's disease, three consecutive negative ring tests on a composite herd sample, four months apart, followed by one negative agglutination test on blood from all animals in the herd are accepted as freedom from infection.

b. Flocculation Test. Hunter and Colbert[55] reported development of a simple, specific test using a *Br. abortus* extract antigen employing either a microscopic slide or macroscopic tube flocculation test.

c. Minoprio Test. Minoprio and Harris[56] (1955) recommended the diagnostic use of a modification of a procedure originally investigated by Signorelli (1941) in humans and Huddleson (1945) in cattle. The test was based on the observation that undiluted serum from individuals infected with *Brucella* had little or no bactericidal activity *in vitro* against *Br. abortus* compared to sera from normal individuals or those suffering from other diseases.

d. Detection by Fluorescent Antibody. Moody, Biegeleisen, and Taylor[57] labelled *Brucella* anti-sera with fluorescein isothiocyanate (FITC) and were able to demonstrate generic specificity. Organisms were detectable in films prepared from cultures containing as few as 2.5×10^3 cells per ml. Inhibition titrations revealed titres similar to agglutinin titres obtained with the corresponding anti-sera, thereby providing a more rapid method of serum titre determination.

e. Opsonocytophagic Test. The *in vitro* phagocytosis of smooth phase *Brucella* organisms by polymorphonuclear leucocytes in fresh citrated whole blood from individuals following *Brucella* infection was noted by Huddleson, Johnson, and Hamann.[58] The test results are recorded as negative, slight (1-20 bacteria per cell), moderate (21-40 bacteria per cell), or marked (over 40 bacteria per cell) with a total of twenty-five cells counted. Phagocytosis by the leucocytes may increase or decrease during the course of the disease, and becomes quite marked following recovery.

f. Intradermal Tests for Dermal Sensitivity. The detection of dermal sensitivity in man and animals by skin tests with antigens prepared from *Brucella* has been investigated by many workers. As yet, a dependable skin test for bovine and porcine brucellosis has not been developed. Meyer and Eddie[59] reported that in goats the intradermal test is more dependable than serologic tests for detecting inapparent and latent infections, if suspensions of killed *Br. melitensis* are employed. Most investigators have failed to obtain a satisfactory correlation between the results of the agglutination test with those of skin tests in animals and in man. Certainly, this cannot be expected because dermal sensitivity persists in the host for a much longer period of time than detectable agglutinins. Furthermore, in the authors' opinion, the specificity of the intradermal reaction is more dependable than that of the agglutination test. Dermal sensitivity is indicative of exposure to infection, but will not differentiate active infection from immunity, a problem which necessitates further research. Many antigens prepared from *Brucella* have been tested, including heat and chemically-killed vaccines, bacterial extracts such as abortin, purified *Brucella* protein (PPB), Brucellin, a preparation derived from liquid media in which *Brucella* have been grown, and Brucellergen, which is a most suitable antigen for human use. It is a nucleoprotein derived from *Brucella* and its uniformity and availability are distinct assets.

In man, the intradermal test is carried out by injecting intradermally 0.1 ml. of Brucellergen diluted 1:5, usually in the skin of the forearm. Observations should be made twenty-four and forty-eight hours after injection. If no reaction occurs, the test is repeated using 0.1 ml. of undiluted Brucellergen. The results of the test are classified as negative or positive, and the degrees of reaction are designated as 1+, 2+, 3+, and 4+. The following classification is recommended for reports of intradermal tests on man.

1+ —Erythema and slight edema, varying from 1.0 to 2.0 cm. in diameter.
2+ —Erythema and edema, 2.0 to 4.0 cm. in diameter.
3+ —Erythema and edema, 4.0 to 8.0 cm. in diameter and lymphangitis, but with no systemic reaction.
4+ —Marked erythema and edema at the site of injection, with lymphangitis and a systemic reaction indicated by one or several of the following symptoms: fever, headache, malaise, arthralgia, and lymphadenitis.

The more marked the reaction, the longer it persists. A 3+ or 4+ reaction may not disappear for from a week to ten days, and occasionally is observed for a longer period.

Patients with marked dermal sensitivity often react with mild symptoms of undulant fever, such as headache, fever, malaise, and muscular pains. With judicious use, Brucellergen seldom causes local necrosis. Repeated use of Brucellergen as a diagnostic agent does not sensitize a patient nor produce agglutinins in the absence of dermal sensitivity. Only one-third of the patients with dermal sensitivity show a rise in agglutinin titre two weeks after a positive test. The agglutinins usually disappear gradually in from six to eight weeks after the test. In general, the host reacts similarly to any *Brucella* antigen used for the intradermal test, but little agreement exists among experts concerning the most suitable antigen.[60]

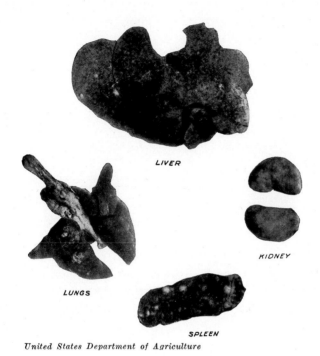

United States Department of Agriculture

Fig. 24. Lesions in guinea pigs caused by *Brucella abortus*.

Animal Inoculation. Frequently, animal inoculation is more successful than a direct bacteriologic examination, particularly if the specimen is excessively contaminated. Guinea pigs are more susceptible to *Brucella* than any other laboratory animal. Hagan,[61] however, has shown that mice are satisfactory and may be substituted for guinea pigs. Milk, cream, blood, and fluid exudates may be injected intraperitoneally or subcutaneously. Blood clots and other tissues should be suspended in broth or in an 0.85-per cent physiologic saline solution and ground prior to injection. At autopsy, which should be carried out approximately four weeks later, an inspection should be made for lesions typical of brucellosis (Figure 24). Cultures are made from the spleen, liver, lymph nodes, and blood, and

an agglutination test made on the blood serum, A positive agglutination test and positive cultures of the organism may be observed
in the absence of gross pathologic changes. Gay and Damon[62] recommend the use of from three to five-day old embryonated eggs for the
isolation of *Brucella* from blood and blood clots. One-half ml. of
the inoculum is injected into the yolk sac of the embryo and at
intervals of from four to five days subcultures on appropriate media
are made by withdrawing a few drops of yolk with a sterile syringe.

BRUCELLOSIS IN ANIMALS

Cattle. Bang's disease in cattle spreads rapidly in a herd, particularly among susceptible, pregnant heifers. At the time of abortion,
the uterine exudate is teeming with organisms which contaminate
food and bedding, and animals ingesting the infected material readily acquire the disease. Cows and bulls become infected by eating
the placenta, licking aborted fetuses and vulvar discharges and by
sucking cows with infected udders. Drinking water contaminated
with infected discharges is a source of infection. Although the disease is chiefly one of the genital organs, it is seldom transmitted by
sexual contact unless the bull's testes and epididymes are infected
making it possible for seminal infection. Other possible modes of
transmission are by artificial insemination which can cause extensive
dissemination of the disease or by permitting the bull to breed several cows in succession without employing proper sanitary measures
after exposure to an infected cow. Infection by way of wounds and
mucous membranes, particularly the conjunctiva, is not uncommon.
Carpenter and Boak[63] have demonstrated that guinea-pigs may be
infected by dropping a culture of *Br. abortus* on the unabraided
skin.

After ingestion of infected material *Brucella* gain entrance to the
blood stream and the lymphatics, thereby becoming distributed to
the tissues. Localization takes place most often in the placental tissue of the pregnant animal, the mammary gland, the reticuloendothelial tissue, lymph nodes, spleen, and liver. It may also localize in
the soft tissues of the joints. The cytoplasm of the cells of the chorionic epithelium, in properly-stained sections or in films, shows
masses of *Brucella* indicating that the organism is chiefly an intracellular parasite.[64] The chorionic tissue reacts to the infection with

inflammation, becomes edematous and thickened, and eventually decreases the fetal circulation which terminates in an abortion. The infection spreads through the placental tissue, and the fetal fluids become contaminated and the fetus becomes infected from swallowing the amniotic fluid. After abortion *Br. abortus* disappears rapidly from the uterus. It localizes in the adjacent lymph nodes and frequently in the udder and in the supramammary lymph nodes. Localization in the mammary gland is responsible for its presence in colostrum and in milk. The udder of many cows remains infected throughout life. The mesenteric lymph nodes and the spleen may yield cultures of *Brucella*. Calves that acquire the infection from milk are comparatively resistant to the infection until puberty. Carpenter[65] observed that soon after *Brucella*-infected milk is withheld from calves the organism can no longer be recovered from the lymph nodes draining the digestive tract. This observation led to the development of calfhood vaccination for the control of Bang's disease. Following invasion of the blood stream of bulls the infection localizes in the testes, epididymes, and seminal vesicles, and the organisms may be present in the semen.

The basic pathologic lesion in brucellosis is that of a granuloma. It is a proliferative lesion similar to the tubercle, except giant cells are usually rare. The lesions vary from 1 to 3.0 mm. in diameter or may be microscopic, comprised chiefly of lymphocytic and endothelial cells which persist for months and years in the tissues of preference. Calcification has not been recognized.

The symptoms in cattle range from inapparent infections to acute illness with fever and abortion. After abortion most animals acquire immunity, appear normal, and fail to show clinical evidence of disease. Many cows still show agglutinins in their blood and discharge *Br. abortus* in their milk either continuously or intermittently. Heifers are most susceptible and abortions in the first pregnancy are more prevalent than in succeeding pregnancies. Only a small percentage of cattle abort a second time. In certain herds, abortion is uncommon but retained placenta constitutes the only evidence of brucellosis. Mastitis is common. Occasionally, hygroma of the knee or other localizations of the infection may be seen (Figure 25). From an economic point of view, the most serious loss from brucellosis is the decreased production of milk, resulting from the disrupted pregnancy and the mastitis. Secondary infection with other bacterial agents often intensifies the initial tissue damage caused by *Brucella*. This is particularly noted in metritis, mastitis, and infections which result in sterility.

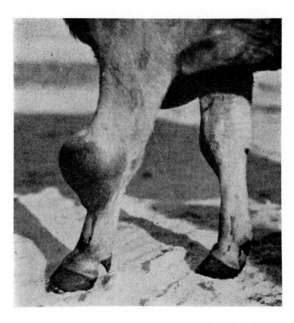

Fig. 25. Hygroma of cow's knee from which *Brucella abortus* was isolated. (Courtesy of Dr. W. L. Boyd, Division of Veterinary Medicine, University of Minnesota. From *Medical Clinics of North America*.)

Swine. The mode of infection and pathogenesis of brucellosis in swine resemble those characteristic of brucellosis in cattle. Certain differences are noted, however. Most strains of *Br. suis* produce abscesses in the tissue, rather than a proliferative granuloma, and the infection localizes more often in the joints and tests. The infection is spread from pig to pig by the ingestion of food contaminated with the organism discharged at the time of abortion. Epidemiologists formerly believed that swine acquire brucellosis from contact with infected cows or dairy products. Although *Br. suis* is pathogenic for cattle and man, *Br. abortus* is practically non-virulent for swine. One of the most frequently observed lesions in swine is arthritis, particularly spondylitis, which often results in a posterior paralysis. Orchitis is likewise very common in boars. But like bovine brucellosis, many herds are infected yet appear normal and serve as carriers of infection to other susceptible hosts.

Goats. The disease pattern of brucellosis in goats caused by *Br. melitensis* is somewhat similar to that caused by *Br. abortus* in cattle and *Br. suis* in swine. The disease is spread among goats by ingestion of contaminated food, by infection of the conjunctival sac, and other mucosal surfaces. Goat's milk is also a source of herd infection.

The absence of clinical reactions in the goat, however, should be emphasized. Abortion is not a conspicuous symptom. Of interest is the failure of the Mediterranean Fever Commission to associate the infection with the interruption of pregnancy. In some breeds of goats, particularly the maltese goat, abortion does occur. In experimentally infected animals fever, malaise, anorexia, diarrhea, and unthriftiness are observed. Roughness of hair coat and decreased milk production are conspicuous signs of chronic infection with *Br. melitensis*. Occasionally, an animal develops arthritis and becomes lame. Mastitis may develop. Most naturally-infected goats show no clinical evidence of disease and even though most infected goats appear healthy, *Br. melitensis* often can be isolated in comparatively large numbers from the blood, urine, and milk. Cultures from milk may reveal as many as 500,000 colonies per ml. The vaginal exudate after apparently normal kidding may contain the organism. Following an acute infection goats acquire an immunity and discharge *Br. melitensis* intermittently as the host-parasite relationship varies. The infection tends to become localized in the lymph nodes of the animal, and many goats remain infected throughout life. Polding[66] has reported the isolation of *Br. melitensis* from the supramammary lymph node seven years after infection. Dermal sensitivity to *Brucella* persists in goats for years. Thus, the skin test is more dependable in detecting infection in goats than in other domestic animals. The diagnosis may be established also by isolation of the causative agent and by the agglutination test.

Horses. Brucellosis in horses manifests itself chiefly as fistulous withers and as poll evil. In the former, infection takes place in the supraspinatus bursa which is located between the supraspinatus ligament and the spines of the second, third, fourth, and fifth thoracic vertebrae (Figure 26). In the latter, the infection localizes in the atlantal bursa located between the supraspinatus ligament and the dorsal arch of the atlas. In either instance abscesses form which are the result of the synergistic action of a complex infection with *Brucella* sp. and *Actinomyces bovis*.[67]

In 1924, McNutt and Murray[68] isolated, for the first time, a strain of *Brucella* from an equine fetus which later was identified as *Br. suis*. This was an unusual finding inasmuch as it is now known that abortion in mares is generally caused by *Salmonella abortus-equi* and by the equine rhinopneumonitis virus (equine abortion virus).

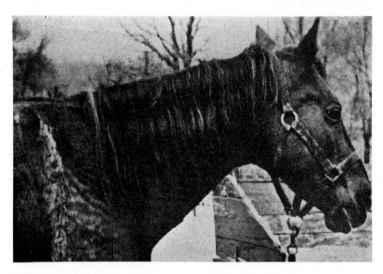

Fig. 26. Horse with fistulous withers from which *Brucella abortus* was recovered. Two children developed brucellosis with serious complications as a result of riding the horse.

In 1928, in France, Rinjard and Hilger isolated *Br. abortus* from horses with bursitis and noted that ten of fifteen horses with either poll evil or fistulous withers had high agglutinin titres for *Brucella*. In 1932, Van der Hoeden[69] made agglutination tests on 424 horses in Holland and observed that approximately 60 per cent were positive. In the United States, Fitch, Delez, and Boyd[70] tested sixty-one horses and forty-eight, or 80 per cent, reacted positively. Carpenter and Boak[71] reported that blood tests were positive on 170, or 48 per cent, of 347 horses in New York City. Only 8 per cent, however, had titres of 1:100 or higher. Although it is not known how horses acquire the infection it is assumed that it results from contact with other species of infected animals. Thus, horses may infect man, particularly horses with abscesses discharging *Brucella*. Carpenter and Boak observed two cases of brucellosis in children with severe complications from riding a horse with fistulous withers due to *Br. abortus.*

Sheep. Little is known in this country of brucellosis in sheep. In certain areas of the world the problem of brucellosis in sheep is not unlike that in goats because usually it is due to *Br. melitensis.* The disease has been reported in France, Africa, Mongolia, and Russia. *Br. abortus* may cause abortion in pregnant ewes. It has been reported in Canada and in France. The organism has been recovered from one flock of sheep in California. Human infections have been traced to sheep milk and to cheese prepared from sheep milk.

BRUCELLOSIS IN MAN—UNDULANT FEVER

Brucellosis in man includes Malta fever, undulant fever, and the forms of generalized chronic illness due to the three species of *Brucella.* In certain patients, only a localized infection may be noted. The sources of human infection are discussed in the section on Epidemiology.

Acute Brucellosis. In man acute brucellosis is characterized by chills, headache, fever, severe night sweats and extreme weakness, symptoms which may persist for from four to sixteen weeks. Often the acute course may last five or six months, during which time the patient loses considerable weight and becomes emaciated. Intermittent fever develops in certain patients at fairly regular intervals in which fever persists for from ten to fourteen days, followed by a two or three weeks' afebrile period. In mild cases the fever may disappear in from ten to fourteen days and never recur. Many cases of inapparent infection occur as indicated by the large number of individuals with dermal sensitivity to *Brucella,* yet have not experienced a febrile illness diagnosed as undulant fever. The temperature may be elevated to 104° or 105° F. but in most cases the range is between 100° and 103° F. Usually it effervesces in the late afternoon or evening, and on reaching its peak, the patient experiences an intensive sweat, often soaking night clothes and bedding to a degree that requires changing. The temperature defervesces and approaches normal in the morning and during the forenoon.

In the acute septicaemic stage cultures from blood and urine are usually positive. The differential blood count shows a leukopenia with a relatively high lymphocytosis. Later, a secondary anemia may develop. Specific agglutinins appear in the blood after two weeks. Not infrequently, the onset of the disease is heralded with symptoms of an upper respiratory infection, such as non-productive cough, pain in the chest, and general muscular pains and aches. The acute phase of the disease may be complicated with general lymphadenopathy, arthritis, cholecystitis, epididymitis, ovaritis, and occasionally with mastitis. A few cases of abortion have been described. If the disease is not cured in the acute stage, chronic brucellosis ensues and may persist for years, occasionally causing marked morbidity and particularly mental depression. A low grade, afternoon fever may persist for months and even years.

In the acute stage a physical examination often shows a lymphadenopathy, splenomegaly, and hepatomegaly. On the other hand, a physical examination may be negative or reveal only signs that are referable to the disease focus. A secondary anemia develops if the course of the disease is prolonged. Although the infection may be caused by any one of the three species of *Brucella;* namely, *Br. abortus, Br. melitensis,* and by *Br. suis,* the course of the disease is, in general, similar. Certain differences may be noted, however. *Br. abortus* is considered to be the least virulent and causes comparatively mild symptoms. *Br. suis* most often initiates an acute septicaemic form of the disease which not infrequently is seen among abattoir workers. The swine strain has a tendency to localize in the joints, particularly the vertebrae, and set up a spondylitis. *Br. meletensis* infection recurs often and follows the intermittent pattern of fever.

Chronic Brucellosis. Many physicians fail to recognize chronic brucellosis as a specific syndrome, yet, many patients who have had an attack of acute brucellosis experience recurrences of symptoms such as arthritis, tenosynovitis, low grade fever, abdominal distress, certain cardiovascular symptoms,[72,73] as well as malaise and depression, which are symptoms often associated with chronic illness of long duration. In a host with latent infection symptoms may recur following physical or mental stress due to an imbalance of the host-parasite relationship. Many patients with such complaints improve when contact with *Brucella* infection has been eliminated, especially antigenic dead *Brucella* present in dairy products. Protection of the sensitized host against exposure to any *Brucella* antigen prevents further allergic symptoms. Thus, chronic brucellosis may be conjectured in a large measure as an allergic reaction to the organism, particularly as it occurs in relation to the consumption of food containing dead *Brucella*. Of particular interest are two experimental studies supporting this point of view. First of all, sediment from pasteurized milk containing dead *Brucella* gave a positive skin test in *Brucella* infected guinea pigs equivalent to that observed with Brucellergen.[74] Secondly, marked cytotoxicity occurred in tissue cultures prepared from infected human or guinea pig spleen when minute amounts of *Brucella* antigen were introduced.[74] When a similar amount of antigen was added to tissue cultures from normal human or guinea pig spleen no cytotoxicity was observed.

PREVENTION AND CONTROL

Animals. The economic losses in the cattle industry and the public health hazards have necessitated active control measures against brucellosis in animals. During the past three decades marked progress has been made in the prevention of the disease in animals. Control procedures vary according to the species of animal and with the sanitary regulations established by the authorities in a particular area. Two entirely different basic principles are employed for the control of brucellosis in animals: 1) the isolation or slaughter of infected animals detected by the blood test; and 2) immunization against the disease by vaccination with living cultures of *Brucella*.

The agglutination test makes it possible to follow with some degree of accuracy an endemic infection in a herd or community. Blood tests are comparatively inexpensive and may be repeated as often as necessary. Control by means of the blood test, however, has been somewhat disappointing because of undependable results encountered with unsatisfactory antigens and because the serum from certain cows will cause non-specific agglutination. On the other hand, early in the course of Bang's disease agglutinins may not be detected. Nevertheless the disease has been satisfactorily controlled in many herds by use of the agglutination test. Success with the blood test requires intelligent cooperative effort on the part of farmers and their neighboring herd owners, with veterinarians, and with the public health authorities. The fact that herds freed from brucellosis by serologic tests have become reinfected, and, in other instances, entire eradication of the disease was not accomplished, have discouraged the use of the method.

Control by vaccination with living strains of *Brucella* alleged to be non-virulent has, in recent years, been extensively employed. Attenuated vaccines are effective in preventing abortion in heifers vaccinated during calfhood from four to eight months of age. The purpose is to establish immunity prior to the first pregnancy. Calves are comparatively resistant to infection before puberty, yet develop sufficient immunity from vaccination to protect them from a natural infection during pregnancy. The prevention of abortion breaks an important link in the chain of infection by eliminating herd exposure to mass infection from the placental tissue, uterine and vaginal discharges teeming with *Brucella* when pregnancy is interrupted.

Most of the research and control programs have been carried out with three vaccines designated as Strain 19, developed by Buck,[75] Strain 45/20 recommended by McEwen and Priestley in England,[76] and a third, "M" or mucoid strain, advocated by Huddleson.[77] Strain 19, a lyophilized agglutinogenic strain of *Br. abortus,* has been in use for approximately thirty years and is currently one of the important measures for bovine brucellosis control in the United States. Five ml. of a standardized suspension is injected subcutaneously into calves from four to eight months of age. The vaccine may cause fever and occasionally an indurated area or abscess at the site of injection. Usually agglutinins for *Brucella* can be demonstrated two weeks after vaccination. The agglutinin titre rises during the next ten or twelve weeks to from 1:100 to 1:400 following which it declines to from 1:25 to 1:50 one year after vaccination. The blood of most heifers returns to negative after termination of their first pregnancy. The vaccine from Strain 19 is the only agent approved for use in the United States by the Agricultural Research Service of the U. S. Department of Agriculture. The Agricultural Research Service has accepted the responsibility of maintaining Strain 19 and is charged with providing stock cultures to manufacturers of the vaccine. The widespread use of calfhood vaccination in the United States from 1935 to 1961 has resulted in the vaccination of 65,859,103 calves. The utilization of calfhood vaccination increased rapidly from the late 1940's to the present. At first only the large dairy states waged active campaigns. California was the first to establish a State-wide calfhood vaccination law in 1947. In 1950, less than 25 per cent of the eligible calves were vaccinated, however, by 1958-'59 over 50 per cent of the eligible calves were being vaccinated. In 1950, 2,255,678 calves were vaccinated, while from 1958 to 1961 over 6 million calves were vaccinated annually. During the same period, 1950-1961, the per cent reactors had decreased from 3.5 to 1.0 per cent.

The vaccine 45/20 of McEwen and Priestley is a rough strain of *Br. abortus,* but is not as effective as Strain 19. Although it was purported to be non-virulent for cattle and non-agglutinogenic, animal passage in guinea-pigs revealed that it gradually acquired virulence. The "M" (mucoid strain) vaccine is only a slightly agglutinogenic strain of *Br. suis* with which Huddleson immunized guinea pigs and cattle against all three species of *Brucella.* Field tests of this vaccine, however, revealed no superiority to Strain 19. In fact, some evidence was obtained indicating greater resistance was imparted by Strain 19.[78] Elberg and Faunce[79] recently developed a living vaccine employing an attenuated strain of *Br. melitensis.* Field trials with this vaccine conducted by Szyres, Blood, Cedro, and Mendy[80] in Argentina revealed no increase in resistance to abortion in vaccinated goats in comparison to unvaccinated controls. Carpenter, Naylor-Foote, Taplin, Lawrence, and Drake[81] have recently been investigating the antigenicity of *Brucella* vaccines inactivated by gamma irradiation from a Co^{60} source.

Although calfhood vaccination only is recommended by public health veterinarians many herdsmen confronted with a severe outbreak of abortion insist that adult animals be vaccinated with Strain 19. The recommended dosage is 5.0 ml. of the vaccine administered subcutaneously, or from 0.2 to 0.4 ml. intradermally. A relative degree of immunity to *Brucella* infection develops but blood tests on vaccinated adult animals become positive and subsequent serologic tests will not differentiate immune from infected cows. Thus, the status of Bang's disease in a herd cannot be determined. The economic value of purebred animals, especially, decreases inasmuch as most breeders prefer to purchase animals free from brucellosis. In many states, adult vaccination is used chiefly among range and beef cattle.

The Agricultural Research Service, U.S. Department of Agriculture, recognizes three alternative plans for the control of brucellosis in individual cattle herds.

> *Plan A:* Testing of cattle, permanent indentification, and prompt disposal of positives, for slaughter only, with or without vaccination of calves.
>
> *Plan B:* Testing of cattle, permanent identification, and temporary retention of positives pending their disposal for slaughter, with vaccination of calves. Positives may be retained in a quarantined herd for a period not to exceed three years from the date retention of positives was started. All Plan B herds should be retested at least every six months.
>
> *Plan C:* Calf vaccination without test of any part of the herd. This plan is to be confined to those herds in which the movement of animals is restricted by special permits issued by the State Livestock Sanitary Authority.

The nationwide Cooperative State-Federal Brucellosis Eradication Program provides a yardstick for measurement of success in the effort to eradicate bovine brucellosis in the United States. The program is built around testing and certification of individual herds as brucellosis-free. Testing progresses from the individual herd to an "area" (usually a county). The latter may be classified as a Modified Certified Brucellosis Area or Certified Brucellosis-Free Area depending on the results of the test. Each of the above classifications may be defined as follows:

Certified Brucellosis-Free Herd. The herd has passed at least two consecutive negative blood tests, with the first clean test and the certifying test not less than twelve months nor more than eighteen months apart. If the first blood test reveals no evidence of infection, the herd may be certified if it passes one additional negative test not earlier than six months nor more than eighteen months later. Where the Ring Test is employed, herds may be initially certified with a minimum of three satisfactory milk tests conducted at not less than ninety day intervals and followed by a negative herd blood test conducted within ninety days after the last negative ring test.

Modified Certified Brucellosis Area. The number of blood test positive cattle does not exceed one percent and the herd infection does not exceed five percent following blood test of all cattle within the area. The area may also qualify following application of two milk ring tests not less than 6 months apart, together with a blood test of all milk reacting herds, such other herds as are not included in the milk test, and herds in which the BRT does not represent a majority of the cattle in the herd. Range and semi-range areas may qualify as the result of a blood test of all dairy cattle, all purebred cattle, and not less than 20 per cent of the range and semi-range cows over three years of age in each herd. The result of the latter two alternatives must each be at least as satisfactory as the result of the complete blood test.

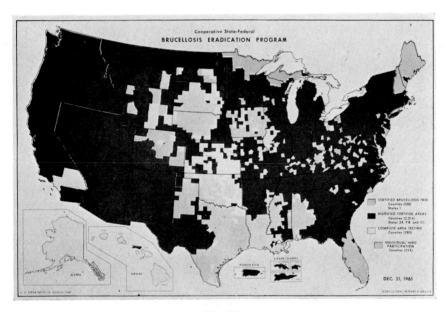

Fig. 27.

Certified Brucellosis-Free Area. The area must be located in a State in which all areas have current Modified Certified Brucellosis Area or Certified Brucellosis-Free Area status. Not more than one per cent of the herds, or one herd, whichever is greater, and not more than 0.2 per cent of the cattle shall have been found to be infected or reactors, respectively, during the eighteen months immediately preceding. All suspect individuals and quarantined herds shall have met sufficient tests to be legally released. All herds of other species of domestic livestock in which brucellosis has been found or suspected have either been tested negative or eliminated, leaving no known foci of infection.

As of December 31, 1961 one State (New Hampshire) and 100 counties have qualified as Certified Brucellosis Free. Twenty-four States, Puerto Rico, and the Virgin Islands and 2,214 individual counties qualified as Modified Certified (Figure 27).

Swine. Control of brucellosis in swine is dependent upon the detection of infected animals by the agglutination test and subsequent slaughter of positive reactors. Inasmuch as disposal by slaughter can be carried out without serious economic loss the procedure becomes practical. Vaccination has not been successful in swine.

The Agricultural Research Service, U.S. Department of Agriculture, has recently adopted recommendations for the eradication of brucellosis in individual swine herds. Three alternative plans are provided for the establishment of Validated Brucellosis-Free Swine herds.

Plan 1. Recommended for commercial herds. If evidence of infection if found, market the entire herd for slaughter and replace with stock from a Validated herd. Following two consecutive negative blood tests 30 to 90 days apart, the herd is eligible for validation.

Plan 2. Recommended for purebred herds desiring to retain valuable blood lines. Separate pigs from sows at forty-two days of age or younger and isolate, then market infected herd for slaughter. Blood test the gilts about thirty days before breeding and save only those which are negative. Breed only to negative boars. Retest the gilts immediately after farrowing and remove reactors. The cycle may need to be repeated. Following two consecutive negative tests not less than ninety days apart the herd is eligible for validation.

Plan 3. Not generally recommended but found useful in herds with few reactors and no clinical symptoms noted.

Remove the reactors from the farm. Retest the herd at thirty-day intervals, removing reactors, until the entire herd is negative. Two negative tests not less than ninety days apart qualify the herd for validation. Should success not be readily achieved, switch to plan 1 or 2.

Swine serum agglutination titres are classified as follows:

Negative Individual
a. Animal from herd of unknown or infected status—no agglutination at 1:25 or higher dilution.

b. Animal from validated herd—incomplete agglutination at 1:100 dilution.

Negative Herd

No animal reacting more than incomplete at dilution of 1:100.

Reactor Individual

Complete agglutination at 1:100 or higher dilution.

Infected Herd

Contains one or more individuals reacting at 1:100 or higher, then any animal in the herd showing complete agglutination at 1:25 or higher shall be considered a reactor.

Goat. The control of caprine brucellosis is difficult because of the limitations of the agglutination test and because vaccination is still an experimental procedure as yet considered unsatisfactory. The intradermal test may be employed to detect infected goats, but its value has not been established. Infected animals should be eliminated. Unfortunately, control measures are often not carried out effectively, particularly in Mediterranean and Latin American countries where goats provide the chief supply of meat and dairy products.

The control of brucellosis in other animals, such as horses, sheep, and chickens, depends for the most part upon their isolation from infected cattle, swine, and goats. Chickens should not be fed infected meat or milk. The agglutination test may be employed in individual herds to detect infected animals which should be isolated or slaughtered.

PREVENTION OF BRUCELLOSIS IN MAN

Pasteurization of milk is the most effective means of preventing human brucellosis. The present standard holding method; namely, 145° F. for thirty minutes or the short time, high temperature, procedure; namely, 161° F. for fifteen seconds, are effective in destroying *Brucella* and rendering milk and dairy products prepared from pasteurized milk safe for human consumption. The effectiveness of pasteurization was demonstrated by Carpenter and Boak[63] who examined by guinea-pig inoculation, 205 samples of milk and cream collected from fifty cities and towns in five states and failed to observe any evidence of infection. The danger of contracting brucellosis from drinking raw cow's and goat's milk cannot be overemphasized. Pasteurization or boiling of milk is just as essential on the farm and in rural areas as in urban areas.

The necessity for pasteurization of milk and for the control of the disease in animals in order to prevent human burcellosis was emphasized approximately thirty-five years ago.

TABLE 24

NUMBER OF CASES OF UNDULANT FEVER REPORTED IN THE UNITED STATES, 1925-1961

1925........ 24	1937........2,675	1949........4,235
1926........ 46	1938........4,379	1950........3,510
1927........ 112	1939........3,501	1951........3,139
1928........ 669	1940........3,310	1952........2,537
1929........ 975	1941........3,484	1953........2,032
1930........1,435	1942........3,228	1954........1,923
1931........1,578	1943........3,734	1955........1,444
1932........1,502	1944........4,286	1956........1,300
1933........1,788	1945........4,959	1957........ 983
1934........2,017	1946........5,887	1958........ 924
1935........2,008	1947........6,321	1959........ 892
1936........2,095	1948........4,991	1960........ 742
		1961........ 580 (preliminary)

During this period public health authorities, physicians, and veterinarians have put forth much effort to prevent human infections. However, through 1947 a steady increase in the annual number of cases was reported in the United States (Table 24). Since then a precipitous decline in the incidence of human brucellosis has occurred (Figure 28). Undoubtedly, pasteurization of milk prevented numerous cases. A variety of other factors must be considered. A decrease in bovine infection has reduced the opportunity for exposure of occupational groups associated with cattle, including husbandmen, veterinarians, and abattoir workers. The improvement of rural hygiene and the shift of population from rural to urban areas may each have played a role. The fact that numerous cases are still reported each year reflects the job remaining to be done in the control of brucellosis. Swine brucellosis, in particular, remains a major economic and public health problem in the United States. Even though gross under-reporting occurs, the current downward trend is encouraging for the control of human brucellosis.

Although pasteurization is essential in the control of human brucellosis it affords protection principally to urban populations. The elimination of brucellosis from cattle, swine, and goats is still the basic problem necessary to protect man from the disease, particularly dairymen and herdsmen who are in contact daily with infected animals. They should observe strict rules of sanitation following milking of infected cows, caring for animals at the time of abortion, and in handling aborted fetuses. Wounds on hands are particularly hazardous and spattering of infected discharges into the eye should be avoided.

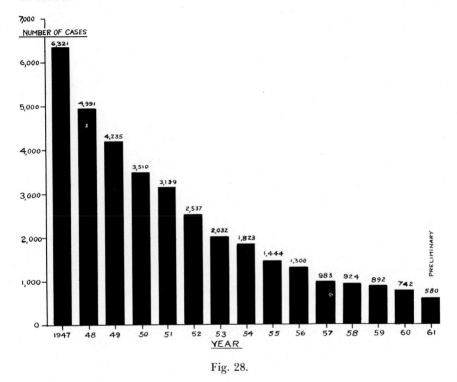

Fig. 28.

Veterinarians should use special care in handling living vaccines and in treating infected animals. Rubber gloves and long-sleeved gauntlets should be worn, especially the latter when removing retained placentas. The prevention of brucellosis among employees of the meat packing industry is difficult, particularly among those working with raw meat. Such employees should be cautioned regarding the dangers of infection and be provided with protective clothing. Wounds on hands and arms should be treated and covered. If possible, only personnel with dermal sensitivity to the *Brucella* should be employed where danger of infection is greatest. Although vaccines for human prophylaxis have been recommended, their value is unknown. Possibly vaccines from killed cultures would provide sufficient protection to warrant use among personnel continuously exposed to the infection. Inasmuch as laboratory workers are prone to accidental infection, protection is effected by pointing out the dangers of infection and how laboratory infections are acquired and prevented. Personnel with dermal sensivity are safer than unsensitized individuals for employment in laboratories where live cultures and experimentally infected animals are under investigation. Vaccines may be recommended to personnel with negative skin tests, but their relative protective value have not been established.

Educational programs are most essential in prevention and control and must be advanced to inform husbandmen of the facts concerning brucellosis. Modern audio-visual techniques serve as valuable tools for teaching prevention of the disease in man and animals.

THERAPY

Animals. As yet, no dependable specific treatment for brucellosis in animals has been discovered. Therapy with the new antibiotics has been investigated, particularly the use of penicillin, chlortetracycline, streptomycin, and chloramphenicol. Furthermore, at present prices their cost would almost prohibit their use if they were effective. Mortality from brucellosis in animals is minimal and although morbidity is serious, the most important aspect of the problem is to render infected animals non-infectious.

Many drugs, particularly sulfonamides and antibiotics, have been evaluated in experimental brucellosis of guinea pigs. Yet, no single effective therapeutic agent has been developed. Several drugs used singly will modify the course of the disease, but only when used concurrently with another drug is an apparent cure brought about. Although *Brucella* cannot be isolated from the tissues of the infected guinea-pig at autopsy, agglutination tests on their blood remain positive. Further evaluation of more combinations of antibiotics and sulfonamides may lead to a more dependable therapy. Once the infection has become well established in the host and the *Brucella* have become established intracellularly in the reticuloendothelial tissues elimination of infection is distressingly difficult.

Man. Carpenter and Boak,[82] in 1936, concluded in a review of the current therapeutic measures for human brucellosis that "a successful

method for the treatment of brucellosis still awaits development."
Many successful and unsuccessful forms of therapy have since been
reported.[83],[84],[85] Favorable results are usually obtained in acute cases
during the first two or three months of illness in which many drugs,
chiefly sulfonamides and antibiotics, ostensibly are effective. The
senior author has observed prontosil, sulfanilamide, and sulfadiazine,
as well as oxytetracycline, streptomycin, chlortetracycline, and
chloramphenicol, to be successful in a few acute cases. But, inasmuch
as brucellosis is usually a self limiting disease in man, evaluation of
therapy is difficult. Certain cases recover in the absence of treatment.
*Of particular interest are two recently observed cases of acute brucel-
losis from which Brucella were isolated who recovered uneventfully
with only bed rest and aspirin.* Evidently many similar cases which
are undiagnosed recover spontaneously. In man, the advantages of
chemotherapy and antibiotic therapy versus symptomatic treatment
have not been clearly defined. Therapy which shortens the course of
the disease is desirable provided toxicity of the drug and sensitivity
from its use are minimal. Based on an appraisal of drugs in experimental and human brucellosis, the concurrent use of comparatively
large doses of streptomycin and sulfadiazine, which was recommended by Eisele and McCullough[85] in 1947, warrants recognition
as effective suppressive therapy. Spink, Hall, and Shaffer[86] have likewise reported favorable results from the simultaneous use of these
two agents. Oxytetracycline and sulfadiazine or oxytetracycline and
gantrisin appear equally effective. Patients should be hospitalized
and observed carefully for toxic effects of such drugs. Combinations
of antibiotics have also been employed successfully especially streptomycin and oxytetracycline, streptomycin and chlortetracycline,
and streptomycin and chloramphenicol.

Therapy with specific biologic agents prepared from *Brucella* is
advocated by a few physicians. Such agents include heat- or chemically-killed vaccines, detoxified cells, chemical fractions of cells
such as Brucellergen and Brucellin, a product composed of a medium
in which *Brucella* have been grown. The antigen is employed on the
one hand to stimulate antibody production while others employ
small doses to hyposensitize the patient. Only minute amounts of
antigenic material should be employed therapeutically because most
are toxic and distress the patient. Although therapy with such agents
is desired by certain patients because they believe their symptoms are

relieved, the psychologic effect of such therapy must not be over-looked. An ideal treatment for human brucellosis in which the infection in the host is entirely eliminated is, as yet, unavailable. It must be borne in mind that chronic brucellosis in man resembles, in many respects, the disease pattern of tuberculosis and that often simple measures such as rest, sunshine, nutritious food, symptomatic therapy, and reassurance adequately restore a patient's health.

An important measure to follow in the case of patients with chronic brucellosis is the elimination of dairy products from the patient's diet in order to decrease consumption of *Brucella* antigen which often activates a patient's symptoms.

ITEMS OF NOTE

1) Brucellosis is a worldwide disease of animals and man in which animals serve as a reservoir of infection for man. The disease is caused by three species of *Brucella*: 1) *Br. abortus* of bovine origin; 2) *Br. suis* of swine origin; and 3) *Br. melitensis* of carprine origin.

2) Brucellosis of cattle, namely, Bang's disease, is most prevalent in the dairy-raising areas of the world, Central Europe, Scandinavia, England, United States, Canada, South Africa, and Argentina. Brucellosis of swine prevails in the hog-raising states of the Midwest and on the West Coast of the United States. Brucellosis of goats and sheep is prevalent in Latin America, the Mediterranean littoral, China, the Phillipines, Russia, and in the Southwestern United States.

3) Many animals show no clinical evidence of the disease, yet are carriers of the infection which our present laboratory tests fail to detect thereby rendering the disease very difficult to eradicate.

4) Man becomes infected from drinking unpasteurized milk or from consuming dairy products prepared from raw milk. Veterinarians, farmers, and employees in abattoirs and in meat packing plants acquire the disease from contact with infected animals and raw infected meat. Laboratory workers often become accidentally infected from cultures and from experimental animals. Symptoms of chronic burcellosis may persist in a hypersensitive patient as a result of consumption of *Brucella* antigens in dairy products even though adequately pasteurized.

5) The prevention of human brucellosis is dependent upon: a)

pasteurization of milk; b) eradication of disease in animals; c) deletion of dairy products from diets of patients hypersensitive to *Brucella* antigens to eliminate allergic symptoms.

6) Brucellosis in animals is controlled by: a) the use of the BRT test in screening dairy herds. b) the use of the blood test and removal or slaughter of infected animals; and c) immunization of calves with non-virulent strains of *Br. abortus,* particularly Strain 19 to prevent abortion during subsequent pregnancies.

REFERENCES

1. BUDDLE, M. B., and BOYES, B. W.: *Australian Vet. J., 29:*145, 1953.
2. STOENNER, H. G., and LACKMAN, D. B.: *Am. J. Vet. Res., 18:*947, 1957.
3. EVANS, A. C.: *J. Infect. Dis., 22:*580, 1918.
4. HUTRYA and MAREK: *Special Pathology and Therapeutics of the Diseases of Domestic Animals,* 2nd English edition, Vol. I. Chicago, Alexander Eger, p. 780.
5. BANG, B.: *Ztschr. Tiermedizin, 1:*241, 1897.
6. MCNEAL, W. J. and KERR, J. E.: *J. Infect. Dis., 7:*469, 1910.
7. SCHROEDER, E. C. and COTTON, W. E.: Twenty-eighth Annual Report of the Bureau of Animal Industry. U.S. Department of Agriculture, 1911, p. 139.
8. SMITH, T. and FABYAN, M.: *Centralb. Bakt., 61:*497 (Abt. 1), 1912.
9. MOHLER, J. R. and TRAUM, J.: Twenty-eighth Annual Report of the Bureau of Animal Industry. U.S. Department of Agriculture, 1911, p. 147.
10. LARSON, W. P. and SEDGWICK, J. P.: *Am. J. Dis. Child., 6:*326, 1913.
11. COOLEDGE, L. H.: *J. M. Res., 34:*459, 1916.
12. TRAUM, J.: Annual Report of the Chief, Bureau of Animal Industry, U.S. Department of Agriculture, 1914, p. 30.
13. BRUCE, D.: *Practitioner, 39:*161, 1887.
14. GENTRY, E. R. and FERENBAUGH, T. L.: *J.A.M.A., 57:*889, 1911.
15. KEEFER, C. S.: *Bull. Johns Hopkins Hosp., 35:*6, 1924.
16. CARPENTER, C. M. and MERRIAM, H. E.: *J.A.M.A., 87:*1269, 1926.
17. CARPENTER, C. M. and BAKER, D. W.: *Cornell Vet., 17:*236, 1927.
18. HUDDLESON, I. F.: *J.A.M.A., 86:*943, 1926.
19. MOORE, V. A. and CARPENTER, C. M.: *Cornell Vet., 16:*147, 1926.
20. EVANS, A. C.: U.S. Pub. Health Service, Hygienic Laboratory Bulletin, 143, 1925.
21. GAGE, E. A. and GREGORY, D. A.: *J.A.M.A., 87:*848, 1926.
22. KNOWLTON, M.: Annual Report, Connecticut State Dept. of Health, 101, 1924.
23. HULL, T. G. and BLACK, L. A.: *J.A.M.A., 88:*463, 1927.
24. HELD, J. R. and HENDRICKS, S. L.: Presentation at A.P.H.A. Ann. Meet., 1961.
25. HENRY, B. S.: *J. Infect. Dis., 52:*374, 1933.
26. CASTANEDA, M. R.: *Proc. Soc. Exper. Biol. & Med., 64:*114, 1947.
27. MEYER, M. E. and CAMERON, H. S.: *J. Bact., 78:*130, 1959.
28. World Health Organization 1953 Joint FAO/WHO Expert Committee on Brucellosis, WHO Tech. Rep. Sero., No. 67, 20.
29. BUDDLE, M. B.: *J. Hyg., 54:*351, 1956.
30. BRAUN, W. and BONESTELL, A. E.: *Am. J. Vet. Res., 8:*386, 1947.
31. HUDDLESON, I. F. and BALTZER, B.: *Science, 112:*651, 1950.

32. STINEBRING, W. R. and BRAUN, W.: *J. Bact., 78:*736, 1959.
33. MEYER, M. E. and CAMERON, H. S.: *Am. J. Vet. Res., 17:*495, 1956.
34. OLITZKI, A. L. and SULITZEANU, D.: *Brit. J. Exper. Path., 39:*219, 1958.
35. CARRERE, L., ROUX, J., and SERRE, A.: *Ann. Inst. Past., Paris, 95:*588, 1958.
36. PHILLIPS, J. H., BRAUN, W., and PLESCIA, O. J.: *Nature, 181:*573, 1958.
37. BENDTSEN, H., CHRISTIANSEN, M., and THOMSEN, A.: *Nord. Vet. Med., 6:*11, 1954.
38. *Ibid: Nord. Vet. Med., 8:*1, 1956.
39. EDWARDS, S.: *Alaska Med., 1:*41, 1959.
40. STOENNER, H. G., HOLDENREID, R., LACKMAN, D., and OSBORN, J. S., JR.: *Am. J. Trop. Med. & Hyg., 8:*590, 1959.
41. BEAL, G. A., LEWIS, R. E., McCULLOUGH, N. B., and CLAFLIN, R. M.: *Am. J. Vet. Res., 20:*872, 1959.
42. CARPENTER, C. M. and BOAK, R. A.: *J. Bact., 27:*73, 1934.
43. STILES, G. W.: *Rocky Mountain M. J., 42:*18, 1945.
44. JORDAN, C. F. and BORTS, I. H.: *J.A.M.A., 130:*72, 1946.
45. CARPENTER, C. M., BOAK, R. A., and CHAPMAN, O. D.: *J. Immunol., 17:*65, 1929.
46. MCALPINE, J. G. and MICKLE, F. L.: *Am. J. Pub. Health, 18:*609, 1928.
47. HARDY, A. V., JORDAN, C. F., BORTS, I. H., and HARDY, G. C.: *Bull. National Institute of Health,* 158, 1931.
48. HARDENBERGH, J. G.: *Certified Milk, 3:*6, 1927.
49. GILMAN, H. L.: *Cornell Vet., 34:*193, 1944.
50. WEED, L. A.: *Am. J. Clin. Path., 27:*482, 1957.
51. PICKETT, M. J. and NELSON, E. L.: *J. Bact., 61:*229, 1951.
52. EISELE, C. W., McCULLOUGH, N. B., and BEAL, G. A.: *Ann. Int. Med., 28:*833, 1948.
53. McCULLOUGH, N. B., EISELE, C. W., and BEAL, G. A.: *J. Infect. Dis., 83:*55, 1948.
54. FLEISCHAUER, G.: *Berl. Tierartzl. Tiermed., 53:*527, 1937.
55. HUNTER, C. A. and COLBERT, B.: *J. Immunol., 77:*232, 1956.
56. MINOPRIO, J. L. and HARRIS, H. J.: *Rev. Med. de Cordoba (Argentina), 43:*428, 1955.
57. MOODY, M. D., BIEGELEISEN, J. Z., JR., and TAYLOR, G. C.: *J. Bact., 81:*990, 1961.
58. HUDDLESON, I. F., JOHNSON, H. W., and HAMAN, E. E.: *Am. J. Pub Health, 23:*917, 1933.
59. MEYER, K. F., and EDDIE, B.: *J. Am. Vet. M.A., 39:*286, 1935.
60. CARPENTER, C. M., DEBOER, C. J., KLEIN, S. J., and TEMPEREAU, E.: *J. Immunol., 65:*331, 1950.
61. HAGAN, W. A.: *J. Exper. Med., 36:*727, 1922.
62. GAY, K. and DAMON, S. R.: *Pub. Health Reports, 66:*1204, 1951.
63. CARPENTER, C. M. and BOAK, R. A.: *Am. J. M. Sc., 185:*97, 1933.
64. SMITH, T.: *J. Exper. Med., 29:*451, 1919.
65. CARPENTER, C. M.: *Cornell Vet., 14:*16, 1924.
66. POLDING, J. B.: Second Progress Report of the Undulant Fever Committee Malta, Research Station, 1939.
67. RODERICK, L. M., KIMBALL, A., McLEOD, W. M., and FRANK, E. R.: *Kansas State College Tech. Bull.,* 63, 1947.
68. McNUTT, S. H. and MURRAY, C.: *J. Am. Vet. M. A., 65:*215, 1924.
69. VAN DER HOEDEN, J.: *Tijdschrift voor Diergeneeskunde, 59:*612, 1932.
70. FITCH, C. P., DELEZ, A. L., and BOYD, W. L.: *J. Am. Vet. M. A., 76:*17, 1930.
71. CARPENTER, C. M. and BOAK, R. A.: *J. Bact., 33:*1, 1937.
72. PEERY, T. M.: *Ann. Int. Med., 49:*568, 1958.
73. KONWALER, B. E., CARPENTER, C. M., and OHNO, S.: *Am. Heart J., 59:*101, 1960.
74. HEILMAN, D. H., RICE, E., HOWARD, D. H., WEIMER, H. E., and CARPENTER, C. M.: *J. Immunol., 85:*258, 1960.

75. BUCK, J. M.: *J. Agricultural Research, Washington, 41:*667, 1930.
76. McEWEN, A. D. and PRIESTLEY, F. W.: Vet. Rec., *50:*1097, 1938.
77. HUDDLESON, I. F.: Michigan Agricultural Experiment Station, *Quart. Bull.* No. 31, 1948.
78. BERMAN, D. T. and IRWIN, M. R.: *J. Am. Vet. M. A., 125:*401, 1954.
79. ELBERG, S. S., and FAUNCE, K., JR.: *J. Bact., 73:*211, 1957.
80. SZYFRES, B., BLOOD, B. D., CEDRO, V. C. F., and MENDY, R. M.: *Zoonoses Res., 1:*145, 1962.
81. CARPENTER, C. M., NAYLOR-FOOTE, A. W. C., TAPLIN, G. V., LAWRENCE, C. A., and DRAKE, C. L.: *Am. Rev. Tuberc. & Pulm. Dis., 79:*374, 1959.
82. CARPENTER, C. M. and BOAK, R. A.: *Medicine, 15:*103, 1936.
83. BLUMGART, H. L. and GILLIGAN, D. R.: *M. Clin. North America, 23:*1193, 1939.
84. LONG, P. H. and BLISS, E. A.: *The Clinical and Experimental Use of Sulfanilamide, Sulfapyridine and Allied Compounds.* New York, Macmillan, 1939, p. 209.
85. EISELE, C. W. and McCULLOUGH, N. B.: *J.A.M.A., 135:*1053, 1947.
86. SPINK, W. W., HALL, W. H., SHAFFER, J. M., and BRAUDE, A. I.: *J.A.M.A., 136:*382, 1948.

Chapter 4

VIBRIOSIS

Charles M. Carpenter, D.V.M., Ph.D., M.D.
William T. Hubbert, D.V.M., M.P.H.

V<small>IBRIOSIS</small> is a disease of animals, primarily cattle and sheep, and of man, caused by *Vibrio fetus*. The disease is characterized in animals by metritis resulting in infertility and a placentitis terminating in either abortion or retained placenta. Vinzent, Dumas, and Picard[1] in 1947 first reported the isolation of a *Vibrio* similar *to V. fetus* from the blood of a woman with placentitis, who aborted. During the past four decades an ever increasing interest has centered on the etiology of abortion and sterility in herds in which no evidence of brucellosis could be detected. Many veterinarians and dairymen believed that the elimination of Bang's disease in cattle would solve the problem of abortion and sterility. Nevertheless, breeding problems similar to those caused by *Brucella* have continued in many herds and research on the etiology of such infections has revealed the causative agent to be *V. fetus*. Extensive studies, especially during the past decade, have demonstrated that the disease is widespread among cattle and sheep. Methods for its detection and treatment have been developed and epidemiologic investigations have been carried out.

HISTORY

Abortion in cattle, sheep, and goats is an old disease which prevailed prior to the Christian Era. References to abortion, particularly in ewes and "she" goats are cited in Genesis.[2] In the 19th century in Lincolnshire, England, a serious outbreak involving 7,000 lambs was reported.[3] Abortion in animals was suspected as a contagious disease long before it was definitely proven. Bang's epoch-making discovery of *Brucella abortus*[4] as the cause of contagious abortion in cattle was a marked step forward, but it has not solved the entire problem inasmuch as abortion and sterility continue to cause losses among cattle and sheep in which infections with *Brucella* can not be detected.

McFadyean and Stockman,[5] appointed by the Board of Agriculture and Fisheries to investigate epizootic abortion in England, first described *Vibrio* as a cause of abortion in sheep and cattle in 1913. They isolated the organism from ovine fetuses and reproduced the disease in pregnant cattle and ewes by intravenous inoculation. In 1918 in the United States, Theobald Smith[6] recovered *V. fetus* from aborting cattle and demonstrated it to be an important cause of bovine abortion. He confirmed the observation that *V. fetus* produced abortion in pregnant cows injected intravenously with the culture, but in addition noted that in certain animals only a placentitis resulted. In the same year, vibrionic abortion in sheep was first observed in this country by Carpenter.[7] In 1924, Welsh and Marsh[8] reported ovine abortion in Montana. Graham and Thorp[9] in Illinois in 1930, and a decade later, 1940, Ryff observed the disease in sheep in Michigan.[10] More recently it has been described in other states and the infection appears to be well disseminated throughout the sheep industry.

Since Smith's[6] first report of vibrionic abortion in cattle, other investigators have observed the disease in herds free from brucellosis. In 1920 Schroeder[11] working in the U. S. Bureau of Animal Industry, and Thomsen[12] in Denmark, each observed four cases of the disease. Gminder[13] in Germany in 1922, and Traum[14] in California one year later, reported cases. The next observation of the disease in cattle was made by Fritz and Barnes[15] in Pennsylvania. Extensive studies on vibriosis in cattle have been carried out recently by Plastridge, Williams, Easterbrooks, Walker, and Beccia[16] following their detection of the infection in Connecticut, particularly in herds free from Bang's disease.

ETIOLOGY

V. fetus, which in earlier reports was often referred to as a spirillum, is a curved rod from 1.5 to 2.0μ long and from 0.2 to 0.3μ wide. A single cell may have one or two spirals and longer forms, which are often observed in older cultures, may have several. They often appear as a number of curved rods attached as in a short chain. The organism is actively motile possessing a single polar flagellum. Smith and Taylor,[17] however, described a tuft of polar flagella on long forms. Granules are sometimes observed in older cultures. The organism is Gram-negative (Figure 29).

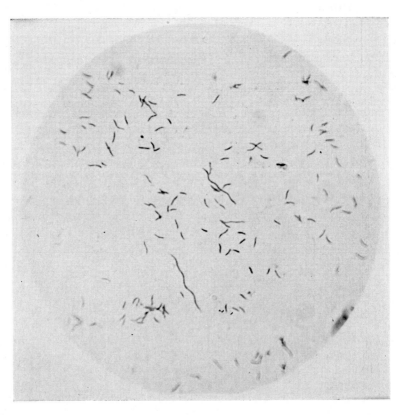

Fig. 29. *Vibrio fetus* (Bovine Strain) 2000x. (From Plastridge, *et al.: Connecticut Agricultural Experiment Station Bulletin* 281.)

Isolation of *V. fetus* presents the same general difficulties encountered in the cultivation of *Br. abortus*. It is microaerophilic, grows slowly at 37° C. on a moist enriched medium containing blood or serum. Kuzdas and Morse[17a] found the temperature range for growth of *V. fetus* to be from 15°C. to 43°C. Thus, original cultures should be incubated in a candle jar or in an atmosphere in which from 5.0—10.0 per cent of the air has been replaced by CO_2. A very fine film of growth appears on serum agar slants which is difficult to observe except by transmitted light. Often the first growth develops in the water of cineresis at the base of the slant and then grows up along the margin of the agar slant forming a white line. In certain tubes growth is observed between the agar and the glass.

Growth in a broth medium is usually scant. Reich, Dunne, Bortree, and Hokanson[18] obtained accelerated, profuse growth in broth culture by aeration with a gas mixture of 5 per cent CO_2, 35 per cent air, 10 per cent H_2, and 50 per cent He. Maintenance of stock cultures is difficult unless frequently transferred to a moist enriched agar medium. Plastridge[19] recommends the use of a semi-solid agar prepared from liver infusion broth containing 0.3 per cent agar. Transfers are carried out at intervals of from four to six weeks. After incubation at 37° C. for three days, the cultures are stored at room temperature in the dark. Huddleson[20] recommends "Thiol" (Difco) medium for cultivation of *V. fetus*. Hansen, Price, and Clements[21] also report excellent results from the use of a thioglycolate broth medium for isolation. They employ a 3 per cent agar prepared from a thioglycolate broth for cultivation of the antigen for the agglutination test.

Carbohydrates are not fermented, indole is not formed, and gelatin is not liquefied. Kiggins and Plastridge,[21a] employing standard manometric techniques, noted significant oxygen uptake only with the addition of pyruvate of all the Embden-Meyerhof substrates tested, whereas rapid oxygen uptake occurred with all members of the tricarboxylic acid cycle tested. Strains of bovine, ovine, and human origin were compared by DiLiello, Poelma, and Faber[22] and were observed to be antigenically related. Bovine strains were catalase-positive, usually H_2S negative, salt-sensitive, and produced no change in plain litmus milk. They produced an alkaline reaction with reduction in enriched litmus milk and raised the pH (8.0) of thioglycollate medium after five days incubation. Ovine and human strains were less fastidious than bovine strains, were weakly H_2S positive, and peptonized enriched litmus milk. Bryans and Smith[22a] considered hydrogen peroxide decomposition and inability to grow in a medium containing 4 per cent NaCl the two most reliable criteria for identification of pathogenic *V. fetus* strains of bovine or ovine origin. In contrast, presence or absence of H_2S production had little correlation with pathogenicity.

Lyophilization of cultures is a suitable means of preservation.

Proom and Hemmons[23] observed two lyophilized ovine strains of *V. fetus* to remain viable for years.

EPIDEMIOLOGY

Most of the information on the epidemiology of vibriosis has been obtained during the past thirty-five years and particularly during the past two decades. The disease is widespread among cattle and sheep. Its detection in England in 1913, the United States in 1918, Denmark in 1920, and Germany in 1922, was followed by reports from Australia in 1943, Sweden in 1946, South Africa in 1948, and in Holland in 1949. Positive blood tests in cattle have been reported from most states including Hawaii, and from Canada. Undoubtedly the disease was introduced into the United States with the importation of cattle from Europe.

The incidence of the disease is unknown, but present day clinical observations, together with the results of the agglutination test, and the isolation of *V. fetus* from animals indicate that the infection is far more extensive than was suspected and, furthermore, is a very important cause of abortion and sterility in cows and sheep. In England, the first record by McFadyean and Stockman[5] reported that in sheep the average abortion rate from vibrionic infection was 23.2 per cent and that 10 per cent of the sheep in infected flocks suffered from sterility. In this country some data have been obtained. Carpenter[7] observed that approximately 50 per cent of the ewes in the flock he examined either aborted or gave birth to premature lambs. Plastridge, Williams, and Petrie[24] noted that the annual abortion rate in twelve herds comprising 363 cows varied from 4.0 to 20 per cent. The average percentage of animals aborting was 12 per cent. In another herd, sixteen or 30 per cent of fifty-four cows and heifers aborted. Among 450 bovine abortions in Connecticut, Plastridge observed 44 per cent of them to be vibrionic. Twenty-three per cent were diagnosed by the isolation of *V. fetus* and 21 per cent by means of the agglutination test. In New York, Roberts, Gilman, and Larsen[25] isolated *V. fetus* from sixteen (11.5 per cent) of 139 bovine fetuses.

Leaver and Hart[26] reported that vibriosis in 1958 was diagnosed in 40 per cent of the infertility problem herds and was found to be present in all the major dairying districts of Victoria, Australia. Data on the number of cases of bovine and ovine vibriosis in the United States reported to the Agricultural Research Service, U.S. Department of Agriculture have been available since July, 1958 (Table 25). These figures reflect an awareness of the presence of vibriosis but represent only a fraction of the total incidence of the disease in domestic livestock. Abortion due to *V. fetus* has been reported in goats by Dobbs and McIntyre.[27] Trueblood and Post[28] isolated the organism from aborted fetuses of antelope, *Antilocapra americana*, in Wyoming. DiLiello, Poelma, and Faber[22] postulated swine may be a reservoir due to the similarity observed in *Vibrio* strains isolated from swine to those from cattle and sheep.

TABLE 25

Vibriosis Reported in the United States (Agricultural Research Service, United States Department of Agriculture Figures)

Year	Cases	
	Cattle	Sheep
1958 (July-Dec.)	1,344	42
1959	2,746	553
1960	1,529	2,216
1961	1,281	1,837

The natural transmission of the disease in cattle and sheep has not been completely traced. Experimentally the introduction of *V. fetus* into the genital canal readily brings about infection which is considered to be the most common mode of infection. Vibriosis may be transmitted by infected bulls and experimentally it has been demonstrated that the disease can be induced during artificial insemination with infected semen.[29,30] Experiments with oral infection have usually failed. Although it has been stated that the disease will spread from infected animals to virgin heifers in the absence of bulls, McEntee, Hughes, and Wagner[31] were unable to infect heifers by repeated exposure of the vulva to very high numbers of organisms during various stages of the estrual cycle. Experimentally, abortion and sterility have been produced both in cattle and sheep by intravenous inoculation of cultures of *V. fetus*. Calves and sexually immature animals are, in general, resistant to infection. Young sexually mature heifers are most susceptible to the infection. No special seasonal occurrence of vibriosis has been noted.

Venereal transmission is apparently not important in ovine vibriosis.[32] Frank, Bailey, and Heithecker[33] fed suspensions prepared from infected fetuses to eleven ewes bred sometime during the previous ninety days. All aborted from nine to fifty-three days after exposure with a mean incubation of nineteen days and *V. fetus* was isolated from thirteen of fifteen fetal lambs. Miller, Jensen, and Gilroy[34] found a bacteremia occurred in 65.3 per cent of forty-nine ewes in the fifth month of gestation following oral administration of a *V. fetus* culture. The bacteremia was detectable from three to fourteen days postexposure.

EXPERIMENTAL INFECTION IN LABORATORY ANIMALS

Lerche[35] reported abortion in guinea pigs following injection of *V. fetus* into the conjunctival sac, the peritoneal cavity, and into subcutaneous tissue. Later studied by Ristic and Morse[36] verified the observations. The latter authors further demonstrated the organism could be cultured from the gall bladder and uterine contents of both gravid and non-gravid guinea pigs as well as from the stomach contents of aborted fetuses. Ristic, Morse, Wipf, and Mc-Nutt[37] demonstrated *V. fetus* in the testes of male hamsters infected by intraperitoneal inoculation. These same hamsters were able to transmit the organism to female hamsters by coitus resulting in uterine infection. No reports of experimental infections in other laboratory animals were noted.

Plastridge and Williams[38] in 1943 cultivated *V. fetus* in embryonated eggs for which it was pathogenic. Studies of the pathologic lesions in the chick embryo were reported by Webster and Thorp.[39] They observed arteriolar lesions in the chorio-allantoic membrane as well as lesions in the embryo, including the cutaneous tissues, liver, kidney, spleen, gizzard, and brain.

VIBRIOSIS IN MAN

Vinzent, Dumas, and Picard,[1] in 1947, reported the isolation of *V. fetus* in a blood culture from a woman who aborted a seven month fetus. She obtained milk from a herd experiencing vibrionic abortion just prior to her illness. Since the initial report 21 additional cases of human infection due to *V. fetus* have been reported (Table 26). Although three of the first four cases reported occurred in women, of the twenty-two cases eighteen were men. The ages ranged from twenty-five to seventy-four with the following distribution: 25-29, two; 30-39, four; 40-49, five; 50-59, five; 60-69, three; 70 or older, one; and unknown, two. Regarding possible sources of infection, thirteen cases reported no known contact with animals or

TABLE 26

REPORTED CASES OF HUMAN VIBRIOSIS

	Age	Sex	Occupation	Symptoms	References
1.	39	F	Housewife	Fever, abortion 7th month, placentitis.	1, 41, 42.
2.	—	M	Laboratory worker	Pustule on cheek.	40.
3.	25	F	Midwife	Abortion 6th month, placentitis.	41, 42.
4.	26	F	Housewife	Fever 5th month pregnancy, normal fetus delivered at term, placentitis.	41, 42.
5.	47	M	Miner	Fever, paralysis.	43.
6.	31	M	Harness maker (Handled cattle from 7 to 15 yrs. of age)	Paralysis, fever.	44, 45.
7.	—	F	—	Positive blood culture only definite fact, although was thought patient suffered from ankylosing arthritis.	45.
8.	40	M	Hotel employee	Fever, phlebitis.	45.
9.	51	M	Metal worker	Fever, paralysis.	45.
10.	44	M	Warehouse worker	Fever, S.B.E.	45, 46.
11.	40	M	Abbatoir worker	Febrile illness resembling brucellosis.	47, 48.
12.	50	M	Painter (worked) on dairy 20 yrs. before)	Fever, hepatomegaly.	48.
13.	39	M	Livestock trucker	Fever, abdominal discomfort.	48.
14.	65	M	Farmer	Fever, diarrhea, splenomegaly, death.	48.
15.	58	M	Shoe repairman	Paralysis, paranoia, fever.	48.
16.	47	M	Janitor	Fever, S.B.E.	48.
17.	31	M	Abattoir worker	Fever, lymph node enlargement, blurred vision, dizzy.	48.
18.	67	M	Sheet metal worker	Thrombophlebitis, fever, cardiac arrhythmia.	49.
19.	58	M	Retired	Chronic thrombophlebitis, fever.	49.
20.	54	M	Longshoreman	Fever, malaise, thrombophlebitis.	50.
21.	68	M	Farmer	Fever.	50.
22.	74	M		Swollen knee joint, positive synovial culture.	51.

consumption of raw milk, or the information was lacking. The remaining nine cases provided the following information: ingestion of unpasteurized milk from a herd infected with vibriosis, one; laboratory exposure to the organism, one; contact with cattle several years earlier, two; farmer, two; transported livestock, one; and abattoir worker, two.

Predominant symptoms were fever, chills, malaise, and occasional headache. Others were pneumonitis with effusion and cough, sub-acute bacterial endocarditis, and thrombophlebitis. Placentitis was the outstanding feature of the disease in women. The prolonged febrile course of the disease was noteworthy, usually lasting from several weeks to several months. Weight loss and paralysis were also observed.

PATHOGENESIS

Obviously, *V. fetus* gains access to the blood stream, but it is not as yet known how or where the invasion occurs. The presence of *V. fetus* is expressed clinically by abortion which either takes place soon after implantation of the fertilized ovum or most frequently during the third, fourth, and fifth months of pregnancy. *V. fetus* localizes in the fetal membranes, particularly in the chorionic villi, causing necrosis, and also in the intercotyledonary areas in which patches of edema develop. The membranes become markedly thick-ened and present a leathery appearance. Grossly the lesions appear similar to those produced by *Br. abortus*. The placentitis, if exten-sive, terminates in abortion as a result of the damage to the fetal circulation. Many fetuses aborted early in the first trimester are expelled with intact membranes (Figure 30). Although the organism

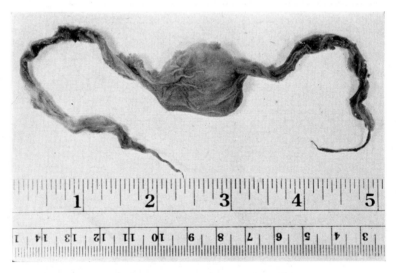

Fig. 30. Bovine fetus with intact membranes aborted fifty days after breeding. (From Plastridge, *et al.: Conn. Agri. Exp. Sta. Bull.* 281.)

is isolated from a relatively high percentage of aborted fetuses few lesions are seen except edema of the subcutaneous tissues and an excess of fluid in the thoracic and peritoneal cavities which may be blood tinged. Meconium is often present in the stomach contents.

Carpenter[7] observed that in ovine abortion macerated fetuses were often expelled with the fetal membrane intact and that the utero-chorionic space of some ewes contained a large amount of mucopuru-lent or tarry exudate. In the liver of ovine fetuses, he observed areas of necrosis from which pure cultures of *V. fetus* were recoverd. Microscopically, the lesions showed marked destruction of the hepa-tic cells and infiltration with polymorphonuclear leucocytes and round cells (Figure 31). Baker and Stone[52] and Ryff[10] reported simi-lar lesions in the liver of ovine fetuses.

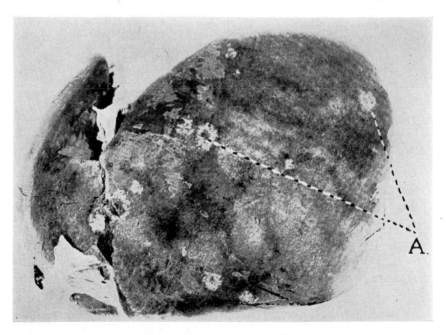

Fig. 31. Necrotic foci in liver of aborted ovine fetus from which *V. fetus* was isolated. (From Carpenter: *Cornell Vet., 9*:191, 1919.)

Subsequent to abortion, the organism may disappear from the uterus and no bacteriologic or clinical evidence of infection is ob-served. On the other hand, a mild chronic metritis may ensue if the infection persists in the genital canal, particularly in the uterus, and prevent conception. In non-pregnant cows a metritis often develops and persists from one to several months or even results in permanent sterility. Salpingitis has been reported and vaginitis has been observed in cows bred to an infected bull. Agglutinins are formed in from three to four weeks after natural infection takes place. In experimentally infected cows agglutinins may be detected as early as two weeks after intravenous inoculation. Thus, an agglutination test serves as an important diagnostic procedure.

DIAGNOSIS

Clinical. Vibriosis should be suspected in brucellosis-free herds in which abortion and sterility occur. Although abortion takes place most frequently during the third, four, and fifth months of pregnancy, it can occur at any time throughout gestation. The pattern of sterility due to *V. fetus* is one of an irregular estrus cycle and a low rate of conception. Inspection of the fetus fails to reveal lesions pathognomonic of vibriosis. Thus, an accurate diagnosis is dependent upon laboratory examinations.

Laboratory. Bacteriologic examinations are carried out employing both films and cultures. *V. fetus* can be detected most often in films prepared from amniotic fluid, placental tissue, and from stomach contents of the fetus. They may be air dried or fixed with gentle heating and stained with Giemsa's stain or with dilute fuchsin. Direct examination of fresh material by darkfield microscopy readily demonstrates the vibrios. Fetal stomach content is the best material for cultures if the cultures are made within a few hours after abortion. If the bacteriologic examination is delayed, proper refrigeration of the fetus is essential in order to prevent contamination and decomposition. Freezing is not harmful to *V. fetus*. Positive cultures are frequently obtained from the fetal lung and the heart's blood. The amniotic fluid should be cultured when available on fetuses expelled with intact membranes. Cultures should also be made from placental tissue, uterine, cervical, and vaginal exudates. Semen may be cultured from bulls if collected in a sterile artificial vagina after special cleansing of the bull's sheath to avoid contamination. Routine cultures for *V. fetus* should be made on blood agar plates and on a thiol broth medium, "Difco," and incubated at 37° C. as previously described. By direct microscopic examination of films Plastridge, Williams, Easterbrooks, Walker, and Beccia[16] detected *V. fetus* in 97 or 65 per cent of 148 specimens. By culturing the same specimens on blood agar they isolated *V. fetus* in 105 or 71 per cent.

Serology. The agglutination test for vibriosis in cattle and sheep is a helpful procedure for detecting infection. Blood for the agglutination test is collected by the same technique employed in brucellosis. Blood should not be tested for two weeks following abortion, however. Serum dilutions of 1:25, 1:50, 1:100, and 1:200 are made in 2.0 ml. of a dependable antigen prepared from *V. fetus*. The tests are read after incubation at 37° C. for forty-eight hours. Inasmuch as the antigen contains both O and H agglutinins and because the blood serum from normal cows contains O agglutinins, agglutination in serum dilutions of 1:25 is considered negative. Agglutination at 1:50 or higher is interpreted as a positive reaction. Some laboratories recommend serum dilutions of 1:100, 1:200, 1:400, and 1:800, and consider that only agglutination of 1:200 or higher is significant. Evidently the quality of the antigen is a most important factor and control tests with positive and negative sera should be carefully observed.

A modification of the agglutination test has been described by Stegenga and Terpstra[53] and designated the "vaginal mucus test" because the agglutinins for *V. fetus* are present in the vaginal mucus of infected cows. The mucus is collected from the vagina with a special pipette and then diluted with sixteen parts of physiologic salt solution. After centrifugation the supernatant fluid is removed and diluted in the antigen in the same manner as serum is employed in a standard agglutination test. Szabo[54] recommended a tampon for collecting the vaginal mucus, a method originated by A. Jepsen and T. Vindekilde of the Royal Veterinary and Agricultural College, Copenhagen, Denmark. The mucus is expressed from the tampon, similarly diluted with physiologic saline solution, centrifuged, and tested for agglutinins as above. Plastridge, Williams, Easterbrooks, Walter, and Beccia[16] have shown that agglutinins for *V. fetus* appear in the blood serum before they may be detected in the vaginal mucus. On the other hand, they may disappear from the blood serum within a few weeks after formation, yet persist in the vaginal mucus for long periods of time.

PREVENTION AND CONTROL

Vibriosis in cattle may be prevented, in general, by the same procedures employed in brucellosis. Good herd sanitation should be practiced. Agglutination tests should be carried out on all sexually-mature males and females added to a vibriosis-free herd. In addition, the vaginal mucus test should be made on the females. A vibriosis-free herd can best avoid infection by raising its own young stock, rather than purchase animals for replacements. Easterbrooks[55] has recommended that in artificial insemination with semen from an infected bull, 500 micrograms of streptomycin be added to each ml. of diluted semen to prevent infection with *V. fetus*. Prophylactic vaccination of heifers with living cultures of *V. fetus* has been investigated,[16] but as yet, insufficient data are available to reliably evaluate its efficacy. An avianized vaccine prepared from *V. fetus* by Osborne[56] has been shown to be agglutinogenic and to provide some protection to a group of experimentally infected heifers.

Elimination of the disease in a herd is dependent upon serologic tests to detect infected animals, following which they should either be isolated from non-infected animals or be removed from the herd. Bacteriologic examinations should be made on placentae and fetuses from aborting cattle and on uterine exudates from sterile animals.

TREATMENT

Non-pregnant, infected cows, as well as animals that have recently aborted should be treated with intrauterine infusions of antibiotics. Chlortetracycline, penicillin, streptomycin, and oxytetracycline have been observed to be effective, particularly in eliminating infection in cows that fail to conceive. Easterbrooks and Plastridge[57] have used successfully 1.0 gm. of streptomycin in 15 ml. of water *in utero* at the time of estrus, followed by breeding at the next estral period. McAuliff[58] recommended the intrauterine injection of 30 ml. of water containing 1.0 gm. of aqueous streptomycin from six to eight hours prior to breeding. McEntee, Hughes, and Gilman[59] reported that a combination of penicillin, streptomycin, and sulanilamide added to semen extender prevented infection in heifers inseminated with contaminated semen. Lank, Seger, and Levy[60] reported intramuscular injections of dihydrostreptomycin sulfate to be successful in eliminating infection in bulls. Ryff and Breen[61] observed streptomycin or oxytetracycline given intramuscularly, and sulfabromo-methazine or oxytetracycline given orally provided some reduction in per cent of abortions during ovine vibriosis epizootics. Inasmuch as vibriosis suddenly appears in a herd of cattle or sheep and then spontaneously disappears within a few months, evaluation of therapy requires experience and a long observation period.

Chloramphenicol, chlortetracycline, and a combination of dihydrostreptomycin and tetracycline were found effective in human infections whereas penicillin failed to be of benefit.

ITEMS OF NOTE

1) Vibriosis is a communicable disease of cattle and sheep caused by *Vibrio fetus*. Twenty-two human infections have been reported, eight in France and the remainder in the United States. Four cases were in women. Placentitis and abortion with fever were the predominant symptoms.

2) The disease is widely disseminated among cattle and sheep in the United States, Great Britain, Scandinavia, Central Europe, and in Australia.

3) *V. fetus* causes abortion, retained placenta, metritis, salpingitis, and vaginitis. Sterility in cattle is also a conspicuous sign of the disease. In sheep, abortion is the outstanding manifestation.

4) Vibriosis is suspected in herds in which abortion and sterility occur in the absence of brucellosis. A specific diagnosis is made by the agglutination test and batceriologic examination of uterine exudates, fetal membranes, and fetal tissues.

5) The mode of transmission of the disease appears to be different in cattle and sheep. Venereal transmission is the main factor in cattle. Ingestion of the organism plays the major role in the latter. How the infection is transmitted to man is not well understood.

6) The control of the disease is dependent upon the introduction of only non-infected animals into vibriosis-free herds. The disease is eliminated from herds by detecting infected animals by means of serologic and bacteriologic tests and by their subsequent isolation or removal.

7) Intrauterine therapy with antibiotics, especially streptomycin, is effective in eliminating *V. fetus* from the genital canal, thereby overcoming sterility and preventing infection that might result in

abortion. Limited research with prophylactic vaccination indicates it may have possible value.

REFERENCES

1. VINZENT, R., DUMAS, J., and PICARD, N.: *Bull. Acad. Nat. Med., 131*:90-92, 1947.
2. *Genesis, XXXI*:38.
3. AXE, J. W.: *J. Roy. Agric. Soc. England,* 2nd series, *21*:199-206, 1885.
4. BANG, B.: *Ztschr. Tiermed., 1*:241, 1897.
5. MCFADYEAN, F. and STOCKMAN, S.: *Report of the Departmental Committee Appointed by the Board of Agriculture and Fisheries to Inquire into Epizootic Abortion,* London, 1913.
6. SMITH, T.: *J. Exper. Med., 28*:701-719, 1918.
7. CARPENTER, C. M.: *Cornell Vet., IX*:191-203, 1919.
8. WELSH, H. and MARSH, H.: *J.A.V.M.A., 65*:203-210, 1924.
9. GRAHAM, R. and THORP, F.: *J.A.V.M.A., 76*:568-573, 1930.
10. RYFF, J. F.: *J.A.V.M.A., 97*:452-453, 1940.
11. SCHROEDER, E. C.: *J.A.V.M.A., 57*:270-281, 1920.
12. THOMSEN, A.: *S. Maanedssdr. Dyrlaeg, 32*:1-9, 1920.
13. GMINDER, A.: Cited by Smith 1923. Original in *Berl. tierärztt. Woch., 38*:184, 1922.
14. TRAUM, J.: *California Agr. Exp. Station Bull.,* 353, 1923.
15. FRITZ, B. S. and BARNES, M. F.: *J.A.V.M.A., 87*:542-558, 1935.
16. PLASTRIDGE, W. N., WILLIAMS, L. F., EASTERBROOKS, H. L., WALKER, E. C., and BECCIA, R. N.: *Storrs Agr. Exper. Station, Bull.,* 281, 1951.
17. SMITH, T. and TAYLOR, M. S.: *J. Exper. Med., 30*:299-312, 1919.
17a. KUZDAS, C. D., and MORSE, E. V.: *Am. J. Vet. Res., 17*:331-336, 1956.
18. REICH, C. V., DUNNE, H. W., BORTREE, A. L., and HOKANSON, J. F.: *J. Bact., 74*:246-250, 1957.
19. PLASTRIDGE, W. N.: *J. Bact., 42*:816-817, 1941.
20. HUDDLESON, I. F.: *J. Bact., 56*:508, 1948.
21. HANSEN, P. A., PRICE, K. E., and CLEMENTS, M. F.: *J. Bact., 64*:5, 1952.
21a. KIGGINS, E. M., and PLASTRIDGE, W. N.: *J. Bact. 75*:205-208, 1958.
22. DILIELLO, L. R., POELMA, L. J., and FABER, J. E.: *Am. J. Vet. Res., 20*:532-536, 1959.
22a. BRYANS, J. T., and SMITH, A. G.: *Cornell Vet., 50*:331-338, 1960.
23. PROOM, H. and HEMMONS, L. M.: 1949. Cited by Levi, M. L., 1950.
24. PLASTRIDGE, W. N., WILLIAMS, L. F. and PETRIE, D.: *Am. J. Vet. Res., 8*:178-183, 1947.
25. ROBERTS, S. J., GILMAN, H. L. and LARSEN, P. H.: *Cornell Vet., 40*:111-124, 1950.
26. LEAVER, D. D., and HART, I. H.: *Australian Vet. J., 36*:460-465, 1960.
27. DOBBS, E. M., and MCINTYRE, R. W.: *Calif. Vet., 4*:19, 1951.
28. TRUEBLOOD, M. S., and POST, G.: *J.A.V.M.A., 134*:562-564, 1959.
29. EASTERBROOKS, H. L. and PLASTRIDGE, W. N.: *J.A.V.M.A., 120*:199-201, 1952.
30. MCENTEE, K., HUGHES, D. E., and GILMAN, H. L.: *Cornell Vet., 44*:376-384, 1954.
31. MCENTEE, K., HUGHES, D. E., and WAGNER, W. C.: *Cornell Vet., 49*:34-40, 1959.
32. FIREHAMMER, B. D., MARSH, H., and TUNNICLIFF, E. A.: *Am. J. Vet. Res., 17*:573-581, 1956.
33. FRANK, F. W., BAILEY, J. W., and HEITHECKER, D.: *J.A.V.M.A., 131*:472-473, 1957.
34. MILLER, V. A., JENSEN, R., and GILROY, J. J.: *Am. J. Vet. Res., 20*:677-679, 1959.
35. LERCHE: *Deutsch. tierarztl. Woch., 30*:484-487, 1927.
36. RISTIC, M., and MORSE, E. V.: *Am. J. Vet. Res., 14*:399-404, 1953.

37. RISTIC, M., MORSE, E. V., WIPF, L. and McNUTT, S. H.: *Am. J. Vet. Res., 15:*309-313, 1954.
38. PLASTRIDGE, W. N. and WILLIAMS, L. F.: *J.A.V.M.A., 102:*89-95, 1943.
39. WEBSTER, H. D., and THORP, F., JR.: *Am. J. Vet. Res., 14:*118-122, 1953.
40. WARD, B. Q.: *J. Bact., 55:*113-114, 1948.
41. VINZENT, R.: *Presse med., 57:*1230-1232, 1949.
42. VINZENT, R., DELAURE, J., and HEBERT, H.: *Ann. de med., 51:*23-68, 1950.
43. AUGUSTE, C., BUTTIAUX, R., and TACQUET, A.: *Arch. mal. app. digest., 43:*861-864, 1954.
44. WEISMANN-HETTER, R., THIBAULT, P., ROBERT-LEVY, and SECOND, L.: *Bull. et mem. Soc. med. Hop. Paris, 70:*835-844, 1954.
45. THIBAULT, P., GAILLARD, J., SECOND, L., and CHATELAIN, R.: *Bull. Acad. nat. med., 139:*95-99, 1955.
46. AUGUIER, L., CHRETIEN, J., and HODARA, M.: *Bull. et mem. Soc. med. d. hop. de Paris, 72:*580, 1956.
47. SPINK, W. W.: *J.A.M.A., 163:*180-182, 1957.
48. KING, E. O.: *J. Infect. Dis., 101:*119-128, 1957.
49. KAHLER, R. L., and SHLEDON, H.: *New England J. Med., 262:*1218-1222, 1960.
50. JACKSON, J. F., HINTON, P., and ALLISON, F., JR.: *Am. J. Med., 28:*986-994, 1960.
51. KING, S., and BRONSKY, D.: *J.A.M.A., 175:*1045-1048, 1961.
52. BAKER, D. W. and STONE, W. S.: *Cornell Vet., XXIX:*32-34, 1939.
53. STEGENGA, T. and TERPSTRA, L. I.: *Tijdschr. v. Diergeneesk, 74:*293, 1949.
54. SZABO, L.: *S. Nord. Vet. Med., 3:*597-608, 1951.
55. EASTERBROOKS, H. L.: *Fertility and Sterility, 2:*430-443, 1951.
56. OSBORNE, J. C.: Proc. Book. *Am. Vet. Med. A.,* 1952, pp. 112-116.
57. EASTERBROOKS, H. L. and PLASTRIDGE, W. N.: *J.A.V.M.A., 117:*388, 1950.
58. McAULIFF, J. L.: *Vet. News, 14:*9-12, 1951.
59. McENTEE, K., HUGHES, D. E., and GILMAN, H. L.: *Cornell Vet., 44:*395-402, 1954.
60. LANK, R. B., SEGER, C. L., and LEVY, H. E.: *J.A.V.M.A., 139:*1316-1318, 1961.
61. RYFF, J. F., and BREEN, H.: *J.A.V.M.A., 139:*665-668, 1961.

Chapter 5

SWINE ERYSIPELAS

Erskine V. Morse, D.V.M., Ph.D.

Swine erysipelas is a communicable disease of hogs caused by *Erysipelothrix insidiosa*. The infection also occurs in a variety of animals, and in birds. Man is relatively resistant, particularly when the organism enters through the gastrointestinal tract. In man it occurs in a cutaneous form and as an acute septicemia. The cutaneous form is referred to as "erysipeloid." Erysipelas in man is caused by streptococci.

HISTORY

Swine erysipelas probably has existed in Europe for many years, but it was confused with hog cholera and its history is not clear. It is said that it was first differentiated as a specific disease in France about 1846. Cartwright in England in 1847 described its chronic form without knowing its true nature. Baker in 1873 published in St. Bartholomew's Hospital Reports an accurate clinical picture of the disease in man. Loeffler in 1882 isolated the causative agent of the disease which he designated as "Bacillus des Schweinerotlaufs." Pasteur in 1883 developed a vaccine for immunizing purposes by passing the organism through rabbits and then making broth cultures. Rosenbach in Germany in 1884 contributed much to the clinical and bacteriologic knowledge of the disease, hence the name for the infection in man, "Rosenbach's erysipeloid." Bang in 1888 and MacFadyean in 1891 found the organism in chronic heart lesions of hogs.

PREVALENCE

The disease is prevalent in Europe, where it is known as "rouget" in France, "rotlauf" in Germany, and "erysipelas" in England. It exists to a considerable extent in Austria, Denmark, Russia, Hungary, and other countries. In England, in 1905, in a small strip of country four miles long by one mile broad, the disease attacked most of the hogs with 80 per cent mortality.

In the United States the existence of the disease had been suspected for many years. As early as 1885 Smith isolated from hogs dead of hog cholera the closely allied mouse septicemia organism of Koch which has been confused with the swine erysipelas organism. Other investigators had similar experiences. In 1920 Ten Broeck found organisms of this group in pigs dead of hog cholera, but failed to differentiate between the two species. It was generally believed therefore that swine erysipelas did not exist in the United States. In 1921, Creech definitely established the fact that the disease did exist in the United States by isolating *Erysipelothrix insidiosa* from several hogs which showed typical symptoms of "diamond skin disease." Klauder, in 1926, again called attention to the disease. In 1930, there was an outbreak in South Dakota, since then swine erysipelas has been receiving more and more attention.

Siebold and Neal as well as Simpson, Wood and Young isolated *Ery. insidiosa* from captive porpoises (dolphins, *Tursiops truncatus* and *Stenella plagiodon*). The first authors described the condition as a septicemia, while the second authors reported the condition to be primarily cutaneous in nature.

THE ETIOLOGIC AGENT

Erysipelothrix insidiosa (Erysipelothrix rhusiopathiae, Bacillus erysipelatous suis, Bacillus rhusiopathiae) is classified by Breed *et al.* among bacteria of the order of *Eubacteriales*. The organism is 0.2 to 0.4 microns wide by 1 to 1.5 microns long, appears as a straight or slightly curved rod (Figure 32). It is not motile and does not form spores. It is easily cultivated on the ordinary laboratory media, aerobically as well as anaerobically, and is gram positive. Long threadlike forms may be seen in old cultures. Smooth (S) and rough (R) forms exist.

The organism is destroyed quickly by boiling water and within a few minutes by the usual disinfectants. The organism is quite resistant to phenol. It is very resistant to drying, in which state it will remain alive in the dark for a month or more, and in the sunlight for ten to twelve days. In salted or pickled meats it will remain alive for three or four months and in putrid material it is capable of retaining its viability and virulence for months.

The organism is widely disseminated, its habitat being dead matter of plant or animal origin. In certain environments it exists in the soil as a saprophyte while it retains virulence. In addition to this source of infection, infection carriers may be found among healthy hogs in erysipelas territory. The organism has been recovered from the slime of fish, from house flies and from putrefying horseflesh. *Erysipelothrix insidiosa* is not the cause of any known disease of fish. A more likely explanation of fish source of human infection is the

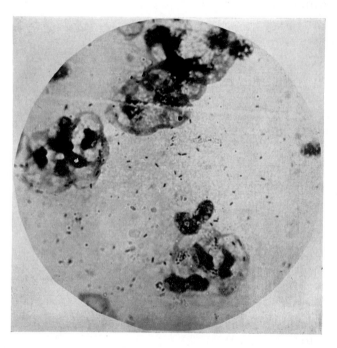

Fig. 32. *Erysipelothrix insidiosa* (bacillus of swine erysipelas) in smear of heart blood from inoculated pigeon. Phagocytoses should be noted. Carbol fuchsin stain; magnification, 1200 times (Klauder).

apparent attraction of slime for the organism. Decaying matter and refuse thrown in the water may serve as a source of the bacterium.

Three strains of *Erysipelothrix insidiosa*—the human, the swine and mouse, have been reported previously. All appear to be variants of a common strain, if not identical.

When the swine erysipelas organism is injected immediately after isolation it is sometimes, but not always, virulent for hogs; when it has grown on artificial culture media for any length of time, or after it has been passed through some of the experimental animals, it loses its virulence and fails to cause disease when injected into pigs. Kolda found that when pure bile was used as a culture medium the virulence *Erysipelothrix insidiosa* was not decreased over a series of transplants, but when bile was mixed with other culture ingredients the virulence diminished. Virulence was decreased as reported by Mantovani when malachite green was added to culture media and, according to Vallée when gonacrine was added. The virulence is increased by passage through pigeons and decreased by passage through rabbits for certain hosts.

THE DISEASE IN ANIMALS

The disease is essentially an affection of swine. The white mouse and the pigeon are very susceptible to artificial injection, dying within three to five days; the rabbit is suscpetible to experimental inoculation, requiring a large amount of virulent culture intravenously to kill it; the guinea pig and the field mouse are immune, as are cattle, dogs, and cats. The horse is supposed to be resistant but there have been reports of human infection among veterinary students dissecting a horse. Christiansen reported an epidemic with high mortality among lambs, due to the organism. At the time of the outbreak there were no sick hogs in the vicinity. Poels found the organism in erysipelas of sheep. Schipp, in 1910, isolated from chickens suffering from enteritis, organisms which could not be distinguished from the swine erysipelas bacillus. Broll, in 1911, recorded an outbreak in which all the fowls in one flock succumbed within a few weeks to this organism.

Pfaff found chickens two to three months old fairly resistant to infection, but in chickens one to three weeks old, the rotlauf bacillus in pure culture caused an epidemic lasting two to five weeks. Jarosch described the organism as the cause of the disease in turkeys, and Poels in the pigeon and fowl. Beaudette and Hudson described epidemics of the disease in turkeys. Rosenwald and Dickinson observed that a swollen, turgid, purplish red caruncle was the most pathognomonic symptom of naturally occurring *Erysipelothrix indisiosa* infection in turkeys (Figure 33). Stiles isolated *Erysipelothrix indisiosa* from a brown rat caught on a dump near a stockyard. Such recovery was also reported by Drake and Hall.

The disease in hogs occurs mostly in animals four to eight months old; young pigs under three months of age are fairly resistant as are also old hogs. This is only a relative immunity, however, and such animals become infected on some occasions.

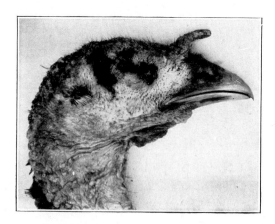

Fig. 33. A swollen turgid purplish red caruncle is the most pathognomonic symptom of naturally occurring *Ery. insidiosa* infection in turkeys (supplied by A. S. Rosenwald and E. M. Dickinson).

The infection in swine is manifested in three forms: a severe, or septicemic form, characterized by constitutional symptoms of septicemia, presence of diffuse areas of erythema and at times vesicles, petechiae and necrosis; a mild form (urticarial form, or "diamond skin" disease), characterized by mild constitutional symptoms and presence of sharply circumscribed quadrangular lesions on the skin, and a chronic form, characterized by polyarthritis and at times by symptoms referable to a vegetative type of endocarditis.

Septicemic Form

In the septicemic form the eruption appears on or about the second or third day of sickness. The animal is obviously sick with high fever. Irregularly shaped patches of erythema (Figure 34) appear, favoring the following regions: ears, snout, axillas, lower surfaces of the thorax and abdomen, inner surfaces of the thighs, groins and perianal region. The surfaces of the erythematous patches may be studded with vesicles. The involved areas are not tender, and the erythema disappears on pressure. At the onset the color is pink or light red; later it is bright red, dark red or purple. The purple color compares with the characteristic purple of the localized cutaneous form of infection (erysipeloid of Rosenbach) in man. In swine the lesions, which are ill defined, may remain localized, but more likely they enlarge and become confluent, affecting the greater part of the

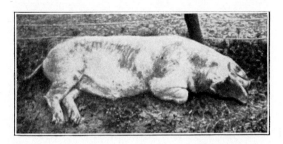

Fig. 34. Irregular shaped patches of erythema in the septicemic form of *Ery. insidiosa* infection (supplied by L. Van Es, Department of Animal Pathology, University of Nebraska, Lincoln, Neb).

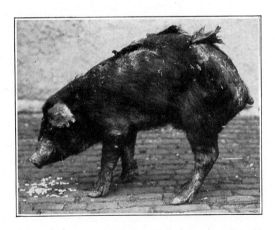

Fig. 35. Sequestration of skin, tail and part of ear after necrosis following septicemic form of infection (from G. L. Dunlap and R. Graham: Swine Erysipelas, Circular 471, University of Illinois, College of Agriculture, 1937).

cutaneous surface. In some cases the erythematous eruption is followed by an outbreak of petechiae. As a complication localized or extensive areas of necrosis—a dry form of gangrene—appear, in which event the dead skin is stiff and leather-like and later is sequestrated. This process may involve the entire back. The ears and tail may be lost through necrosis (Figure 35). If the animal does not die of sepsis or other complication, necrotic areas become cicatrized.

Moussu mentioned the occurrence of a hematoma-like swelling of the ears, violaceous in color, which undergoes necrosis (Figure 36).

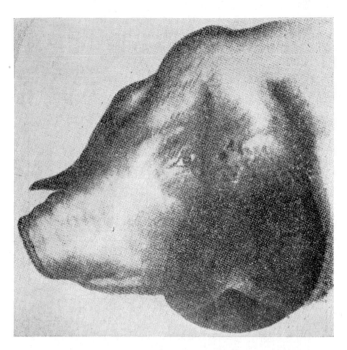

Fig. 36. Showing hematoma-like swelling of the ears, violaceous in color, which undergoes necrosis in the septicemic form of infection. (From Moussu, G.: *Maladies du porc.* Paris, Vigot Freres, 1931.)

Mild, or Urticarial, Form ("Diamond Skin" Disease)

The eruption in this form is unlike that in the severe or septicemic form. Constitutional symptoms are mild and according to Van Es and McGrath rapidly improve after the appearance of the eruption. Cutaneous lesions may go unnoticed until the animal is slaughtered, scalded and cleaned. The eruption is characterized by the appearance of a few to a hundred or more variously shaped lesions that may form bizarre designs (Figure 37). The eruption is generally described as consisting of raised wheals. Wheals are early lesions which through central clearing and peripheral extension form irregularly shaped macules, which regress and leave scaly bor-

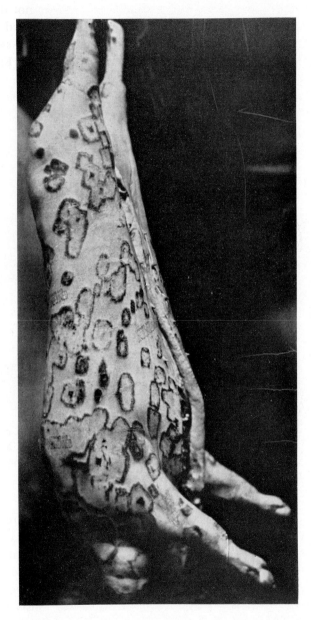

Fig. 37. An eruption of "diamond skin" disease, presenting the curious pattern of eruption peculiar to this disease. (Supplied by the Bureau of Animal Industry, United States Department of Agriculture, Washington, D. C.)

ders. The wheals are raised, variously shaped and slightly edematous. Other early lesions are spots and ill defined blotches. The color in the early eruptive stage is bright red or pink, later becoming dark red, purplish red and brownish red in the regressing stage. The shade of red of some lesions is not uniform throughout. Klauder (1944) has observed the center to be darker than the periphery. Apparently through central clearing, extension and joining of lesions, a pattern is produced the conformation of which is remarkable and unique among disease of the skin, both in man and in animals. Although the disease is called "diamond skin" disease, rhomboidal configuration (Figure 38) is not always conspicuous and at times is

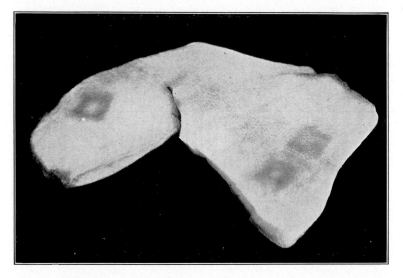

Fig. 38. Rhomboidal lesion which gives rise to the name "diamond skin" disease (Klauder).

absent. Quadrangular, rectangular and oblong lesions are common and may join in such manner to form a steplike pattern. The bizarre designs that the eruption may present sometimes show square lesions containing a smaller square concentrically or eccentrically placed and circinate, oval or square lesions with a central discoid lesion (bull's eye) (Figure 37).

The lesions vary from about 2 to about 8 cm. in diameter. They are artificial in appearance, as though produced by a brand or as if stuck on the skin (Figure 37).

The final stage of the eruption may be presented as desquamation, usually at the periphery, and as dark brown adherent crusts.

Chronic Form

The chronic form usually is subsequent to a previous mild attack of the disease and is characterized by polyarthritis and vegetative endocarditis. There is first noticed an increased respiration with sometimes a cough, followed in a day or two by discoloration beginning at the tops of the ears and spreading along the ventral surface of the body. Death results in one to two weeks.

Infection is spread from hog to hog directly. Ingestion is the common route of infection. A considerable number of animals may be "carriers" harboring the organisms either in the intestinal tract or throat. Ten Broeck isolated such bacilli from the tonsils of five out of sixteen pigs examined. Other workers in Europe previously had had similar experiences. Bauermeister in 1901 isolated the organism from the tonsils of five normal hogs out of sixteen examined; Van Velzen in 1907 found it in the tonsils of three out of elevent pigs examined; Pitt found it in 56 per cent of tonsils of fifty hogs, and in 40 per cent of glands of the ileocecal valve of sixty-six hogs.

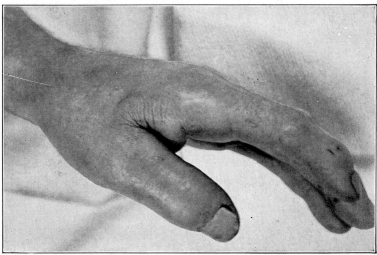

Klauder

Fig. 39. Human infection with the organism of swine erysipelas (Klauder).

THE DISEASE IN MAN

The infection in man may be found in the following three forms: 1) a mild, rather localized, cutaneous infection, which may be accompanied by mild arthritic symptoms, usually involving the fingers (Figures 39 and 40); 2) a diffuse or generalized cutaneous erup-

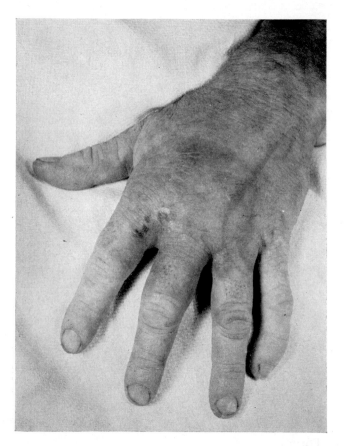

Fig. 40. Showing sharply marginated erythema and vesicles which were hemorrhagic (on index finger adjacent to site of inoculation). The patient was an abattoir worker who cut his hand when cutting products of swine (Klauder).

tion, with arthritic and constitutional symptoms and negative blood culture (Figure 41); and 3) a septicemic form with endocarditis, positive blood culture, and with or without cutaneous lesions (Figures 42 and 43). In addition arthritis (Düttman, Brind, and Wüthrich), meningitis (Dumont and Cotoni) and intracranial abscess (Torkild-sen) have been attributed to the infection.

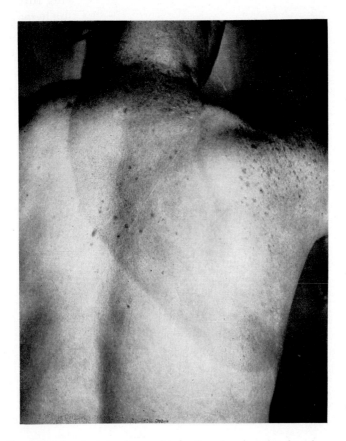

Fig. 41. Generalized cutaneous form of infection showing the sharply marginated advancing border. Wave-like areas of erythema would appear and disappear (Klauder).

Localized Form (Erysipeloid of Rosenbach)

The eruption occurs at the site of inoculation, usually the hand, and is invariably caused by injury, which may be trivial. The disease arose out of occupation in 88 of 100 cases which Klauder (1938) reported. The source of infection of these 100 patients is found in their occupation, as shown in Table 27. There was a history of injury at the site at which the infection first appeared in all but five in this series.

TABLE 27

SOURCE OF INFECTION, OR OCCUPATION, OF 100 PATIENTS WITH ERYSIPELOID*

Occupation and Remarks	Cases
Abattoir	58
Fish, retail	11
Tallow, grease, fertilizer	7
Veterinary students (dissecting horse)	6
Butchers, retail	3
Fishermen, pleasure	3
Bakers (lard)	2
Clam Opener	1
Food handler	1
Furrier (unfinished pelt)	1
Rabbit (removing skin)	1
Opossum (carry animal)	1
Weaver	1
Dressmaker	1
Housewife (cleaning fish)	1
Fish (handling)	1
Kitchen worker	1

*88 of these patients were infected through injury in the course of employment and were claimants under workmen's compensation laws.

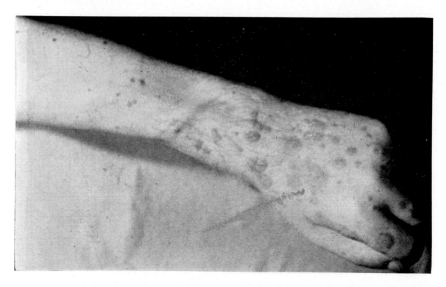

Fig. 42. Purpuric spots and purplish disciform lesions in the septicemic form of infection (Klauder, Kramer and Nicholas).

"Blubber finger," "sealers finger," or "speckfinger" is an erysipeloid condition observed as an occupational disease of persons engaged in the dressing of seals. Workers in Scandanavian countries,

Alaska and adjacent areas have been affected. The exact etiological agent has not been delineated according to Svenkerud, Rosted and Thorshaug. It has been suggested that *Ery. insidiosa* may be at least one cause.

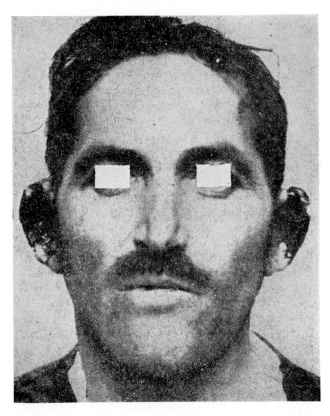

Fig. 43. Auricular involvement in the septicemic form of infection. At onset the ears were swollen, purplish red and painful, resembling traumatic hematoma. Later part of the ears became necrotic and sequestrated as shown in the illustration. (From Fiessinger, N. and Brouet, G.: *Présse méd., 42:*889-892, 1934.)

The incubation period of erysipeloid is from one to three days. The disease is of variable severity, with or without localized arthritic or constitutional symptoms. The first symptoms is pain at the site of inoculation, followed by swelling and erythema (Figures 39 and 40). The most distinctive feature of the disease, of considerable diagnostic import, is the purplish red color of the erythema. The erythema slowly progresses, producing another distinctive feature, a sharply defined, slightly elevated zone, which extends peripherally as the central portion fades away. The involved area is swollen and tense, as though fluid had been injected intracutaneously. If the finger is involved, the swelling and tenseness make movement difficult. At times one or a few vesicles which may be hemorrhagic may occur early at site of the erythema (Figure 40).

Another characteristic of the disease is its migratory nature: new purplish red patches appear at remote areas. If the infection originally involved one finger, eventually all the fingers and the dorsum of the hand, or the palm, or both may become affected, the erythema appearing and disappearing, or extension may take place by continuity. The disease may completely disappear at the areas first involved, at the time when other areas are affected. The disease involutes without desquamation.

The appearance is not that of a pyogenic infection, with which the condition is frequently confused. The color of the erythema is different, there is no pitting on pressure, and suppuration never occurs. Although itching and tingling are frequently present, pain is the most conspicuous subjective symptom. It is throbbing and burning in character, often preventing sleep.

The mildness or severity of the infection usually suggests its source, which, in turn, governs the virulence of the organism. In the studies of Klauder, Righter and Harkins (1926) infection was more severe when contracted from a fish source. The virulence of the organism isolated from this source was greater than that isolated from sources as shown in the studies of Klauder and Harkins (1931).

At times, fever, mild constitutional symptoms, lymphangitis, and adenitis occur. Stiffness of the joints of the involved finger is a common symptoms of erysipeloid. Such stiffness cannot be attributed entirely to the tenseness of the swollen finger, since it persists after the swelling disappears. Sometimes, there is an associated dull pain in the finger joints, as well as in the wrist, the elbow and even the shoulder. Arthritic symptoms may persist after the skin becomes normal. Klauder observed these symptoms to persist for as long as eight months.

Erysipeloid invariably spreads only on the hand. Extension above the wrist is unusual. The disease tends towards spontaneous retrogression. In the 100 patients which Klauder reported (1938), the duration of the disease, for the majority, was about three weeks.

Infection with erysipeloid confers no immunity, since second attacks occur. This is, perhaps, consistent with inconstant result of agglutination tests conducted with the serum of patients with erysipeloid. In Klauder's experience, such a test is unreliable as a diagnostic aid in the localized form of the disease. Others (Stiles, Ehrlich, Ingram and Stuart) have found it of diagnostic value in severe generalized form of infection.

In the United States Klauder (1926) observed that the disease was widespread among commercial fishermen along the Atlantic coast from Maine to Florida. The affliction is called "fish poisoning." It is thought that possibly the organisms are already on the hands and other parts of the body from the mud and slime in which fishermen work, and that injury to the skin makes infection possible. A similar circumstance applies to the infection among abattoir workers whose hands are contaminated from infected swine. Fishermen in fresh waters are less subject to the disease but infection from this source occurs.

Sheard and Dicks reported the disease among fishermen and processors of crayfish in Western Australia. Lawson encountered an epidemic of 210 cases among employees of a button factory where cattle bones were utilized.

Diffuse or Generalized Eruption

The eruption, as later discussed, is variably manifested and may have certain morphologic features that compare with the mild form of infection in swine. Cases of this type of eruption comprise cases in which the eruption progressed from the site of inoculation, becoming diffuse or generalized, or appeared at areas remote from the site of inoculation. Such cases have been notably reported by Sieben, Domrich, Richter, Gottron, Schreiner, Chevallier and co-workers, Schölzke, Natusch, Krieger, Habersang, and Ehrlich. The majority of these patients had constitutional symptoms of variable severity with fever. In addition some had articular pains. The duration of the infection (including recurrences) was variable, in some patients, months. Blood culture (if made) was negative, and recovery ensued in all.

Klauder (1934) reported the case of a man who had at the onset a typical erysipeloid of one finger from a fish as the source of infection. The entire finger became involved, and the infection spread across the dorsum of the hand, affecting all the fingers and eventually the palm. About five months from the onset the infection spread beyond the wrist and gradually involved the skin of the forearm and arm. The infection continued to spread until at the end of a year it had extended over the cutaneous surface from scalp to soles, exempting only the genitalia. At no time, however, was the entire cutaneous surface involved; the extension was wavelike, with the advancing border always sharply marginated, appearing as a red or pink band or erythema (Figure 41). The skin posterior to the advancing border gradually became normal. At times the border showed finger-like projections. In addition, large circinate and oval lesions with clear centers would appear and disappear at varying periods over the entire body.

There were cutaneous relapses which were without subjective symptoms and which would regress without desquamation. There were constitutional symptoms, polyarthritis, and negative blood culture. *Ery. insidiosa* was recovered from two different cutaneous lesions and at different intervals. All treatment was without avail. The patient was partially incapacitated, became depressed and committed suicide twenty-nine months after the onset of the infection.

In the case reported by Richter and by Domrich and in one case by Natusch's review, the eruption was presented as bandlike areas of erythema which progressed in wavelike fashion over the arms and back. In Domrich's patient the eruption spread over the entire body. The illustration in his paper showing five wavelike bands of erythema was similar to that of the eruption in Klauder's patient (Figure 41).

The eruption in the patient reported on by Chevallier and his co-authors comprised large violaceous patches with irregular margins on the extremities and trunk. The surfaces of some of the patches were covered with vesicles. The lesions regressed with desquamation.

In Sieben's patient the eruption at its onset on the back comprised red spots with a papule in the center. These lesions enlarged, becoming confluent. The centers of the patches were scarlet red and were sharply marginated from the pale red discoloration toward the periphery. Other patches appeared scattered over the trunk and extremities. There were two bluish red spots on the forehead, their surfaces covered with vesicles.

Krieger (a veterinarian) reported the case of his own infection. His thigh was accidentally punctured with a needle containing pure culture of *Ery. insidiosa*. The following day the site of injury became red, and the area of redness gradually enlarged. Other bright red patches of variable size appeared, tending to confluence. In the course of ten days the entire anterior surface of the thigh was affected.

Erysipeloid appeared at the site of injury to the left hand of the patient reported by Schölzke. A few days later lesions of the disease appeared on the right hand and still later on the left cheek. In the course of ten months there were six recurrences, each confined to the left hand.

A veterinarian, Habersang, reported the case of a butcher who had eaten freely of raw sausage made from the flesh of hogs that were subjected to emergency slaughter on account of septicemic form of *Ery. insidiosa* infection. A few days later he had a temperature of 104° F., headache and dizziness. Two or three days later an eruption appeared, first on the chest and abdomen, becoming generalized in the ensuing eight days. It was described as typical rhomboid wheals measuring 1 to 2 cm. in length, bluish red and of hemorrhagic character. The eruption regressed with considerable degree of desquamation. There was no history of wound infection. The physician who treated the patient diagnosed *Ery. insidiosa* infection, though there was no bacteriologic confirmation.

The patient reported by Ehrlich was a farmer, who prior to onset of eruption and illness had slaughtered a "sick" hog (subsequently diagnosed as having swine erysipelas). The eruption at onset on the right hand and forearm comprised redness with edema, vesicles and bullae. Subsequently, the face, ears and left hand became similarly involved. There was stiffness and pain in one shoulder, the patient felt ill and had fever. Still later violaceous erythema appeared on the trunk and elsewhere and clusters of papules which coalesced to form circumscribed placques. Some of the cutaneous lesions retrogressed with scaling and desquamation. Diagnosis of erysipelothrix infection was established by rising titers of agglutinins in the patient's serum and by the presence of the organism in stained sections of a cutaneous lesion.

Septicemic Form

The occurrence of this form of infection has been definitely established by positive blood culture (Prausnitz, Fiessinger and Brouet)
and, in addition, by necropsy demonstration of endocarditis and
recovery of the organism in the endocardial vegetations (Russell and
Lamb, Klauder, Kramer and Nicholas). Probably instances of septicemic infection, lacking, however, in bacteriologic and necropsy
demonstrations, have been reported occurring in veteriarians accidentally inoculated with culture of the organism (Gunther, Spitzer).

Cardinal symptoms of the septicemic form of infection in swine
are an eruption, symptoms referable to the joints, and endocarditis.
This triad occurs in human beings. Of these symptoms the eruption
and also monocytosis* doubtless have more diagnostic value.

The patient reported by Russell and Lamb, however, had no cutaneous lesions, and no portal of entry of infection could be demonstrated. The patient was a lobster fisherman, who presented a hospital course of sepsis with endocarditis. Death occurred after three
months' illness. Antemortem blood culture revealed *Ery. insidiosa.*
Vegetative endocarditis of the aortic and mitral valves was found at
necropsy.

The patient reported on by Klauder, Kramer and Nicholas was
a butcher who cut his finger on a bone. Although these authors did
not see the patient at the time, evidence suggested a severe form of
erysipeloid with necrosis of bone. The patient resumed work. Four
months after injury he became weak and incapacitated. On admis-
sion to the hospital he had constitutional symptoms, fever, anemia
and an eruption. Scattered over the extremities and trunk there were
purpuric macules, varying in diameter from 0.5 to 4 mm.; the color
varied from shades of red to purple. The macules on the trunk faded,
and they were followed by a new outbreak of purplish macules with
smooth nonelevated surfaces on the dorsa of the hands and on the
forearms (Figure 42). Here the lesions were disciform, varying in
diameter up to about 5 cm., and some became confluent; others were
somewhat rounded with irregular borders. Around the elbows and
ankles the eruption consisted of discrete spots. There were purpuric-
like linear lesions that followed some creases on the palms and palmar surfaces of the fingers; concomitant with these palmar lesions

_____

*The significance of monocytosis and the relation of *Ery. insidiosa* to *Listerella
monocytogenes* infection has been discussed by Klauder, Kramer and Nicholas.

there were swelling, tenderness and pain of the carpal and metacarpal joints of both hands.

Of the limited number of patients reported on with septicemia the eruption has been described as "purpuric spots," "bluish red" lesions and "red spots."

Prausnitz' patient was a ten-year-old child. There were bluish red spots on different parts of the body, articular pains and a clinical picture of sepsis with endocarditis. Blood culture disclosed *Ery. insidiosa*. Death resulted after an illness of six months. Necropsy was not performed.

Fiessinger and Brouet's patient presented an eruption similar to that of the patient of Klauder, Kramer and Nicholas. Infection, apparently arising from the gastrointestinal tract, was accompanied with constitutional sympoms, fever, anemia and leukopenia with monocytosis. Blood culture revealed *Ery. insidiosa*. The eruption was described as red spots on the trunk and extremities, becoming confluent in places and forming large placques. Purpuric spots appeared on the face. A distinctive feature was auricular involvement, a replica of that occurring in swine* and resembling the involvement of the caruncle of turkeys (Figure 33). The ears were swollen, purplish red and painful, the lesion resembling a traumatic hematoma. Part of the ears became necrotic and sequestrated (Figure 43).

Another possible instance of auricular involvement in a human patient is the case mentioned by Natusch in his review of reported cases of the infection in veterinarians. A veterinarian cut his finger when inoculating swine with pure culture of the organism. Vesicles occurred at the site of injury with constitutional symptoms; fever was absent. A few days later the right side of the head became red and a bluish red swelling of the lobe of the right ear appeared; later the left side of the head and the lobe of the left ear became similarly affected. The day following an injection of immune serum these symptoms improved and then gradually disappeared.[†]

---

*The diagnosis of *Ery. insidiosa* septicemia was facilitated through a veterinarian student who called attention to the similarity in the appearance of the ears to that of an illustration in Moussu's volume (see Figure 45) showing auricular involvement of a swine with sepicemic form of infection.

†In discussing this case Natusch was undecided whether these symptoms were caused by erysipelas or *Ery. insidiosa* infection. In view of subsequent reports and in consideration of the source of infection and of the result of injection of immune serum, it appears most likely that the auricular involvement was an expression of *Ery. insidiosa* infection.

In the questionably identified fatal cases of septicemia in veterinarians (two cases reported by Gunther and one by Spitzer) no cutaneous symptoms were described other than local cutaneous infection—erysipeloid.

The eruption in human beings is, therefore, purpuric in type, and the distinctive features of it are: formation of placques, purpuric linear lesions on the creases of the palms and fingers, and hematoma-like swelling of the ears. The eruption in human beings (in so far as has been reported) does not compare with the diffuse, large, ill defined patches of erythema that occurs in the septicemic form of infection in swine. It compares, however, with petechial lesions that occur in swine and more particularly with auricular involvement. Such involvement in human beings is a unique cutaneous symptom (if frozen ears are excluded) and of diagnostic import.

TREATMENT

Penicillin was effective in treatment of mice with septicemic form of *Erysipelothrix insidiosa* (Heilman and Herrell, Klauder and Rule 1946), and in the experimentally produced infection in pigeons (Van Es, Olney and Blore). The sulfonamide compounds had little or no effect in treatment of infected mice (Porter and Hale, Klauder and Rule 1944), although in Klauder and Rule's study (1949) there was evidence of a synergistic action of sulfanilamide and penicillin.

Klauder and Rule studied the effects of aureomycin, oxytetracycline ("terramycin") and ilotycin in treatment of the experimentally induced infection in mice. The results were inferior to those obtained with penicillin. Next to penicillin, aureomycin and streptomycin were the two most effective. Studies of other investigators also showed superior effect of penicillin in contrast to other antibiotics in the treatment of the experimental infection of mice, pigeons, and turkeys.

Penicillin therapy of the infection in all its forms is the method of choice. However, antiserum still remains the treatment of choice in swine. In the localized form although cure has been reported from less than one million units (Mechin, Marchini) larger doses are desirable. Goodwin treated eight cases employing doses varying from 1 million units and less to about 2 million units. In two cases a total dose of about 3 million and 5 million units were required in treatment of recurrence of the disease after minimum doses had been administered. Ehrlich gave 8 million units in treatment of the generalized form of the infection. Bothe successfully treated one patient with the localized form with terramycin ointment and two other patients with such ointment combined with oral administration of terramycin given for a few days. Miani employed streptomycin administered intramuscularly in the treatment of fourteen patients with erysipeloid. He administered either one gram daily or 0.5 grams twice daily, or 0.1 gram every three hours. Cure was obtained in three to four days.

The septicemic form should be treated with massive doses of penicillin. Conjoint treatment with a sulfonamide compound could be employed for synergistic action. If necessary immune serum could also be used.

Prior to the use of penicillin the localized form of infection was treated by splinting the affected hand, application of dry or moist heat and a constant wet dressing of 12 per cent ichthammol in alcohol.

PREVENTION

The prevention of swine erysipelas in hogs can be accomplished by vaccination. Pasteur originally used living organisms attenuated by passage through rabbits, two doses of the material being administered, the second of which was more virulent than the first. Sometimes, however, such living virus initiated the disease in healthy animals. The method has been modified, therefore, so that immune serum is given to the animal at the same time that the living culture is given. Immune serum is likewise efficacious in curing the disease if it is given early.

The preventon of the disease in man depends upon painstaking care by those persons who come into contact with infected hogs, and by fishermen and others handling dead animal matter, that abrasions of the skin do not become contaminated.

ITEMS OF NOTE

1) Swine erysipelas is primarily a disease of hogs and poultry.
2) Few other animals are susceptible to infection.
3) The causative organism is widely disseminated, its habitat being dead matter of plant or animal origin.

4) Man is infected through abrasions of the skin and rarely by ingestion.

5) The prevention of the disease in hogs may be accomplished by vaccination plus immune serum.

6) The prevention of the disease in man requires precaution as to cuts and abrasions by those who come into contact with hogs and by fishermen and others handling dead animal matter.

ACKNOWLEDGMENT

The material in this chapter, for the most part, was prepared by the late Dr. Joseph V. Klauder for the previous edition. The present author has revised and edited this material as necessary to bring it up to date for the Fifth Edition.

REFERENCES

BEAUDETTE, F. R. and HUDSON, C. B.: *J.A.V.M.A., 88:*475-487, 1936.

BOTHE, F. A.: Surgical Clinic, Presbyterian Hospital, Philadelphia, personal communication.

BREED, R. S., MURRAY, E. G. D. and SMITH, R. N.: *Bergey's Manual of Determinative Bacteriology.* Sixth edition. Baltimore, Williams and Wilkins, 1957.

BRIND, A. I.: *Novy khir. Arkhir, 47:*177-181, 1940.

CHEVALLIER, P., COLIN, P., LEVY-BRÜHL, M., MORICARD, R. and ELY, Z.: *Bull. Soc. franc. dermat. et syph., 38:*1477-1487, 1931.

CHRISTIANSEN, M.: *Abst. Exper. Stat. Rep., 44:*583, 1921.

CREECH, G. T.: *J.A.V.M.A., 59:*139-150, 1921.

DOMRICH, H.: *Zentralbl. Chir., 59:*593-597, 1932.

DRAKE, C. H. and HALL, E. R.: *Am. J. Pub. Health, 37:*846-848, 1947.

DUMONT, J. and COTONI, L.: *Ann. Inst. Pasteur, 35:*625-633, 1921.

DÜTTMANN, G.: *Beitr. klin. chir., 123:*461-470, 1921.

EHRLICH, J. C.: *Arch. Int. Med., 78:*565-577, 1946.

FIESSINGER, N. and BROUET, G.: *Presse méd., 42:*889-892, 1934.

GOODWIN, M. A.: *Brit. M. J., 1:*765-766, 1950.

GOTTRON, H.: *Deliberationes Congressus Dermatologorum Internationalis.* Leipzig. Johann Ambrosius Barth. *1:*529-548, 1939.

GÜNTHER, G.: *Wien. klin. Wchnschr., 35:*1318-1320, 1912; *Tierärztl. Zentralbl., 26:*141, 1903.

HABERSANG: *Berl. tierärztl. Wchnschr., 42:*243, 1926.

HEILMAN, F. R. and HERRELL, W. E.: *Proc. Staff Meet. Mayo Clin., 19:*340-345, 1944.

INGRAM, J. T. and STUART, R. D.: *Brit. J. Dermat., 46:*303, 1934.

KLAUDER, J. V.: *J.A.M.A., 86:*536-541, 1926.

KLAUDER, J. V., RIGHTER, L. L. and HARKINS, M. J.: *Arch. Dermat. & Syph., 14:*662-678, 1926.

KLAUDER, J. V. and HARKINS, M. J.: *J.A.M.A., 96:*1205-1209, 1931.

KLAUDER, J. V.: *Dermat. Wchnschr., 98:*613-619, 1934.

KLAUDER, J. V.: *J.A.M.A., 111:*1345-1348, 1938.

KLAUDER, J. V., KRAMER, D. W. and NICHOLAS, L.: *J.A.M.A.*, *122*:938-943, 1943.

KLAUDER, J. V.: *Arch. Dermat. & Syph.*, *50*:151-159, 1944.

KLAUDER, J. V. and RULE, A. M.: *Arch. Dermat. & Syph.*, *49*:27-32, 1944.

KLAUDER, J. V. and RULE, A. M.: *J. Invest. Dermat.*, *7*:329-335,1946.

KLAUDER, J. V. and RULE, A. M.: *J. Invest. Dermat.*, *12*:335-338, 1949.

KLAUDER, J. V. and RULE, A. M.: *Arch. Dermat. & Syph.*, *69*:570-576, 1954.

KOCH, R.: Investigations into the etiology of traumatic diseases. New Sydenham Society, London, 1880.

KOLDA, J.: *Rev. gen. Med. Vet.*, *33*:293-312, 1924.

KRIEGER, A.: *Berl. tierarztl. Wchnschr.*, *29*:289, 1913.

LAWSON, G. B. and STINNETT, M. S.: *South. M. J.*, *26*:1068-1070, 1933.

LOEFFLER: *Arb. a. d. kaiserlich. Gesundheits*, *1*:46, 1885.

MANTOVANI, G.: *Gior. batteriol. e immunol.*, *39*:203, 1948.

MARCHINI, E.: *Acta med. ital.*, *3*:183, 1948.

MECHIN, R.: *Arch. Inst. Pasteur*, *28*:103-104, 1950.

MIANI, G.: *Dermatologia*, *1*:285, 1950.

MOUSSU, G.: *Maladies du Porc.* Vigot Frèes, Paris, 1931.

NATUSCH, E.: *Beiträge zur Kenntnis des Schweinerotlaufs, Inaug. Dissert.* Berlin, S. Karger, 1910.

PFAFF, F.: *Abstr. Exper. Stat. Rep.*, *49*:81, 1923.

PITT, W.: *Centralbl. Bakt.*, *45*:33, 111, 1907.

PORTER, J. R. and HALE, W. M.: *Proc. Soc. Exper. Biol. & Med.*, *42*:47-50, 1939.

PRAUSNITZ, C.: *Centralbl. Bakt.* *85*:362-365 (Abt. 1), 1921.

RICHTER, W.: *Dermat. Wchnschr.*, *94*:45-48, 1932.

ROSENWALD, A. S. and DICKINSON, E. M.: *Am. J. Vet., Res.*, *2*:202-213, 1941.

RUSSELL, W. O. and LAMB, M. E.: *J.A.M.A.*, *114*:1045-1050, 1940.

SCHIPP, C.: *Deutsch. tierartzl. Woch.*, *18*:97, 1910.

SCHREINER: Cited by Gottron.

SCHÖLZKE, K. H.: *Med. Klin.*, *33*:1299-1300, 1937.

SEIBOLD, H. R. and NEAL, J. E.: *J.A.V.M.A.*, *128*:537-539, 1956.

SHEARD, K. and DICKS, H. G.: *M. J. Australia*, *2*:352-354, 1949.

SIEBEN, H.: *Med. Klin.*, *21*:129-130, 1925

SIMPSON, C. F., WOOD, F. G. and YOUNG, F.: *J.A.V.M.A.*, *133*:558-560, 1958.

SMITH, T.: *U. S. Dept. Agri. Bureau Animal Indus.* 2nd Annual Report, 196, 1886.

SPITZER: *Ztschr. Fleisch. Milchhyg.*, *16*:66, 1906.

STILES, G. W.: *Am. J. Vet. Res.*, *16*:243-245, 1944; *J.A.M.A.*, *134*:953-955, 1947.

SVENKERUD, R. R., ROSTED, A. F. and THORSHAUG, K.: *Nordisk. Vet. Med.*, *3*:147-169, 1951.

TEN BROECK, C. J.: *Exper. Med.*, *32*:331, 1920.

TORKILDSEN, A.: *Bull. Hyg.*, *18*:1013, 1943. *Abs. Acta Chir. Scandinav.*, *89*:89-96, 1943.

VALLÉE, M.: *Revue path. comp.*, *45*:417, 1945.

VAN ES, L. and MCGRATH, C. B.: *Coll. Agri., Univ. Nebraska Res. Bull.*, *84*:1936.

VAN ES, L., OLNEY, J. F. and BLORE, I. C.: *Uni. Nebraska Coll. Agri., Agri. Exper. Sta. Res. Bull.*, 141 Lincoln, Nebraska, October 1945.

WÜTHRICH, A.: *Beitr. klin. Chir.*, *174*:98-103, 1942.

Chapter 6

SALMONELLA FOOD INFECTIONS

G. M. Dack, Ph.D., M.D.

Salmonella food infections are caused by one or another of the *Salmonella* bacteria, of which approximately six hundred and fifty serotypes have been reported (Clarenburg *et al.*) Salmonellae are widespread in nature and are found in the intestinal tract of mammals, birds and reptiles.

HISTORY

Food infection is as old as civilization itself. From his earliest creation, down through the ages, man apparently acquired considerable knowledge concerning what was good to eat and what to let alone. By the fourth century B.C., it was recognized that the bodies of animals dying a natural death were not fit for food, for Moses commanded that ". . . You must not eat anything that has died a natural death . . ." Moses was not particularly concerned about the ethics of the matter, however, for he permitted that ". . . You may give it to any alien residing in your community to eat, or sell it to a foreigner. . . ." (Smith *et al.*).

Food poisoning mentioned by Hippocrates, Horace, Ovid and other ancient writers was often of a different nature, usually having to do with poisonous mushrooms or other poisonous foods. When foods implicated in outbreaks of food poisoning were fed to experimental animals, frequently no ill effects followed. The foods were then extracted chemically and the extracts injected parenterally into animals, often producing profound effects with diarrhea and death. Such poisonous products obtained from putrefying matter were given the name "ptomaines" by the Italian toxicologist Selmi in 1870 (Dack). There is no evidence, however, that these toxic amines cause illness when eaten either by man or animals and the term ptomaine should be discarded. Many of these outbreaks were without doubt due to the staphylococcus enterotoxin which causes no illness when fed to most experimental animals in the amounts naturally occurring in foods.

Salmon and Smith, in 1885 isolated *Salmonella choleraesuis (B. cholerae suum, Bact. suipestifer,* the hog cholera bacillus) from hogs suffering from cholera, which was thought to be the cause of the disease. Since this was the first organism of the group to be described, the whole group had been named *Salmonella* in recognition of its discoverer.

Gärtner, in 1888, reported the illness of fifty-seven persons who had eaten the flesh of a cow that had been killed because it was sick. One man who consumed nearly two pounds of the raw meat died in thirty-five hours. From the organs of the man, as well as from the meat he had eaten, Gärtner isolated the causative agent, *S. enteritidis (B. enteritidis,* the Gärtner bacillus).

De Nobele, in 1889, isolated *S. typhimurium (S. aertrycke, B. aertrycke, B. pestis cavae,* the mouse typhoid bacillus) from a food poisoning outbreak.

Much confusion has existed in the identification and nomenclature of Salmonella organisms. Different names have been applied to the same organism isolated in different countries, or the same name has been used to describe different organisms. It was many years before *Salmonella* typing centers were established and accurate identification made available.

PREVALENCE

Accurate figures concerning the prevalence of food infection in the United States are lacking. Compulsory reports of such instances are not required; many of the reports taken from the daily press are wholly unfounded and few of the actual outbreaks are carefully studied.

Statistics regarding the causative agents in outbreaks of food poisoning are usually inaccurate. Food samples submitted for investigation are often unsatisfactory, having been stored improperly or too long before culturing. Undoubtedly only a small number of cases of food infection which occur in family groups are reported, whereas when large gatherings of people are afflicted the attention of the public is called to the episode. This is due to the fact that the symptoms may be mild, or if severe, of short duration. Previous to 1930,

laboratory workers investigating the causative agents of food poisoning outbreaks were concerned principally with *Salmonella* or *Clostridium botulinum,* and they overlooked those outbreaks due to
staphylococci. Even now, the proof of staphylococcus enterotoxin
in a food is difficult, and staphylococci are often reported as the
causative organism without adequate evidence. Due to the above
reasons we have no accurate knowledge concerning the prevalence
of bacterial food poisoning.

In England and Wales for the years 1954-1959 there were 20,179
incidents of *Salmonella typhimurium,* 3,267 endogenous and 4,287
exogenous salmonellae. The endogenous types were common in the
United Kingdom before 1940 and the exogenous types unrecognized
or uncommon. The increase in endogenous types has been irregular
but the exogenous types have increased regularly each year (Ministry of Health, 1960).

Many serotypes of salmonellae have been reported in the Netherlands. Of 173 strains from bone and fish meal forty-six different
serotypes were found of which thirteen had never before been encountered in that country.

Seeliger, in reviewing food-borne infections and intoxications in
Europe, makes the statement "Even more important than the im-
ports of contaminated egg products were the quantities of imported
fish-, blood- and bone meal from tropical countries. This type of
animal food was found to contain a tremendous number of *Salmonella* species. A glance at the German import statistics shows,
however, that the origin of these products was the decisive factor,
and not the quantity alone."

THE ETIOLOGIC AGENTS

Salmonella organisms are serologically related small gram-negative,
non-sporeforming, motile rods—with a few exceptions, such as *S.
pullorum* and *S. gallinarum* which are non-motile—which grow well
on culture media and ferment many sugars with acid and gas (with
some exceptions).

They have been variously known as the paratyphoid group, the
Gärtner group, the hog cholera group, the enteritidis group, the
intermediate group and the *Salmonella* group. More than 650 serotypes of the germs have been isolated and classified into different

groups on a biochemical and serological basis. A classification on the basis of host susceptibility is not possible at the present time.

New types are being discovered with the progress of years and are being added to the different groups. It has been customary to name a new type after the place where the organism was first isolated. Some of the *Salmonella* types, which have caused gastroenteritis in man and which have been found in healthy or diseased animals are listed in Table 28. Many of the types have been en-

TABLE 28

OUTBREAKS OF FOOD-BORNE ILLNESS DUE TO SALMONELLA REPORTED TO THE NATIONAL OFFICE OF VITAL STATISTICS OF THE UNITED STATES PUBLIC HEALTH SERVICE FOR THE YEARS INDICATED

Salmonella Serotype	1957		1958		1959		1960	
	Outbreaks	Cases	Outbreaks	Cases	Outbreaks	Cases	Outbreaks	Cases
S. adelaide			1	1				
S. anatum	2	387						
S. bareilly	1	45	1	1				
S. blockley					3	77		
S. bredney					2	92	1	51
S. california					1	1000		
S. chester	1	70						
S. dublin			1	30				
S. enteritidis			1	3	1	49	1	23
S. group							1	3
S. group C					1	400		
S. group E							1	3
S. heidelberg	1	12	1	24	1	3	4	112
S. infantis			1	1				
S. manhattan							4	11
S. montevideo			1	2			1	10
S. newington					1	35		
S. newport	5	442					1	5 (1 death)
S. oranienburg					3	122	1	6
S. paratyphi B	1	3						
S. pullorum	1	19						
S. reading	(312 sporadic—nationwide) (3 outbreaks—nationwide)							
	1	1	2	3				
S. sandiego	1	32	1	5				
S. St. Paul					1	130		
S. serologic type D			1	4				
S. taksony							1	122
S. tennessee	3	61						
S. typhimurium	14	494			9	455	4	168

countered but a few times. Bornstein (1943) considers all types of Salmonella pathogenic for man, although all have not yet been isolated from human sources.

The typhoid bacillus is related to the *Salmonella* organisms serologically, falling into group D, and is called *Salmonella typhi*. It is rarely found in animals (one instance). *S. paratyphi* A (the paratyphoid A bacillus) is included in group A and *S. paratyphi* B (the paratyphoid B bacillus) is in group B. The occasions when they have been found in animals are exceptional.

Salmonella organisms grow rapidly in most foodstuffs without producing much evidence of their existence. Koser found that all types multiplied rapidly in the liquor of several cooked vegetables, with the exception of highly acid sauerkraut. In fruit juices a rapid destruction of the organisms took place. In several meat products the organisms exhibited a marked ability to spread from the original point of inoculation throughout the foodstuff, although this occurred only under optimum conditions. Damon and Leiter had a similar experience, finding that under ordinary household conditions, the organisms will multiply to a considerable extent in twenty-four to seventy-two hours, producing such slight changes in color and odor as to be readily overlooked. Segalove and Dack found that *Salmonella enteritidis* experimentally inoculated into dehydrated beef and pork grew scantily in only one pork sample at the lowest salt concentration (0.28 per cent) when adjusted to 50 per cent moisture. Growth occurred in both beef and pork samples adjusted to 60 per cent moisture where the salt in the dehydrated product was less than 2 per cent. In all cases the salt content represents that of the dehydrated samples before hydration.

ANIMALS RESPONSIBLE FOR FOOD INFECTIONS

Poultry

Many *Salmonella* types have been isolated from poultry and egg products. Barnes considers the domestic fowl as "the main animal reservoir of organisms affecting man." He lists twenty types of *Salmonella* in which the domestic fowl is the chief reservoir (Table 29).

The hen is commonly infected with *S. pullorum* which is transmitted to the egg. Human infections have been reported by Mickle and his co-workers and by Edwards and Bruner. Commercial egg preparations have been found to contain *S. senftenberg* and *S. paratyphi* B. (Rubenstein et al.) The duck is infected with several varieties of *Salmonella* organisms, and Snapper has reported human

TABLE 29

Salmonella ORGANISMS WHICH HAVE CAUSED GASTRO-ENTERITIS IN MAN AND WHICH HAVE BEEN ISOLATED FROM ANIMALS. FROM BORNSTEIN[9]

GROUP B

S. typhimurium...............natural pathogen of animals
S. heidelberg.................from a pig
S. chester....................from a normal hog
S. san diego.................from fowl and swine
S. saint paul.................from turkeys
S. reading...................from swine
S. derby.....................from swine, fowl and ruminants
S. bredeney..................from fowl, hogs and ruminants
S. schleissheim...............pathogen for animals

GROUP C 1

S. cholerae suis..............pathogen for animals, secondary invader in hog cholera
S. thompson..................from hog and fowl
S. montevideo................from various animals
S. oranienburg...............epizootics in quails and chickens
S. braenderup................from a fatal diarrhea
S. bareilly...................from chicken, swine and carnivores

GROUP C 2

S. newport...................from various animals
S. muenchen..................from hogs and other animals
S. litchfield.................from fowl
S. morbificans...............from a diseased cow
S. glostrup..................from a diseased hog

GROUP D

S. enteritidis................pathogen for animals
S. dublin....................pathogen for animals
S. panama....................from fowl and swine

GROUP E 1

S. london....................found in healthy and diseased animals
S. give......................found in fowl and swine
S. anatum....................pathogen for various animals
S. meleagridis...............found in fowl and swine

GROUP E 2

S. newington.................pathogen for fowl, found in swine and rodents
S. new brunswick.............from fowl, hogs and ruminants

GROUP E 3

S. senftenberg...............from fowl and swine

GROUP F

S. kentucky..................from chicken with enteritis and from camels
S. aberdeen..................from fowl
S. rubislaw..................from fowl
S. wichita...................from swine and turkey
S. worthington...............from fowl and swine
S. hvittingfoss..............from animals
S. cerro.....................from hog and fowl
S. urbana....................from enteritis in a hog and from diseased chicken

outbreaks caused by duck eggs. Turkeys were found to harbor twenty-three types of *Salmonella,* among the most common of which were *S. pullorum* and *S. typhimurium.* (Pomeroy et al.) Turkey eggs harbored the former organism from 8 per cent of the birds examined. Goose eggs and pigeon eggs used in the preparation of salads and puddings have caused human *Salmonella* infections. Dried eggs were shipped in large quantities to Europe during World War II. Of samples from the United States, Canada and Argentina, 9.9 per cent of 7,584 examined were found to contain Salmonella comprising 33 types. The ten most common types were as follows:

Type	No. isolated
S. oranienburg	245
S. montevideo	139
S. meleagridis	117
S. tennessee	90
S. bareilly	82
S. anatum	30
S. typhimurium	30
S. newport	24
S. senftenberg	8
S. london	6

Of these thirty-three types, twenty-two including the six most common, had not been encountered before 1941 in Great Britain in cases of human infections. There was an increase in the number of *Salmonella* outbreaks in England in 1943 and a further increase in 1944. During the latter part of 1942, 1943 and 1944, outbreaks of food poisoning in Great Britain were due partly to the old *Salmonella* types and partly to twenty-four new types. Of the new types the six commonest in order were the same six that headed the list of the dried-egg types. From these facts the British concluded that dried eggs were probably responsible for a considerable proportion of the greatly increased number of food poisoning outbreaks occurring during the years 1943 and 1944. (Med. Res. Council).

Sweden had a similar experience to Great Britain. In Sweden it is compulsory to report all *Salmonella* cases to the Medical Board and it was observed that the incidence of *Salmonella* infections was low until 1945 when a considerable increase occurred. Lundbeck and his co-workers made the following statement . . . "The wave of *Salmonella* infections during the years 1946-1948 was caused by dry egg products imported from the U.S.A. and South American countries. This conclusion is based on the following observations. First, nine strains previously not recognized in Sweden were found in specimens from patients. All but one of these strains were demonstrated in the imported egg products. Second, 12,300 samples of egg products were examined bacteriologically, and *Salmonella* bacteria were demonstrated in 28.1% of packages from the U.S.A. The corresponding percentage for South American countries was 26.6. In all, seventeen different types were recognized.Third, there was a relationship between the quantities of imported egg products and the number of *Salmonella* infections." . . .

Gibbons and Moore isolated *Salmonella* organisms from twenty-eight of 380 samples of Canadian egg powder. On twenty-one samples *Salmonella* counts were made and thirteen contained less than one organism per gram; seven, between one and ten and one, fifty-four organisms per gram.

Schneider examined 901 samples of high quality egg powder and found that thirty-two or 3.18 per cent contained *Salmonella* species. Of 797 lots processed with the aid of a preheater and multistage drying, only thirteen or 1.63 per cent contained *Salmonella*. In 104 lots spray-dried without the aid of a preheater, nineteen or 18.27 per cent of the samples tested contained *Salmonella*.

Solowey, McFarlane, Spaulding and Chemera isolated *Salmonella* from samples of spray-dried whole egg powder obtained from 100 dehydration plants between September 1943 and January 1945. Of 5,198 samples they found 3,590 to contain *Salmonella*. From some plants no *Salmonella* were found in specimens, whereas from others 71 per cent of the samples were positive. They isolated fifty-two types, five of which comprised 73 per cent of the isolations: *S. Pullorum, S. oranienburg, S. montevideo, S. tennessee* and *S. anatum*.

Hinshaw, McNeil and Taylor isolated 561 *Salmonella* strains from 353 avian outbreaks caused by twenty-three types, of which twenty-one were types found in man.

Watt (1945) traced an outbreak of salmonellosis to shell eggs and isolated *S. montevideo* from two cases of shell eggs obtained on a merchant vessel.

Gaumont from 1948 through the first six months of 1950 examined 245 birds originating from industry, farms, flocks, or families of Northern France and the channel regions and isolated 41 strains of

Salmonella with an incidence of 16.7 per cent. *S. gallinarum* (23 strains) and *S. pullorum* (13 strains) were the most common types encountered.

Swine

Hogs have been found to harbor many types of *Salmonella* organisms. Salmon and Smith considered *S. choleraesuis* to be the cause of hog cholera, but it has since been shown that it is a secondary invader in hog cholera. It is an ordinary inhabitant of the intestinal tracts of hogs, to which no significance is attached under normal conditions. When the resistance of the animal is lowered it takes on special pathologic significance as a secondary invader. Jordan (1918) isolated *S. choleraesuis* and *S. paratyphi* B from the organs of diseased hogs. He obtained no *Salmonella* organisms from the organs of 291 normal swine.

Cherry and his co-workers in Lexington found ten samples infected in 170 samples of market pork. The organisms were *S. typhimurium, S. derby, S. senftenberg, S. anatum, S. bredeney, S. give, S. newington* and *S. newport*. Rubin, Scherago and Weaver studied mesenteric lymph glands in a thousand hogs in groups of twenty-five each. There were 242 cultures of *Salmonella* isolated, falling into thirteen types. Other workers have had similar experiences. Savage and White (1925) encountered *S. enteritidis* twice and *S. choleraesuis* once from porcine sources in thirty-one epidemics of food poisoning which were carefully studied.

The mesenteric lymph nodes of 503 healthy pigs were examined for the presence of *Salmonella* by Clarenburg, Vink and Huisman who, using selective media, tetrathionate broth and brilliant green agar found the bacteria in fourteen animals (2.78 per cent) but not in the feces.

Hardy and Galton examined fecal cultures from live hogs on twenty-eight farms. *Salmonella* infection was prevalent in hogs from two farms, both with epidemic diarrheal disease; it occurred sporadically on six and on twenty farms no infected animals were found. In contrast, the proportion of positives was 25 per cent in a series of tests on live animals taken at the abattoir before slaughter. Examination of swabs taken from relaxed sphincter after death revealed about twice the number of positives as compared with those obtained from the struggling live animals. These authors also reported *Salmonella* in fresh pork sausage purchased on the open market. The contamination of fresh pork was explained by the rapid spread of infection among hogs a few hours or days before slaughter and the wide dissemination of *Salmonella* within the abattoirs.

Hobbs reported finding two strains of *S. typhimurium* and one of *S. anatum* from 1146 pig carcasses.

In Bradford, England during the years 1954-1956 McDonagh and Smith isolated 706 *Salmonella* cultures from 2,861 specimens of liver, spleen or lymph glands of pigs slaughtered at the Bradford abattoir. Three hundred and ninety-five were *S. typhimurium,* 6 *S. bovis morbificans,* 301 *S. derby,* 1 *S. manhattan,* 2 *S. muenchen* and 1 *S. anatum.* The pigs presented no signs of illness although human *Salmonella* infections in Bradford over the same period were closely related to the abattoir findings.

Newell *et al.* in northern Ireland took cecal swabs from 489 pigs killed in two bacon factories and found a *Salmonella* isolation rate of 2 per cent. They isolated *Salmonella* organisms from twenty-three out of 100 samples of cecal feces and from only six of 100 cecal swabs taken from the same animals. Three per cent of meat samples from these pigs and 70 per cent of sausage samples from this meat contained *Salmonella.* Rectal swabs from 162 pigs on five farms producing infected pigs showed *Salmonella* in 9 per cent of those examined. Twenty-four per cent of pig-meal samples taken from these farms contained *Salmonella* and the same *Salmonella* types were found in the meal at the mill and in fish meal and bone meal before mixing.

Cruz in Costa Rica isolated 18 different serotypes of *Salmonella* from the liver, spleen, mesenteric lymph nodes and feces of 150 apparently healthy pigs.

Clarenburg and Kampelmacher during the years 1946-1958 typed 21,162 *Salmonella* strains. Of this number, 219 were from pigs representing twenty serotypes while 250 strains were from bone meal and fish meal isolated from 1955-1958. These 250 strains represented 58 serotypes. The eight most common types in the bone and fish meal were in order of frequency, *S. bareilly, S. newington, S. senftenberg, S. typhimurium, S. anatum, S. oranienburg, S. montevideo* and *S. schwarzengrund.*

Leistner *et al.* examined seventy-five fecal specimens of pig feces at the farm level and found only two positive for *Salmonella*. An examination of litter from fifteen trucks resulted in no samples positive for *Salmonella*. Thirty-one samples of holding pen litter were examined for six companies and twenty-nine samples were positive for *Salmonella* representing thirteen serotypes. In an examination of sixty-one samples of rendered animal by-products forty-seven contained *Salmonella* representing twenty-nine serotypes. They observed that the incidence of *Salmonella* was greater in pigs that were held for a few days in the holding pens before slaughter. *Salmonella* were not recovered from mesenteric lymph nodes of ten pigs which were not held over as compared to finding them in the mesenteric lymph nodes of seven of twenty-five pigs held for a few days before slaughter.

Cattle

Cattle may suffer from puerperal fever, diarrhea, septicemia, uterine inflammations and the like, caused by *Salmonella* organisms. Gärtner isolated *S. enteritidis* from the meat of a cow that had been slaughtered because it was sick. McWeeney encountered the same organism in beef stew that apparently was contaminated after cooking. Savage and White (1922) isolated it three times from bovine sources in thirty-one food poisoning outbreaks. It occurs occasionally as an inhabitant of the intestinal tract of cattle.

Uhlenhuth reported the occurrence of *Salmonella* organisms in the intestinal tract of healthy calves and cattle, but Jordan's (1925) study on the intestinal contents of fifty-two normal cattle, killed at the Union Stock Yards in Chicago, showed no organisms that fulfilled all the requirements of the food poisoning group. Friesleben examined the intestinal contents of 100 cattle with similar results.

Cherry, Scherago and Weaver examined sixty-four samples of beef in the markets of Lexington, Kentucky and found three which contained *Salmonella* organisms. If the hamburger was excluded (which may have contained some pork), there was only one sample in forty that was infected. This contained *S. senftenberg*.

Sutherland and Berger encountered an epidemic among 162 persons in England due to *S. dublin* in milk. The cow suffered from gastroenteritis.

Schroeder and Dale report forty-seven cases, eleven of which were confirmed in the laboratory in an outbreak following the use of certified milk contaminated with S. *dublin.* Subsequent sampling of the milk revealed no S. *dublin.* Fecal samples taken from 398 cows in the dairy revealed S. *dublin* in three animals. Two of these cows although not ill were proven to be active carriers. The cases occurred between Oct. 29 and Nov. 4, 1958. An unusually high coliform count was recorded for the milk which was bottled and distributed on Oct. 28, 1958.

Sheep

Sheep are subject to infection with S. *typhimurium,* and several European epidemics have been reported from such animals. The famous "mutton strain" was isolated from a man in Newcastle in 1911. Several epidemics of disease in sheep as well as food poisoning epidemics in man have been caused by organisms identical with the "mutton" type. Sheep are of less importance than cattle or hogs in food poisoning. Cherry and his co-workers found no *Salmonella* organisms in eleven samples of market lamb.

Rodents

Rodents are extremely susceptible to infection with *Salmonella* organisms. Friesleben found 52 per cent of wild mice and 19 per cent of wild rats carrying such organisms in their intestines. Meyer found 58 infected animals among 775 wild rats examined, twenty-eight with S. *enteritidis* and thirty with S. *typhimurium.* Zwick and Weichel found twenty-eight out of 177 mice carried such organisms. Verder isolated S. *typhimurium* from the spleen of one rat out of 114 examined.

Welch, Ostrolenk, and Bartram examined 420 specimens of rat droppings collected from all regions in the United States. Only five showed *Salmonella* organisms. Rat droppings kept at room temperature remained infective for 148 days. Transfer of infection from an infected rat or mouse to cage mate did not take place in the experience of these investigators. Price-Jones found S. *enteritidis* in the liver and spleen of rats forty-eight hours after they were fed these organisms. Two months later 10 per cent of the animals were carriers and a few of these remained carriers when examined after five months. Such carriers were capable of starting new epidemics among other rats.

Guinea pigs have been found infected with S. *typhimurium*. A few instances of infection in rabbits have been reported. Neither guinea pigs nor rabbits, however, are relatively important compared to rats and mice.

Other Animals

Other animals harbor organisms of the *Salmonella* group but their relation to food poisoning is of less significance.

The horse has been responsible for several outbreaks of *Salmonella* food poisoning in Germany, through the use of horse meat as food. The horse is commonly infected with S. *abortus equi*, but human infections from this source are probably rare. S. *muenster* was isolated in Germany from one human case that consumed raw horse meat.

The dog carries S. *enteritidis* (Torrey et al.) and S. *anatum*, (Craigie) as does also the cat. (Craigie; Mori; Krumwiede *et al.*) Bruner and Moran report on 2,788 cultures of *Salmonella* from thirty-two animal species other than man or fowls studied during a period of sixteen years at the Kentucky Experiment Station. The majority of the strains (2,119) were from swine with 103 strains from dogs second on the list. Wolff, Henderson and McCallum reported results of examination of rectal swabs from 100 dogs in a veterinary clinic, an animal shelter and a crowded unsanitary private kennel in Michigan. Sixteen different *Salmonella* types were isolated from eighteen of the dogs; one dog yielded five different types in six rectal swabbings tested. The diet of the animals in the most heavily infected institution included a supply of rejected candled eggs. Many of the *Salmonella* types isolated were those commonly found in poultry and eggs in the United States. Cruickshank and Smith in a survey made in London found salmonellae in the feces of five of 500 dogs (1.0 per cent); seven of 500 cats (1.4 per cent) and three of 133 pigeons (2.25 per cent). The organisms from the dogs were S. *newport*, S. *typhimurium* and a Salmonella of doubtful identity; from the cats, S. *typhimurium*, S. *anatum*, S. *montevideo* and S. *paratyphi* B; from the pigeons, S. *typhimurium*.

Watt and DeCapito examined rectal swabs from 1,156 dogs which were community contacts of known human infections and found 3.4 per cent to be carrying salmonellae. Of 625 cats similarly tested,

3.0 per cent were found to be carriers. Other workers have made large surveys on dogs which were hospitalized or impounded and reported from 1.0 to 18.0 per cent of the animals with positive cultures. (Galton *et al.*)

Jordan included in his collection of food poisoning organisms a culture of *S. choleraesuis* isolated from the mesenteric gland of a monkey and a culture of *S. typhimurium* isolated from the spleen of a skunk.

EXPERIMENTAL HUMAN SALMONELLOSIS

The fact that a large number of samples of spray-dried whole egg powder were found to contain *Salmonella* types raised the question of the pathogenicity of some of these types for man. The majority of textbooks of bacteriology have described *S. pullorum* as non-pathogenic for man. In addition to *S. pullorum,* the types of *Salmonella* found in egg powder represented many species. Although some of these species were recognized as pathogenic for man, the question of whether those strains found in egg powder were pathogenic still remained unanswered.

Since the mere finding of an organism in the stools does not constitute proof of its etiological role in causing illness, it was considered desirable to test the pathogenicity of *S. pullorum* for man and also that of some of the other types found in spray-dried whole egg powder. Such a study was made by Drs. N. B. McCullough and C. Wesley Eisele with strains provided by Dr. M. Solowey. The tests were made on human volunteers in a penal institution under ideal sanitary conditions.

Three strains each of *S. pullorum, S. meleagridis* and *S. anatum,* and one strain each of *S. bareilly, S. derby* and *S. newport* were tested. All strains produced illness when sufficient numbers were fed. Infective dosages ranged from 125,000 to several billion *(S. pullorum)* with wide variation in the infective dose occurring from strain to strain of the same species. The cases varied from mild brief enteritis to serious prostrating disease. The incubation period ranged from four hours to seven days with the greater number falling within the usually recognized incubation period of seven to seventy-two hours. Many cases of asymptomatic carrier states were produced, some persisting for many weeks.

With the strains studied a rise in serum agglutinin was not regularly found following illness and when present the titre was as a rule low.

In reinfection experiments with *S. meleagridis* and *S. anatum* some increased resistance to infection was demonstrated, but the immunity was not of a high order.

The dosage of *S. pullorum* required to produce illness was manyfold greater than that for the other species. The experimental subjects had all received repeated immunization against typhoid. In view of the somatic relationship between *S. pullorum* and TAB vaccine, possible cross-immunity due to this vaccine may have influenced the results with this species.

SALMONELLA INFECTION IN MAN

Salmonella food poisoning in man is an infection rather than an intoxication (Dack). Filtrates of cultures and heated meat cultures of *S. typhimurium* and *S. enteritidis* when fed to human volunteers fail to produce symptoms. Living organisms in sufficient numbers are necessary to cause infection. The incubation period is usually seven to twenty-four hours, though sometimes it is less and sometimes as long as several days; in general, the larger the number of infecting organisms, the shorter the period of onset of symptoms. The onset is sudden, with headache and a chill and often with vomiting. Nausea, abdominal pains and severe diarrhea are characteristics of the infection. The temperature is elevated at first. The symptoms rapidly diminish after a few days. Mortality does not exceed one or two per cent of the cases (Table 30).

The severity of the symptoms varies in different outbreaks, depending upon the size of the infecting does and the type and pathogenicity of the *Salmonella* strain. All members of the group cause gastro-intestinal upsets with identical symptoms. All age groups of people are susceptible to *Salmonella* infection. Among 425 cases of gastro-enteritis in Massachusetts caused by these organisms, *S. typhimurium* was the most common cause (Rubenstein *et al.*). Thirtynine per cent of patients infected with *S. typhimurium* were under ten years of age. These figures are in accord with the findings of Barnes (Table 31) as well as others.

Bornstein (1942) studied 429 *Salmonella* cultures isolated from

TABLE 30

SYMPTOMS OF SALMONELLA FOOD POISONING COMPARED WITH FOOD INTOXICATIONS.
FROM DACK[3]

Symptoms	Botulism Intoxication	Staphylococcus Intoxication	Salmonella Infection
Incubation period	Average 1 or 2 days	1 to 6 hours Average 2½ to 3 hours	7 to 72 hours
Onset	Gradual	Sudden	Sudden
Vomiting	About 1/3 of cases	Common	Common
Diarrhea	Uncommon	Severe	Severe
Constipation	Common	Absent	Absent
Abdominal pain	Absent	Present	Present
Temperature	Subnormal	Variable	Elevated at first
Prostration	Absent at first	Acute	Present
Nervous system	Double vision, difficulty in swallowing, in speech and in respiration	Not involved	Not involved
Duration of symptoms	Protracted and progressive. Convalescence slow	5 to 6 hours or longer	Rapidly diminishing after few days
Mortality	65 per cent of cases	Practically nil	1 or 2 per cent of cases

TABLE 31

TYPES OF SALMONELLA ORGANISMS LISTED IN ORDER OF FREQUENCY FOUND IN MAN
(BARNES[13])

Type	Human Outbreaks	Animal Outbreaks
S. paratyphi B	51	Fowls 4; others 2
S. typhimurium	50	Fowls 472; others 105
S. newport	33	Fowls 19; others 7
S cholerae suis	30	Swine 272; others 32
S. panama	20	Fowls 6; others 1
S. montevideo	17	Fowls 11; others 3
S. oranienburg	13	Fowls 28
S. san diego	13	Fowls 3; others 1
S. bareilly	11	Fowls 47; others 7
S. anatum	10	Fowls 44; others 12
S. enteritidis	8	Rodents 12; others 7
S. bredeney	7	Fowls 27; others 6
S. give	6	Fowls 18; others 7
S senftenberg	4	Fowls 15; others 4
S. meleagridis	3	Fowls 15; others 1
S. oregon	3	Swine 5; others 2
S. derby	2	Fowls 33; others 9
S. saint paul	2	Fowls 1
S. thompson	2	Fowls 1
S. pullorum	2	Fowls 492; others 3
S. newington	2	Fowls 18; others 4

man and found *S. typhimurium* in 37 per cent. Mickle and his co-workers encountered *S. typhimurium* in 34 per cent of human *Salmonella* cases. Edwards and Bruner found it in 17 per cent of human cases and in 47 per cent of *Salmonella* cultures isolated from animals. Seligman found 369 of 1,000 human cases of *Salmonella* infection with nineteen deaths due to *S. typhimurium.*

Outbreaks due to *S. choleraesuis* are relatively common (Table 31). This type constituted 13 per cent of Bornstein's (1941) cultures of *Salmonella* from human cases, 2 per cent of Mickle's cultures and 8 per cent of Edward's. Seligman reported ninety cases of infection caused by *S. choleraesuis* with sixteen deaths in 1,000 salmonellosis patients. In another survey, fifty-four cases of *S. choleraesuis* were reported in 1,916 human cases (Seligman *et al.*).

S. enteritidis, although first associated with food-borne infections (1888), is not found as often as many of the other *Salmonella* organisms. Bornstein (1942) found *S. enteritidis* constituted only 4 per cent of 429 *Salmonella* cultures from human cases; Mickle, Edwards and Seligman each had a figure of 3 per cent. In cultures of *Salmonella* from animals, Edwards found it constituted 2 per cent of the total.

The severity of the disease in man caused by salmonellae may vary from mild gastro-intestinal disturbances to invasion of the tissues and blood stream with the organisms such as occurs in typhoid fever. Some types of salmonellae are more likely to produce severe diseases than others.

Sometimes, following bacteremia, the organisms locate in regions other than the intestinal mucosa. Bornstein (1943) includes among pathologic conditions found in this way endocarditis, percarditis, meningitis, osteomyelitis, arthritis, rhinopharyngitis, sinusitis, pneumonia, pleurisy, peritonitis, cholecystitis, pyelonephritis and abscesses.

D'Albora, Ingegno and Edson reported nineteen cases of broncho-pneumonia following an outbreak of 350 cases of gastro-enteritis due to *S. montevideo.* Other investigators have found that severe infections with blood stream invasion with salmonellae sometimes follows gastro-enteritis due to *Salmonella.*

More than thirty types of Salmonella have been implicated in severe salmonellosis in man (Barnes).

EPIDEMIOLOGY

The epidemiology of salmonellosis is not well understood. A possible explanation for the finding of: (1) *Salmonella* in animal products, (2) a low incidence of *Salmonella* in the feces of swine on the farm, (3) the failure to find *Salmonella* in the litter of trucks hauling swine to market, (4) the very high incidence of *Salmonella* in the litter in holding pens at the abattoir, and (5) the presence of *Salmonella* in the intestinal tract of swine at the time of slaughter may be as follows. Swine receiving small numbers of *Salmonella* in feed may excrete large numbers of *Salmonella* of the serotypes represented in the feed for a few days or weeks after the initial exposure. However, by the time they go to slaughter the carrier condition has largely disappeared. When entering the holding pens a few carrier animals may introduce serotypes of *Salmonella*. Contact with animals from other farms which have not had past experience with the new serotypes will make *Salmonella* excreters of these animals. Thus, the litter of the holding pens becomes heavily seeded with serotypes of *Salmonella* which find new host animals.

Meat products from infected animals are often, but not always, the cause of salmonellosis. For instance, human infections with S. *choleraesuis* are rare on farms where hog cholera (with associated infection with S. *choleraesuis*) is common. Even consumption of pork from such hogs does not necessarily produce illness. The same condition exists in regard to the consumption of poultry and eggs from flocks infected with S. *pullorum*.

Bengtsson *et al.* and Lundbeck *et al.* describe an outbreak of S. *typhimurium* in Sweden involving 8,845 cases with at least ninety deaths in the summer of 1953. There was an unusually warm spell of weather at the time of the outbreak and a strike involved the packing house associated with the outbreak. It was concluded that an outgrowth of bacteria must have taken place in the carcasses although no clear cut details were elicited to explain the episode.

Hobbs in England has called attention to boneless meats, carcass meats, meat and bone meals for fertilizers and animal feeding stuffs as providing sources for *Salmonella* contamination.

Couper, Newell and Payne describe an outbreak of typhoid fever traced to canned ox-tongue. In this outbreak thirty patients had typhoid fever and two were carriers. This outbreak was traced to a

6-lb. can of ox-tongue sold after slicing in a store for sandwich meat. At the factory where this can was prepared, raw sewage polluted river water was used for cooling the cans. A few months later a 6-lb. can of corned beef from the same factory caused the illness of twenty-five of the twenty-six persons at risk (Ministry of Health, 1956). *Salmonella newport* was isolated from the twenty-five patients, from the butcher who handled the meat (he had no symptoms), from the meat sold to the customers and from the meat remaining in the can. As some meat was eaten immediately after the can was unsealed there is no doubt about the contents being contamined before the can was opened. Surgalla and Dack inoculated corned beef with *S. enteritidis* and found that good growth occurred without eliciting signs of spoilage (gas or off odors or color).

From the above outbreaks of *S. typhi* from a can of ox-tongue and *S. newport* from a can of corned beef it is evident that very small leaks in a can may admit a single pathogenic contaminant when the retorted cans are cooled in sewage-polluted water. Following this experience the canning factory uses only potable chlorinated water in cooling cans coming from the retort.

Seeliger mentions an outbreak of *Salmonella bareilly* infection involving 6,000 people in Germany and traced to Camembert cheese (Bonitz). Seeliger states "This cheese was apparently contaminated by a healthy carrier of *S. bareilly* who lived on a farm where swine were fed with batches of fish meal known to contain *S. bareilly.*"

Two outbreaks have occurred from bakery goods in England. Joan Taylor reports an outbreak in the Midlands in which a number of people over a wide area were ill over a two week period. Illnesses involved six serotypes of *Salmonella* and were traced to the eating of cakes and trifles distributed from a single factory. Ultimately infection was traced to American egg albumen powder which was dusted throughout the bakery. A second outbreak occurred in the industrial area of Yorkshire in customers of a bakery (Ministry of Health, 1960). In this outbreak numerous serotypes, *S. oranienburg, S. anatum, S. schwarzengrund, S. infantis, S. enteritidis, S. orion, S. thompson* and *S. typhimurium* were isolated from the cases. Those ill had eaten custards, trifles and cream confectionery. Over 400 persons were ill and over 100 symptomless excreters were detected. The source was stated to be probably egg albumen of American origin, but some cases may have arisen from contaminated English frozen egg.

In the author's laboratory Mrs. Golda Lippitz examined the egg powder in 6 packages of angel food cake mixes in January of 1960. These packages had been purchased in the open market in Chicago. From one package the egg powder was found to have 15,000 *Salmonella montevideo* per gram. Since the powder is diluted 1-3 this represents approximately 50,000 Salmonella per gram.

Kunz and Ouchterlony reported five cases of salmonellosis in hospital patients who had been fed by tube dried inactive brewers yeast. From three patients *S. oranienburg,* from two *S. montevideo* and from one *S. senftenberg* was isolated. The dried yeast was contaminated with all three serotypes.

Desiccated coconut from Ceylon has been found contaminated with food poisoning types of salmonellae and also *S. paratyphi* B.

Two outbreaks in the United States have been traced to watermelon (Gaylor et al.) One outbreak in Upton, Massachusetts consisted of seventeen primary cases among five families and two secondary cases. *S. miami* was recovered from sliced melon in two of the homes, from all of the stools submitted and from the shelf in the store where the slicing knife was kept. The melons came from Florida where *S. miami* is common.

Flies have been implicated as mechanical carriers of *Salmonella* organisms. Gwatkin and Mitchell showed that flies carried S. *pullorum* from chicken droppings. Ostrolenk and Welch also implicated the house fly in the spread of *Salmonella* organisms, while Braun found that the mosquito, *Culex pipiens,* was a vector. Parker and Steinhaus demonstrated that the wood tick, *Dermacentor andersoni,* transmitted *S. enteritidis* experimentally.

Commercial "rat viruses" usually contain the enteritidis organism. Several human epidemics were traceable to such products (Jordan). Spray reports an outbreak involving 123 cases due to contamination of milk with a commercial rat virus.

Human carriers sometimes are responsible for food poisoning epidemics. D'Albora, Ingegno and Edson report such an outbreak involving 350 cases due to *S. montevideo* from a carrier in the kitchen who contaminated rice pudding. The carrier state, while it may exist for a considerable time, is usually regarded as of short duration after infection.

Rubenstein found that convalescents showed *Salmonella* organisms in the stools in 43 per cent of 711 cases after the fourth week from onset, 18 per cent after the eighth week and 11 per cent after the tenth week. Sixteen cases were permanent carriers, none of which were among the *S. typhimurium* cases.

Sulkin and Pike in their survey of laboratory acquired infections reported only nine infections and salmonellosis ranked fourteenth in their list of bacterial infections. Typhoid fever on the other hand ranked fourth with fifty-eight cases. Ante mortem inspection of food animals is carried out in the slaughter houses where meat is prepared for sale in interstate commerce. Under such conditions where apparently healthy animals are slaughtered, the carrier incidence in these animals must be appreciable because products subjected to these inspections cannot be considered free from salmonellae. Why then is there not more salmonellosis in our population? Most meat and egg products are cooked before serving although in many instances the cooking may not be adequate to destroy all salmonellae in the products. As pointed out previously in the experiments of McCullough and Eisele with human volunteers fed salmonellae, the pathogenicity of the strain is important and is directly reflected in the number of organisms (dosage) required to cause illness. In instances where illness did not follow the feeding of small numbers of the salmonella strain many individuals became carriers. Under such circumstances man may play a role in propagating strains of animal origin.

In order to have cases of salmonellosis it is necessary to have sufficient numbers of organisms to cause illness. The number required depends upon the type or species and the individual strain within the type. Although large outbreaks of *Salmonella* food poisoning are in the minority, the amount of salmonellosis occurring in individual homes is unknown.

Neter reported transmission of salmonellosis from a mother who became a convalescent carrier of *S. oranienburg* to a premature infant who after delivery was immediately taken to a premature nursery and did not have further contact with the mother. A careful history indicated that the mother had a very mild diarrhea one week prior to delivery. Neter found salmonellae in the nasopharynx and throat of children suffering from salmonellosis. In a study of forty-three children clinically recovered from salmonellosis twenty-six were still carrying the organism at the time of discharge from the hospital.

Mackerras and Pask in Brisbane, Australia estimated a *Salmonella* carrier rate of about 3.5 per cent in children under the age of two years. They pointed out the extremely low pathogenicity of all species of salmonellae for children and suggested that pathogenicity is associated either with dosage of salmonellae or, more probably, with selection by passage of virulent mutants.

PREVENTION OF FOOD INFECTIONS

Animal products such as meat scraps, bone meal and fish meal as well as vegetable products used in animal feeds appear to be commonly contaminated with salmonellae (Ministry of Health, 1959). In rendering, these products are cooked which should free them from viable salmonellae. Therefore, viable *Salmonella* must enter as contaminants after cooking. Since these products are commonly used in high protein feeds for poultry, swine and other domestic animals, particularly young animals, it is important that they should be *Salmonella* free to avoid cycling *Salmonella* back to the farm. Prevention obviously involves improvement in sanitation in rendering plants avoiding recontamination of cooked products with the raw products. It is important to keep the cooked and raw product operations separated as well as personnel handling these products.

The evidence cited in this chapter would also point to the holding pens in abattoirs as a source of infection of animals coming from the farm to slaughter. Sanitation measures should be taken to prevent the build-up of *Salmonella* serotypes in holding pens.

Great advances have been made in processing broken out eggs, frozen eggs and dehydrated egg products. Pasteurization and other methods of treatment have been developed which reduce the numbers of *Salmonella* so that egg products may be purchased which are comparatively free from these microorganisms. Progress in this direction should eventually lead to processing methods which should eliminate the *Salmonella* hazard.

Hogs, cattle or sheep which are sick should not be used for food. The emergency slaughter of sick animals is not generally practiced in the United States and careful inspection of regularly established abattoirs eliminates many diseased animals. Adequate cooking of meat and poultry is a safeguard. Eggs should not be eaten raw. Foods in markets and bakeries, as well as in the home must be kept free from rodents which may contaminate food directly with droppings. Flies and other insects that carry infection mechanically from rat droppings or other dejecta must be prevented access to food supplies. Persons who handle pets should wash their hands thoroughly before eating or preparing food. The same precautions, but perhaps to a lesser extent, should be observed in regard to human carriers as for other enteric infections.

ITEMS OF NOTE

1) There are approximately 650 types of *Salmonella* organisms, all which possibly may cause gastro-enteritis in man.

2) The usual period of incubation in *Salmonella* food poisoning is seven to seventy-two hours, although in a few instances it may be as short as four hours or as long as seven days.

3) Infection of the blood stream sometimes follows gastro-enteritis. *Salmonella* organisms travel from the blood stream to other parts of the body where they may localize in the tissues.

4) The number of *Salmonella* organisms ingested (dosage) is an important factor which determines whether or not illness will follow.

5) Ingestion of small numbers of salmonellae which fails to cause infection may give rise to carriers of the strain.

6) Dosage required to cause infection is dependent upon: (1) the immune state of the host, (2) the type or species of *Salmonella*, and (3) the specific strain within the type or species.

7) The domestic fowl is an important reservoir of *Salmonella* organisms. The hog, cow, sheep or rat are the other animals usually associated with this type of food poisoning.

8) The house fly is a mechanical carrier of *Salmonella* organisms.

9) Prevention consists in the proper cooking and refrigeration of meat products and eggs from healthy animals and in the protection of food supplies from contamination by flies and rats.

REFERENCES

BARNES, L. A.: *U. S. Naval Med. Bull., 33*:105; *43*:939, 1944.

BENGTSSON, E., HEDLUND, P., NISELL, A., and NORDENSTAM, H.: *Acta Medica Scad., 153*:1, 1955.

BONITZ, K. *Zentralblatt fur Bakteriologie, Parasitenkunde, Infektionskrankheiten und Hygiene*, I. Orig. 168, pp. 244-256, Gustav Fisher Verlag, Stuttgart, 1957.

BORMAN, E. K., WHEELER, K. M., WEST, D. E., and MICKLE, F. L.: *Am. J. Pub. Health,* 33:127, 1943.

BORNSTEIN, S., SAPHRA, I., and STRAUSS, L.: *J. Infectious Dis.,* 69:59, 1941.

BORNSTEIN, S.: *New York State J. Med., 42*:163, 1942.

BORNSTEIN, S.: *J. Immunol., 46:*439, 1943.

BRAUN, H., and CASPARI, E.: *Tuerk. tib. cem. mec., 4:*264, 1938.

BRUNER, D. W., and MORAN, A. B.: *Cornell Vet., 39:*53, 1949.

CHERRY, W. B., SCHERAGO, M., and WEAVER, R. H.: *Am. J. Hygiene, 37:*211, 1943.

CLARENBURG, A., and KAMPELMACHER, E. H.: *Veral. en medel, betr. Volks-gezondh.,* No. 1, 1960.

CLARENBURG, A., VINK, H. H., and HUISMAN, W.: *Antonie Van Leeuwenhoek, 15:*14, 1949.

COUPER, W. R. M., NEWELL, K. W., and PAYNE, D. J. H., *Lancet, 270:*1057, 1956.

CRAIGIE, J. E.: *J.A.V.M.A., 105:*33, 1944.

CRUICKSHANK, J. C. and SMITH, H. W.: *Brit. M. J., 2:*1254, 1949.

CRUZ, E. DE LA: *Rev. Biol. Trop., 6:*27, 1958.

DACK, G. M.: *Food Poisoning.* The University of Chicago Press, 1956, 3rd Edition.

D'ALBORA, J. B., INGEGNO, A. P., and EDSON, J. N.: *J.A.M.A., 129:*10, 1945.

DAMON, S. R., and LEITER, L. W.: *Am. J. Hygiene, 7:*27, 1927.

DE NOBELE, J.: *Ann. Soc. Med. Gand., 77:*281, 1899.

EDWARDS, P. R., and BRUNER, D. W.: *J. Infectious Dis., 72:*58, 1943; *Ibid, 83:*220, 1948.

FRIESLEBEN, M.: *Deutsche med. Wchschr., 53:*1589, 1927.

GALBRAITH, N. S., HOBBS, B. C., SMITH, M. E., and TOMLINSON, A. J. H.: *Monthly Bull. Ministry Health & Public Health Serv., 19:*99, 1960.

GALTON, M. M., SCATTERDAY, J. E., and HARDY, A. V.: *J. Infectious Dis., 91:*1, 1952.

GARTNER, A.: *Correspondenzbl. d. allg. aerztl. Ver. v. Theuringen, 17:*233, 1888.

GAUMONT, R.: *Ann. Inst. Pasteur, 3:*140, 1950.

GAYLER, G. E., MACCREADY, R. A., REARDON, J. P., and MCKERNAN, B. F.: *Public Health Reports, 70:*311, 1955.

GIBBONS, N. E., and MOORE, R. L.: *Canad. J. Res., 22:*48, 1944.

GWATKIN, R., and MITCHELL, C. A.: *Canad. Public Health J., 35:*281, 1944.

HARDY, A. V., and GALTON, M. M.: *Am. J. Trop. Med. & Hyg., 4:*725, 1955.

HINSHAW, W. R., MCNEIL, E., and TAYLOR, T. J.: *Am. J. Hygiene, 40:*267, 1944.

HOBBS, B. C.: *Ann. Conf. of Assoc. of Public Health Inspectors held at Eastbourne,* Sept. 17-20, 1957.

JORDAN, E. O.: *J. Infectious Dis., 22:*252, 1918.

JORDAN, E. O.: *J. Infectious Dis., 36:*309, 1925.

KOSER, S. A.: *J. Infectious Dis., 31:*79, 1922.

KRUMWIEDE, C., VALENTINE, E., and KOHN, L. A.: *J. Med. Res., 39:*449, 1919.

KUNZ, L. J., and OUCHTERLONY, O. T. G.: *New England J. Med., 253:*761, 1955.

LEISTNER, L., JOHANTGES, J., DIEBEL, R. H., and NIVEN, C. F., JR.: *Proc. Thirteenth Research Conf., Amer. Meat Inst. Foundation, Univ. of Chicago,* 1961.

LUNDBECK, H., PLAZIKOWSKI, U., and SILVERSTOLPE, L.: *J. Applied Bact. (Great Britain), 18:*535, 1955.

MACKERRAS, J. M., and PASK, V. M.: *Lancet, 257:*940, 1949.

MCCULLOUGH, N. B., and EISELE, W. C.: *J. Infectious Dis., 88:*278, 1951; *Ibid, 89:*209, 259, 1951; *J. Immunol., 66:*595, 1951.

MCDONAGH, V. P., and SMITH, H. G.: *J. Hygiene, 56:*271, 1958.

MCWEENEY, E. G.: *Brit. M. J., 1:*1171, 1909.

*Med. Res. Council Spec. Rep. Ser. (London), 260:*29, 1947.

MEYER, K. F., and MATSUMURA, K.: *J. Infectious Dis., 41:*395, 1927.

*Ministry of Health and the Public Health Laboratory, Monthly Bulletin 15:*265, 1956; *18:*26, 1959; *19:*224, 1960.

NETER, E.: *Am. J. Public Health, 40:*929, 1950.

NEWELL, K. W., McCLARIN, R., MURDOCK, C. R., MacDONALD, W. N., and HUTCHINSON, H. L.: *J. Hygiene, 57:*92, 1959.

OSTROLENK, M., and WELCH, H.: *Am. J. Public Health, 32:*487, 1942.

PARKER, R. R., and STEINHAUS, E. A.: *Public Health Reports, 58:*1010, 1943.

POMEROY, B. S., and FENSTERMACHER, R.: *Am. J. Vet. Res., 5:*282, 1944.

PRICE-JONES, C.: *J. Path. Bact., 30:*45, 1927.

RUBIN, H. L., SCHERAGO, M., and WEAVER, R. H.: *Am. J. Hygiene, 36:*43, 1942.

RUBENSTEIN, A. D., FEEMSTER, R. F., and SMITH, H. M.: *Am. J. Pub. Health, 34:*841, 1944.

SALMON, D. E., and SMITH, T.: *Rep. Com. Agr., Wash., D.C.,* 1885.

SAVAGE, W. G., and WHITE, P. B.: *J. Hygiene, 21:*258, 1922-23.

SAVAGE, W. G., and WHITE, P. B.: *Med. Res. Council, Spec. Rep. Ser., 91:* 1925.

SCHNEIDER, M. D.: *Food Res., 11:*313, 521, 1946; *Food Technology, 15:*349, 1951.

SCHROEDER, R. J., and DALE, M. B.: *63rd Annual Proceedings United States Livestock Sanitary Associations,* December, 1959.

SEELIGER, H. P. R.: *Bull. World Health Organ. 22:*469, 1960.

SEGALOVE, M., and DACK, G. M.: *Food Res., 16:*118, 1951.

SELIGMAN, E., SAPHRA, I., and WASSERMANN, M.: *Am. J. Hygiene, 38:*226, 1943; *J. Immunol., 54:*69, 1946.

SMITH, J. M. P. and GOODSPEED, E. J.: The Complete Bible; An American Translation, The University of Chicago Press, 1939. *Deuteronomy, 14:*21.

SNAPPER, J.: *Am. J. Digest. Dis., 11:*8, 1944.

SOLOWEY, M., McFARLANE, V. H., SPAULDING, E. H., and CHEMERDA, C.: *Am. J. Pub. Health, 37:*971, 1947.

SPRAY, R. S.: *J.A.M.A., 86:*109, 1926.

SULKIN, S. E., and PIKE, R. M.: *Am. J. Pub. Health, 41:*769, 1951.

SURGALLA, M., and DACK, G. M.: *Food Res., 10:*108, 1945.

SUTHERLAND, P. L., and BERGER, F. M.: *Brit. M. J., 1:*488, 1944.

TAYLOR, J.: *Royal Society of Health Journal, 80:*253, 1960.

TORREY, J. C., and RAHE, A. H.: *J. Med. Res., 27:*291, 1912-13.

UHLENHUTH, P.: *Med. Klin., 48:*1823, 1908.

VEDER, E.: *Am. J. Pub. Health, 17:*1007, 1927.

WATT, J.: *Public Health Report, 60:*835, 1945.

WATT, J., and DE CAPITO, I.: *Am. J. Hygiene, 51:*343, 1950.

WELCH, H., OSTROLENK, M., and BARTRAM, M. T.: *Am. J. Pub. Health, 31:*332, 1941.

WOLFF, A. H., HENDERSON, N. D., and McCALLUM, G. L.: *Am. J. Pub. Health, 38:*403, 1948.

ZWICK and WEICHEL: *Arb. aus dem Kaiserl. Gesundheitsamte, 33:*250, 1910.

Chapter 7

LISTERIOSIS

Robert Graham, B.S., D.V.M.

LISTERIOSIS IS A specific infectious and often fatal disease of sheep, cattle, rabbits, guinea pigs, and chickens. In ruminants it is characterized by symptoms involving the central nervous system though in rodents it assumes a septicemic form. In chickens the principal lesions are in the myocardium. It has also been reported in the canary, capercaillie, fox, pig, goat, chinchilla, raccoon, lemming, ferret, and vole, as well as in man. The disease in man is accompanied by disturbances of the central nervous system.

HISTORY

Nyfeldt (1940) in his historical account of the discovery of *Listeria monocytogenes* stated that Hulphers first observed and cultivated the organism in Sweden in 1911. Murray, Webb, and Swann isolated the organism in rabbits and guinea pigs in 1926 in England and gave it the name *Bacterium monocytogenes* because the disease was characterized by an increase in the number of circulating monocytes. Recognizing the causative organism of "Tiger river disease" in rodents to be a new genus, Pirie (1927) in South Africa gave it the name *Listerella* and suggested the specific name *hepatolytica* because of the liver lesions it produced. When an exchange of cultures showed that the organisms isolated by Pirie and by workers in England were the same, Pirie withdrew the name *hepatolytica* in favor of the earlier name *monocytogenes*. After Becker (1939) pointed out that the generic name *Listerella* had already been used for a mycetozoon, Pirie (1940) suggested that new name *Listeria,* be used. This name, however, was not adopted at the time because it had already been given to a certain plant group. The name was changed to *Listeria monocytogenes* by Pirie (1948).

Listeria was first recognized as a cause of disease in domestic animals by Gill (1931) when he isolated the organism from sheep in New Zealand and gave the name "circling disease" to the encephalitis which it caused. Goodpasture reported the disease in rabbits in Tennessee in 1924, but the relation of this strain of *Listeria* to that isolated by other investigators was not established.

To date the causative organism has been isolated in the United States from twelve different animal species as well as man from twelve hosts in Germany, Uruguay, Argentina, Scotland, Italy, Denmark, Norway, France, Australia, Russia, England, New Zealand, South Africa, Sweden, Holland, Puerto Rico, Wales, Canada, and India (see Table 32).

Experimental studies on epizoology and immunology have not established the avenues of infection and the mode of transmission has not been determined. Little progress has been made in immunizing susceptible animals. Drew (1946) reported the occurrence of two immunological groups within the genus *Listeria* based upon results of precipitation reactions. King and Seeliger (1958) reported that four serological types of *Listeria monocytogenes* were found among 100 strains isolated in the United States. Of the 100 strains, seventy-one were type 4b, twenty-four were type 1, four were type 4a, and one was type 3.

TABLE 32

REPORTS ON SPONTANEOUS LISTERIOSIS

Host	Observer	Date Report Was Pub-lished (a)	Place of Origin or Study	Type of Disease
Rabbit	Goodpasture	1924	Tennessee	Encephalitis
	Murray, Webb and Swann	1926	England	Generalized infection
	Paterson	1940	England	Generalized infection
	Henricson	1943	Sweden	Generalized infection
	Jansen and Hurk	1945	Holland	Abortion
Guinea pig	Murray, Webb and Swann	1926	England	Generalized infection
Gerbille	Pirie	1927	South Africa	Generalized infection
Sheep	Gill	1931, '33, '37	New Zealand	Encephalitis
	Doyle (b)	1932	Indiana	Encephalitis
	Ten Broeck		New Jersey	Encephalitis
	Jungherr	1937	Connecticut	Encephalitis
	Graham, Dunlap, and Brandly	1938	Illinois	Encephalitis
	Morin	1938	Illinois	Encephalitis
	Biester and Schwarte	1939	Iowa	Encephalitis
	Paterson	1939, '40	England	Abortion

TABLE 32

REPORTS ON SPONTANEOUS LISTERIOSIS—*(cont'd)*

Host	Observer	Date Report Was Published (a)	Place of Origin or Study	Type of Disease
Sheep, *Cont.*	Graham, Hester, and Levine	1940	Illinois	Encephalitis
	Olafson	1940	New York	Encephalitis
	Pallaske	1940	Germany	Encephalomyelitis
	Cross	1941	Colorado	Encephalitis
	Henderson	1941	Illinois	Encephalitis
	Hoffman	1941	California	Encephalitis
	Jensen and Gay	1941	Illinois	Encephalitis
	Grini	1942	Norway	Encephalitis
	Hoffman and Lenarz	1942	California	Encephalitis
	Muth and Morrill	1942	Oregon	Encephalitis
	Belin and Lagriffoul	1943	France	Generalized infection
	Pomeroy, Fenstermacher, and Andberg	1943	Minnesota	Encephalitis
	Pothmann	1944	Germany	Encephalitis
	Spencer, Hoyt, and Whitehair	1944	Wisconsin	Encephalitis
	Cheng	1945	Michigan	Encephalitis
	Pounden and Edgington	1947	Ohio	Encephalitis
	Ryff and Lee	1948	Wyoming	Encephalitis
	Gray, Nelson, and Thorp	1949	Michigan	Generalized infection
	Jensen and Mackey	1949	Colorado	Encephalitis
	Stoenner, Mencimer, and Foster	1949	Utah	Encephalitis
	Viswanathan and Avyar	1950	India	Encephalitis
	Gray, Johnston, and Thorp	1951	Michigan	Encephalitis
	Gray, Stafseth, and Thorp	1951	Michigan	29 cases
	Gray, Stafseth, and Thorp	1951	Michigan	Encephalitis
	Olson, Rollins, Bagdonas, Blore and Segre	1953	Nebraska	67 cases
	Young	1956	Shetland	Encephalitis
	Watson and Hunter	1958	England	Multiple necrotic foci on liver
	Weide, Lagrace, Frank, Sanger and Bell	1960	Ohio	Encephalitis
Goat	Olafson	1940	New York	Encephalitis
	King	1940	New Jersey	Encephalitis
	Gifford and Eveleth	1942	Arkansas	Encephalitis
	Kaplan and Lager	1945	Massachusetts	Encephalitis
Cattle	Mathew (b)	1928	Indiana	Encephalitis
	Jones and Little	1934	New Jersey	Encephalitis
	Fincher (b)	1935	New York	Encephalitis
	Graham, Dunlap, and Brandly	1938	Illinois	Encephalitis
	Graham, Hester, and Levine	1939, '40	Illinois	Abortion

TABLE 32

REPORTS ON SPONTANEOUS LISTERIOSIS—(*cont'd*)

Host	Observer	Date Report Was Published (a)	Place of Origin or Study	Type of Disease
Cattle, *cont.*	Graham, Hester, and Levine	1940	Illinois	Encephalitis
	Biester and Schwarte	1941	Iowa	Encephalitis
	Harbor	1941	Wales	Generalized infection
	Peterson	1941	England	Hepatitis
	Schwarte and Biester	1942	Iowa	Encephalitis
	Evans and Sawyer	1942	Vermont	Abortion
	Poppensiek	1944	Maryland	Encephalitis
	Hatch	1945	Virginia	Encephalitis
	Boucher	1946	Pennsylvania	Encephalitis
	Cole	1946	Ohio	Encephalitis
	Pounden, Bell, and Mairs	1947	Ohio	Encephalitis
	Jensen and Mackey	1949	Colorado	Encephalitis
	Sellers, Pomeroy, Sautter, Pint, and Schrafel	1949	Minnesota	Meningo-encephalitis
	Svenkerud	1950	Norway	Encephalitis
	Gray, Stafseth, and Thorp	1951	Michigan	23 cases
	Ferguson, Bohl, and Ingalls	1951	Ohio	Abortion
	Jones	1954	England	Encephalitis
	Gray, Lassiter, Webster, Huffman and Thorp	1956	Michigan	6 calves, focal necrosis of the liver and gastroenteritis (septicemia)
	Young and Firehammer	1958	Montana	Abortion
	Smith and Sundquist	1960	Iowa	Encephalitis
	Osebold, Kendrick, and Njoku-Obi	1960	California	Abortion (3 herds)
Pig	DeBlieck and Jansen	1942	Holland	Necrotic foci in liver
	DeBlieck and Jansen	1943	Holland	Generalized infection
	Pomeroy, Fenstermacher, and Andberg	1943	Minnesota	Encephalitis
	Slabospits'kii	1938	Russia	Pox-like
	Biester and Schwarte	1940, '41	Iowa	Encephalitis
	Kerlin and Graham	1945	Illinois	Diarrhea
	Rhoades and Sutherland	1948	Illinois	Generalized infection
	Hemboldt, Jacobs, and Case	1951	Connecticut	Paralysis
	Hale	1959	Georgia	Generalized infection
	Jarrett, McIntyre, and Thorpe	1959	Scotland	Generalized infection
Horse	Jones (d)	1940	Virginia	Periodic ophthalmia
	Grini	1943	Norway	Generalized infection
	Svenkerud	1948	Norway	Generalized infection
Fox	Cromwell, Sweebe, and Camp	1939	Illinois	Distemper-like

TABLE 32

REPORTS ON SPONTANEOUS LISTERIOSIS—(*cont'd*)

Host	Observer	Date Report Was Published (a)	Place of Origin or Study	Type of Disease
Fox, *cont.*	Jensen and Pepperkamp	1947	Holland	Generalized infection
Man	Atkinson (e)	1917	Australia	Meningitis
	Dumont and Cotoni	1921	France	Meningitis
	Baldridge, Rohner and Hausmann (e)	1926	United States	Infectious mononucleosis
		1929, '32	Denmark	Infectious mononucleosis
	Nyfeld	1934	Norway	Meningitis
	Tesdal (e)			
	Schultz, Terry, Brice, and	1934, '38	California	Meningitis
	Gebhardt	1934, '35, '36	Connecticut	Meningitis
	Burn	1935	Scotland	Meningitis
	Gibson		Connecticut	Meningitis
	Allen (f)	1936	Massachusetts	Meningitis
	Carey			
	Poston, Upchurch and Booth	1937	North Carolina	Meningitis
	Schmidt and Nyfeldt	1938	Denmark	Infectious mononucleosis
		1938	Italy	Meningitis
	Cislaghi (g)			
	Pons and Julianelle	1939	Missouri	Infectious mononucleosis
	Porzecanski and de Baygorria	1939	Uruguay	Meningitis and otitis media
	Wright and Macgregor	1939	Scotland	Meningitis
	Wagner and Porter (h)		Iowa	Meningitis
	Savino	1940	Argentina	Meningo-encephalitis
	Fisher	1941	Uruguay	Meningo-encephalitis
	Handelman, Rotonde, Scott, and	1946	Kentucky	Meningitis
	Knighton	1948	Puerto Rico	Generalized infection
	Felsenfield	1948	Australia	Meningitis
Chicken	Stanley		New Jersey	Generalized infection
	Ten Broeck (c)	1937, '39	England	Generalized infection
	Paterson		England	Generalized infection
	Watkins (i)	1940	Germany	Generalized infection
	Pallaske	1941	New York	Generalized infection
	Cole			
	Hurt, Levine, and Graham	1941	Illinois	Generalized infection
	Hoffman and Lenarz	1942	California	Generalized infection
		1944	Germany	Generalized infection
	Pathmann			
	Jensen and Pepperkamp	1947	Holland	Generalized infection
		1950	Canada	Generalized infection
	Bigland	1951	North Dakota	Newcastle virus and Listeria isolated from brain
	Bolin and Turn			

TABLE 32

REPORTS ON SPONTANEOUS LISTERIOSIS—(*cont'd*)

Host	Observer	Date Report Was Published (a)	Place of Origin or Study	Type of Disease
Chicken, cont.	Thompson	1954	Washington, D. C.	Cirrhosis of the liver
Dog	Cox	1945	Alabama	Listeria in 4 dogs suspected of rabies
	Chapman	1947	Oregon	Encephalitis
Canary	Bigland	1950	Canada	Generalized infection
Capercaillie	Lilleengen	1950	Sweden	
Chinchilla	Shalkop	1950	Washington, D. C.	Generalized infection
	Smith	1955	Iowa	Generalized infection
	Leader and Holte	1955	Washington	Generalized infection
Lemming	Plummer and Byrne	1950	Canada	Generalized infection
Raccoon	Gifford and Jungherr	1947	Connecticut	Septicemia
Ferret	Morris and Norman	1950	Washington, D. C.	Possible carrier
Vole	Levy	1948	England	Generalized infection
Skunk	Osebold, Shultz, and Jameson	1957	California	Generalized infection
Turkey	Belding and Mayer	1957	Michigan	Focal necrosis of liver and encephalitis

(a) These reports are listed in the bibliography. (b) Did not identify as listeriosis but it was probably this disease. (c) Observation reported by Seaston (1935). (d) Relation of this strain of *Listeria* to that isolated by other investigators is not certain. (e) Classified organism as a diphtheroid, but it may have been *Listeria*. (f) Observation reported by Burn (1936). (g) Did not isolate *Listeria*. (h) Observation reported by Porter and Hale (1939). (i) Observation reported by Paterson (1939).

Seeliger and Sulzbacher (1956) investigated the antigenic relationships between the different serotypes of *Listeria monocytogenes* and *Staphylococcus aureus*. Reciprocal cross-reactions were demonstrated with serotypes 1, 2, and 3 of *Listeria monocytogenes* and many *Staphylococcus aureus* strains.

ETIOLOGY

The causative organism, *Listeria monocytogenes,* is a Gram-positive rod, 1 by 0.5 microns (see Figure 44). In hanging-drop preparations the species exhibits a rather peculiar tumbling motility that appears to be characteristic. All strains isolated at the Illinois Experiment Station are beta-hemolytic and grow well at 37° C. as well as at room temperature. Heavy growth in dextrose broth at room temperature, first noted by Paterson (1939), is sometimes helpful in recognizing *Listeria* species.

The morphologic and biochemic characters of *Listeria* have been studied by Seastone (1935), Webb and Barber (1937), Schultz, Terry, Brice, and Gebhardt (1938), Barber (1939), Biester and Schwarte (1939), Julianelle (1940, 1941B), Graham, Hester, and Levine (1940B), Cole (1941) and Harvey and Faber (1941B). Probably the most extensive study is that of Harvey and Faber, who reported the characteristics of fifty strains of *Listeria* from animal and human sources. More recently investigations have been conducted on specific growth requirements of organisms by Porter and Pelczar (1941) and Hunter (1942).

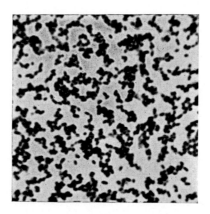

Fig. 44. Causative organism of listeriosis *Listeria monocytogenes* (magnified 1200x). *(Illinois Agri. Exper. Sta. Bull. 499.)*

The organism grows quite well on plain agar (see Figure 45); small colonies, bluish by transmitted light, can be distinguished in twenty-four hours. The organism grows still better on blood agar with a clear hemolytic zone, which helps to differentiate the colonies. *Listeria* strains ferment rhamnose, dextrose, levulose, lactose, maltose, sucrose, trehalose, dextrin, and salicin with acid production. Other sugars such as arabinose, raffinose, inulin, dulcitol, mannitol, sorbitol, and inositol were not attacked. Galactose was only occasionally attacked. Some sugars are fermented slowly. A selective method for the isolation of *Listeria monocytogenes* from mixed bacterial populations has been described by McBride and Girard (1960).

Lesbouyries (1943) confirmed the value of the ocular test proposed by Anton (1934). Olson and Boden (1944) reported a method of staining by which it was possible for the same preparation to diagnose more than one kind of infection including *Spirilla, Bacillus abortus, Listeria,* pyogenic bacteria, *Streptococci* and *staphylococci*.

Gray, Stafseth, Thorp, Sholl, and Riley (1948) reported that refrigeration of bovine brain tissue suspension for five weeks to three months before culturing yields a higher percentage of recoveries of *Listeria*. It is possible that bovine brain tissue may contain a growth-inhibiting factor which is sensitive to lower temperatures. This technique presents the possibility that listeriosis in cattle may be more frequent than the results with usual cultural methods would indicate.

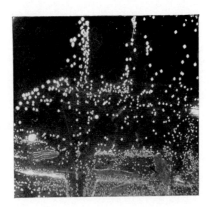

Fig. 45. Culture of *Listeria* from medulla of a cow naturally infected. The culture was incubated for forty-eight hours at 37 degree C. on plain agar. (*Illinois Agri. Exper. Sta. Bull. 499.*)

SEASONAL INCIDENCE

Listeriosis in ruminants usually occurs in winter and early spring, when animals are confined in feedlots. In Illinois, New York, and other states reported outbreaks have occurred from December through June, although one case in dairy cattle in Illinois occurred early in July. Gray, Stafseth, and Thorp (1951) reported listeriosis which occurred July 16, and Spencer, Hoyt, and Whitehair (1944) reported a case which occurred August 10. Although the disease has occurred in sheep that had been on pasture as long as four weeks, losses usually subside and the clinical disease disappears after animals are placed on pasture. These facts indicate that crowding may favor transmission of the disease. Dry feeds during the winter may lower resistance sufficiently to allow the organism to gain a foothold and possibly the lack of some essential nutrient in the ration so alters the defensive mechanism, particularly the nasal mucous membrane, as to favor infection.

EPIZOOTIOLOGY

Sporadic outbreaks reported in different sections of the United States suggest the widespread distribution of this disease, but knowledge of the reservoir and the method by which the disease is spread from animal to animal is not known.

Gill (1931, 1933, 1937) suggested that the sheep nasal fly, *Oestrus ovis,* might be the transmitter of the disease, but this has not been confirmed. The absence of the larvae in some affected sheep, together with the occurrence of the disease in cattle and in spring lambs, suggests that other factors may be involved in the transmission.

TABLE 33

LOSSES FROM LISTERIOSIS IN OUTBREAKS AMONG SHEEP IN ILLINOIS*

Outbreak No.	Animals in Herd	Animals Dead		Outbreak No.	Animals in Herd	Animals Dead	
		Number	Per Cent			Number	Per Cent
1............	300	30	10.0	4.......	180	12	6.7
2............	100	8	8.0	5.......	300	101	33.5
3 (1st year)...	800	40	5.0	6.......	—	—	—
(3rd year)...	894	57 (a)	6.4	7.......	—	12–15	—
(4th year)...	1,025	46	4.5				

(a) Exclusive of 31 lambs born during the outbreak.
*Illinois Agricultural Experiment Station Bulletin 499.

On an Illinois farm, an outbreak of ovine listeriosis occurred one winter when there were many rats in the barns. The next winter there were relatively few rats, and listeriosis did not occur. The disease reappeared the next winter when the rats were again numerous. On another farm where ovine listeriosis occurred, no livestock had been kept for several years previous to the time when the disease appeared, but on this farm, too, the buildings were overrun with rats. Olafson (1940) suggested that the rat might be the carrier of the disease. The Illinois Agricultural Experiment Station examined five live rats and two dead ones from a farm where the disease occurred. At autopsy no gross lesions were observed in any of the rats. The heart blood, liver, pharynx, and colons of all seven rats and the lungs of two were cultured on plain agar plates, but listeria was not recovered. However, the possible relation of rats to spontaneous outbreaks of the disease merits further study. Bolin and Turn (1951) pointed out the possibility that swine and fowl may be carriers of the disease. They believe that every effort should be made to keep species separated when losses occur. Morris and Norman (1950) suggest that the organism may be harbored by apparently healthy animals. Observations made by Osebold, Shultz and Jameson (1957) during an epizootic of listeriosis in California indicated that raccoons and skunks may be involved in outbreaks of the disease. They noted a population decline among raccoons and skunks preceding and during the time that the ruminants were affected. No raccoons could be obtained for study, but *Listeria* was isolated from a skunk that was collected during the outbreak.

TABLE 34

LOSSES FROM LISTERIOSIS IN OUTBREAKS AMONG CATTLE IN ILLINOIS*

Outbreak No.	Animals in Herd	Animals Dead		Outbreak No.	Animals in Herd	Animals Dead	
		Number	Per Cent			Number	Per Cent
1........	68	3	4.4	6..........	40	3	7.5
2........	—	1 (abortion)		7 (1st herd)..	173	5	2.9
3........	15	2	13.3	(2nd herd).	110	2	1.8
4......	30	2	6.7	8..........	20	1	5.0
5......	—	1	—				

*Illinois Agricultural Experiment Station Bulletin 499.

Observations indicate that in ruminants the disease does not sweep rapidly through the herd. Ordinarily less than 10 per cent of the herd may be affected. Isolated single cases have also been observed. While the morbidity is thus relatively low, the mortality in affected animals is very high. Few animals that show marked symptoms of the disease recover. Young animals are more susceptible than adults, and the disease seems to run a more rapid course in them. Sheep are apparently more susceptible than cattle, since the death losses among sheep are higher and death often follows a shorter period of illness. Eveleth, Goldsby, Bolin, Holm, and Turn (1953) reported that outbreaks of ovine listeriosis were often associated with the introduction of purchased animals. They also stated that in nearly all cases some radical change in management usually preceded the outbreaks.

The recurring nature of the disease was observed by Osebold, Kendrick, and Njoku-Obi (1960) in a herd of cattle where the *Listeria* organism was isolated during succeeding calving periods.

The avenues of infection in ruminants have not been determined, but it is possible that *Listeria* enter the nasal passages. This supposition is partially supported by the fact that experimental listerellosis, similar in all its aspects to the natural disease, is not ordinarily produced by intravenous or subcutaneous inoculation or by feeding. Experimentally the natural syndrome has occasionally followed the intranasal instillation of viable cultures at the Illinois Agricultural Experiment Station. In support of intranasal infection, Pons and Julianelle (1939) reported that an organism which was probably *Listeria* was isolated from the throat of a girl whose blood contained *Listeria* while Gill (1933) reported that repeated drenching of sheep with the culture by way of nostril resulted in meningitis and encephalitis. Asahi, Hosoda, and Akiyama (1957) demonstrated that *Listeria monocytogenes* may invade the oral or nasal mucous membranes. On the other hand, Julianelle (1940) reported that spraying the culture into the noses of rabbits and monkeys failed to produce the disease; whereas feeding the culture to mice in place of drinking water caused death in all cases. The results of a study by Gray, Singh and Thorp (1956) established the oral route as a possible mode of entry for *Listeria monocytogenes* and revealed that exposure by this method may cause intrauterine infection in pregnant sheep and goats.

Roine, Raitio and Vartiovaara (1953) produced listeriosis in the guinea pig by feeding aureomycin. They concluded that by suppressing certain strains of bacteria, aureomycin permits the active growth of other organisms such as *Listeria* which normally play only a subordinate part in the intestinal flora. Further investigation is needed to establish the mode of infection.

Olafson (1940) observed that outbreaks of listeriosis occurred in animals being fed silage, but he also noted that outbreaks had occurred in animals which had not been fed silage. This observation was confirmed by Graham, Levine, and Morrill (1943). Ryff and Lee (1948) reported an outbreak of listeriosis in 240 feeder lambs which had been feed corn silage for three weeks when the first cases began to develop. Olson, Bagdonas, Rollins and Blore (1953) found that there was no clear cut effect of continuous feeding of silage on development of listeriosis in sheep. A series of abortions in a range herd of beef cows following shortly the commencement of silage feeding was reported by Young and Firehammer (1958). Gray (1960) isolated *Listeria monocytogenes* from the viscera of a nonpregnant mouse and the fetuses of a pregnant mouse fed poor-grade silage thought to have initiated death and abortion in range cattle.

Gray (1960) reported that a culture of *Listeria monocytogenes* isolated from the brain of an infected sheep from a flock fed contaminated silage and cultures isolated from this silage were all serological type 4b, establishing a definite epidemiological relationship.

DIFFERENTIAL DIAGNOSIS

The isolation and identification of *Listeria monocytogenes* is regarded as conclusive evidence of the malady. Histopathologic changes marked by perivascular infiltration is suggestive of *Listeria* encephalitis. Myocardial and hepatic degeneration in chickens and rodents also suggest *Listeria* infection, but the isolation of *Listeria monocytogenes* is required in confirming a diagnosis.

Serologic tests have proved of no value in detecting infected animals. This disease, however, can generally be detected in ruminants by careful study of the history and symptoms. Other diseases which cause nervous symptoms might be confused with listerellosis. Therefore bacteriologic examination is required to confirm clinical diagnosis. Shannon (1951) contends that the early recognition of the disease in animals affected (swine, sheep, cattle, foxes, man) may prevent its becoming a serious public health problem.

THE DISEASE IN ANIMALS

The clinical symptoms and pathologic lesions associated with listerellosis vary with the host species. In the rabbit, guinea pig, and gerbille a generalized septicemic infection associated with a circulating monocytosis and necrotic foci of the liver is characteristic. In the chicken the disease is characterized by focal but massive necrosis of the myocardium. Thompson (1954) observed an advanced cirrhosis of the liver of a chicken from which *Listeria* was isolated.

Belding and Mayer (1957) isolated *Listeria* from two turkeys in which there was a scarcity of visceral lesions.

In experimentally induced listeriosis in turkey poults, Malewitz, Gray and Smith (1957) report that the first symptom observed was drooping of the head followed by nervous symptoms, hunched position and finally almost complete paralysis. The fox from which *Listeria* was isolated by Cromwell, Sweebe, and Camp (1939) suffered from a distemper-like disease. In swine, Biester and Schwarte (1940) described an encephalitic form of the disease, and deBlieck and Jansen (1943) and Rhoades and Sutherland reported a septicemic form. Kerlin and Graham (1945) isolated the organism from a pig's liver. Bolin and Eveleth (1951) isolated *Listeria* from the liver of a pig dying from lye poisoning. Helmboldt, Jacobs, and Case (1951) reported an encephalitis in swine due to *Listeria* characterized by paralysis and dyspnea. Cox (1945) cultured the organism from four dogs suspected of rabies. Hofman and Lenarz (1943) isolated *Listeria* from a chicken with lesions of lymphomatosis. Jones (1940) reported isolation of *Listeria*-like organisms from the organs of fourteen out of twenty-seven cases of equine periodic ophthalmia, but their taxonomic relation to *Listeria* seems inconclusive. Webb (1935) inoculated rabbits with *Listeria* intravenously in producing pseudotubercle lesions.

Listeriosis in ruminants is usually manifested by an encephalitis or encephalomyelitis. Meningitis may also be present. Bovine abortion unaccompanied by cerebral disturbances has been reported by Graham, Hester, and Levine (1939, 1940A) and by Evans and Sawyer (1942) and by Ferguson, Bohl, and Ingalls (1951) and in sheep by Paterson (1939A, 1940D). Ferguson Bohl, and Ingalls (1951) suggested that in two cases of abortion in cows there were circumstances which might indicate that there were in each case some factors in addition to *Listeria* which could have been involved, such as violence or injury. Gray, Lassiter, Webster, Huffman and Thorp (1956) reported the isolation of *Listeria monocytogenes* from the livers of six calves less than nineteen days of age. The predominant symptoms were general weakness and loss of weight, and the most consistent lesions at necropsy were hepatic necrosis and gastroenteritis. The encephalitic syndrome in sheep and cattle is preceded by symptoms of dullness and impaired vision. In fact in some outbreaks the first observed symptom has been refusal to come to the feeding racks, though not all affected animals exhibit symptoms of inappetence. High temperatures may be noted in the first stages of the disease. The animal walks into feed bunks or other objects or close to them before observing them. In some outbreaks the first

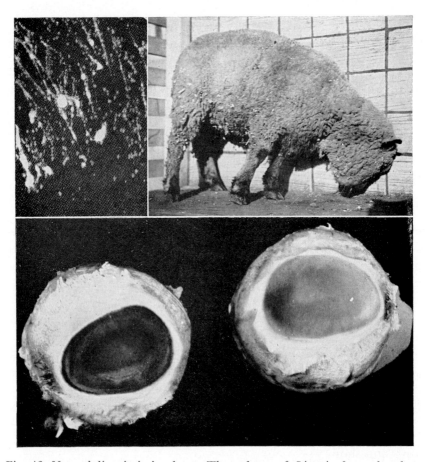

Fig. 46. Natural listeriosis in sheep. The culture of *Listeria* from the sheep medulla (upper left) was incubated forty-nine hours at 37° C. The large white masses are medulla tissue. The eye of the sheep shown below to the right is affected with keratitis; the other is normal. *(Illinois Agri. Exper. Sta. Bull. 499.)*

observed symptom may be a staggering, unsteady gait. As the disease progresses the animals begins to circle either to the right or the left and to push or lean against solid objects (see Figure 46). Circling is especially characteristic of the disease in sheep and cattle. Torticollis may be observed. If the head is placed in normal position, it returns to the side as soon as released. Because of the increasing numbers of animals exhibiting central nervous symptoms of undiagnosed etiology, Boucher (1946) suggested that brain cultures for the presence of *Listeria* be made whenever possible.

A mucous nasal discharge is noted in some animals. Quite frequently one ear droops and in some cases the animal drools stringy

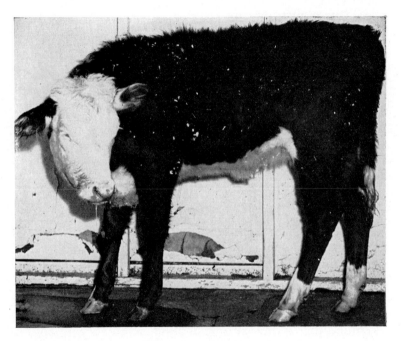

Fig. 47. Feeder calf affected with listeriosis. Note the drooling and the drooped ear. *(Illinois Agri. Exper. Sta. Bull. 499.)*

saliva and shows apparent paralysis of the pharynx (see Figure 47). The animal, though able to drink slowly, may be unable to eat.

Conjunctivitis and opacity of the cornea of the eye have been noted (see Figures 46 and 48). As the disease progresses, the affected animal is unable to rise. Some animals perform running movements while lying on their sides. In sheep this causes the wool to come off and decubital sores to appear on the shoulder and hip. The animal becomes progressively weaker accompanied by coma, lasting several hours or a few days before death. The results of studies conducted by Olson, Rollins, Bagdonas, Blore and Segre (1953) on sixty-seven natural cases of listeriosis in sheep indicate that *Listeria monocytogenes* is not always localized or limited to the central nervous system.

In experimental listeriosis the nature of the histopathologic changes depends to some extent upon the route of infection. Olson, Cook, and Blore (1950) noted variation in reaction of sheep following experimental exposure. The method of exposure, together with the possibility of previous contact with the organism, was mentioned in explanation of the variation. Segre, Olson, Marsh and Blore

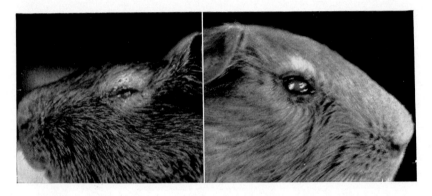

Fig. 48. Guinea pigs after suprajunctival exposure to *Listeria*. Both guinea pigs have conjunctivitis; the one to the right has keratitis also. *(Illinois Agri. Exper. Sta. Bull. 499.)*

(1956) found that several antimetabolites, when administered in an attempt to alter the tricarboxylic acid cycle, failed to influence the course of experimental listeriosis in young chickens. Virulence of the organism may also be a factor, as pointed out by Schwarte and Biester (1942). When microscopic lesions are present, they follow a rather constant pattern according to the organ affected. Lesions produced by the natural infection among ruminants are largely limited to the central nervous system (Figure 49). In the central nervous system the disease is characterized by perivascular infiltration with cells among which lymphocytes and monocytes predominates, focal areas of infiltration, or necrosis and infiltration with neutrophiles. Some of the foci fulfill all the requisites for true suppuration. Whether the cells found in the perivascular infiltrations are recorded as predominately lymphocytes or monocytes may depend upon the organism and the host. The foci of neutrophilic infiltration may or may not have vascular relations. Olafson (1940) considers this lesion the most characteristic of the infection, since it is said to contain the bacteria; the perivascular infiltrations do not.

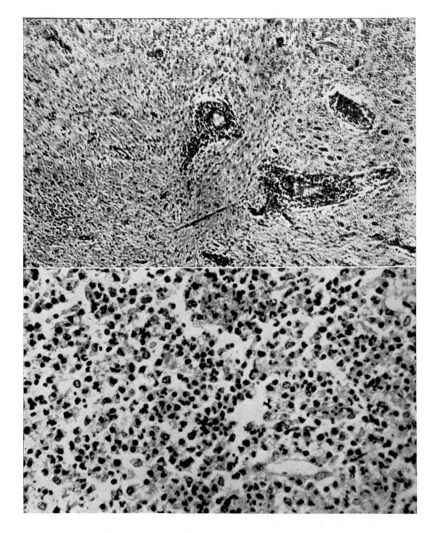

Fig. 49. Brain stem from a sheep naturally infected with listeriosis. Perivascular infiltration with lymphoid and mononuclear cells and necrosis of neurons are shown above magnified 100x. Below is shown focal cellular reaction in which neutrophiles predominate (magnified 300x). *(Illinois Agri. Exper. Sta. Bull. 499.)*

A study of the reaction of lymphatic tissue of rabbits to repeated injections of *Listeria* was made by Conway (1939).

Less constant lesions are focal and perivascular edema or hemorrhage, or both, and degenerative changes in the nerve cells and tracts. Cell inclusions have not been observed. This fact and the fact that attempts to reproduce the disease with bacteria-free filtrates from infected tissues have failed would indicate that a filtrable virus is not a factor in listeriosis. That there is some unrecognized factor in natural infection is suggested by the difficulty with which the infection is produced experimentally. Olson and Segre (1956) reported the isolation of a nonbacterial listeriosis-enhancing agent from a sheep kept on the premises where an attack of listeriosis had occurred. They concluded that listeriosis-enhancing agent plays a definite role in aiding the entrance of *Listeria* and in the pathogenesis of the infection. The distribution of lesions in the brain suggests the possibility of spread by way of the meninges, canal systems, and vessel sheaths. The results of studies made by Asahi, Hosoda and Akiyama (1957) suggested that in naturally occurring encephalitic listeriosis, *Listeria monocytogenes* invades the oral or nasal mucous membranes and travels along the trigeminal nerve to the brain stem.

On the other hand, neuropathic examination of 15 natural cases of ovine listeric encephalomyelitis by Cordy and Osebold (1959) indicated that lesions first developed in association with the smallest vessels. They reported that the lesions bore no relationship to meningeal or ependymal surfaces nor to cranial nerve roots.

Liver lesions when present in cases of listeriosis in rodents are noted as discrete foci of necrosis, sometimes preceded by visible fatty changes in the cells (Pirie, 1927) and later surounded by hepatic cells showing fatty changes (Webb and Barber, 1937). Necrosis is thought to appear in the hepatic cells surrounding Kuppfer cells which have ingested numerous organisms, according to Webb and Barber (1937) and Bianchi (1930). The foci of necrosis enlarge and often become infiltrated with neutrophiles or mononuclear cells, or both. Bloom (1928) observed necrotic foci in suprarenals, liver, spleen, and occasionally in lymph glands in rabbits.

Myocardial lesions (Figure 50) consist of necrosis of the heart muscle and cell infiltrations among which mononuclears usually predominate.

Eye lesions consist of conjunctivitis, which may be catarrhal or follicular in nature; keratitis, characterized principally by destruction of epithelium and mild infiltration with leucocytes, mainly neutrophiles; and extension of the capillary system into the substantia

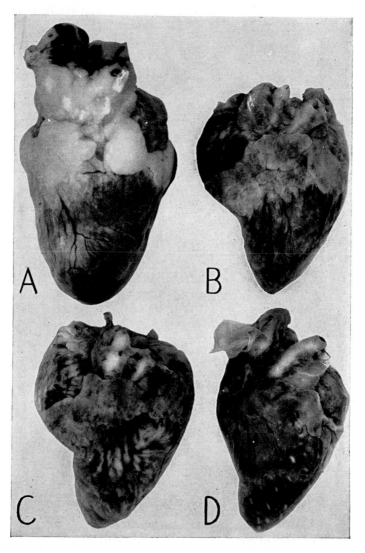

Fig. 50. Massive and focal necrosis of the myocardium. Heart A is normal, Hearts B and C show massive necrosis and Heart D focal necrosis in chickens that died following intravenous inoculation with *Listeria*. *(Illinois Agri. Exper. Sta. Bull. 499.)*

propria of the cornea. Other lesions have seldom been observed or have not been well described.

Gray (1958) reported that in a few instances *Listeria monocytogenes* has been associated with mastitis in cows.

Listeria monocytogenes was isolated by Osebold, Kendrick and Njoku-Obi (1960) from the mammary gland secretions of a cow following abortion.

THE DISEASE IN MAN

Listeriosis in man has been reported in California, Connecticut, Iowa, Kentucky, Missouri, and North Carolina, and in the following countries: Argentina, Australia, Denmark, France, Italy, Scotland, Holland, Puerto Rico and Uraguay. The mode of transmission is not known.

The relationship of *Listeria* to human and veterinary medicine was described by Nyfeldt (1940) although the role of infected animals in the epidemiology of human cases has remained obscure. Stoenner, Mencimer, and Foster (1949) reported that three sheep that had died of listeriosis were skinned by herdsmen, using no precautions, and yet no infection resulted.

In man the disease always involves the central nervous system. In thirteen of the reported cases, it was associated with meningitis; in four cases, with infectious mononucleosis; and in two cases, with meningo-encephalitis.

Among the histopathologic changes described in human listeriosis by Burn (1936) and Wright and Macgregor (1939) the more prominent and constant changes were: suppurative leptomeningitis, focal areas of necrosis in the liver, focal pneumonia and bronchiolitis, and splenic engorgement. Also observed in the brain were hemorrhages and perivascular infiltration with neutrophiles, lymphocytes, and plasma cells.

Nyfeldt (1929, 1932) and Schmidt and Nyfeldt (1938) reported the isolation of *Listeria* from a number of cases of infectious mononucleosis of which it was believed to be the cause. Pons and Julianelle (1939) obtained true *Listeria* from a single case of infectious mononucleosis, but further study by Julianelle (1940, 1941A) indicates that the association was probably incidental. In a controlled experiment, Janeway and Damnin (1941) found no relationship between the organisms of *Listeria* and infectious mononucleosis in humans as judged by agglutination reaction. Subsequently Nettle-ship (1942) reported that infectious mononucleosis in man is caused by a filtrable virus. Some evidence that *Listeria* may be responsible for certain syndromes diagnosed as infectious mononucleosis (gland-ular fever) has been offered by Stanley (1949).

Gray (1960) has presented evidence which indicates that listeriosis may be a cause of repeated abortion in women and mental retarda-tion in young children.

PREVENTION AND CONTROL

No universally effective preventive measures are known. Isola-tion of sick animals seems effective in some herds; in others, the dis-ease may fail to subside until the animals are turned out on pasture. Thus it is quite evident that the epizootiology of listeriosis deserves further investigation, with special reference to the carrier feature, the natural reservoir of infection and the mode or modes of trans-mission. Experimental vaccines and antiserums have been employed experimentally in natural outbreaks and experimentally in guinea pigs and rabbits with irregular and unfavorable results. Pothman (1944) attempted to produce agglutins in chickens but failed. Ose-bold and Sawyer (1955) successfully immunized seventeen sheep against *Listeria monocytogenes* by the subcutaneous inoculation of virulent live culture.

EXPERIMENTAL THERAPY

In general, sulfonamides, penicillin, and streptomycin therapy have given indifferent or poor results in listeriosis. Marshall (1940) reported that the sulfanilamide group was effective. Jensen, Rue, and Mackey (1949) found that late in an outbreak in cattle, when many cases were found before prostration developed, the results of treatment with penicillin and sulfanilamide were favorable. Graham, Levine, and Morrill (1943) suggested that sulfonamides may be of value in treating cattle and sheep but only if administered very early and in large doses. Reporting a case of human listeriosis, Handleman, Rotonde, Scott, and Knighton (1946) reported that penicillin was without effect. Ryff and Lee (1948) reported that streptomycin, sulfathiazole, and sulfamerazine were of little or no value, while sodium sulfapyridine and penicillin appeared promising.

On the basis of *in vitro* and *in vivo* experiments in rabbits, Gray, Stafseth, and Thorp (1950) found that streptomycin used on *Listeria* was contraindicated. *In vitro* studies by Foley, Epstein, and Lee (1944) demonstrated that penicillin was ineffective, while Felsenfeld, Volini, Ishihara, Bachman, and Young (1950) found that *Listeria* was sensitive to low levels of aureomycin, neomycin, and polymycin D. Gray, Thorp, and Laine (1950) reported that aureomycin inhibited the organism *in vitro* and that it was also very effective *in vivo*. Zink, deMello, and Burkhart (1950), after conducting comparative *in vitro* sensitivity tests made by the tube-dilution method of Dornbush and Pelcak (1948), reported that a strain of *Listeria monocytogenes* was very sensitive to aureomycin and resistant to terramycin, penicillin, chloromycetin, and streptomycin. These authors also reported that aureomycin gave 100 per cent protection against experimental infection in mice when the antibiotic was given in daily doses of 5 milligrams per kilogram of body weight for four days. Long, Bliss, Scheonbach, Chandler, and Bryer (1950) recognized the value of aureomycin in treating listeriosis.

Santi and Serembe (1950), in studies on absorption, distribution, and elimination of aureomycin, reported that there was a concentration of 10 micrograms per gram of brain five minutes following intravenous administration of 40 milligrams per kilogram of body weight to rabbits or guinea pigs while, after thirty minutes, a concentration of only 1 microgram was present. After one hour, no trace of the drug could be demonstrated in the brain. From their findings, it is suggested that one daily dose administered to an animal seven days after the onset of the disease, with manifest central nervous system involvement, could not be expected to maintain a therapeutic concentration at the site of infection. Gray (1958) reported that although some animals, especially cows, with listeric encephalitis may respond to therapy with terramycin or aureomycin there is always danger that the animal may continue to show evidence of brain damage. It appears that in animals the brain lesions are so far advanced before symptoms are shown that, although growth of the bacterium may be arrested, complete recovery is not possible.

Sulfonamides may be of value in treating cattle and sheep but only if administered very early and in large doses. Once encephalitic symptoms develop it is probably too late to institute therapy with much hope of success. The problem then becomes one of recognizing new cases and starting treatment as early as possible. The most promising approach in detecting new cases is a study of the body temperatures of apparently normal animals in affected herds, since the temperature is usually elevated in the initial stages of the disease.

ITEMS OF NOTE

1) Listeriosis is a specific bacterial septicemia in rodents and chickens. In man it is characterized chiefly by meningitis, in ruminants and swine by encephalitis. Abortion in cattle and sheep has also been reported as due to *Listeria,* and premature birth has been experimentally induced by inoculating pregnant ruminants with viable cultures of *Listeria.*

2) In its usual encephalitic form the clinical symptoms make it possible to recognize affected animals easily. Listeriosis can be confirmed by bacteriologic examination of the medulla at autopsy.

3) Listeriosis occurs most commonly in winter and early spring when animals are closely confined. The disease appears to be of worldwide distribution and apparently is increasing in frequency. It has even been suggested by some authors that listeriosis may continue to spread until someday it will assume the importance of brucellosis as a public health problem.

4) Sulfonamides administered in large doses have on occasion given encouraging results, but only when administered very early and in large doses. Of all the drugs employed in treating listeriosis, aureomycin seems preferable. No specific effective preventive measures are known. Sanitation and isloation of the affected animals, and good pasture in season are apparently helpful in checking the spread of the disease in some outbreaks.

5) The causative organism, *Listeria monocytogenes,* is Grampositive and rod-shaped. It is approximately 0.5 by 1 micron, is characterized by a tumbling type of motility, and causes beta hemolysis. Growth occurs quite well at room temperature as well as 37° C.

6) In experimental listeriosis in cattle, sheep, rabbits, guinea pigs, swine, and chickens, the distribution of lesions varies with the route of inoculation. Conjunctivitis and keratitis, which are occasionally observed in the natural disease in ruminants, may be quite readily induced in rabbits and guinea pigs by supraconjunctival inoculation. This characteristic of *Listeria* is an aid in identifying the organism.

7) Histopathologic studies indicate that the essential character of the lesion in a given tissue is the same in the experimental infection as in the naturally incurred disease. In the brain, lesions are likely to be more numerous in the white than in the gray matter and are constituted mainly by focal infiltrations of neutrophiles and by perivascular infiltration of lymphoid and mononuclear cells. In animals which develop systemic infection, foci of necrosis and infiltration with lymphoid and mononuclear cells may be observed in the liver and heart.

8) Attempts at immunization of rabbits, guinea pigs, chickens, and sheep against listeriosis by means of killed (and in some cases living) *Listeria* cultures were unsuccessful.

9) Attempts at immunization of rabbits, guinea pigs, sheep and cattle against listeriosis by means of antisera were unsuccessful. In some cases the administration of antiserum apparently rendered the animals even more suceptible to experimental infection.

REFERENCES

ANTON, W.: *Zentrabl. Bakt., 131*:89-103, Abt. 1, Orig., 1934.
ASAHI, O., HOSODA, T., and AKIYAMA, Y.: *Am. J. Vet. Res., 18*:147-157, 1957.
ATKINSON, E.: *M. J. Australia, 1*:115-118, 1917 (cited by JULIANELLE, 1940).
BALDRIDGE, C. W., ROHNER, F. J. and HANSMAN, G. H.: *Arch. Int. Med., 38*:413-448, 1926.
BARBER, MARY: *J. Path. & Bact., 48*:11-23, 1939.
BECKER, E. R.: *Rep. to Com. on Nomenclature at Third Internatl. Cong. for Microbiol.,* New York, 1939.
BELDING, R. C. and MAYER, M. L.: *J.A.V.M.A., 131*:296-297, 1957.
BELIN, M. and LAGRIFFOUL, A.: *Bull. acad. vétér., 16*:376, France 1934 (abstracted in *Bull. Inst. Pasteur., 44*:37).
BIANCHI, L.: *Haematology, 11*:163-188, 1930.
BIESTER, H. E. and SCHWARTE, L. H.: *J. Infect. Dis., 64*:135-144, 1939.
—— *J.A.V.M.A., 96*:339-342, 1940.
—— *U. S. Livestock Canit. Assoc. Rep.,* 1940, pp. 42-47.
—— *North Am. Vet., 22*:729-734, 1941.
BIGLAND, C. H.: *J. Comp. Med., 14* (10):319-324, 1950.
BLOOM, W.: *Arch. Path., 6*:995, 1928. *Folia Haematol., 37*:1-62, 1928.
BOLIN, F. M. and TURN, JENNY: *North Dakota Agric. Exp. Sta. Bimonthly Bull., 8*: No. 3, 107-108, Jan. and Feb., 1951.
BOLIN, F. M. and EVELETH, D. F.: *J.A.V.M.A., 118*:7, 1951.
BOUCHER, W. B.: *J.A.V.M.A., 109*:213, 1946.
BURN, C. G.: *Soc. Exper. Biol. & Med. Proc., 31*:1095, 1934.
—— *J. Bact., 30*:573-591, 1935.
—— *Am. J. Path., 12*:341-348, 1936.
CAREY, B. W., JR.: *Pediatrics, 8*:626-629, 1936.
CHAPMAN, MERWYN P.: *North Am. Vet., 28*:532-538, 1947.

CHENG, CING-TUAN: A thesis submitted to the School of Graduate Studies, Michigan State College, 1945. (Cited by GRAY, STAFSETH and THORP, 1951).

CISLAGHI, F.: *Pediatria, 46:*637-641, 1938 (cited by JULIANELLE, 1940).

COLE, CLARENCE R.: *J.A.V.M.A., 109:*216-217, 1946.

COLE, R. K.: *Poultry Sc., 20:*28-31, 1941.

CONWAY, E. A.: *Arch. Path., 25:*200-227.

CORDY, D. R. and OSEBOLD, J. W.: (1959) *J. Infect., Dis., 104:*164-173.

COX, BENJ. F.: *Auburn Vet., 1:*98-99, 1945

CROMWELL, H. W., SWEEBE, E. E. and CAMP, T. C.: *Science, 89:*293, 1939.

CROSS, FLOYD: *Colo. Farm. Bull., 3:* No. 3, 9, 1941.

DE BLIECK, L. and JANSEN, JAC.: *Tijdschr. V. Diergencesk, 69:*575, 1942.

DE BLIECK, L. and JANSEN, JAC.: *J. Microbiol. & Serol., 9:*93-103, 1943.

DORNBUSH, A. C. and PELCAK, E. J.: *Ann. New York Acad. Sc., 51:*318-320, 1948

DOYLE, L. P.: *J.A.V.M.A., 81:*118, 1932.

DREW, RUTH M.: *Proc. Soc.,* XBM *61:*30-33, 1946.

DUMONT, J. and COTONI, L.: *Ann. Inst. Pasteur, 35:*625-633, 1921.

EVANS, W. M. and SAWYER, J. E.: *Cornell Vet., 32:*448-449, 1942.

EVELETH, D. F., GOLDSBY, A. I., BOLIN, F. M., HOLM, G. C., and TURN, J.: *Vet. Med., 48:* 321-323, 1953.

FELSENFELD, OSCAR: *Puerto Rico J. Pub. Health & Trop. Med., 24:*1-4, 1948.

FELSENFELD, O., VOLINI, I. F., ISHIHARA, S. J., BACHMAN, M. C. and YOUNG, V. M.: *J. Lab. & Clin. Med., 35:*428-433, 1950 (cited by ZINK, DE MELLO and BURKHART, 1951).

FERGUSON, L. C., BOHL, E. H. and LINGALLS, W. L.: *J.A.V.M.A., 118:*10-11, 1951

FINCHER, M. C.: *Cornell Vet., 25:*61-63, 1935.

FISCHER, J. T.: *Arch. urug. med., 18:*156-170, 1941 (not seen).

FOLEY, E. J., EPSTEIN, J. A. and LEE, S. W.: *J. Bact., 47:*110-111, 1944.

GIBSON, H. J.: *J. Path. & Bact., 41:*239, 1935.

GIFFORD, REBECCA and EVELETH, D. F.: *J.A.V.M.A., 101:*413-417, 1942.

GIFFORD, REBECCA and JUNGHERR, ERWIN: *Cornell Vet., 37:*39-48, 1947.

GILL, D. A.: *Vet. J., 87:*60-74, 1931.

—— *Vet. J., 89:*258-270, 1933.

—— *Australia Vet. J., 13:*46, 1937.

GOODPASTURE, E. W.: *J. Infect. Dis., 34:*428-432, 1924.

GRAHAM, R.: *J.A.V.M.A., 95:*289-292, 1939.

—— DUNLAP, G. L. and BRANDLY, C. A.: *Science, 88:*171-172, 1938.

GRAHAM, R., DUNLAP, G. L. and LEVINE, N. D.: *Cornell Vet., 30:*268-290, 1940.

—— HESTER, H. R. and LEVINE, N. D.: *Science, 90:*336-337, 1939.

—— *J. Infect. Dis. 66:*91-96, 1940.

—— *Cornell Vet., 30:*97-111.

—— *Ohio State Vet. M. A. Proc.,* 58th Ann. Mtg., 1941.

—— and LEVINE, N. D.: *J.A.V.M.A., 102:*365-367, 1943.

GRAHAM, R. LEVINE, N. D. and MORRILL, C. C.: Bull. 499, *Univ. Ill. Agric. Exper. Sta.,* pp. 99.

—— MORRILL, C. C. and LEVINE, N. D.: *Cornell Vet., 30:*291-298, 1940.

GRAY, M. D., STAFSETH, H. J., THORP, F., JR., SHOLL, L. B. and RILEY, W. R., JR.: *J. Bact. 55:*471-476, 1948.

GRAY, M. L., JOHNSTON, R. L. and THORP, FRANK, JR.: *MSC Veterinarian* 2, 3, 108 and 136, 1951.

GRAY, M. L.: *Arch. Pediat. 76:*488-492, 1959.

GRAY, M. L.: Beiheft 1 zum *Zentralblatt fur Veterinarmedizin*, 1958.

GRAY, M. L.: *J.A.V.M.A.*, *136*:205-208, 1960.

GRAY, M. L.: *Science, 132*:1767-1768, 1960.

GRAY, M. L., LASSITER, C. A., WEBSTER, H. D., HUFFMAN, C. F., and THORP, F., JR.: *Vet. Med.*, *51*:316-318 and 335-336, 1956.

GRAY, M. L., NELSON, R. N., and THORP, FRANK, JR.: *J.A.V.M.A.*, *115*:103-104, 1949.

GRAY, M. L., SINGH, C. and THORP, F., JR.: *Am. J. Vet. Res.*, *17*:510-516, 1956.

GRAY, M. L., STAFSETH, H. J. and THORP, FRANK, JR.: *J.A.V.M.A.*, *115*:171-173, 1949.

GRAY, M. L., STAFSETH, H. J. and THORP, FRANK, JR.: *J.A.V.M.A.*, *118*:242-252, 1951.

GRAY, M. L., THORP, F., JR. and LAINE, S. L.: *Bact. Proc.*, *1950*:93 (cited by ZINK, DE MELLO and BURKHART, 1951).

GRINI, OLA: *Norsk. Vet.-tidsskr.* 417-428, 1942. (Cited by GRAY, STAFSETH and THORP, 1951).

GRINI, OLA: *Norsk. Vet.-tidsskr.* 97-104. 1943. (Cited by GRAY, STAFSETH and THORP, 1951).

HALE, M. W.: *J.A.V.M.A.*, *135*:324-325, 1959.

HANDLEMAN, N. I., ROTONDE, C. C., SCOTT, E. P. and KNIGHTON, H. T.: *Pediatrics, 28:* 210-213, 1946.

HARBOR, A. E.: *Vet. J.*, *97(12)*:401-407, 1941.

HARVEY, P. C. and FABER, J. E.: *J. Bact.*, *41*:45-46, 1941.

—— *J. Bact.*, *42*:677-687, 1941.

HATCH, RAY D.: *J. Bact.*, *49*:110-111, 1945.

HELMBOLDT, C. F., JACOBS, R. E. and CASE, L. I.: *Vet. Met.*, *46(9)*:347-449, 1951.

HENDERSON, J. A.: *North Am. Vet.*, *aa*:545-546, 1941.

HENRICSON, T.: *Svenska Vet. Tidskr.*, *48*:1-9, 1943 (abstracted in *Vet. Bull.*, *13*:312).

HOFFMAN, H. A.: *J.A.V.M.A.*, *98*:234-235, 1941.

HOFFMAN, H. A. and LENAR, C.: *J.A.V.M.A.*, *100*:340-342, 1942 (abstracted in *Vet. Bull.*, *12*:483).

HURT, R. H., LEVINE, N. D. and GRAHAM, ROBERT: *Am. J. Vet. Res.*, *2*:279-280, 1941.

HUNTER, S. H.: *J. Bact.*, *43*:629-640, 1942.

JANEWAY, C. A. and DAMNIN, G. J.: *J. Clin. Investigation*, *20*:233-239, 1941.

JANSEN, J. and HURK, G. F.: *Tijdschr. Diergeneesk*, *70*:106-114, 1945.

JANSEN, JACOB and PEPPERKAMP, C. W.: *Tidschr, Diergeneesk.*, *72*:319-320, 1947 (abstracted in *J.A.V.M.A.*, *114*:255, 1949).

JANSEN, JACOB and PEPPERKAMP, C. W.: *Tidschr. Diergeneesk.*, *72*:3219-320, 1947 (abstracted in *J.A.V.M.A.*, *114*:255, 1949).

JARRETT, W. F. H., McINTYRE, W. I. M. and THORPE, E.: *Vet. Rec.*, *71*:225-226, 1959.

JENSEN, G. W. and GAY, W. J.: *North Am. Vet.*, *22*:601-605, 1941.

JENSEN, RUE and MACKEY, D. R.: *J.A.V.M.A.*, *114*:420-424, 1949.

JONES, E. W.: *Vet. Rec.*, *66*:296-298, 1954.

JONES, F. S. and LITTLE, R. B.: *Arch. Path.*, *18*:580-581, 1934.

JONES, T. C.: *Am. J. Vet. Res.*, *1*:54-56, 1940.

JONES, T. C.: *Am. J. Vet. Res.*, *3*:45-71, 1942.

JULLIANELLE, L. A.: *Ann. Int. Med.*, *14*:608-620, 1940.

—— *J. Bact.*, *42*:367-383, 1941.

—— *J. Bact.*, *41*:44-45, 1941.

—— *J. Bact.*, *42*:385-394, 1941.

—— and MOORE, ELIZABETHS *Am. J. Path.*, *18*:813-825, 1942.

—— and PONS, C. A.: *Soc. Exper. Biol. & Med. Proc.*, *40*:362-363, 1939.

—— *Soc. Exper. Biol. & Med. Proc.*, *40*:364-365, 1939.

JUNGHERR, ERWIN: *J.A.M.A.*, *91:*73-87, 1937.

KAPLAN, MARTIN M. and LAGER, A. E.: *Vet. Med.*, *40:*199-202, 1945.

KERLIN, D. L. and GRAHAM, ROBERT: *Proc. Soc.*, *XBM 58:*351-352, 1945.

KING, E. O. and SEELIGER, H. P. R.: *J. Bact.*, 77 No. 1:122-123, 1959.

KING, L. S.: *Am. J. Path.*, *16:*467-478, 1940.

LANG, F. J.: *Folia Haematol*, *36:*383-389, 1928.

LEADER, R. W. and HOLTE, R. J. A.: *Cornell Vet.*, *45:*78-84, 1955.

LESBOUYRIES, G.: *Rec. Med. Vet.*, 119-145, 1943. (*Bull. Inst. Pasteur, 44:*37.)

LEVI, G. M. and PENATI, F.: *Arch. sc. med.*, *58:*773-796, 1934.

—— *Haematology*, *16:*317-343, 1935.

LEVY, M. L.: *Vet. J.*, *104:*310-312, 1948.

LILLEENGEN, K.: *Abst. Exper. Sta. Rec.*, *59:*313-314, 1950 (Cited by GRAY, STAFSETH and THORP, 1951.)

LONG, P. H., BLISS, E. A., SCHEONBACH, E. B., CHANDLER, C. A. and BRYER, M. S.: *Lancet*, *258:*1139-1145, 1950. (Cited by ZINK, DE MELLO, and BURKHART, 1951.)

MALEWITZ, T. D. GRAY, M. L. and SMITH, E. M.: *Poult. Sci.*, *36:*416-419, 1957.

MARSHALL, E. K., JR.: *Science*, *91:*345-350, 1940.

MATHEWS: *J.A.V.M.A.*, *73:*513-516, 1928.

MCBRIDE, M. E. and GIRARD, K. F.: *J. Lab. & Clin. Med.* 55 No. 1:153-157, 1960.

MORIN, L. N.: *A.V.M.A.J.*, *93:*32, 1938.

MORRIS, J. A. and NORMAN, M. C.: *J. Bact.*, *59:*313-314, 1950.

MORRIS, M. C. and JULIANELLE, L. A.: *Am. J. Ophth.*, *18:*535-541, 1935.

MURRAY, E. G. D., WEBB, R. A. and SWANN, M. B. R.: *J. Path. & Bact.*, *29:*407-439, 1926.

MUTH, O. H. and MORRILL, D. R.: *J.A.V.M.A.*, *100:*242-243, 1942.

NETTLESHIP, A.: *Soc. Exper. Biol. & Med. Proc.*, *49:*116-117, 1942.

NYFELDT, AAGE: *Compt. rend. Soc. biol.*, *101:*590-592, 1929.

—— *Folia Haematol.*, *47:*1-144, 1932.

NYFELDT, AAGE: *Scandinav. Vet. Tidskr.*, *30(3):*280-285, 1940.

NYFELDT, A.: *Vgesk. laeger*, *102:*773-774, 1940 (abstracted in *QCI Med.*, *29:*765).

OLAFSON, PETER: *Cornell Vet.*, *30:*141-150, 1940.

OLSON, AAKE and BODEN, OCH BARBRO: *Scandinav. Vet. Tidskr.*, *34(7):*416-422, 1944.

OLSON, C., JR., BAGDONAS, W., ROLLINS, C. L. and BLORE, I. C.: *Am. J. Vet. Res.*, *14:*202-208, 1953.

OLSON, CARL, JR., COOK, R. H. and BLORE, IDA C.: *J.A.V.M.A.*, *116:*306-307, 1950.

—— *Am. J. Vet. Res.*, *11:*29-40, 1950.

OLSON, C., JR., ROLLINS, C. L., BAGDONAS, V., BLORE, I. C. and SEGRE, D.: *J. Infect., Dis.*, *93:*247-256, 1953.

OLSON, C. and SEGRE, D.: *Am. J. Vet. Res.*, *17:*235-242, 1956.

OSEBOLD, J. W., KENDRICK, J. W. and NJOKU-OBI, A.: *J.A.V.M.A.*, *137:*221-226, 1960.

OSEBOLD, J. W. KENDRICK, J. W., and NJOKU-OBI, A.: *J.A.V.M.A.*, *137:*227-234, 1960.

OSEBOLD, J. W. and SAWYER, M. T.: *Proc. Am. Vet. M. A.*, 92nd Ann. Meet. 189-195, 1955.

OSEBOLD, J. W., SHULTZ, G. and JAMESON, E. W., JR.: *J.A.V.M.A.*, *130:*471-475, 1957.

PALLASKE, G.: *Berl., Tierärztl. Wchnschr.*, *(Sept. 13):*441-445 (abstracted in *Vet. Bull.*, *12:*571), 1940.

PATERSON, J. S.: *Vet. Rec.*, *49:*1533-1534, 1937.

—— *Vet. Rec.*, *51:*873-876, 1939.

—— *J. Path. & Bact.*, *48:*25-32, 1939.

—— *Berl. Tierärztl. Wchnschr.*, *(Sept. 12):*441-445 (abstracted in *Vet. Bull.*, *12:*571), 1941.

—— *Ztschr. Infektionskrank, Parasitare Krank, u. Hyg. der Haustiere, 59:*125-145 (abstracted in *Vet. Bull., 13:*312), 1943.

—— *J. Path. & Bact., 51:*427-436, 1940.

—— *J. Path. & Bact., 51:*437-440, 1940.

—— *J. Path. & Bact., 51:*441-442, 1940.

—— *Vet. J., 96:*327-332, 1940.

—— Personal communication (1941).

PENATI, F. and LEVI, G. M.: *Haematology, 16:*261-275, 1935.

—— *Haematology, 16:*409-419, 1935.

PIRIE, J. H. H.: A New Disease of Veld Rodents. *South African Inst. Med. Res. Pub., 3:*163-186, 1927.

—— *Science, 91:*383, 1940.

—— *Nature* (London), *145:*246 (abtracted in the *Vet. Bull., 10:*325, 1940).

PLUMMER, P. J. G. and BYRNE, J. L. (reprint): *Canad. J. Comp. Med.,* 214-217, 1950.

POMEROY, B. S., FENSTERMACHER, REUEL, and ANDBERG, W. G.: *Cornell Vet., 33:*269-273, 1943.

PONS, C. A. and JULIANELLE, L. A.: *Soc. Exper. Biol. & Med. Proc., 40:*360-361, 1939.

POPPENSIEK, GEORGE C.: *J.A.V.M.A., 105:*147-148, 1944.

PORTER, J. R. and HALE, W. M.: *Soc. Exper. Biol. & Med. Proc., 42:*47-50, 1939.

—— and PELCZAR, M. J., JR.: *J. Bact., 42:*141, 1941.

PORZECANSKI, B. and DE BAYGORRIA, C.: *Arch. Soc. biol. Montevideo, 9:*98, 1939. (Cited by PATTERSON, 1939).

POSTON, M. A., UPCHURCH, S. E. and BOOTH, M.: *Pediatrics, 11:*515, 1937 (cited by PATERSON, 1939).

POTHMAN, EMILIE: *Deutsche tier. Woch. u. Tier. Rundsch., 52/50:*127-129, 1944.

POUDEN, W. D., BELL, D. S. and MAIRS, R. E.: *J.A.V.M.A., 111:*128-129, 1947.

POUNDEN, W. D. and EDGINOTON, H. B.: *J.A.V.M.A., 110:*107, 1947.

REZZESI, F. D.: *Haematology, 14:*239-258, 287-314, 1933.

RHOADES, HARRY E. and SUTHERLAND, A. K.: *J.A.V.M.A., 112:*451-452, 1948.

ROINE, F., RAITIO, A. and VARTIOVAARA, U.: *Nature, Lond., 172:*767, 1953.

RYFF, J. F. and LEE, A. M.: *Am. J. Vet. Res., 9:*147-151, 1948. (Abstracted in *J.A.V.M.A., 113:*600, 1948.)

SANTI, R. and SEREMBE, M.: *Arch. internat. pharmacodyn, 81:*493-499, 1950. (Cited by ZINK, DE MELLO and BURKHART, 1951.)

SAVINO, E.: *Inst. Bact. (Argentina), Rev., 9:*587-592, 1940 (not seen).

—— *Inst. Bact. (Argentina), Rev., 9:*593-601, 1940 (not seen).

—— and VILLLAZON, N. MORALES: *Semana Med., 1:*732-736, 1941 (not seen).

SCHMIDT, VIGGO and NYFELDT, AAGE: *Ugesk. laeger., 100:*336, 1938. (Cited by PATERSON, 1939.)

SCHOENING, H. W. and CREECH, G. T.: *J.A.V.M.A., 82:*503-508, 1933.

SCHULTZ, E. W., TERRY, M. D., BRICE, A. T., JR. and GEBHARDT, L. P.: *Soc. Exper. Biol. & Med. Proc., 31:*1021-1023, 1934.

—— *Soc. Exper. Biol. & Med. Proc. 38:*605-608, 1938.

SCHWARTE, L. H. and BIESTER, H. E.: *Am. J. Vet. Res., 3:*165-176, 1942.

SEASTONE, C. V.: *J. Exper. Med., 62:*203-212, 1935.

SEGRE, D., OLSON, C., MARSH, C. L. and BLORE, I. C: *Am. J. Vet. Res., 17:*299-302, 1956.

SEELIGER, H. P. R. and SULZBACHER, F.: *Canad. J. Microbiol., 2:*220-231, 1956.

SELLERS, A. F., POMEROY, B. S., SAUTTER, J. H., PINT, L. H. and SCHRAFEL, C. E.: *J.A.V.M.A., 114:*69-73, 1949.

SHALKOP, W. T.: *J.A.V.M.A., 116:*447-448, 1950.

SHANNON, WM. H.: *J.A.V.M.A., 109:*382, 1951.

SLABOSPITS, KIL, T. P.: *Zap. Kiev. Vet. Inst., 1:*39-49, 1938 (abstracted in *Vet. Bull. 12:* 367).

SMITH, H. C.: *Vet. Med., 48:*294-295, 1953.

SMITH, H. C. and SUNDQUIST, E.: *Vet. Med., 55* No. 4:70-73, 1960.

SPENCER, G. R., HOYT, H. H. and WHITECHAIR, C. K.: *J.A.V.M.A., 105:*195-197, 1944.

STANLEY, N. F.: *Australian J. Exper. Biol. & M. Sc., 27:*133-142, 1949.

STANLEY, NEVILLE F.: *M. J. Australia, 2:*205-208, 1948.

STOENNER, H. G., MENCIMER, F. R. and FOSTER, R. S.: *J.A.V.M.A., 115:*174-175, 1949.

SVENKERUD, R. R.: *Norsk. Vet-Tidsskr., 60:*321-340, 1948. (Cited by GRAY, STAFSETH and THORP, 1951.)

SVENKERUD, R. R.: Personal communication to GRAY, M. L., 1950.

TESDAL, M.: *Acta med. Scandinav., 83:*351-358, 1934. (Cited by JULIANELLE, 1940.)

THOMPSON, C. H., JR.: *Am. J. Vet. Res., 15:*130-132, 1954.

VISWANATHAN, G. R. and AYYAR, V. VENKATARAMA: *Indian Vet. J., 26:*395-402, 1950. (Cited by GRAY, STAFSETH and THORP, 1951.)

WALLBACK, GUNTER: *Arch. Anat. Micros., 30:*275-294, 1934.

WATSON, W. A. and HUNTER, D.: *Vet. Rec., 70:*1189, 1958.

WEBB, R. A.: *J. Path. & Bact., 41:*214-215, 1935. (Abstracted in *Biol. Abstr., 10:*11331.)

WEBB, R. A. and BARBER, MARY: *J. Path. & Bact., 45:*523-539, 1937.

WEIDE, K. D., LAGRACE, A., FRANK, N. A., SANGER, V. L. and BELL, D. S.: *Vet. Med. 55:* No. 1, 42-46, 1960.

WITTS, L. J. and WEBB, R. A.: *J. Path. & Bact., 30:*687-712, 1927.

WRIGHT, H. A. and MACGREGOR, A. R.: *J. Path. & Bact., 48:*470-472, 1939.

YOUNG, S.: *Vet. Rec., 68:*459-461, 1956.

YOUNG, S. and FIREHAMMER, B. D.: *J.A.V.M.A., 132:*434-438, 1958.

ZINK, A. DE MELLO, G. C. and BURKHART, R. L.: *Am. J. Vet. Res., 12:*194-198, 1951.

Chapter 8

GLANDERS

W. E. JENNINGS, D.V.M.

Glanders (farcy) is a highly communicable disease of solipeds (horses and species akin thereto). The disease also affects man through occupational contact with diseased animals and through handling infective material and laboratory cultures of the causative organism. Other species of animals occasionally infected are ferrets, moles, field mice, cats and dogs. Guinea pigs and hamsters are reported to be almost universally susceptible. The causative organism of the disease is known as *malleomyces mallei (Pfeifferella* or *Loefflerella mallei* or *Actinobacillus mallei).*

HISTORY OF THE DISEASE

The disease is one of the oldest known. It is mentioned in the writings of Hippocrates between the years 450 B.C. and 425 B.C., and by Aristotle a century later. The word "malleus" originated from Aristotle and is derived from the Greek word meaning malignant disease or epidemic. Glanders was described during the fourth century (A.D.) as a contagious disease. During the seventeenth and eighteenth centuries it was generally regarded as an infectious disease. However, even as late as the middle of the nineteenth century, some in influential positions did not subscribe to the infectious nature of the disease. Consequently, the regulations for the eradication of the disease were relaxed or suspended with a resultant marked increase in its incidence.

Solleysel (stable master to Louis XIV), between 1667 and 1682, expressed the view that glanders could be transmitted through the air. Caspard de Saunier in 1734 regarded the contagion as being either conveyed by direct contact or indirectly through contaminated harness, water troughs and feed mangers. In 1797, Viborg in Denmark published a systematic description of glanders in which he referred to the presence of an infectious substance in the nasal discharge and material from pulstules and ulcers of the skin. He considered glanders and farcy to be the same disease transmissible through direct contact and indirectly through contaminated harness, mangers and water troughs.

White (1842), in a published treatise on clinical glanders, convincingly declared it to be a contagious disease. Likewise, Gerlach (1868) and Bollinger (1874) demonstrated beyond doubt that glanders resulted only from direct or indirect contact with an affected animal. Inoculation tests by Rayer (1837) and Leblanc (1838) proved conclusively the contagious nature of the disease. The causative organism—*Malleomyces mallei*—was isolated in pure culture, identified and proven to be the etiologic agent, by Loeffler and Schutz in Germany in 1882 and in the same year in France, by Bouchard, Charrin and Capitan.

DISCOVERY OF MALLEIN TEST

In 1890, Helman in St. Petersburg and Kalning in Dorpat, and Leonard Pearson in the United States, all working independently, prepared mallein from pure cultures of the organism. This substance incited a reaction when injected into animals affected with the disease. Thus was discovered the mallein test as a method of diagnosis for the disease. Control and ultimate eradication of glanders was, thereby, made possible.

INCIDENCE OF GLANDERS IN HORSES

Glanders was widely prevalent in most countries until about 1924 when it became far less frequent. Glanders still persists in varying incidence in many countries in Central Europe, Russia, Asia and Africa. It was spread widely during World War I in Germany, Russia and most countries of Central Europe. The prevalence and distribution of glanders have always increased during and following all major wars in different parts of the world when conditions favored distribution of infected animals. Effective methods of control under war conditions were employed by the Allied Forces during World War I. An effective control program has been in force in the United States and Canada since 1905, and consequently, the disease is practically nonexistent in these countries.

ETIOLOGY

The causative agent, the glanders bacillus, known originally as *Bacillus mallei* and later as *Pfeifferella mallei* and *Loefferella mallei*, is now generally referred to as *Malleomyces mallei* or *Actinobacillus mallei*. It is a small gram negative, nonsporeforming, nonmotile rod without capsule or flagella. In young cultures the cells are long and slender. Older cultures are quite pleomorphic; cells varying in shape and size from coccoid forms to long, slender, sometimes branching filaments. Usually the longer rods are distinctly beaded. The shorter rod may appear to be bipolar due to the presence of granules in each end of the cell. The organism grows well, but slowly, on ordinary media. Glycerol added to such media enhances the growth. On potato media characteristic growth which begins to appear in two days is honey-colored and becomes luxuriant and slimy, and tends to increase in thickness and darken in color until it becomes dark brown.

Pini[1] in 1957, stated that in a malachite green-fuchsin medium colonies of *Malleomyces mallei* grew in twenty-four hours with a characteristic blue color surrounded by a violet-red color. On thionin agar, which is violet in color, the colonies are greyish white surrounded by bluish zones. Thionin may be replaced by parafuchsin, in which case the *M. mallei* colonies are surrounded by a zone of discoloration while the rest of the medium is red. These media were satisfactorily used for the isolation of *M. mallei*. Wetmore and Gochenour[2] readily distinguished in 1956 members of genus *Malleomyces* from *Pseudomonas pyocyanea* by lack of growth of *Malleomyces* on SS agar, desoxycholate agar, sodium azide agar and cetyltrimethyl ammonium bromide agar, and when incubated at 21° C. In 1953 murase *et al.*[3] showed that growth of *M. mallei* was enhanced by addition of 0.05-0.1% defibrinated horse blood to the culture medium.

SPECIES SUSCEPTIBLE

Horses, mules, asses and other members of the soliped family are very susceptible to glanders. Man, though less susceptible than members of the horse family, can readily contract the disease. Ferrets, moles, mice, camels, cats (wild and tame) and dogs are less susceptible to infection. Sheep, swine, pigeons and cattle show high resistance. Guinea pigs and hamsters are reported to be almost universally susceptible, dying of a fulminating infection after twenty-four hours following a massive inoculation, and within three weeks after a smaller one.

RESISTANCE OF THE ORGANISM

Hagan and Bruner[4] state that the organism possesses only slight resistance to drying, heat and chemicals. Outside the body it probably cannot exist longer than two or three months even under most favorable conditions. Miller *et al.*[5] in their experimental work proved that the organism can remain viable for at least four weeks when suspended in tap water. They further proved that viability and virulence of cultures were well preserved over periods of at least three to six months by lyophilization.

MODE OF TRANSMISSION

Glanders is usually spread from diseased to healthy animals either directly or indirectly. Infection is acquired from the discharges of the respiratory tract or from exudates of skin lesions. Infection by indirect means results from contamination of mangers, troughs, utensils, harness, water buckets and the like, with the discharges. Close cohabitation either in stables or in pastures favors spread of the disease.

The organism is present in the nasal discharges and exudates from pustules and ulcers (farcy buds) which appear in lymph nodes and along the course of the lymphatics on the legs and other parts of the body. The organism gains entrance into the body by the following three routes:

1) *By ingestion into the digestive tract.* This is regarded as the most common mode of infection resulting from the consumption of feed or water contaminated with discharges either from respiratory tract or skin ulcerations.

2) *By inoculation through the skin.* Slight abrasions of the skin or mucous membrane which are contaminated with discharges either from skin lesions or from the respiratory tract of glandered animals.

3) *By inhalation into the respiratory tract.* This is not considered the usual mode of infection of animals.

Though some differences of opinion exist relative to the mode of infection, it is rather generally believed and accepted that natural infection through ingestion is more common and far more important than through inhalation.

Infection in man results from direct or indirect contact with diseased animals, their tissues and cultures of the organism.

Laboratory infections of man with this organism are rather frequently observed. Such infections are usually acquired by inoculations through the skin. Infection by inhalation is less common.

Carnivora are usually infected by eating meat from glandered animals. This is particularly true in carnivora in zoological parks which subsist in large part on horse meat.

Miller *et al.*[6] proved in their studies that hamsters are easily infected by inoculation by intraperitoneal, subcutaneous and respiratory routes. Oral administration of the organism gave irregular results. Their studies further indicated that hamsters were most susceptible of all laboratory animals and were, therefore, the laboratory animal of choice in working with this disease. Guinea pigs proved to be only moderately susceptible.

TYPES OF INFECTION

Hutyra, Marek and Manninger[7] state that infection in solipeds occurs in the majority of cases from ingestion of food and water which is contaminated with secretions and excretions from the nose and lungs with exudates from ulcers of glandered animals. They further state that infection can take place through the intact mucous membrane. Infection is more likely to occur, however, when superficial lesions are present in the buccal mucosa and that of the intestinal tract. Infection is also facilitated by catarrh of the mucous membranes.

Udall[8] states that after the organism enters the digestive tract by means of contaminated feed or water, the infection is carried by the circulatory systems from pharyngeal or intestinal mucosa to the lungs. Localization occurs in the lungs with formation of primary lesions. Experimental studies reveal that fever is evidenced shortly after artificial feeding of infected material. This would indicate the presence of infection in the circulation. Most authorities agree that the seat of primary lesions in practically all cases is the lungs. Hagan and Bruner[4] state that there is apparently considerable organ immunity in the intestinal tract, spleen and liver. The lungs are in most cases involved irrespective of the manner by which the organism gains entrance to the body. Localization in the nasal mucosa and in the lymph nodes and lymphatics of the skin (farcy) are observed in addition to the primary lesions in the lungs.

Studies were conducted by Miller *et al.*[6] on the virulence of several strains of *Malleomyces mallei*, their infectivity by various portals of entry and a comparison of susceptibility of several common species of laboratory animals. Their work revealed that strains of very low virulence produced subacute or chronic infection in hamsters. Moderately virulent strains produced acute fulminating infections in hamsters and ferrets, but only subacute or chronic infection in guinea pigs. Highly virulent strains produced acute fulminating forms of the disease in both hamsters and guinea pigs.

Experimental studies by Hu *et al.*[9] in 1958 revealed that intravenous or intratesticular inoculation of glanders bacilli caused acute toxemia and rapid death in sheep and goats. Subcutaneous injection was also lethal but the infection was less acute. Cattle resisted infection by all three routes and although there was extensive destruction of testicle after intratesticular injection, the cattle did not die. They concluded that virulence of strain has much to do with type of disease produced. This is a possible explanation for occurrence of all gradations of the disease in horses.

MORBID ANATOMY

Considerable differences exist in the susceptibility of the individual organs. The lungs, mucous membrane of the air passages and nose, lymph nodes and lymphatic plexus of the skin are frequently involved in the order shown. Less frequently infected are the spleen, liver, testes, bone marrow and periosteum. The lesions in the lungs and upper respiratory tract are most constantly observed.

Lesions of Respiratory Tract. The lungs contain tubercle-like nodules or a diffuse catarrhal pneumonia. The nodules are often referred to as nodular glanders. Acute or chronic forms of nodular lung glanders are observed. The nodules may be few or many in number. The nodules are easily recognized by their characteristic histologic structure which is accurately and fully described by Duval and White[10] and McFadyean.[11] Frothingham[12] describes these as follows: The acute nodule, varying usually in size from one to four millimeters, has a small dark red foci of hemorrhagic pneumonia.

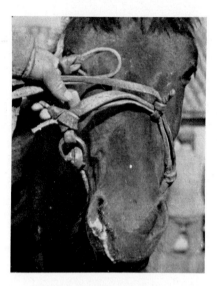

Fig. 51. Clinical case of glanders. Profuse, purulent nasal discharge is characteristic symptom.

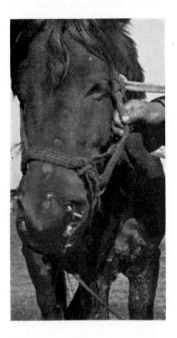

Fig. 52. Clinical case of glanders. Pulmonary and cutaneous forms of the
disease characterized by profuse, viscid nasal discharge and nodules, abscesses and
ulcers along the course of the lymphatics, respectively.

In the more advanced stage the nodule becomes grey with a yellow-ish center and surrounded by a red zone. The chronic nodules are well organized and show an area of central necrosis with some calci-fication. A strong connective tissue wall surrounds the calcified zone.

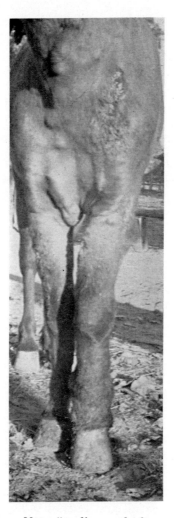

Fig. 53. Clinical glanders. Note "cording and abscessation" along course of lymphatics and emphysematous swellings of the limb.

On preliminary examination these may be confused with parasitic nodules which may be differentiated by noting the more uniform structure of the parasitic nodules and their reaction to stain with hematoxylin. Quite frequently well defined glanderous pneumonic areas with suppurating foci discharging into the bronchi are observed in the lung. Lung glanders is usually chronic.

Lesions of the upper air passages in the form of nodules and ulcers are commonly observed. These may result from rupture of lung nodules into the bronchi with the infective material being carried upward into the trachea, larynx, nasal septum and turbinate bones. Lesions in the upper respiratory tract of animals can occur also by direct metastasis from the portal of entry. Well defined lesions are often observed in the upper respiratory tract with few or none observed in the lungs. Lesions in the upper respiratory passages first appear as submucosal nodules. These break and form shallow ulcers which exude a thick, sticky, purulent, highly dangerous exudate which is the characteristic nasal discharge of glanders (Figures 51 and 52). Healed ulcers appear as irregular, radiating, star-shaped masses which are raised somewhat above the surrounding tissue.

Skin Lesions. Lesions of the skin are frequently observed in glandered animals. This form of glanders is known as farcy. These consist of nodules, pustules, and ulcers which can occur over any part of the body but are most frequently observed on the legs (Figures 53 and 54). These nodules usually appear in chains occurring along the course of the lymphatics. Initially the lesions appear as nodules or "farcy buds" which tend to break down and form crater-like ulcers discharging a thick, viscid, and sticky pus heavily laden with the glanders organism. Skin lesions per se are very infrequently, if ever, observed. Such cases usually show lesions in the lungs. McFadyean[11] who had extensive experience with this disease in England states that "no case of glanders with lesions elsewhere than in the lungs and with those organs healthy has ever been recorded."

Lesions of the Lymphatics. Lymph nodes such as the submaxillary, axillary, inguinal, broncial, and retropharyngeal are frequently the seat of lesions. Ofttimes, these are not abscessed but show only enlargement and induration.

Lesions in Other Organs. Lesions of glanders are observed occasionally in other organs such as the mucosa of the digestive tract, liver, spleen, testicles, brain, spinal cord, and bones.

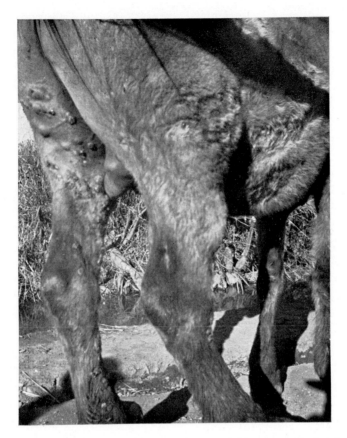

Fig. 54. Clinical glanders. Nodules, abscesses and ulcers over both hind limbs and in abdominal region. Orchitis frequently complicates such cases.

SYMPTOMS AND COURSE IN HORSES

Glanders in the horse may be either acute or chronic though the latter is by far more common. The acute form is more commonly observed in mules and donkeys. Length of the incubation period depends upon intensity of the infection. It appears to be shorter in the mule and donkey. Infection is usually slow, from several days in a very small percentage of cases, to several weeks or months. Lesions may occur in less than five days after artificial inoculation. The highly variable incubation period has resulted in an arbitrary classification of two forms of the disease, clinical and nonclinical or latent glanders.

Clinical cases are recognized by definite symptoms commonly known as the "cardinal signs of glanders": 1) a chronic nasal discharge from one or both nostrils with or without visible ulceration of the nasal septum; 2) chronic enlargement and induration with or without suppuration along lymphatics and in lymph nodes, most frequently the submaxillary; 3) presence of nodules (farcy buds), pustules, and ulcers on the skin of the legs most frequently, and other parts of the body. Unilateral swelling of submaxillary lymph nodes is frequently observed. Acute glanders begins with chills and a high fever—106°F. This is characterized by ulcers of the nasal mucosa which spread rapidly. Inspiratory dyspnea may result from edema of the glottis. Secondary skin glanders is characterized by formation of nodules, abscesses, and ulcers. Death results within one week. This acute form is the type commonly observed in the ass and donkey. Murase *et al.*[13] in 1953 observed that nasal discharge due to glanders was present in twenty-nine out of the one thousand horses examined in Manchuria. The further noted that sixteen pregnant mares which reacted to the intrapalpebral and complement-fixation tests gave birth to healthy foals which at the age of two or three months, reacted to the complement-fixation test but not the intrapalpebral test. The foals remained free from infection during the eight months period of observation.

Nonclinical or latent cases are usually pulmonary in type. The lesions occur in the lungs in the form of tubercle-like nodules and suppurating foci. In latent cases the affected animal may show only slight labored breathing which may pass unnoticed. Such cases often spread the infection through respiratory secretions for a period of several months before showing recognizable symptoms. These cases are far more numerous than clinical cases and can be detected only by the application of the mallein test. The insidious nature of the disease accounts for the widespread occurence of this disease when large numbers of horses are assembled for military operations and are in close contact in corrals and stables.

Hutyra, Marek and Manninger[7] classify clinically three different forms of the disease—pulmonary, nasal and cutaneous. For practical purposes it should be considered that the three forms tend often to merge into one another and all forms are frequently observed to coexist in the same case of the disease. Glanderous orchitis is rather frequently observed in male animals. A general state of malnutrition and gradual emaciation is observed commonly in advanced and progressive cases of the disease.

DIAGNOSIS IN HORSES

The importance of making an early and accurate diagnosis cannot be overemphasized. By so doing it is possible to control the disease and retard or prevent its further spread in groups of animals. Several methods are employed in the diagnosis of glanders.

1) **Physical Examination.** Diagnosis of this disease can be made by observation of various clinical symptoms which are present in well advanced cases. Some of these are pathognomonic of the disease. Some symptoms, however, may be confused with other diseases in which cases a differential diagnosis must be made.

2) **Post-mortem Lesions.** Lesions described above are characteristic of the disease. Autopsy findings permit an accurate diagnosis of the disease to be made.

3) **Isolation of the Organism.** Organism may be cultured from open or preferably closed lesions using those culture media which are suitable for the growth of the organism.

4) **Inoculation of Guinea Pigs and Hamsters.** Injection of the organisms intraperitoneally will produce characteristic lesions in male guinea pigs. The number of *Malleomyces mallei* in the inoculum and their virulence will determine the severity of the lesions. Moderate doses usually produce a localized peritonitis involving the scrotal sac which becomes enlarged and painful. Involvement of testicles follows and the entire organs become a caseous mass which breaks through the skin covering the scrotal sac. This is known as the Strauss reaction and is characteristic of the reaction produced by this organism in male guinea pigs.

Miller *et al.*[6] state that strains of low virulence produce a subacute or chornic infection in hamsters. Highly virulent strains of *M. mallei* produce acute fulminating forms of the disease in both hamsters and guinea pigs causing death usually in two to four days. Other investigators have observed similar responses including a generalized peritonitis when inoculum consisted of large numbers of organisms.

5) **Serologic Tests.** (a) *Complement-fixation test.* This is the most accurate of serologic tests used in the diagnosis of glanders. It was first applied about 1909 by Schutz and Schubert in the diagnosis of glanders. It was introduced into the United States shortly thereafter

by Mohler and Eichorn.[14] Its accuracy is reported to be approximately 90-95 per cent. Zeljiko and Bas-Luketic[15] employed the conglutination test for glanders in a modified form in 1954—using 2 per cent instead of 5 per cent red blood cells. It was considered of value for the routine examination of mule sera, of horse sera containing non-specific, complement-fixing antibodies and also for use in conjunction with complement-fixation test in the case of horse sera.

(b) *Agglutination test.* McFadyean[16] in 1896 first used this method for detection of glanders. In studies made by New York City Health Department it was reported about 85 per cent accurate. Frequently sera of horses affected with chronic glanders or in a debilitated condition give negative or inconclusive results. Reactions in dilutions of 1 to 1000 are usually considered to be positive evidence of infection with glanders.[17] Jager[18] described in 1954 application of the hemagglutination test to the diagnosis of glanders in horses. Twelve out of eighteen cases were positive to this test, compared with only eight positive to other serological tests.

(c) *Precipitation test.* Some investigators state that this test has proven to be quite reliable. Its efficacy in the diagnosis of glanders does not appear to be any greater than that of the agglutination test. Positive reaction to the test is generally considered to be indicative of glanders but a negative reaction does not exclude the disease.

6) **Mallein Tests.** These are the methods most commonly employed in the diagnosis of glanders. Mallein, which is produced by growing the organism on glycerol broth and removing the organisms by filtration, is a very valuable agent for diagnosis of glanders. Its injection into normal animals occasions little noticeable response. In glandered animals which are hypersensitive to it, the substance produces a marked reaction and response indicative of intoxication.

Delpy[19] suggested in 1954 that mallein be standardized by the intrapalpebral injection of 0.25 ml. of a 1:10 dilution of the test material into one eye and a similar dose of the standard into the other eye, of three groups of horses, one of proven cases, one doubtful and one negative. The results are then compared at twenty-four and forty-eight hours. Fras[20] evaluated in 1955 samples of mallein either by establishing the highest dilution of specific hyperimmune serum capable of agglutinating red blood cells sensitized with a fixed amount of mallein or by establishing the smallest amount of mallein, necessary to sensitize sheep corpuscles sufficiently to agglutinate, when fixed amounts of serum were added. Results were compared with those obtained with standard mallein. Ciortea *et al.*[21] in 1958 published results on their studies indicating that specificity of mallein was improved by growing *m. mallei* on a medium consisting of equal proportions of glycerine peptone broth, Sauton's medium containing 0.4 gram per cent of citric acid and brewers' yeast or on a medium consisting of equal proportions of glycerine peptone broth, Sauton's medium containing asparagine and yeast or on a combination of equal parts of glycerine peptone broth and yeast or on a combination of equal parts of glycerine peptone broth, Sauton's medium containing 0.8 per cent of citric acid and Sauton's medium containing succinic acid instead of asparagine.

Mallein is employed by three methods for diagnosis of glanders:

a) *Intrapalpebral test.* The intrapalpebral test is the most accurate method and is the method most commonly used. This test has been the official test for glanders of the United States Army during the past quarter century. Only in those suspicious or inconclusive reactions to this test is the complement-fixation test employed. Captain Goodall[22] of the South African Veterinary Corps in 1915 reported superiority of the intradermic mallein test. Maurase *et al.*[23] in 1952 compared the reactions of intrapalpebral and complement-fixation tests at different stages of glanders. Those horses which reacted to both tests had active circumscribed lesions, from which they isolated the causal organism; in general, symptoms were slight. Those which reacted to the intrapalpebral test alone tended to have chronic infection. The test consists of injection of 0.1 cc. of concentrated mallein into the skin of the lower lid ¼ inch from the palpebral fissure and equal distance from the medial and lateral canthi (Figure 55). Specific reaction to the test consists of a marked edematous swelling which pits on pressure. In addition, a purulent conjunctivitis, photophobia, pain and general depression are observed. Variations in severity of reaction to the test are observed. Test is read forty-eight hours after injection of the mallein. Reactions to the test often persist for several days thereafter (Figure 56).

b) *Opthalmic test.* This test does not interfere with serologic diagnosis of the disease as further confirmed by recent studies of Stehlik and Zarzycki.[22] For this and other reasons it has replaced the subcu-

taneous test for diagnosis of glanders. This method consists of in-
stilling concentrated mallein in liquid or tablet form into the conjunctival sac. Positive reaction is evidenced by a purulent exudate
in the conjunctival sac in from six to twelve hours after administra-

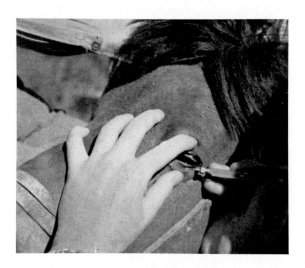

Fig. 55. Proper method for administration of palpebral (intradermic) Mallein
test. 25 gauge ¼ inch needle and ½ cc. hypodermic syringe are used.

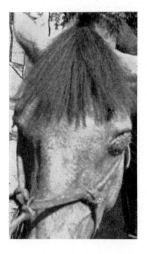

Fig. 56. Typical positive reaction to palpebral (intradermic) Mallein test. Note
swelling, discharge and photophobia. Such reactions often persist for several
days.

tion. The opthalmic test has been replaced by the intrapalpebral test in many countries.

c) *Subcutaneous test.* This test consists of administration subcutaneously of 2.5 ml. of dilute mallein in the neck region. In glandered animals a definite post-injection rise in temperature is evidenced in from eight to twelve hours and a distinct painful swell-

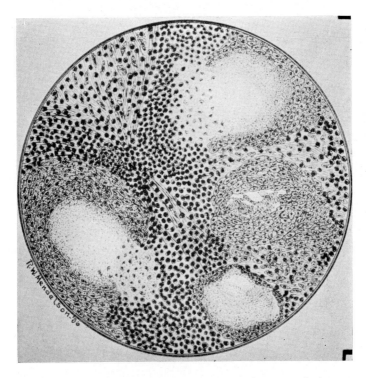

Fig. 57. Biopsy of a section of tissue showed granulomatous lesions—masses of epithelioid cells with central necrosis and abundant leucocytic infiltration. Giant cells are not observed. (Courtesy of Lt. Col. Ralph W. Mendelson, USAF (MC). Published in July, 1950, issue *United States Armed Forces Medical Journal.* Reprinted by permission.)

ing at point of injection. This method has been replaced in practically all countries by other methods such as the intrapalpebral and ophthalmic tests which do not influence subsequent serodiagnosis of the disease should such diagnosis be necessary.

Studies by Murase *et al.*[25] in 1952 revealed that an average of 15 per cent of one thousand horses in Manchuria reacted to both the intrapalpebral mallein test and the complement-fixation test for glanders. The horses were tested every two months during a period of sixteeen months. The highest incidence of reactors occurred during March-July, and in geldings and older horses. Murase *et al.*[26] in 1953 concluded that, for the purposes of epidemiological survey, the complement-fixation test should be used in conjunction with the intrapalpebral test. This disease may be confused clinically with such diseases as epizootic lymphangitis, lymphangitis, strangles, nasal catarrah, and purulent sinusitis resulting from alveolar periostitis and the like. Differential diagnosis of the disease is accomplished effectively by mallein tests, isolation of the organism from the lesions, serologic determinations, and animal inoculations (Figure 57).

CONTROL

McFadyean[27] states that recoveries to this disease in animals have apparently occurred in a small percentage of cases. Therapeutic treatment of glanders is not advisable or indicated since it tends to assist in the further spread of the disease and nullifies the control program for glanders. The only method which has proven effective for the control and eradication of the disease is early diagnosis of the disease and immediate destruction of animals affected with the disease.

Diagnosis is usually accomplished by the routine—usually every three weeks—of the intrapalpebral or ophthalmic (conjunctival) tests using serologic tests where necessary and indicated. Prompt destruction and proper disposal by deep burial or cremation of affected animals is essential. This should be followed immediately by thorough, effective disinfection of stables, troughs, and other places where glandered animals have been kept and the disinfection of all equipment. It is imperative that all contact and exposed animals be retested at routine short intervals—usually every three weeks—until it has been definitely determined that the infection has been entirely and effectively eliminated. Under this method glanders has been practically eradicated from many countries such as the United States, Canada, and Great Britain. In those areas and countries such as Asia and Africa and some parts of Europe in which such a program has not been instituted or employed effectively, the disease still prevails and constitutes a menace to health of animals and man as well.

GLANDERS IN MAN

Though the disease in horses has been known and recognized from early times (by Hippocrates circa 450 B.C.), the disease in man was not definitely known or described until the early part of the last century. This is known as the Travers case which was reported in 1830 and describes the disease in a veterinary student who became infected while dissecting a donkey affected with glanders in London, England. Since then, the disease has attracted more attention. Many authentic cases have been reported in medical and veterinary literature. William Hunting,[28] Chief Veterinary Inspector to the London County Council, published in 1908 a comprehensive treatise on glanders in the horse. In that report he described ten cases of the disease in man which occurred between 1903 and 1905. Robins[29] of the Royal Victoria Hospital in Montreal published a comprehensive monograph in May, 1906, dealing with chronic glanders in man. This report includes 156 cases which had been covered in the literature prior to that time. Bollinger published a report covering 120 cases of human glanders. In Manitoba two cases were observed and described by McGilvray in 1905 and 1906. S. H. Gaiger,[30] a veterinary pathologist at the Punjab Veterinary College in India, became infected while autopsying a glandered horse. During the two-year period of illness which followed, Gaiger underwent forty-five operations including the amputation of an arm. A graphic account of his illness was published by him after his recovery.

The Department of Health in the City of New York reported four hundred and six cases occurring in the five-year period from 1920 to 1924. The control of the disease in horses resulted in a rapid decrease in the incidence of the disease in man. In 1918, following the conclusion of World War I, the incidence of human glanders in Russia is reported to have been for a time appallingly high due to lack of control of the disease in horses.

SOURCES OF HUMAN INFECTION AND TRANSMISSION

Man is not highly susceptible to glanders though numerous infections have occurred in persons caring for glandered animals. Infections usually occur from occupational contact as in stablemen or from treating animals and conducting autopsies of glandered animals as in veterinarians. Laboratory workers rather frequently contract the infection from handling of cultures of the organism and handling laboratory animals artificially infected with *Malleomyces mallei*. The majority become infected through abrasions of the skin or mucous membrane—either by the nasal discharge or secretion from pustules of the skin of an affected animal. Transmission of infection may also occur through the eyes and possibly through the nose and mouth when an animal coughs or snorts directly into a person's face. Transmission from one person to another has been reported while caring for other humans affected with the disease. This occurs most commonly when adequate precautions are not taken to prevent infections or from lack of recognition and appreciation of exact nature of the disease.

SYMPTOMS AND COURSE IN MAN

Period of incubation in the majority of cases averages from one to five days. Cases have been reported in which the exact length of the incubation period was unknown but considered to be several

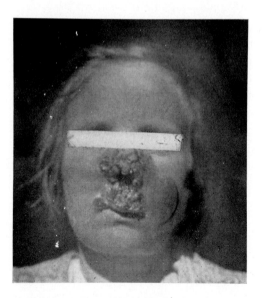

Fig. 58. Human glanders. Disease contracted directly from horse. Smears from lesions revealed infection with *M. mallei*. (Courtesy Lt. Col. Ralph W. Mendelson, USAF (MC). Published in July, 1950, issue *United States Armed Forces Medical Journal*. Reprinted by permission.)

months. Such prolonged incubation periods possibly should be regarded as latent cases of the disease. Within a few days following infection prodromal constitutional disturbances develop manifested by fever, malaise, fatigue, loss of appetite, jaundice, nausea, headache and rheumatic pains in the legs. Shortly thereafter definite physical signs develop such as erysipelatous swelling on the face and limbs or painful nodules and phlegmonous inflammation (Figures 58, 59 and 60).

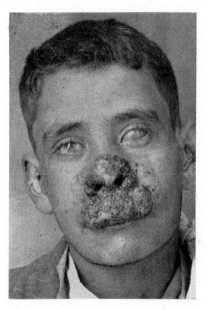

Fig. 59. Human glanders. Disease apparently contracted from horse dying of undetermined cause. Infection manifested first in eye causing ocular lesions. Later followed by mucopurulent nasal discharge and ulceration. (Courtesy of Lt. Col. Ralph W. Mendelson, USAF (MC). Published in July, 1950, issue *United States Armed Forces Medical Journal*. Reprinted by permission.)

The nodular eruption increases rapidly and soon is followed by a general pustular eruption of the skin over the face and on the legs, arms and other parts of the body (Figure 61). There is also nasal involvement in which the nasal mucosa becomes reddened and swollen, followed by a mucopurulent, viscid discharge from the nose. The nasal discharge is sometimes streaked with blood. This is associated with ulceration of the nasal septum and other parts of the nasal structure. Lymphatic involvement is also common and in the course of which the cervical, submaxillary, axillary and inguinal glands may be swollen. The final stage of the disease is that of a severe pyemia characterized by appearance of suppurating pustules covering the body, muscular abscessation, metastatic pneumonia, diarrhea, emaciation and fatal collapse. These symptoms characterize the typical course of acute glanders in man, lasting

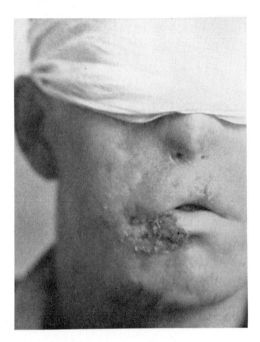

Fig. 60. Human glanders. Lesion had persisted for several months prior to submission for treatment. Bacteriologic examination revealed typical *M. mallei.* (Courtesy of Lt. Col. Ralph W. Mendelson, USAF (MC). Published in July, 1950, issue *United States Armed Forces Medical Journal.* Reprinted by permission.)

usually from two to four weeks. In latent or chronic cases the symptoms are quite similar in character but are prolonged over a greater period of time, extending to months and occasionally several years in the form of a pyemia from which a few have ultimately recovered. Glanders in man can best be described as an intensely painful and loathsome disease from which few recover.

Womack and Wells[31] in 1949 state that human infection presents a varied clinical picture characterized by formation of granuloma-

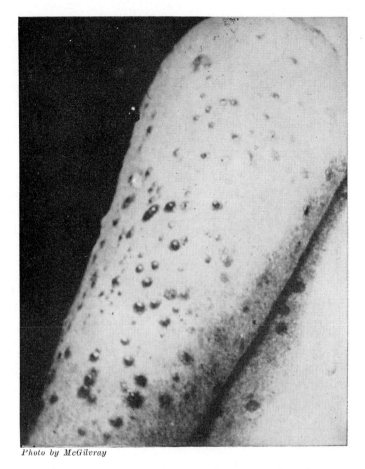

Photo by McGilvray

Fig. 61. The pustular manifestation on the arms of a human case of generalized glanders.

tous lesions in the skin and subcutaneous tissues, chronic ulceration of mucous membranes with profuse discharges from the nose, mouth and throat or pulmonic and pleuritic manifestations. Clinical picture may be complicated by metastatic hematogenous spread to meninges, bones, joints and abdominal viscera. They further state that the disease may run an acute, fulminating fatal course or it may persist chronically with remissions and exacerbations for as long as fifteen years. A few recover spontaneously, the majority die. Howe and Miller[32] in 1947 reported on six cases of human glanders which resulted from infections contracted in the laboratory. They describe two forms of the disease in man: 1) acute or chronic systemic form; and 2) cutaneous type. The acute systemic type is described as rapid in onset and often fatal in ten to thirty days. Bronchopneumonia or lobar pneumonia with or without bacteremia or a generalized pyemia is observed in this type. Four of these cases resulted from handling of strains of relatively low virulence; the remaining two were exposed to a more virulent strain. These investigators state that pulmonary lesions were present in five of the six cases, suggesting the main route of infection through the respiratory tract. X-ray studies of the lung lesions in four cases suggested early stage of lung abscess. In the fifth case x-ray examination of the lungs revealed diffuse lesions—similar to those of pneumonitis.

Mendelson[33] in 1950 reports on four cases of the chronic form of the disease. He states that acute cases may become chronic cases and chronic cases exhibit acute exacerbations. Mendelson warns against the working with cultures of the organism except under most meticulous bacteriologic technique. Each of the four patients had a history of contact with either horses or donkeys. Mendelson states that nasal passages appear to be the portal of entry for the infection although in one of the four cases the eye was apparently the site of the primary lesion.

DIAGNOSIS IN MAN

In suspected cases of glanders inquiry should be made into the patient's possible contact with a glandered animal or a case of human glanders. Further investigation should be made of the patient's contact on autopsy of glanders cadavers (horses, mules, etc.) and tissues therefrom and laboratory work with cultures of *Malleomyces mallei* or laboratory animals artificially infected with this organism. Early diagnosis of the disease is most important to permit proper precautions being taken by those caring for the patient affected with glanders.

It is rather difficult, if not impossible to make a positive diagnosis on clinical findings alone. History of contact of patient with horses, donkeys or mules may be very suggestive. Mendelson[33] states that the disease must be differentiated from syphilis, tuberculosis, epithelioma and a variety of other diseases including granuloma inguinale, lymphogranuloma inguinale and mycotic lesions.

Glanders may be mistaken for the following diseases and be incorrectly diagnosed:

During the prodromal stage: typhoid fever, rheumatism, jaundice.

During the various stages of pustular eruption: smallpox, tuberculosis, syphilis, erysipelas, lymphangitis, pyemia, yaws, melioidosis.

The following methods of test may be used for the diagnosis of glanders in man:

1) **Blood Serum Tests.** The complement-fixation test, the agglutination test. Studies made by Cravitz and Miller[34] in 1950 indicate that the agglutination test is more sensitive than the complement-fixation test for detection of glanders in humans. Further the complement-fixation test proved to be of greater value in differentiating between infection with *Malleomyces mallei* and *Malleomyces pseudomallei*.

2) **Mallein Skin Tests.** Fairly high percentage of human cases give a positive reaction to skin test using injection of 0.1 ml. of commercial mallein in a dilution of 1 to 10,000.

3) **Isolation of M. mallei.** Bacteriologic examination can be made of suspected pus and cultures made to isolate the organism.

4) **Inocluation of Laboratory Animals.** Inject suspected material from a lesion intraperitoneally into male guinea pig or hamster. Male guinea pig will show usually typical Straus reaction. Hamsters are laboratory animals of choice.

TREATMENT IN MAN

Several methods of therapy have been used and others explored in the treatment of glanders in man. Older methods of therapy include use of: 1) autogenous vaccines; 2) mallein; 3) other products of the organism such as "Farase"; 4) immune serum; and 5) therapy with heavy metals. Iodides and quinine have been used in handling chronic forms of the disease. Surgical treatment of abscesses and cauterization of ulcers are frequently employed. Palliative treatment may be used in conjunction with other types of therapy.

Miller *et al.*[35] in 1948 reported on results of their studies testing various sulfonamides and antibiotics in vitro and in laboratory animals artificially infected. They concluded that sodium sulfadiazine was very effective in treatment of acute experimental glanders in hamsters. Prolongation of therapy from seven to twenty days increased the rate of recovery from 50 per cent or less to approximately 100 per cent. Streptomycin and penicillin were without significant effect in the treatment of glanders in hamsters. Howe and Miller[32] in 1947 reported very effective results in the treatment of six human cases of laboratory infection with sulfadiazine. Womack and Wells[31] in 1949 stated that penicillin therapy was ineffective. They further indicated that streptomycin appeared to be valuable therapeutically in the treatment of this disease. Further investigation should be made of the use of other antibiotics in the treatment of glanders in man. Studies by Sirmon and Marcia[36] in 1956 indicated that sulfathiazole exerted a bacteriostatic action on *M. mallei* which, compared with other gram negative bacilli, was less sensitive to chloramphenicol and nitrofuran. Streptomycin and aureomycin had a marked effect. Penicillin, p-aminosalicylic acid and isoniazid were inactive.

In 1956, Tezok[37] reported on treatment of three human cases each infected with a different strain of the organism in Ankara during the first half of 1956. Diagnosis was confirmed by cultural and serological methods and by animal inoculation. All patients recovered after supportive antibiotic therapy.

First strain was remarkably sensitive to penicillin, tetracycline, oxytetracycline and chlortetracycline;

Second strain was sensitive to chlortetracycline, oxytetracline and streptomycin;

Third strain yielded to chlortetracycline, streptomycin, oxytetracline, but not to penicillin.

Nemoto *et al.*[38] in 1956 reported on results of their in vitro and in vivo studies of *M. mallei*. The organism was inhibited in vitro by 0.75ug. aureomycin, 3.1 ug. terramycin, 3.1 ug. dihydrostreptomycin, and 2.5 ug. chloramphenicol. In vivo tests were carried out on guinea pigs with tetramycin, aureomycin and dihydrostreptomycin. Animals in the untreated control group showed Strauss reaction and died within fifteen days, after inoculation. In the treated groups Strauss reaction was observed at varying periods (no mortality attributable to the organism was reported). Dhanda *et al.*[39] in 1958 reported on their in vitro and in vivo studies of *M. mallei* using sulphathiazole, sulphadimidine and sulphadiazine. These three agents inhibited growth of *M. Mallei* in vitro and also prevented infection of male guinea pigs when administered at 100 mg. daily for seven consecutive days, the treatment starting immediately after inocluation of a lethal dose of the organism. MirChamsy *et al*[40] reported that their studies in 1954 revealed that *M. mallei* is sensitive in vitro to aureomycin, chloramphenicol and terramycin, but seven daily oral doses of 500 mg./Kg. had no effect on infection in guinea pigs. A sulphonamide-resistant strain in guinea pigs resisted treatment with sulphadiazine but was sensitive to "tetrasulphamide" (a mixture of four sulphonamides). Eghbal *et al.*[41] in 1953 reported on results of treatment of a case of glanders. The patient—a groom aged forty—was successfully treated for glanders with sulphonamides, having been given sulphathiazole, sulphadiazine and also "sulfatriad" and "tetrasulfamide" (the latter being formulations containing mixtures of certain sulphonamides), in combination with "anamorve" (a formalized culture). The authors stated that two different strains of the glanders bacillus were isolated from this case. They were both resistant to penicillin but sensitive to streptomycin, chloramphenicol, aureomycin and terramycin, but they stated that these antibiotics had no therapeutic action in the experimental infection in the guinea pig. One strain was sensitive to sulphadiazine while the other was not, but it was not curative in infected guinea pigs, which were, however, cured with "tetrasulfamide."

PREVENTION AND CONTROL IN MAN

Prevention of glanders in man is concomitant with control of the disease in horses. When glanders is suspected in horses, elimination of all effected animals should be accomplished and effective control measures instituted. Compulsory notification of the existence of the disease, routine mallein testing of all animals in the group and those exposed to the disease and immediate destruction and proper disposal of all glandered animals and disinfection of premises, have proven to be highly effective in the elimination of the disease. Attendants in charge of horses should be cautioned against the careless handling of horses showing a chronic nasal discharge or an eruption of pustules and ulcers of the skin, particularly of the legs. Laboratory workers should exercise due care and extreme caution in handling diseased tissues, laboratory cultures of the organism and artificially infected laboratory animals. Cultures of *Malleomyces mallei* should be regarded as highly infectious since a considerable number of laboratory workers have contracted the disease by this method. In handling human patients affected with glanders attendants should exercise every precaution, while feeding, handling and dressing the patient and in the proper and effective sterilization of instruments, bandages, garments, bedding and table utensils. The prevention of the disease in man depends essentially on the eradication of the disease in horses by those methods proven effective. Glanders is no longer a prevalent disease of animals and man in North America—a striking and noteworthy accomplishment in the suppression of a disease transmitted from animals to man.

ITEMS OF NOTE

1) Glanders is primarily a disease of the horse, ass and mule.

2) The disease was widely prevalent in most countries until 1924. It is frequently observed still in many countries in Europe, Asia and Africa.

3) It has been eradicated in the United States and Canada by early detection and destruction of infected animals.

4) The disease in man results usually from occupational contact with horses.

5) Prevention of the disease in man depends in large part if not entirely—upon eradication of glanders in horses.

REFERENCES

1. PINI, A.: Isolation of Pfeifferella mallei on malachite green-fuchsin agar and on thionin agar. *Vet. ital. 8:*103, 1957.
2. WETMORE, P. W. AND GOCHENOUR, W. S., JR.: Comparative studies of the genus *Malleomyces* and selected *Pseudomonas* species. I. Morphological and cultural characteristics. *J. Bact. 72:*79, 1956.
3. MURASE, N., JURAKU, A., TIEN, J. AND SHIMIZU, F.: Epizootiological observations on glanders of horses in Manchuria. IV. Studies on the diagnosis and control, *Jap. J. Vet. Sci. 15:*157, 1953.
4. HAGAN, W. A. AND BRUNER, D. W.: *The Infectious Diseases of Domestic Animals,* Fourth Edition, Ithaca, Comstock, 1961.
5. MILLER, W. R., PANNELL, L., CRAVITZ, L., TANNER, W. A. AND INGALLS, M. S.: *J. Bact., 55:*115, 1948.
6. MILLER, W. R., PANNELL, L., CRAVITZ, L., TANNER, W. A. AND ROSEBURY, T.: *J. Bact. 55:*127, 1948.
7. HUTYRA, F., MAREK, J. AND MANNINGER, R.: *Special Pathology and Therapeutics of the Diseases of Domestic Animals.* 5th Edition, Chicago, Alexander Eger, 1946.
8. UDALL, D. H.: *The Practice of Veterinary Medicine,* 5th Edition, Ithaca by Author, 1947.
9. HU, T. P., KUNG, C. D. AND AU, B. H.: Studies on experimental infection of cattle, sheep and goats with glanders bacilli. *Acta vet. zootech sinica, 3:*36, 1958.

10. Duval and White: *J. Exper. Med.*, 9:352, 1907.

11. McFadyean, J.: *J. Comp. Path. & Therap.*, 17:295, 1904.

12. Frothingham: *J. Med. Res.*, 1:331, 1901.

13. Murase, N., Juraku, A., Tien, J. and Shimizu, F.: Epizootiological observations on glanders of horses in Manchuria. III. Investigations of nasal glanders, newly infected horses and colts born of the infected mares. *Jap. J. Vet. Sci.*, 15:147, 1953.

14. Mohler, J. R. and Eichhorn, A.: U.S. Dept. Agr., Bur. Animal Ind., Bul., 136, 1911.

15. Zeljiko, M. and Bas-Luketic, L.: The Conglutination test for the diagnosis of glanders. *Vet. Arhiv.* 24:52, 1954.

16. McFaydean, J.: *J. Comp. Path & Therap.*, 9:322, 1896.

17. Moore and Taylor: *J. Infect. Dis.*, Supp. No. 3:85, 1907.

18. Jager, S.: The use of the hemagglutination test for the diagnosis of glanders using sheep erythrocytes sensitized by extracts of Pfeifferella mallei. *Mag. Allator. Lapja.* 9:49, 1954.

19. Delpy, L. P.: Standardization of mallein at the Hessarek Institute, Iran. *Arch. Inst. Hessarek.* 8:36, 1954.

20. Fras, A.: Evaluation of mallein by hemagglutination. *Vet. Arhiv.* 25:195, 1955.

21. Ciortea, G., Marcea, E., Nitoiu, I., and Birzu, I.: Improvement of the diagnostic value and specificity of mallein by culture of the glanders bacillus on new media. *Lucr. Stiint. Inst. Pasteur, Bucuresti*, 3:365, 1958.

22. Goodall, Captain: *J. Comp. Path. & Therap.*, 28:281, 1915.

23. Murase, N., Juraku, A., Tien, J. and Shimizu, F.: Epizootiological observations on glanders of horses in Manchuria. II. Studies on the relation between immunological reactions and pathological observations. *Jap. J. Vet. Sci.*, 14:175, 1952.

24. Stehlik, Z. and Zarzycki, J.: Effect of the conjunctival mallein test in horses on subsequent intradermo-palpebral and subsequent mallein tests, and on complement-fixation. *Med. Vet.*, Varsovie, 14:5, 1958.

25. Murase, N., Juraku, A., Tien, J. and Shimizu, F.: Epizootiological observations on glanders of horses in Manchuria. I. Studies on the seasonal changes of the rate of infection. *Jap. J. Vet. Sci.*, 14:157, 1952.

26. Murase, N., Juraku, A., Tien, J. and Shimizu, F.: Epizootiological observations of glanders of horses in Manchuria. III. Investigations of nasal glanders, newly infected horses and colts born of the infected mares. *Jap. J. Vet. Sci.*, 15:147, 1953.

27. McFadyean, J.: *J. Comp. Path. & Therap.*, 13:55, 1900.

28. Hunting, W.: *Glanders, A Clinical Treatise.* London, H. & W. Brown, 1908.

29. Robins, G. D.: *Glanders, Studies from the Royal Victoria Hospital*, Montreal, Canada. 2:1906.

30. Gaiger, S. H.: *J. Comp. Path. & Therap.*, 26:233, 1913; 29:26, 1916.

31. Womack, C. R. and Well, E. B.: *Am. J. Med.*, 6:267, 1949.

32. Howe, C. and Miller, W. R.: *Ann. Int. Med.*, 26:93, 1947.

33. Mendelson, R. W.: *U.S. Armed Forces Med. Jour.*, 1:781, 1950.

34. Cravitz, L. and Miller, W. R.: *J. Infect. Dis.*, 86:52, 1950.

35. Miller, W. R., Pannell, L. and Ingalls, M. S.: *Am. J. Hyg.*, 47:205, 1948.

36. Sirmon, E. and Marcia, D.: Bacteriostatic action of antibiotic and chemotherapeutic agents on Pfeifferella mallei. *Prob. Epiz. Microbiol.*, Inst. Pat. Igien, Anim., Bucuresti, 5:51, 1956.

37. Tezok, F.: Three glanders strains isolated from three patients in 1956 and differing with regard to sensitivity to antibiotics. *Absts. of Proc. VIIth Int. Cong. Microbiol., Stockholm*, 344, 1958.

38. NEMOTO, H., YAMAGUCHI, M., AZUMA, R. AND KAWANISHI, Y.: Therapeutical study of experimental glanders with antibiotics. *Abstr. Proc. Suiyokai*, Tokyo-14, 1956.
39. DHANDA, M. R., GANGULEE, P. C. AND BENERJI, T. P.: Effect of sulphonamides in experimental glanders. *Indian. Vet. J. 35:*342, 1958.
40. MIRCHAMSY, H., NAZARI, F. AND SADEGH, A.: Treatment of glanders in guinea pigs with antibiotics and sulphonamides. *Inst. Hessarek. 8:*50, 1954.
41. EGHBAL, M., RAFYI, A., MIRCHAMSY, H. AND FARVAR, B.: Successful treatment with sulphonamides of glanders in a human being. Development of resistance to sulphonamides during treatment. *Pr. Med. 61:*1535, 1953.

Chapter 9

RABIES

Ernest S. Tierkel, V.M.D., M.P.H.

ETIOLOGY

THE ETIOLOGIC agent of rabies is a filterable virus with a predilection for nervous tissues, as a rule. The virus is approximately 125 millimicrons in diameter; thus, it lies about halfway in the scale of virus particle sizes—between the largest group, e.g., psittacosis, lymphogranuloma-venereum, and the smallest known animal viruses, e.g., foot-and-mouth disease. The virus can be destroyed by the addition of varying concentrations of formalin, phenol, bichloride of mercury, mineral acids and bases, certain quaternary ammonium compounds and other disinfectants to suspensions of infected tissue. Rabies virus remains viable for long periods of time when bits of infected tissue are stored in 50 per cent glycerol-saline or pure glycerol at 4°C; at this temperature, lyophilized suspensions will also keep. Another preferred method of storage is freezing of suspensions and storage at −30° to −60°C. The keeping qualities of the virus in the frozen state are greatly enhanced if 20 per cent tissue suspensions are prepared, and substances high in protein or amino acids are added, such as serum, albumin, sterile milk, or egg yolks.

Resistance of the virus to physical and environmental influences is variable and depends in large measure on the breaking up of the infected host tissue. Generally, however, it can be described as being quite labile. It is destroyed easily by sunlight and heat, and its infectivity becomes negligible when exposed to ordinary environmental conditions of light, heat, and air. This property has a practical application in that fomites have not been known to play a role in the transmission of the virus. For this reason, it is not felt necessary to carry out extensive disinfection of rooms, furnishings, or any objects which might have become contaminated with the saliva of a rabid animal.

In 1804, by transmission experiments in dogs, Zinke first demonstrated rabies virus in saliva. The first positive demonstration that the agent of rabies in man and dogs was the same occurred in 1813 when Magendie and Breschet were able to infect dogs with saliva from a human patient. In the 1880's, Pasteur's classical work opened a new vista in methods of working with the virus in the laboratory. It was this work which established the modification of viruses by serial passage through a definite tissue system of an animal species. Pasteur gave the term "street virus" to the rabies virus as it occurs in nature. He was able to modify this virus by intracerebral serial passages in rabbits. The incubation period became shorter with succeeding passages until it reached a point where this period became fixed and so he named this newly modified agent "fixed virus." In contrast to the long and variable interval of the street virus, the fixed virus, as a rule, does not have the ability to form Negri bodies and is more strictly neurotropic in character. Since it has become more highly adapted to neural tissue, fixed virus has lost its tropism for salivary gland tissue even when introduced by the peripheral route.

The standard measurement of the ability of rabies to multiply and destroy nerve tissues in the living animal is carried out by intracerebral inoculation of varying dilutions of suspensions of infected tissue into young adult laboratory white mice. Tenfold dilutions are used and the 50 per cent mortality end point in the inoculated mice, or the mouse intracerebral titers, is calculated by the method of Reed and Muench (1938). This mouse titration is a valuable tool in the laboratory and has practical application for selecting isolates of fixed virus within a sufficiently high titer for use as a seed virus in the production of rabies vaccines, for testing the potency of vaccines, and for carrying out serum neutralization tests. Since fixed virus in mice has lost the vagaries which are characteristic of street virus, titration standards can be established with fairly reasonable consistency for the performance of these tests.

Either naturally or artificially infecting an animal with the rabies virus stimulates the production of specific antibodies, which may be detected by complement fixation (CF) or serum neutralization (SN) tests. The complement fixation test is generally not used because of the difficulty of obtaining good, stable, standard antigens from infected tissues, and because the CF antibodies do not persist very long. Serum neutralizing antibodies, however, persist for much longer periods and the SN test is the serologic test of choice for confirmatory identification of the virus, and for determining antibody levels in man and animals for epidemiologic purposes, and for measuring the antigenic response of vaccines. The serum neutralization test is carried out by the mixing of serum with suspensions of virus, and titration values are obtained by using a constant quantity of standard fixed virus with serial dilutions of serum, or by using a constant quantity of serum with serial dilutions of virus. The former method is gaining greater acceptance as a tool for determining titers of antibody in human and animal populations. The virus dilution technique is more desirable for confirmatory identification of the virus with known, stock, immune sera.

The mouse is the animal of choice in rabies experiments, but others, such as guinea pigs, hamsters, rabbits, and dogs, are frequently used. Hamsters are gaining in popularity because of their high degree of susceptibility by peripheral routes of infection (Koprowski, 1949). Adaption of the virus to chicken embryos was accomplished by Kligler and Bernkopf (1938) by the chorioallantoic route, and later by Dawson (1941) by intracerebral inoculation of the embryo. Koprowski and Cox (1948) were able to effect serial passage of the virus in chicken embryos by yolk sac inoculation. This yolk sac technique was used by Powell and Culbertson (1950) for adapting the virus to duck embryos. Kissling (1958) adapted rabies virus to hamster kidney tissue culture; although there was evidence of virus multiplication, cytopathogenic effects were not detected consistently. Kaplan *et al.* (1960) adapted the virus to chicken embryo tissue culture monolayers whose presence interferred with the growth of superimposed western equine encephalomyelitis virus. Atanasiu and Lepine (1959) adapted it to glial cell tumor tissue culture and Fernandes and Pomerat (1960) to CNS tissue culture from newborn kittens.

Unlike most other pathogenic animal viruses, distinct or separate immunologic types or strains of rabies virus have never been identified with the presently known means for establishing such differences. This is rather remarkable when one considers the vastly different clinical picture elicited in man and animals succumbing to vampire bat rabies compared to that of cases due to transmission from the usual vectors such as dogs, foxes, and skunks. Thus, virus strains isolated from cases of vampire bat-transmitted rabies in Latin America are immunologically indistinguishable from strains isolated from dog- or fox-transmitted rabies by cross-protection, CF or SN tests.

CLINICAL FEATURES

In Man

The incubation period of rabies is extremely variable and generally long. In man, this averages from thirty to sixty days with a range of two weeks to five months. In rare instances, human cases have been reported where the incubation period was as short as ten days and as long as eight months. The early stages of the disease are marked by prodromal symptoms of headache, malaise, slight elevation of temperature, nervousness, and anxiety. In the majority of cases, there is a sensation of tingling, pain, or burning around the site of the bite. This occurs quite early in the course of the disease. As the disease progresses, there is an increase in anxiety and nervousness with development of increased sensory reactions, excitability, hyperesthesia, and generalized pressor syndrome. There is an increased tendency to move, and the patient often lashes about in bed. The symptom most often associated with human rabies is the

TABLE 35

Human Rabies Deaths in the United States 1961

Locality	Date Died	Age	Sex	Nature of Exposure	Incubation Period	Length of Illness	Treatment	Biting Animal
1. Harlan County, Kentucky	1/6/61	53	F	Bitten on leg	52 days	7 days	14 doses vaccine— next morning	fox
2. Imperial County, California	1/20/61	76	M	Five-inch wound on right wrist	31 days	13 days	14 doses vaccine— 7 days later	dog
3. Powell County, Kentucky	6/27/61	74	M	Bitten on left thumb	39 days	5 days	14 doses vaccine— 2½ weeks later	fox

so-called hydrophobia or "fear of water" phenomenon. This is due to the painful spasms of the pharyngeal muscles upon swallowing of fluid. Subsequent conditioned reflexes related to swallowing will similarly cause these pharyngeal spasms-hence, the tendency of the patient to shun fluids brought to him.

By the same token, he avoids swallowing his saliva, which often drools from his mouth. Although these swallowing symptoms are not constant, they occur frequently enough to make them the most characteristic of the disease in man. The increased anxiety is often associated with a feeling of impending death. As the excitation phase develops, there may be convulsive seizures. In rare cases, maniacal symptoms and violence with biting, kicking, and sudden lashing of the body may be elicited. Generally there are relatively relaxed periods between those of excitation during which the patient is quite lucid. Most patients die during the height of an episode of excitation, but in some the disease may progress to generalized paralysis, and the patient may expire in prostration.

In Animals

Dogs. In all species of lower animals clinical rabies presents a similar picture. The average incubation period in dogs is three to eight weeks, but, as in man and in other susceptible animals, this can be extremely variable. In dogs it has ranged from ten days to six months. It is rarely less than two weeks or more than four months. The clinical course of the disease in dogs can be divided into three phases, the prodromal, the excitative, and the paralytic. The term "furious rabies" refers to animals in which the excitative phase is predominant and "dumb rabies" to those cases in which the excitative phase is extremely short or absent and the disease progresses quickly to the paralytic phase. In the prodromal stage, which lasts two to three days, the animal may exhibit a subtle change in temperament. High-strung dogs may become more affectionate than usual, whereas ordinarily affectionate animals may shy away from their owners and become snappy and irritable. During this phase, there is a slight rise in temperature, dilation of the pupils, and a sluggish corneal reflex. The excitative phase, which lasts from three to seven days, is the one during which signs of the disease are most easily recognized. The dog becomes increasingly irritable, restless, and nervous. In the early part of this stage it may shun people and hide in dark places, under furniture, or in closets. It shows exaggerated response to sudden stimuli of sight and sound. Excitability, photophobia, and hyperesthesia may become apparent. It may snap at insects and imaginary objects. Often there is a tendency to eat unusual things like sticks, straw, stones, and soil. Restlessness increases, and the animals get an urge to move and roam. At this time, it may begin to wander aimlessly through town and countryside, all the time becoming more irritable and vicious; it is at this stage that the animal is most dangerous because of its tendency to bite anything that is encountered, be it man, animal or inanimate

A   **B**

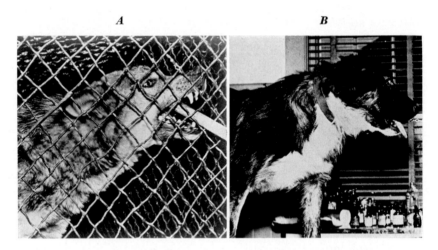

Fig. 62A. Canine rabies at clinical height of the disease. (Photograph courtesy Marvin Carter, Memphis-Shelby County Health Dept., Memphis, Tenn.)
Fig. 62B. Paralysis of jaw muscles in a case of canine rabies. (Photograph courtesy Marvin Carter, Memphis-Shelby County Health Dept., Memphis, Tenn.)

object. If the animal is confined at this stage of the disease, it will bite at chains or the bars of cage or kennel, breaking its teeth, inflicting severe trauma on its oral tissues. In most cases, there is a characteristic change in bark caused by paralysis of the laryngeal musculature. As in man, there is difficulty in swallowing, due to spasms, and eventual paralysis of the muscles of deglutition, causing the animal to drool saliva. Sometimes heavy, rapid respiration through the mouth will cause frothing of the drooling saliva. Convulsive seizures and muscular incoordination are apparent toward the end of this stage. If the animal does not die during one of the convulsive seizures, it enters into the paralytic stage, during which the disease progresses from muscular incoordination to paralysis of the entire body, thence to coma and death. The clinical course of the disease characterized by the excitative phase may last as long as ten days, including the prodromal phase, but rarely as long as twelve days.

The paralytic stage begins almost immediately if the excitative phase is either quite short or entirely absent. The clinical course of the paralytic stage is less spectacular and therefore is often difficult to diagnose. This is the form referred to as dumb rabies. The most characteristic sign of this form of the disease is the so-called "dropped jaw" caused by paralysis of the muscles of mastication, making it impossible for the animal to eat or drink. Paralyzed, too, are the pharyngeal muscles, causing drooling of saliva. Often the animal emits a choking sound which leads the owner to believe there is a bone stuck in the throat. In their attempt to remove the "bone," many dog owners scratch their hands on the dog's teeth, thus allowing the infective saliva to come into contact with these, as well as preexistent, wounds or abrasions of the skin. After initially affecting the head and neck region, the paralysis soon becomes generalized over the body, and death ensues from the second to the fourth day after onset.

Cats. The disease in dogs and cats is similar, generally characterized by viciousness and excitation. Swift movements and erratic behavior are more marked in rabid cats than in dogs, and their bites are considered dangerous because they are generally of the deep puncture type.

Farm Animals. Rabies in cattle generally assume a furious form. As this stage of the disease becomes apparent, there is restlessness, nervousness, and there may be some indication of pruritis. The animal becomes aggressive and will move about violently, paw, and butt into other animals and objects. In some cases, the affected animal cannot retain saliva. The most striking signs are fits of bellowing, general straining, and tenesmus. Although they may thrash about violently, they rarely bite. As the disease enters the paralytic stage, the first signs are weakness in the hind legs followed by paralysis which takes over the muscles of locomotion. Death comes after a period of complete paralysis and prostration.

As in cattle, rabies in horses and mules is characterized by excitation. They become very restless, excitable, and vicious. They often kick, paw, and bite other animals, moving objects, and sometimes themselves. Frequently the ears stand erect, and the lips are drawn back with loss of saliva. Dysphagia is marked. Paralysis soon extends from head and neck region to muscles of locomotion, and death ensues after the animal becomes recumbent and prostrate.

Rabies in sheep and swine is not seen as often as in other live-stock, although the clinical course is similar, with restlessness, nerv-ousness, hyper-excitability, and spasms of muscle groups followed by paralysis and death.

PATHOLOGY

Rabies elicits no gross characteristic pathologic alterations which can be seen during postmortem examination. The histopathologic lesions of the central nervous system are inflammatory in nature and are very much like those seen in other infections. As a rule, there is more damage to the pons, medulla, brain stem, and thalamus than to other parts of the brain. This is probably associated with the fact that the virus is contained in greatest concentration in these parts. The changes which can be seen include nuclear and cytoplasmic degeneration of the neurons, neuronphagia, and diffuse gliosis. Often, one can see evidence of petechial hemorrhage around the blood vessels as well as perivascular, lymphocytic cuffing found in so many infections of the central nervous system. The well-differen-tiated accumulation of glial cells (so-called Babes nodules) which one sometimes sees throughout the brain, and the marked neuronal degeneration and lymphocytic infiltration in the dorsal root and cranial nerve ganglia cannot be considered pathognomonic since these changes may be seen in other encephalitic diseases.

In 1903, Adelchi Negri reported the pathognomonic lesion of rabies, a characteristic inclusion body which bears his name. The Negri body is found in the cytoplasm of the neurons. It is generally rounded, acidophilic, has a mottled matrix and, with most differen-tial red-blue stains, has characteristic basophilic internal granules. Examination of brain tissue for the presence of Negri bodies has evolved as an important standard procedure in the laboratory diag-nosis or rabies.

Over the years, the pathogenesis of rabies has been widely studied. The evidence of most experimental investigation shows the virus traveling from the point of entry in the area of the wound along nerve trunk pathways in a centripetal direction to the central nervous system. Infection in the salivary glands depends upon the virus traveling in a centrifugal direction to the salivary glands via nerve trunk routes. The spread of the virus by neural pathways is thought to be related to the degeneration of the myelin sheaths and general demyelination which is seen in the white matter in various stages of the disease.

DIAGNOSIS

Rabies is diagnosed by recognition of the characteristic clinical, pathologic, and virologic features. The animal suspected of being rabid should be captured and confined and the disease should be allowed to progress until fatal termination. The premature killing of such animals will reduce the accuracy of the laboratory diagnosis,

A   *B*

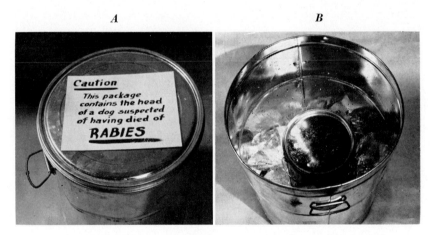

Fig. 63A. Container for shipping animal head covered and labeled.
Fig. 63B. Double container with ice for packing specimens.

since the development of Negri bodies in the brain is directly related to the length of clinical illness in rabies. If circumstances necessitate destruction of the animal, care should be taken not to mutilate the head, since damage to the brain will render it less useful for diagnosis. After decapitation in the field, the head should be cooled promptly and kept cold; wherever possible, it should be delivered by messenger or by express freight via rail, air or road. It should be put into a tin or other suitable water tight metal container which should be closed tightly. This receptacle, in turn, should be put into a large, watertight, metal container, cracked ice being put between the inner and outer container (Figures 63A and B). The package should be clearly labeled and shipped to the laboratory with utmost dispatch. The use of dry ice in packing the head should be avoided if microscopic diagnosis is desired, since freezing the specimen often distorts and tears the brain tissue; furthermore, the time required to thaw causes delay in diagnosis.

A   *B*

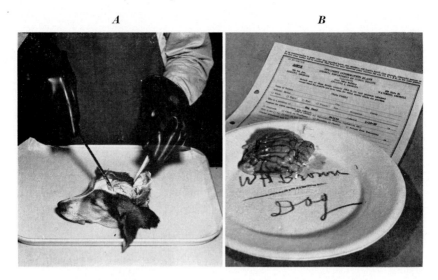

Fig. 64A. Calvaria reflected so that brain can be removed.
Fig. 64B. Brain placed on paper plate.

When heads of animals are submitted for examination, this information is desirable: The species and breed of the animal, and whether it was in contact with other animals; whether the animal died or was killed, and, in the latter case, the means used for killing; whether the animal was confined and observed for any time before death, and, if so, for how long; signs of rabies, if any; history of vaccination against rabies; and names and addresses of persons bitten, if any.

MICROSCOPIC EXAMINATION OF BRAIN TISSUE

Either histologic sections of brain tissue blocks or fresh tissue applied to a slide by impression or smear technique may be micro-

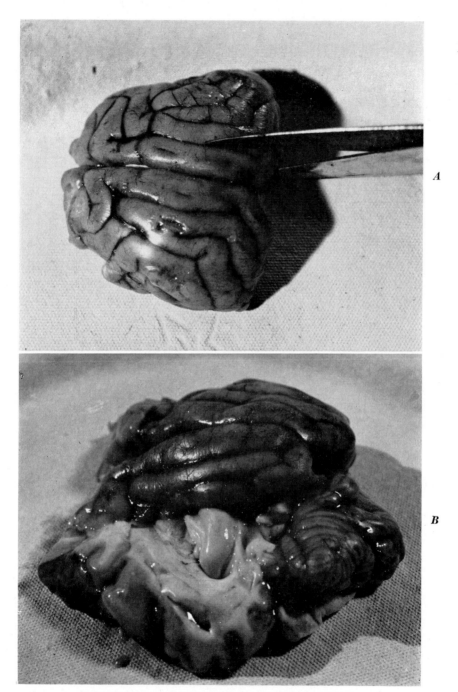

A

B

Fig. 65A. Site of incision for locating Ammon's horn.
Fig. 65B. Dog brain with left cerebral hemisphere dissected to show Ammon's horn bulging from the floor of the lateral ventricle.

scopically searched for Negri bodies. For histologic sections, the staining techniques which have given the best results are those of Schleifstein (1937), Stovall and Black (1940), or Lillie's (1948)

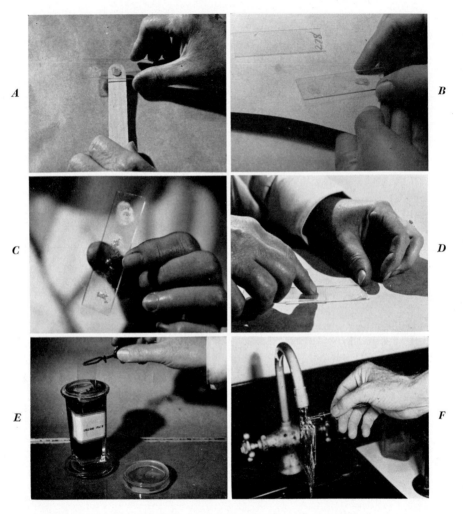

Fig. 66A. Impression method of slide preparation from specimen on tongue depressor.

Fig. 66B. Impression method of slide preparation from specimen on paper towel.

Fig. 66C. Several impressions made on a slide.

Fig. 66D. Smear method of slide preparation.

Fig. 66E. Slide plunged rapidly into Sellers' stain while tissue films still moist.

Fig. 66F. Rinsing freshly stained slide with tap water.

modification of Stovall's method. Most diagnostic laboratories are not equipped to prepare histologic sections and, indeed, experience has shown that this cumbersome practice is not necessary. A film of fresh brain tissue, properly applied and stained, is just as accurate for purposes of diagnosis and is manifestly simpler, quicker, and less costly.

For the impression or smear technique the choice of stain is Sellers' (1954b), the preparation of which he recently modified to employ stock solutions of one per cent methylene blue (dye content not less than 85 per cent) and one per cent basic fuchsin (dye content not less than 92 per cent), each in chemically-pure, acetone-free, methyl alcohol. The working stain is made up of two volumes of the methylene blue stock solution and one volume of the basic fuchsin.

The Negri body in Sellers' stain is well differentiated in a magenta or heliotrope (purplish pink) color with well-demonstrated dark-blue to black, basophilic, internal bodies. All parts of the nerve cell stain blue, and the interstitial tissue stains rose-pink. Erythrocytes stain copper color (orange-tinged red) and can be easily differentiated from the magenta-tinged red of the Negri bodies.

The Negri body varies in shape, although it is generally rounded. Its size also varies greatly, usually within the limits of 0.24 to 27.0 microns.

The position of the Negri body within the neuron is intracytoplasmic. Classically, it is found between the nucleus and one corner of the neuron or in the prolongation of the cell body. However, it should be stressed that the intracytoplasmic position of the Negri body can be expected with reasonable consistency only in histologic sections of the brain. In the simpler tissue application techniques, the histologic pattern is disturbed, thus making the nerve cell outline difficult to discern, and one may very often see well-formed Negri bodies which appear to be entirely outside the neuron. Thus, in the impression or smear techniques, the intracellular position of the Negri body is not required as a diagnostic criterion; Negri bodies which satisfy the requisites of morphologic identification whether they seem to appear inside or outside the neurons, are sufficient to establish a positive diagnosis.

Its internal structure is the most striking characteristic of the Negri body. The matrix of the Negri body has an acidophilic staining reaction, and contained within are small inner bodies (Innerkorperchen), basophilic granules which stain dark blue to black. The size of these inner granules generally varies from 0.2 to 0.5 micron. Rarely, an orderly arrangement of the inner granules, as in a rosette design, may be seen. For purposes of diagnosis, it is sufficient to recognize these granules as part of the inner structure of the Negri body, regardless of their number or pattern of distribution. Although Negri bodies may be found in any portion of the gray matter rich in neurons, they are most often found in the hippocampus (Ammon's horn) and are often abundant in the cerebellum and cerebral cortex. These are the three areas examined routinely.

Because of certain similarities, other types of inclusion bodies are sometimes mistaken for Negri bodies. This is particularly true of the dog, fox, skunk, cat, and laboratory white mouse. In the brains of dogs, foxes, skunks, and other wild carnivores, the acidophilic inclusion bodies of canine distemper or of Rubarth's disease (canine infectious hepatitis, fox encephalitis) are occasionally encountered. These inclusions seem to occur more often in the thalamus and lentiform neclei than in the hippocampus. By the same token, the brains of nonrabid cats and laboratory white mice occasionally contain nonspecific acidophilic inclusion bodies when presented for rabies diagnosis. These nonrabies inclusions all have the same staining characteristics with Sellers' stain and cannot be differentiated from one another with the techniques described above. However, the important thing is that these nonrabies inclusions, as a group, can be differentiated from Negri bodies with the use of Sellers' stain by using the following criteria as a guide for distinguishing them. Negri bodies have a very definite internal structure characterized by basophilic inner granules, a heterogenous or mottled matrix, are not highly refractile, and have a definite purplish tinge. The nonrabies inclusions lack an internal structure, have a homogenous or smooth matrix, are highly refractile, and are somewhat more acidophilic, giving a pinker appearance (Tierkel and Neff, 1957).

Electron microscopy and cytochemistry have been employed to determine the nature of the Negri body. In the electron microscopy studies, Hottle *et al.* (1951) found no particles in the Negri body which could be recognized as elementary bodies of the virus. Lepine and Croissant (1951) observed the Negri body as a cellular reaction around the virus particles. In cytochemical studies, Wolman and Behar (1952) observed small Feulgen-positive, basophilic inclusions which grew in size and, in subsequent daily specimens, became amorphous, acidophilic, and Fuelgen-negative, suggesting the inclusions to be virus particle aggregates.

In 1958, Goldwasser and Kissling reported the Negri bodies are of viral origin, on the basis of their studies of rabies virus antigens with the fluorescent antibody technique.

VIRUS ISOLATION

Negri bodies are not always demonstrable in the brains of rabid animals, so virus isolation on these Negri-negative specimens must be attempted using laboratory mice. Surveys of rabies cases have shown that 10 to 15 per cent of the cases proved positive by mouse inoculation had been missed by direct microscopic examination of

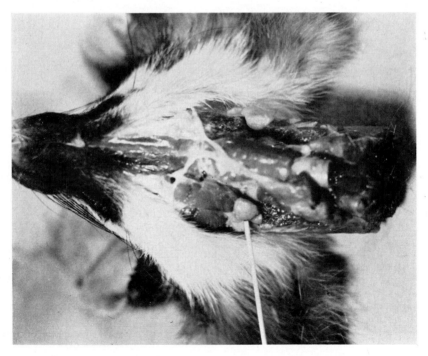

Fig. 67. Exposure of submaxillary salivary gland.

the brain for Negri bodies (Johnson, 1942; Leach, 1938; Damon and Sellers, 1941).

The white mouse is the preferred animal because it costs little, making it possible to use several animals for one specimen, and be-

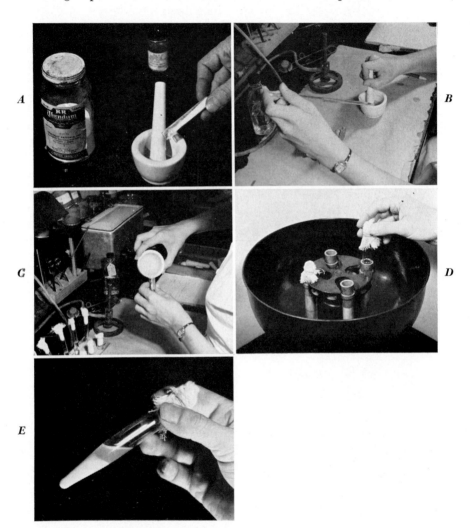

Fig. 68A. Addition of abrasive to facilitate grinding of salivary gland tissue.
Fig. 68B. Addition of diluent to finely ground tissue.
Fig. 68C. Pouring tissue suspension into centrifuge tube.
Fig. 68D. Centrifugation of tissue suspension.
Fig. 68E. Appearance of tissue suspension after centrifugation.

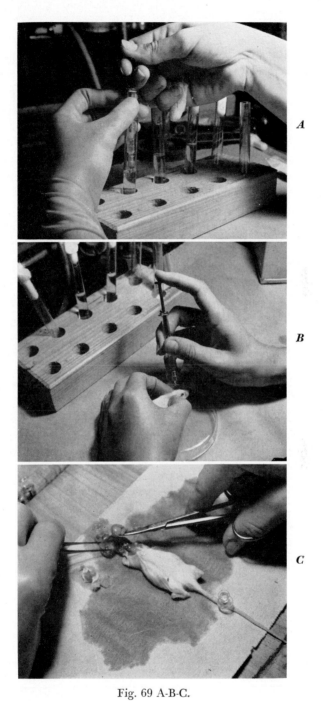

Fig. 69 A-B-C.

Fig. 69A. Drawing supernate fluid into syringe for mouse inoculation.

Fig. 69B. Intracerebral inoculation of mouse.

Fig. 69C. Removal of mouse brain.

cause of the relatively short incubation period of street virus infection together with the constant and typical signs and consistent production of Negri bodies (Webster and Dawson, 1935). The test is carried out by the intracerebral inoculation of .03 ml of a 10 to 20 per cent suspension of tissue into each of five mice per specimen. Tissue sections from hippocampus, cerebral cortex, cerebellum, and the pons-medulla area are pooled for preparing the suspended inoculum; thorough sampling of these areas on both side of the brain is important because of the possible variability of virus distribution.

Contaminated or decomposed specimens treated with antibiotics can be injected into animals without affecting the virus. Emulsions to which are added 500 to 1000 units of penicillin and 2 mg of streptomycin per ml of tissue suspension, or their equivalents with other antibiotics, are ready for inoculation after thirty minutes at room temperature.

Diagnosis of rabies in an animal does not always mean that saliva is infective; therefore, the mouse inoculation test of the submaxillary glands of biting animals, for the presence of virus, provides definitive evidence of whether or not a bite has entailed a risk. Virus isolation from salivary glands also provides important epidemiologic information.

In cases where other viral encephalitides may be suspected, the serum neutralization test is valuable as a specific confirmatory procedure. In these cases, suspensions of the tissue in question are mixed with immune stock anti-rabies serum and tested in mice with the usual negative and immune controls.

FLUORESCENT ANTIBODY TEST

After the work of Goldwasser and Kissling in 1958, the fluorescent antibody test was used on a series of naturally infected salivary glands by Goldwasser *et al.* (1959) and on brain specimens sent into health department laboratories for rabies diagnosis by McQueen *et al.* (1960). Facets in the development and refinement of the test were made by Carski (1960) and Wilsnack (1960). The test is being adopted as a diagnostic tool by an increasing number of laboratories, particularly in the United States and Israel. The test allows direct, visual observation of specific antigen-antibody reaction. It is based on the microscopic examination of tissue specimens for specific fluorescent staining when the tissue has been placed in contact with conjugate, the name given to antirabies serum which has been "tagged" by the addition of a fluorescent dye. Examination of the slide containing a simple impression of the suspected tissue after fixing, staining and washing, is similar to any other microscopic examination, except that ultra-violet light source and a specialized system of filters and condensors are used. Investigations of the fluorescent antibody test have shown that this diagnostic method, when properly executed, can establish a highly specific diagnosis on test specimens within a few hours and that there is a high degree of correlation between this test and the mouse inoculation test. Those who have developed this new and useful technique point out that exacting standards of performance, equipment, and reagents are necessary and these are related to adequate training and proficiency of the diagnostician.

INCIDENCE TRENDS AND DISTRIBUTION

In the United States, there were 3,470 laboratory confirmed cases of rabies during calendar year 1961. There were 594 reported in dogs, 217 in cats, 2,174 in wildlife, 482 in farm livestock and three in man. There was an increase of thirteen cases over the total number of cases reported for the previous year and a decrease of 103 cases in dogs.

In 1961, there was a substantial decrease of rabies in foxes. One-third fewer cases were reported than in 1960. The southeastern states, which long have been areas of high fox rabies, are now virtually free of it.

Reported skunk rabies cases increased by 73 per cent in 1961. This sharp rise is not due to a single regional epidemic but to 100 per cent increases in the number of rabid skunks reported in each of three widely separated foci of skunk rabies in California, Texas and Iowa.

The number of rabid bats in 1961 was 186 as compared to 88 for the previous year. These cases came from twenty-eight States. A number of these, such as Massachusetts, Montana, New Jersey, Utah, Oregon and Washington, seldom report rabies in terrestrial animals.

States showing substantial increases over their 1960 cases were California, Illinois, Iowa, South Dakota and Texas. Marked de-

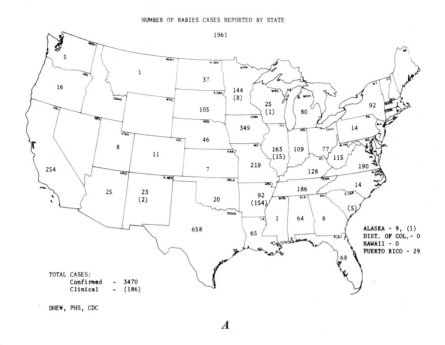

A

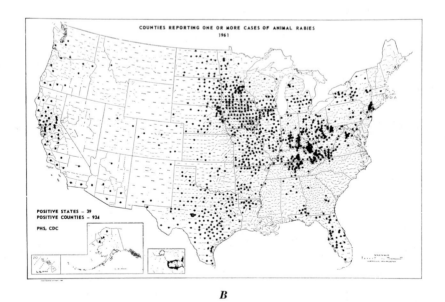

B

Fig. 70 A-B.

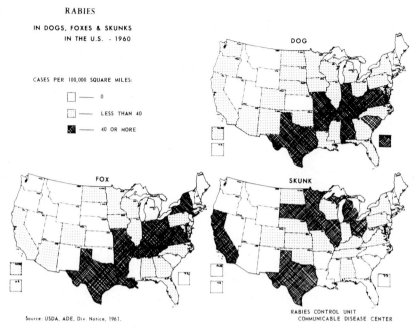

RABIES

IN DOGS, FOXES & SKUNKS
IN THE U.S. - 1960

CASES PER 100,000 SQUARE MILES:

☐ —— 0

▥ —— LESS THAN 40

▨ —— 40 OR MORE

DOG

FOX

SKUNK

Source: USDA, ADE, Div. Notice, 1961.

RABIES CONTROL UNIT
COMMUNICABLE DISEASE CENTER

Fig. 70 C.

creases from the previous year occurred in New York, Alabama, Georgia, Arkansas, Ohio, New Mexico and Alaska.

There were three human rabies deaths in 1961. One resulted from a dog bite in California near the Arizona State line and the Mexican border and the other too from bites of rabid foxes in eastern Kentucky (Table 36).

In 1946, a national rabies-control program was begun by the Communicable Disease Center, U. S. Public Health Service, consisting of research, technical consultation, and training activities. Dur-

TABLE 36

REPORTED CASES OF RABIES IN THE UNITED STATES*

Year	Dogs	Wildlife	Cats	Farm Livestock	Man	Total
1946	8384	956	455	1055	22	10,872
1956	2592	2079	371	794	10	5,846
1961	594	2174	217	482	3	3,470

*Agricultural Research Service, U.S. Department of Agriculture and Communicable Disease Center, U.S. Public Health Service.

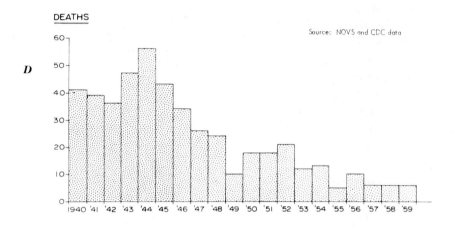

REPORTED HUMAN RABIES DEATHS

in the U.S.; 1940-1959

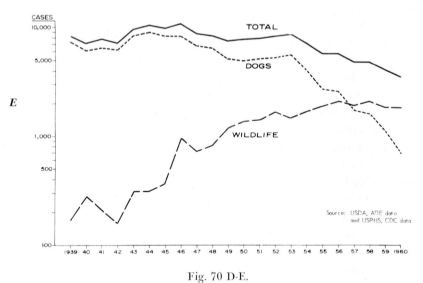

RABIES in the U. S.

1939 – 1960

Fig. 70 D-E.

ing the fifteen-year period since that time, thirty-three State health departments have established veterinary public health programs with the development of organized rabies control activities. Progress achieved in control during these past fifteen years is reflected in the annual, nationwide, reported cases as shown in Table 36. The total number of cases in 1946 was 10,872.

This declined steadily to 3,470 cases in 1961, a decrease of more than two-thirds. Similarly, human deaths have dropped from twenty-two in 1946 to three in 1961, a decrease of 86 per cent. The decline in total number of animal cases is due to the remarkable decrease in the number of canine cases. These went from 8,384 in 1946 to only 594 cases (93 per cent decrease), in spite of a greatly increased dog population. This is eloquent testimony to the success of organized rabies-control programs throughout the country and the wide acceptance of canine rabies vaccination during this fifteen-year period. In sharp contrast to the decrease in canine rabies, the reported number of wildlife cases has doubled.

Canada remained relatively free of rabies for a period of about 10 years until a small focus of infection was discovered in the Northwest Territory in 1947. By 1952-53, the disease had swept south from the arctic region and set off a serious epizootic of wildlife and dog rabies in the province of Alberta and in parts of British Columbia and Saskatchewan. By 1957, this western Canadian region was rid of the disease and the following year new heavily affected areas, principally fox rabies, were reported from the province of Ontario where the bulk of the problem remains today.

In a recent survey by the Pan American Health Organization, incidence data from 1958 was received from twenty-two areas in the Western Hemisphere. From these areas 7,724 cases of rabies in animals were diagnosed and reported. More than 100 cases were reported in each of the following countries: Argentina, Brazil, Canada, Chile, Peru, and the United States. Guatemala, Nicaragua, and Venezuela reported more than fifty cases each. Although no information was provided for Mexico, a report sent to the World Health Organization indicated that in 1958, 747 captured animals in the Federal District were positive for rabies. Similarly eighty-one positive animal cases were reported by the National Institute of Hygiene of Ecuador. Dogs have been most often incriminated as the source of rabies in other animals and man. The other animal most often reported with this disease in the Americas is the cow. Uruguay reports that it has been rabies-free for more than twenty years. Brazil, Mexico, French Guiana, and Trinidad have reported incidents involving the transmission of rabies by bats.

In 1958, 186 human cases of rabies were reported in the Americas. In five countries, ten or more human rabies deaths were reported, namely, Brazil, Colombia, Mexico, Peru and Venezuela.

The latest global rabies report (1958) prepared by the World Health Organization from 170 services in seventy-five countries disclosed that rabies is present in fifty-two countries and absent in twenty-three countries.

Rabies was reported present in animals in Algeria, Bechuanaland Protectorate, Brazil, Bulgaria, Burma, Cambodia, Canada, Chile, Czechoslovakia, Dominican Republic, Egypt, Ethiopia, Finland, France, French Equatorial Africa, French West Africa, Germany, Ghana, Greece, Guatemala, British Guiana, French Guiana, Honduras, India, Indonesia, Iran, Israel, Italy, Kenya, Libya, Madagascar, Mexico, Morocco, Mozambique, Nigeria, Nyasaland, Pakistan, Philippines, Poland, Northern and Southern Rhodesia, Somaliland Protectorate, Sudan, Tanganyika, Thailand, Tunisia, Turkey, Uganda, Union of South Africa, United States, Viet Nam and Yugoslavia.

The following countries reported rabies not present: Australia, Basutoland, Belgium, North Borneo, China (Taiwan), Denmark, Guadeloupe, Hong Kong, Iceland, Ireland, Japan, Luxembourg, Federation of Malaya, Martinique, Netherlands, New Zealand, Norway, Portugal, Singapore, Sweden, Switzerland, United Kingdom, and Uruguay.

A total of 947 human rabies deaths (82 in treated and 845 in untreated persons) were reported from sixty-five countries. The greatest toll of human lives was reported from India, the Philippines, Mexico, Thailand and Egypt. The total number of persons who received vaccine treatment in these sixty-five countries was 487,728 and paralytic side reactions attributable to the vaccine occurred in forty-nine persons.

The reports from sixty-nine countries indicated that the dog can be considered to be the main vector of the disease in most countries. Wild animals, however, have begun to play an increasingly important role in the transmission of the disease. For instance, the fox is more important than the dog as a vector of the disease in Canada, Poland and Germany. In the United States, skunks have been shown to be important vectors and bats are important in Latin America. In Iran rabid wolves are the greatest source of rabies. The Iran Pasteur Institute reports, from 1949 to 1958, 443 persons were bitten by wolves with thirty-nine rabies deaths.

EPIDEMIOLOGICAL CHARACTERISTICS

Rabies is principally a disease of such carnivorous or biting animals as dogs, foxes, skunks, wolves, cats, and coyotes, although all warm-blooded animals are susceptible. The disease is ubiquitous in character. It is found in the arctic regions, as well as the temperate and tropical countries of both hemispheres. Climate and season have no direct influence on its occurrence, and it may be present in enzootic or epizootic proportions during any time of the year. Incidence in animals is highest during those times of the year when movement and contact among them is greatest and, in the United States, this is generally during the autumn shuffle of fox populations when family groups break up, or during late winter or spring when wild carnivores move about in search of food and mate.

Rabies virus entering a wound is ordinarily a prerequisite to infection. Practically all cases of rabies occur as the result of virus-laden saliva entering a wound caused by the bite of a rabid animal. It is possible also for infection to occur when infected saliva comes into intimate contact with pre-existing, fresh, open wounds. This danger is present when owners try to remove what seems to be a "bone in the throat" of a choking rabid dog, or try to relieve what appears to be "choke" signs in a rabid cow. Instances of infection due to other means, such as indirect exposure via fomites, are so rare as to be negligible. There are no reports in the medical literature of alimentary tract infection, which is not possible unless there are frank abrasions of the gastro-intestinal mucosa.

Feeding rabies virus suspensions to laboratory animals has failed to be infective. Similarly, negative results have been obtained after feeding experimentally infected white mice to susceptible dogs and foxes which could later be infected successfully by parenteral routes. Although the milk of rabid cows has been reported occasionally to contain rabies virus, ingestion of infected milk is not considered a bona fide exposure. Arthropods play no role in the transmission of rabies, and, indeed, there is no evidence of viremia in animals infected naturally or artificially (Bell *et al.*, 1957; Kissling, 1957).

Very recently, studies carried out by the Communicable Disease Center demonstrated that rabies virus was transmitted by a non-bite route to foxes and coyotes in a bat cave in Texas. The findings support consideration of an airborn medium, such as an aerosol, as the method of transmission in this instance (Constantine, 1962).

Natural vector animals' emitting virus in sufficient quantity via saliva makes possible the natural spread of rabies. Virus is found in the salivary glands in animals dead of rabies in 54 to 90 per cent of the cases; the prevalence is slightly higher in foxes and skunks than in dogs. The titer of virus in positive salivary glands varies from a trace to as high as $10^{6.8}$. In dogs, the excretion of virus in saliva occurs after onset of clinical disease but since the prodromal signs are so difficult to observe, a few days may elapse between isolation of saliva from daily test samples and the appearance of classical, frank signs of rabies. For this reason, it is recommended that biting animals in which rabies is suspected be confined under clinical observation for ten days. This period allows for a generous margin of safety; if the confined animal remains clinically well during this period, it is certain that it was not infectious at the time of the bite.

Rabies is fatal. No man has recovered from the disease after clinical symptoms have begun. The same can be said for lower animals, although a few cases have been reported in which dogs have recovered from the disease after signs of rabies developed (Starr *et al.*, 1952). However, these are so rare as to be classified as medical curiosities. Occasionally workers have observed residual paralysis and/or recoveries in laboratory animals following peripheral routes of infection.

Soave *et al.* (1961) reported that a guinea pig inoculated intramuscularly with rabies street virus survived for five months, but developed paralysis in the inoculated limb and died of rabies thirteen days after initiation of a course of ACTH inoculated subcutaneously every forty-eight hours in ten unit doses.

Depending upon the part of the world where the exposure occurs and upon the type of biting animal, attack rates in man vary from 3 per cent to 50 per cent. A world-wide average of 15 per cent is most widely accepted as the rate of rabies deaths among untreated persons bitten by rabid animals. Although accurate figures are not available, there seem to be species differences in relative susceptibility to infection. Among domestic animals, cattle are observed to be one of the most susceptible species in the wide host range. Factors which influence the probability of infection are the presence and quantity of virus in the saliva of the biting animal, the severity of the bite, and the possible interposition of clothing. Thus, bites in the region of the head, neck, and face are the most dangerous, next the extremities (hands, feet, arms, legs), and least the trunk. Length of incubation period in the rabies victim is likewise related to factors of body site and of virus entrance; cases characterized by unusually short incubation periods most often occur following severe exposures, particularly in the region of the head. These factors are now believed to be governed by differences in relative richness of peripheral nerve supply in various parts of the body rather than by distance from the central nervous system.

Rabies is more infective to younger than older animals, which is probably also true in man. In the 15-year period 1946 to 1959, more than half the total human rabies deaths in the United States were in children under fifteen years of age. Of course, the great opportunity for severe exposures in children contributes heavily to this preponderance. It is difficult to assess the relative importance of possible increased, inherent susceptibility in the lower age groups.

WILDLIFE RABIES

In Terrestrial Animals

Wildlife rabies (sylvatic) and dog rabies (urban) are the two epidemiologic types of rabies that can be recognized throughout the world (Johnson, 1948). There are no antigenic differences between these types; they are classified in this manner on the basis of natural spread of the disease. In certain rural areas where rabies is enzootic, this epidemiologic differentiation may not always be so discrete. Factors which influence the presence of both types simultaneously in a given area are the amount or degree of contact between wild species and domestic dogs, and the relative population size and immunity status of both groups.

With the success of the control of dog rabies, attention has been centered on what seems to be an increase in the spread of the disease among various species of wildlife. Besides the very obvious effect of wild animal rabies in causing livestock losses, there are also public health aspects of the sylvatic rabies problem. Of primary significance are the reported, direct exposures of man to rabid wild animals. During the past several years, 20 per cent of the human rabies deaths in the United States have been caused by the bites of rabid wild animals, principally foxes and skunks. Observations

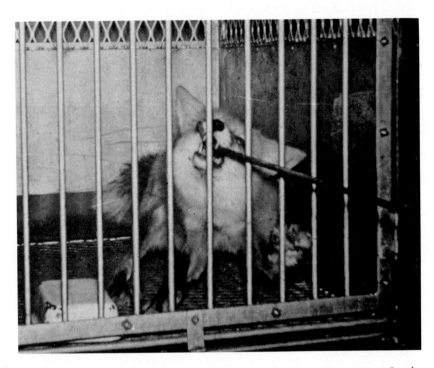

Fig. 71. Red fox exhibiting signs of rabies. (Photograph courtesy Stephen Richards, North Dakota Game and Fish Dept., Fargo, North Dakota.)

of rabies in these wild species indicate that very often the disease spills over into canine populations, where the hazard is greater because of man's closer association with dogs. There is general agreement that if rabies is to be eventually eradicated or brought down to a controllable minimum, the reservoir of the virus in the country's wild fauna must necessarily be included in scientifically devised control operations.

Presently in the United States, the principal wildlife vectors of the disease are the grey fox (genus Urocyon), the red fox (genus Vulpes), the small spotted skunk (genus Spilogale) and the large striped skunk (genus Mephitis). The fox rabies areas can be found along the Appalachian Range, southward from New York State to Georgia and northern Florida, and westward along the southern tier of states to western Texas. Contiguous with this is the fox rabies area which lies roughly between the Ohio River and the Great Lakes. Skunk rabies is active in an area which extends from Oklahoma and Missouri northward into the states of the upper Mississippi and Missouri River Valleys. There is also a sizable, enzootic skunk rabies area in the central valley of California. In 1958, there was evidence of an eastward spread of skunk rabies areas from the Great Plains states, to cause an overlapping of skunk and fox rabies in Illinois, Indiana, Ohio and Kentucky. In 1961, Texas became a third important focus of skunk rabies along with California and the north-central states with Iowa as the hub.

The current high incidence of fox rabies in the United States seems to have begun in 1940, and the great increase in skunk rabies in the upper Mississippi and Missouri Valleys seems to be only about seven or eight years old. To be sure, fox rabies was reported in Massachusetts about 1800, in Alabama in 1890; and skunk rabies in Kansas in 1871. Mari Sandoz, in her book *The Buffalo Hunters* (1954), gives a fascinating account of an outbreak of skunk rabies in 1871 in the Arkansas River Valley of Kansas and the Great Plains of eastern Nebraska and western Iowa. She tells of the skunks, which ordinarily were "harmless, even sociable creatures," becoming furious and "charging in, snapping at everything, their small teeth, sharp and deadly," attacking camps of buffalo hunters through the region. She describes many of the biting incidents involving campers. She writes, "There were sixteen fatal cases of hydrophobia in the region . . ." and it was stated that in one area all cases of bites from rabid skunks except one were fatal. She tells of panic among the hunters and traders, and of the disastrous effect the situation had on the buffalo hide industry. These were all sizable outbreaks, and there can be no doubt that there have been many other waves of the disease which probably were related to cycles of population density-contact in these species.

Even though coyote rabies ravaged the mountains and prairies of the Far West several decades ago, the current U.S. rabies picture has not incriminated the coyote to any appreciable extent. The only important focus of raccoon rabies in recent years has been reported from Florida.

Endemic rabies in arctic foxes has plagued the islands and mainland of Alaska, the Yukon, and the Northwest Territories of Canada. Fox and wolf rabies has swept southward through western and central Canada in the past few years, creating one of the largest rabies problems in the history of the country.

In the Spring of 1950, mongooses of Puerto Rico were incriminated as the principal vectors in an epizootic of rabies, with dogs and farm animals responsible for secondary transmission. This was the first major rabies outbreak in the western hemisphere attributed to the Indian mongoose.

At present Western Europe, especially Germany, is experiencing outbreaks of fox rabies. The important vector of Eastern Europe is still the wolf. Wolf rabies extends down the Caucasus to the Caspian Sea; in Iran, attacks by rabid wolves are still responsible for large losses in human lives.

The mongoose has not been reported as a serious vector of rabies in India, although it abounds in its native land and, as mentioned above, has been the principal transmitter of rabies in Puerto Rico. There, the jackal is the important wild vector. The jackal is also the principal sylvatic transmitter of the disease in the Eastern Mediterranean region and in Eastern and Central Africa. A wide variety of meerkats and mongooses keeps the disease going in the South African veld.

The Communicable Disease Center (CDC) at present has many research projects underway to study the natural behavior of rabies in wildlife. Preliminary results of these investigations have shown that there may be some evidence that subclinical immunizing infection occurs in wild animals in nature. Serum antiviral substances (neutralization of at least 32 LD_{50} of rabies virus by undiluted serum) has been found in twelve out of 262 (4.6%) fox bloods tested, eleven out of 196 (5.6%) raccoon sera, two out of 185 (1.8%) oppossum sera, five out of 27 (18.5%) bobcat sera, and seven out of 48 (14.5%) skunk sera. These animals came from areas with a recent history of fox rabies outbreaks; this is in contrast to completely negative antibody results by SN tests from nearly 300 animals taken from known rabies-free areas. There may be evidence of a relationship between demonstration of antibodies and time of the outbreak on the epizootic curve. In 670 individuals of all species tested, 1.6 per cent showed antibodies before an epizootic peak, whereas 5.2 per cent were serologically positive after an epizootic peak, and 5.1 per cent were serologically positive in enzootic areas.

Seventy-five percent of the submaxillary glands of naturally infected foxes contain rabies virus. In no instance have salivary glands been found infected without concurrent infection of the central nervous system, indicating that the fox is not capable of transmitting the disease as a symptomless carrier. Their transmitting potential, however, is a great one, as evidenced by the fact that experimentally infected foxes were shown to experience long periods of illness, and that daily testing showed saliva to contain rabies virus for long periods of time, in one individual for seventeen days. Other observations in experimentally infected foxes include those on incubation periods ranging from twelve to sixty-two days with an average of 26.5 days, periods of observable clinical illness from one to fifteen days with an average of 4.6 days, virus isolation from salivary glands of eighteen out of twenty-four foxes, from saliva swabs of fifteen out of twenty-four, and positive saliva swabs from seven out of twenty-four animals one to three days before classical, clinical signs were observed.

A rabies virus survey of over 1000 small wild rodents trapped in high enzootic and epizootic fox rabies in New York and Georgia revealed no evidence of infection, confirming previous reports that these species do not serve as reservoirs of the disease in the wild.

Using an isolant of rabies virus from a fox, it was found that foxes are greater than two logs more susceptible to intramuscular infection than skunks (Table 37). The same study demonstrated that when infection does occur in skunks the frequency of virus-positive salivas is greater and the amount of virus in saliva is greater than in

TABLE 37

CALCULATED DOSES OF AN ISOLANT OF STREET RABIES VIRUS NECESSARY TO KILL 50% OF VARIOUS SPECIES OF WILD ANIMALS INOCULATED PERIPHERALLY

	Foxes	*Skunks*	*Raccoons*	*Opossums*
Number of MLD_{50}	<5	500	1,000	>80,000

From: Sikes, R. K., and Tierkel, E. S. (1961).

infected foxes. Thus, when they do become infected, skunks are more efficient transmitters of the virus than are foxes (Sikes and Tierkel, 1960).

Helmboldt and Jungherr (1955) reported canine distemper in wild carnivores which exhibited clinical signs simulating rabies.

In Bats. The first scientific report of the transmission of rabies by bats was published in 1921 by Haupt and Rehaag who described their observation during an outbreak of a severe paralytic disease of cattle in Brazil in 1916. In Trinidad, eighty-nine persons died, between 1929 and 1935, of a disease characterized by an ascending paralysis. The early cases were diagnosed as bulbar poliomyelitis. At the same time, an epizootic of a fatal paralytic disease in cattle was occurring which was thought at first to be botulism. The work of Pawan and Hurst (Hurst and Pawan, 1931, 1932; Pawan, 1936a, b) is a well-documented, epidemiologic classic in the establishment of this outbreak of fatal paralytic disease in man and cattle as rabies caused by the bites of infected bats. The principal vector involved in the outbreaks was the vampire bat (Desmodus rotundus murinus), and this species remains as the most important vector of rabies in many parts of Latin America today. Vampire bats are found from northern Argentina and southern Brazil northward to about 100 miles south of the Rio Grande River in Mexico. The vampire bats of Trinidad came over from the northern coast of South America. They are not known to occur in the United States or in the eastern hemisphere. The vampire bat is hemophagous in nature, i.e., it depends for its existence on the ingestion of blood. With their highly adapted, sharp incisor teeth, they inflict small, crater-like wounds in the skin of their victim and lap the escaping blood with a long, well-developed tongue. They have been shown on occasions to transmit rabies as true, symptomless carriers.

Vampire bat rabies continues to be a great problem in most of the South American countries and Mexico. Malaga-Alba (1958) stated that vampire bat rabies is the most frequent cause of death in South American native cattle and estimated the losses during 1956 to be about one million head of livestock, constituting an economic loss of about eighty million dollars. The hazard of human attacks by vampire bats is present when persons sleep out of doors or in unscreened buildings in enzootic areas; the vampire bat will feed on man when livestock sources of blood meals are not readily available. A total of 117 human deaths have been reported from Trinidad, Mexico and British Guiana (Pawan, 1936b; Malag-Alba and Campillo Saenz, 1957; Nehaul, 1955). Programs for the destruction of vampire bats by dynamiting and gassing caves, bat-proofing buildings and tree hollows, have proved temporarily successful in some countries; these measures seem to have been most successful in Trinidad but almost impossible to carry out in some of the rugged mountain areas of the Sierra Madre mountain ranges in Mexico. The most effective method for controlling the disease in livestock in recent years has been vaccination of cattle with high egg passage (HEP) Flury-chicken embryo vaccine. In Mexico alone, over five million head of cattle have been vaccinated with the HEP Flury-strain vaccine in mass immunization programs; these programs have reduced paralytic cattle rabies to occasional sporadic cases in the enzootic areas (Malaga-Alba, 1958, Camargo, 1955).

In the vampire bat rabies areas of Latin America over the years investigators have found evidence of rabies in a variety of nonhemophagous bats; several species of frugivorous and insectivorous bats have been found infected during outbreaks of bat rabies. Bat rabies in the United States was unknown until June 1953 when the virus was isolated from a yellow bat (Dasypterus floridanus) which had bitten a child near Tampa, Florida. This episode aroused great interest, prompting surveys and surveillance activities through the country. Since the first reported case in Florida, about 500 cases have been diagnosed in bats from thirty-six States in widely diverse geographic areas of the United States (Figure 74A) and from one province in Canada (British Columbia), and from Yugoslavia and Turkey in the eastern hemisphere. Four species of tree-living or solitary bats and twenty species of colonial or cave-dwelling bats have been implicated thus far. All are of the insectivorous variety. The greatest number of isolations have been made from the Mexican free-tailed bat (*Tadarida brasiliensis mexicana*) in the southwestern United States. The largest number of isolations have been made in Texas, New Mexico, and Florida in extensive surveys. The remaining rabid bats were reported from smaller survey areas, and isolated cases diagnosed in public health laboratories and reported through the usual channels, reflecting an increasing awareness of the presence of bat rabies among disease-control authorities and the general public.

Episodes involving the biting of human beings have accounted for about 200 of the positively diagnosed bat rabies cases in the U.S. Thus far, there have been five human rabies deaths attributed to transmission from rabid insectivorous bats in the United States (Table 38). One occurred in Big Spring, Texas in 1951 and was investigated retrospectively and reported by Sulkin and Greve in 1954. The biting had occurred when a woman picked up a moribound bat along the roadside. In two human deaths attributed to bat transmitted rabies, evidence points to contracting the disease in a

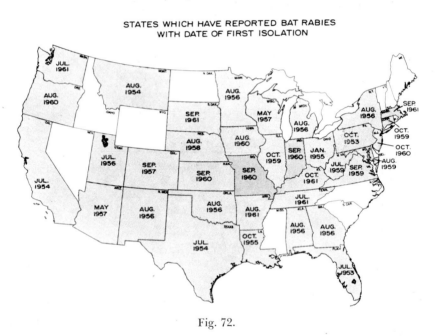

STATES WHICH HAVE REPORTED BAT RABIES
WITH DATE OF FIRST ISOLATION

Fig. 72.

Texas bat cave and in both of these cases no known history of a bite could be elicited. The earlier case (1956) was in a Texas state health department scientist who had been working in the cave on a bat rabies research project. The other case occurred in 1959 when a mining engineer spent some time in the cave on a prospecting assignment for a bat guano mining company. A case reported in 1959 from Wisconsin occurred after a man was bitten on the lobe of the ear; the biting bat was captured but discarded before laboratory tests could be made on the animal. The remaining case was the only one thus far which could be unquestionably

TABLE 38

U.S. Human Rabies Deaths Which Have Been Attributed to Exposure by Bats

Year	Locality	Age	Sex	Nature of Exposure	Length of Illness	Incubation Period	Treatment
1951	Big Spring, Texas	41	F	Bite, hands, forearm	8 days	16 days	None
1956	Austin, Texas	41	M	Unknown, worked with rabid bats	3 days	Unknown	None
1958	Butte County, California	53	F	2 bites on fingers	11 days	55 days	Serum, systemically, 14 doses vaccine 4 days after bite
1959	Los Angeles County, California	54	M	Unknown, probably bats in Texas caves	9 days	Unknown	None
1959	Richland County, Wisconsin	44	M	Bite on ear lobe	6 days	22 days	None

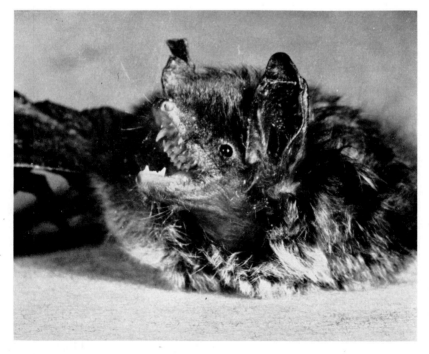

Fig. 73. Agitated signs of rabies exhibited by an infected eastern pipistrel bat.

attributed to the bite of a known rabid bat; this occurred in Butte County, California in 1958 (Lennette *et al.,* 1959, Humphrey *et al.,* 1960). In this case, a woman was bitten when she picked up a moribund silver-haired bat *(Lasionycteris noctivagans)* in her backyard. Rabies virus was isolated from the bat. Two months later, the woman became ill and died after symptoms strongly suggestive of rabies. Rabies virus was isolated from her brain at autopsy by the California State Health Department.

The epidemiologic significance of the bat rabies findings is now the subject of extensive investigations. A few observations from the early phases of these studies may be of interest here. It has been possible to infect experimentally several species of animals, including bats, with virus isolated from naturally infected bats by peripheral routes, but in most instances this has been accomplished with difficulty. (Stamm *et al.,* 1956; Enright *et al.,* 1955; Burns *et al.,* 1956, Kleckner, 1958). It is of interest that experimentally infected bats often exhibit furious signs of the disease. Attempts thus far to transmit the disease by inducing known rabid bats with infectious saliva to bite adult animals in the laboratory have failed (Burns *et al.,* 1958; Constantine, 1957). However, Bell in 1959 and Constantine in 1960 succeeded in transmitting rabies to suckling mice and hamsters through the bites of infected bats.

The problem of asymptomatic rabies is one of many in the epizootiologic puzzle of the disease in insectivorous bats. It is well established that their chiropteran cousins, the vampire bats in Latin America, are capable of transmitting the disease for long periods of time without showing signs of illness. Some have suggested that this symbiotic host-virus relationship may be present in the insectivorous bats as well. During studies by the Communicable Disease Center in caves of the southwestern United States, rabies virus was isolated from 0.5 per cent of a sample of 2,478 apparently normal bats tested in pools of three and four, and 14.6 per cent of 199 individually tested bats, which were collected in flight. Rabies virus was collected from the salivary gland but not from the central nervous system in five of the thirteen rabid bats in the first sample, and fourteen of the twenty-nine rabid bats in the second sample; these bats remained clinically normal until killed for testing. The data, thus far, though suggestive, are not sufficiently conclusive to prove asymptomatic carriers in U.S. insectivorous bats. On the basis of these observations, however, it is recommended that all bat bites be considered as potential rabies exposures.

The most recent CDC study has indicated evidence of airborne transmission of rabies to wild native carnivores held in a bat cave. A number of animals including dogs, cats, foxes, coyotes, ringtails and skunks were held in cages in Frio Cave, a large limestone bat cave near Uvalde, Texas, for about four weeks. Four types of cages were used, one being constructed with plastic mesh and glycerinated spun-glass pad "moats" in such a way that neither mammal nor arthropod could penetrate it. All of the ten coyotes and all of the twelve foxes distributed in all four of the cages became ill and died with clinical rabies which was confirmed by laboratory diagnostic and specific identification tests (Table 39).

TABLE 39

RABIES STATUS OF COYOTES AND FOXES IN FRIO CAVE IN FOUR TYPES OF CAGE
ENCLOSURES

Cage Group	Type of Animal	Rabies Deaths	Days of Exposure
I	coyotes	2/2	27
	gray foxes	2/2	
II	coyotes	2/2	27
	gray foxes	2/2	
	silver foxes	2/2	
III	coyotes	2/2	27
	gray foxes	2/2	
IV	A. coyotes	2/2	24
	gray foxes	2/2	
	B. coyotes	2/2	30
	gray foxes	2/2	

From: Constantine, D. G. (1962).

PREVENTION AND CONTROL

Local wound treatment

Once the clinical disease develops, there is no known treatment for rabies. Specific treatment of exposed persons is carried out by local treatment of the wounds as well as immunospecific, biologic therapy (Pasteur treatment). In persons bitten by rabid or suspected animals, the wound should be thoroughly irrigated as soon as possible with soap or detergent solution (Shaughnessy and Zichis, 1943,

1954). In deep, narrow, puncture-type wounds which cannot be cleansed efficiently with soap or detergent solutions, it may be necessary to use strong mineral acids such as nitric acid. Laboratory experiments have shown good results with topical applications of the wound with 2 per cent aqueous solutions of quaternary ammonium compounds such as Zephiran chloride. On the basis of epidemiologic observation suggesting a relationship between sutured bite wounds and the development of rabies, immediate suturing of these wounds is contraindicated. Experimental evidence in laboratory animals has shown that infiltration of hyperimmune rabies antiserum into the tissues around and beneath the bite wound, when this is feasible is effective in the preventive of rabies (Erzogovac, 1956; Perez-Gallardo *et al.*, 1957).

Immunization

In Man. A variety of human post-exposure rabies vaccines have been in use over the years, the most widely used of which was the Semple vaccine (1919), a phenolized fixed virus, and an ultra-violet, irradiated, fixed virus vaccine, each of which is given in fourteen divided subcutaneous doses, one dose being given daily. Some swelling and pain may occur about the point of injection. An adequate level of immunity develops about fourteen days after treatment is initiated. Both the Semple and ultraviolet, irradiated vaccines are suspensions of infected, central nervous system tissues containing inactivated or "dead" virus. A similar, inactivated, CNS virus vaccine is that of Hempt (1925) which is treated with ether and phenol, and is used in some European countries.

Following administration of a prescribed series of rabies vaccine prepared from nervous tissue there is an occasional occurrence of postvaccinal encephalitis, and neurologic and paralytic complications. These reactions are believed to be tissue-specific, isoallergic phenomena which apparently are not related to the rabies antigen present, but rather to some encephalitogenic component of the nervous tissue in the vaccine. They occur most frequently after the seventh inoculation and most often in persons who have had previous Pasteur treatment. Reports on the frequency of these complications vary as follows: one in 527 (Cook *et al.*, 1955), one in 600 (Pait and Pearson, 1949), one in 2025 (Applebaum *et al.*, 1953), one in 7200 (Sellers, 1948), one in 8500 (McKendrick, 1940). In the meantime, the promiscuous administration of antirabic inoculations should be discouraged by exercising sound judgment in weighing each dog bite case on its individual particular circumstances. The Fourth Report of the Expert Committee on Rabies, World Health Organization (1960) includes a detailed chart which should serve as a valuable guide in establishing indications for vaccine treatment of exposed persons.

Within the past several years a vaccine propagated in embryonated duck eggs has been developed to avoid the use of nerve tissue. This is a single-passage, fixed-virus vaccine grown in developing duck embryos which has been inactivated by addition of beta-propiolactone. This duck embryo vaccine has been shown to elicit good serum neutralizing antibody response and is now being marketed under license in the United States for human use (Peck *et al.*, 1955, 1956; Greenberg and Childress, 1960). Serum neutralization studies have shown that a single, 0.2 ml, intradermal dose of avian embryo vaccine has produced good antibody response in volunteers with a history of previous Pasteur treatment (Fox *et al.*, 1955, 1956, 1957; Koprowski, 1956; Tierkel, 1958, 1961; Sharpless *et al.*, 1957, Fox, 1958). Thus, there is indication that booster inoculations of this material may be shown to be adequate for post-exposure vaccination in persons previously treated, i.e., those in whom the hazard of postvaccinal complications would be greatest if a series of nervous tissue vaccines were used. This work suggests that prophylactic pre-exposure booster inoculations at certain specified intervals can be recommended for high-risk groups such as veterinarians, laboratory workers, dog wardens, predator control specialists, etc. Serum antibody studies now in progress in human volunteers indicate that a series of 3 deep subcutaneous inoculations of 1 ml of duck embryo vaccine, spaced one month apart, prepares the individuals to respond to a booster inoculation of the same dose and route, about six months after the primary series.

Over the years, one of the very real problems in the specific biologic therapy of exposed persons was the ineffectiveness of vaccine in severe bite cases, especially in those cases involving the region of the head, when the incubation period was too short to allow for the development of active, immuno-specific protection. This problem has now largely been alleviated by the production of hyperimmune rabies antiserum which can be administered to confer sufficient passive immunity during the critical early period before the vaccine can stimulate active protection. Convincing experimental evidence in challenge-tested laboratory animals, and in antibody studies in man has established its value when followed by the usual course of vaccine. These findings were collaborated by a limited field trial sponsored by the World Health Organization in Iran, where only one out of thirteen persons died of rabies after being severely bitten by a rabid wolf in the region of the head and treated with serum and a course of vaccine, whereas three out of five individuals bitten similarly by the same wolf and treated with a course of vaccine alone succumbed to rabies (Baltazard and Bahmanyar, 1955). One serum injection of 0.5ml/kg of body weight is given as soon as possible, preferably within seventy-two hours of the bite, followed immediately by a course of at least fourteen inoculations of vaccine. There is evidence that interference of active immunity may occur when more than one dose of antiserum or less than twelve doses of vaccine are administered (Habel, 1957). As an added precaution against the possibility of interference, the last report of the WHO Expert Committee on Rabies (1960) recommends that two additional inoculations of vaccine should be administered on the tenth and twentieth day respectively after completion of the usual vaccine series when this is preceded by hyperimmune serum. Since this is a horse serum product, precautions should be taken to avoid serious anaphylactic shock. A fore-warning can be obtained by skin-testing the patient for sensitivity. The less severe delayed reaction (serum sickness) has been reported in an estimated 50 per cent of persons treated with hyperimmune antiserum from eight to twelve days after serum administration. Antihistamines should be available in the event serum sickness occurs.

In Canines. A practical vaccine for dogs was not developed and used successfully in the field until the early 1920's, even though much of Pasteur's original work with vaccines was with the canine disease. This was the vaccine of the Japanese workers Umeno and Doi (1921), a phenolized, rabbit brain product. This success stimulated interest in dog vaccination in the United States, but the production of canine vaccines in the next two decades was sporadic, with no clear-cut picture of antigenic efficacy of the vaccines used. It was not until Habel (1940) developed a standard, mouse potency test for Semple-type vaccines that intrinsic improvement in vaccines occurred. The Semple-type vaccine used for dogs is a 20 per cent heat-inactivated and phenol-treated, fixed-virus, brain emulsion of equine, caprine, or ovine origin for inoculation in single doses of 5 ml. It is known variously as phenolized, nervous tissue or Semple vaccine. The first significant experimental contribution to our knowledge of the duration of immunity in dogs following rabies vaccination was made by Johnson (1945) of the Rockefeller Foundation.

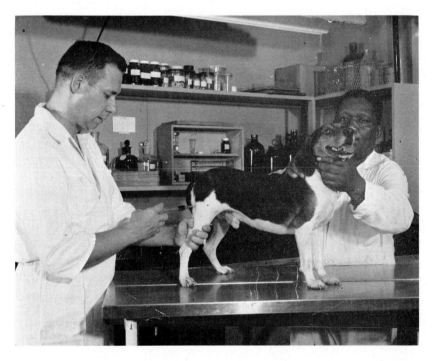

Fig. 74. Intramuscular administration of Flury chicken embryo rabies vaccine.

The result of this work indicated excellent protection in dogs for one year after a single dose of phenolized vaccine. It was on the basis of this work and subsequent field trials that the single-dose method of canine rabies vaccination was put into universal practice as an integral part of rabies control programs.

In recent years one of the most important advances in the field of rabies immunization has been the development of a modified, living-virus vaccine (Flury strain) produced in chicken embryos (Koprowski and Cox, 1948). The strain of virus in this vaccine was named after a young human rabies patient in Georgia from whom it was isolated at autopsy (Leach and Johnson, 1940). The isolated virus was passaged serially by Johnson through 136 one-day-old chicks by the intracerebral route, and was subsequently adapted to chicken embryos by the yolk sac route of inoculation by Koprowski and Cox (1948). It was observed that continuous serial passage of this strain through embryonated chicken eggs attenuated the virus and rendered it nonpathogenic for laboratory animals and dogs after forty to fifty egg passages, when inoculated peripherally. It was further seen that the virus became so modified in character that it thrived in the entire, developing chicken embryo, and could be isolated from all of the embryonic tissues. The fact that it could be inoculated safely by peripheral routes and that its pantropic character in the embryonated egg made the entire embryo a rich source of virus, led to tests of the immunizing power of the egg-adapted Flury strain. A preliminary study of Tierkel *et al.* (1949) and expanded trials by Koprowski and Black (1950, 1952) showed the strain to have a high level of immunizing capacity in dogs. Comparative duration of immunity experiments in dogs at the Communicable Disease Center, U.S. Public Health Service, have shown the Flury-strain, chicken-embryo vaccine to be significantly superior to the older types of inactivated-virus, nervous-tissue vaccines for periods of at least three and one-fourth years between vaccination and experimental exposure (Tierkel *et al.*, 1953) (Table 40).

Field experience with this vaccine has corroborated the results of the controlled tests (Kaeberle, 1958). The reports of the Expert Committee on Rabies of the World Health Organization, in 1954 and 1957, recognized that the chicken-embryo LEP vaccine (Flury strain) produces excellent immunity in dogs for at least three years following a single intramuscular injection (in the posterior thigh muscles), and recommended the use of this vaccine in mass-immunization programs. The vaccine contains modified, live virus cultivated at fortieth to fiftieth passage level and is now often referred to as LEP, Flury-strain vaccine to differentiate it from the Flury-strain vaccine produced from the 180th to 190th or high egg passage (HEP) vaccine for use primarily in cattle and man. The canine LEP vaccine is prepared as a 33 per cent whole-embryo emulsion for intramuscular inoculation of single doses of 3 ml. It is felt that

TABLE 40

COMPARATIVE RABIES MORTALITY RESULTS IN DOGS CHALLENGED WITH STREET VIRUS 39 MONTHS AFTER VACCINATION WITH A SINGLE DOSE OF ONE OF THREE DIFFERENT RABIES VACCINES*†

Vaccine	Nature of Vaccine Preparation	Dose and Route	Rabies Mortality Ratio	Per Cent Mortality
Chick embryo (Flury strain)	33% whole embryo emulsion; living modified virus	3 ml i. m.	0/30	0
Phenolized (Semple type)	20% brain tissue; equine origin; inactivated by heat and phenol	5 ml i. m.	8/34	23.6
Ultra-violet Irradiated	20% brain tissue; equine origin; inactivated by u-v irradiation	5 ml i. m.	7/30	23.3
Nonvaccinated Controls	—	—	31/36	86.1

*Challenge inoculation: 0.2 ml. of a 1:40 dilution of salivary gland street virus in each masseter muscle (total challenge dose 0.4 ml.).
†Tierkel, E. S., Kissling, R. E., Eidson, M. E., and Habel, K. (1953).

the use of the intramuscular route of inoculation is important since, by this method of injection, studies were carried out on the duration of immunity which established the high protective level of chicken-embryo vaccine. The work of Johnston *et al.* (1957) confirmed this point when it showed the intramuscular route to be superior to the subcutaneous route in eliciting immunogenic response to chicken-embryo vaccine.

Further studies have shown that pups can be vaccinated success-fully as early as three months of age, although the animals in these experiments were challenged after relatively short postvaccination periods (Kissling and Eidson, 1955; Kaeberle, 1958; Dean, 1956a) (Table 41). For this reason it is recommended that pups be vac-

TABLE 41

EFFECTIVENESS OF RABIES VACCINE IN PUPS AT VARIOUS AGE LEVELS*, †

Age at Vaccination in Weeks	Rabies Mortality Ratio	Per Cent Mortality
5–7	11/18	61.0
8–10	10/16	62.5
11–16	3/16	18.7
Controls	26/28	93.0

*Pups vaccinated intramuscularly with chicken embryo vaccine and challenged five months later in the masseter muscles.
†Kaeberle (1958).

cinated at three months and revaccinated at one year of age. The vaccination of puppies under three months of age with LEP Flury vaccine is not recommended; during the period before this age they should be kept indoors, in yard enclosures, or leashed. Thus, in areas which have successfully eliminated rabies, but are faced with the constant danger of its reintroduction, a prophylactic regimen for dogs can be visualized as being somewhat similar to smallpox vaccination in human populations; dogs are vaccinated with chicken-embryo vaccine at three months and one year of age, followed by booster vaccinations three to four years later. It should be emphasized, however, that this procedure by no means precludes the necessity of carrying out intensified, mass canine vaccination campaigns in areas of enzootic or epizootic rabies.

Very recently, Kissling (1958) has reported on the early experimental stages of a strain of rabies virus adapted to hamster kidney-tissue culture after approximately the fortieth serial passage. This strain has an infectivity titer high enough after inactivation to give protection and it has passed the Habel mouse potency test. It has not, as yet, been tested in dogs.

In Animals Other than Canines. Cats may be effectively vaccinated with phenolized, nervous-tissue vaccine. Because there have been a few reports of vaccine virus infection in cats following the use of LEP Flury vaccine, this product is presently not recommended for use in cats (WHO Expert Committee on Rabies, 4th Report, 1960). In a recent study carried out by the New York State Health Department, phenolized vaccine and both LEP and HEP Flury vaccine showed significant protection in adult cats; protection with the phenolized vaccine was greater than that induced by either LEP or HEP Flury chicken-embryo vaccines (Dean, 1956b; Kaeberle, 1958). In this study, challenge inoculation was done only seventy days after vaccination and there is no information available on the comparative duration of immunity from these vaccines in cats. The same studies also indicated that there is limited evidence suggesting that kittens may be protected by the three vaccines. Vaccination of kittens under six months of age is not recommended. Although rabies in cats occurs in enzootic areas, this species is not considered an important vector of the disease. There is no evidence that rabies persists among cats in areas where the disease in dogs and wildlife vectors has been successfully eliminated. For this reason, cats are rarely included in mass vaccination programs. However, when rabies occurs in cats it is clearly a public health menace, and cat owners are encouraged to have their animals vaccinated.

In cattle, phenolized vaccines have been used sporadically throughout the years. There is little or no information on the efficacy of this vaccine outside of informal field observations on individual cases and herds by practicing veterinarians. Outside of the vampire bat rabies areas of Latin America, experience in pre-exposure vaccination practices in cattle is meager. In one study (Gomez *et al.*, 1955), it was found that a single dose of 30 ml of 33 per cent of chloroform-inactivated, nervous-tissue vaccine protected cattle challenged one year after vaccination, whereas 15 ml of the same vaccine did not.

The success of Flury, living-virus, chicken-embryo vaccine in dogs led to trials in cattle. The early use of the LEP Flury vaccine in cattle seemed to show that it could be used effectively to protect against subsequent exposure to rabies (Schroeder *et al.*, 1952; Starr *et al.*, 1954; Gomez *et al.*, 1955). However, field use of the LEP vaccine showed it to be capable of causing inoculation infection with paralysis and sometimes death in cows. Because of these observations, the use of LEP Flury vaccine was discontinued in this highly susceptible species. This experience prompted the development of the high egg passage (HEP), Flury vaccine which proved innocuous for all species of animals tested. Indeed, it no longer could bring down young adult mice by intracerebral inoculation, and intracerebral titrations of this virus, now being produced from 180th to 190th serial, egg passage material, must be carried out in suckling mice. Laboratory controlled experiments and field trials with the HEP Flury vaccine in cattle indicated that intramuscular injection of a minimum dose of 3 ml of a 33 per cent suspension protects cattle against challenge inoculation (Starr *et al.*, 1954; Koprowski, *et al.*, 1955; Carneiro *et al.*, 1955). In its 1960 report, the WHO Expert Committee on Rabies recommended the use of HEP vaccine in cattle and suggested that a second dose of vaccine, administered thirty days after the first, may result in a booster effect and provide more complete protection. Pre-exposure vaccination of cattle is most widely practiced by official agencies in the heavily infected, vampire bat rabies areas of Latin America where it presently serves as the most effective measure of controlling bovine, paralytic rabies. Although individual herd owners have been having their valuable cattle vaccinated in highly enzootic sylvatic rabies areas of the United States, mass vaccination of cattle, as an official state-wide program, has not been adopted as an economically feasible policy (Dean, 1956c).

Besides cattle, other species of animals have been shown to be susceptible, occasionally, to vaccine virus infection by the LEP, Flury vaccine. Because it has been used with safety in dogs, veterinarians have administered this vaccine to skunks and foxes which had been tamed as household pets and have found that these wild species will occasionally succumb to LEP, Flury vaccine. Studies carried out in these vaccine-infected animals failed consistently to demonstrate infection of salivary glands or "reversion" of the modified virus to a natural or virulent state. In view of this experience, it is recommended that wild pet animals, such as skunks, be vaccinated with HEP, Flury vaccine or phenolized nervous-tissue vaccine. Data on controlled experiments concerning antigenic efficacy of rabies vaccine in species other than dogs, cats, and cattle are grossly insufficient at this time.

Postexposure Vaccination of Animals. Vaccination of dogs following exposure to a rabid animal, although practiced for many years, has little practical value since, in many cases, too much time will have elapsed between exposure and opportunity for vaccination. Data on the efficacy of experimental postexposure vaccination of dogs and other animals with phenolized nervous-tissue vaccine are practically nil except for a few older European studies, the results of which are inconclusive. Flury, chicken-embryo vaccine administered to two groups of dogs, three days and four days respectively after exposure, gave no significant protection (Koprowski and Black, 1954). On the other hand, significantly better results were obtained when hyperimmune antiserum was given, followed by three-dose courses of Flury vaccine. The need for immunization of dogs after being bitten is diminishing with the expanding mass vaccination programs and the increasing number of pre-exposure canine vaccinations reported throughout the country. The principal value of post-exposure vaccination now is its use as a single inoculation booster in previously vaccinated dogs bitten by rabid animals.

Post-exposure vaccination of other domestic animals is practiced sporadically, and dosage regimens, particularly in the larger farm animals, vary according to the experience of the veterinarian; they are at best used on an empirical basis because of the dearth of experimental data.

RABIES CONTROL METHODS
IN PUBLIC HEALTH PROGRAMS

The ultimate solution to the rabies problem is predicated on the control and eventual elimination of the disease from animal populations. This may be accomplished by the setting up of transmission barriers, e.g., by animal vaccination, elimination of stray dogs, and the reduction of excessive numbers of wildlife vectors. Extensive laboratory research and field projects have proved that these techniques may be applied successfully to eradicate the disease from a given area, if integrated into a carefully planned and well-executed program.

Local. Field demonstrations have proved that local programs work best on a county-wide basis, or on a multi-county unit basis, according to the extent of the health jurisdiction. Local control should include the following basic activities: (1) *Mass vaccination of dogs.* This should be carried out intensively on a schedule that aims at the vaccination of all owned dogs within the shortest possible time. In the face of a serious outbreak, at least seventy per cent of the entire dog population of the county should be vaccinated within a two to three week period. This is best carried out by enlisting all of the veterinarians of the region in an organized canine-vaccination campaign. Temporary dog-vaccination clinics can be operated during the campaign in strategically located points throughout the district or municipality chosen on the basis of population concentrations and geographic distribution of cases. Dramatic demonstrations of the effectiveness of mass immunization programs have been reported in several countries of the world, such as Malaya (Wells, 1954), Israel (Kaplan *et al.,* 1954), United States, and others. In the U.S.A., a number of mass immunization campaigns have been effective in eliminating rabies in large cities. Excellent examples of these were the campaign in Memphis in 1948 with 23,000 dogs (Tierkel *et al.,* 1950) and Houston in 1954, with 45,000 dogs (Tierkel, 1956) vaccinated within a single week. (2) *Elimination of all stray dogs.* Mass vaccination will not reach the stray or ownerless dog, a factor which remains a potential threat in the transmission of rabies. An efficiently conducted program requires the operation of a local pound or humane shelter where stray animals may be kept for a few days and, if unclaimed at the end of that period, destroyed humanely. Collection of strays should be carried out by teams of

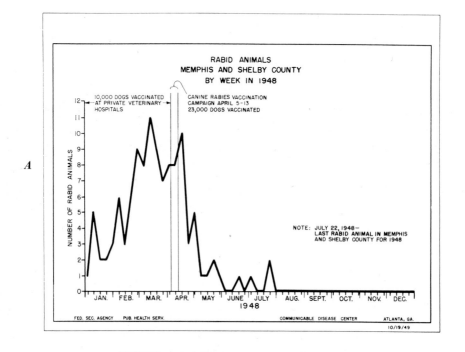

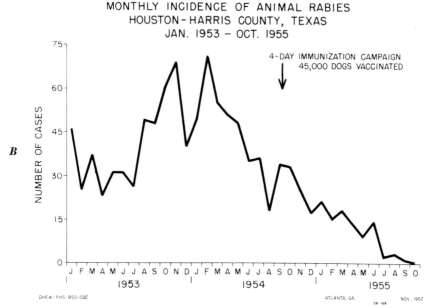

Fig. 75A-B.

dog wardens and assistants in properly equipped trucks. Personnel responsible for this activity should be qualified and trained, and their position should be established on the same general basis as for sanitarians and other members of the health department. Licensing or registration of all dogs is often a valuable adjunct. If properly enforced, it identifies the ownerless strays, helps to defray the expense of control activities, and may serve as the basis of a reasonably accurate dog census. (3) *Reduction of excess numbers of wildlife vectors.* Outbreaks of rabies in wild animals occur generally when the population of the species becomes particularly dense in an area. Organized trapping and poisoning programs are the most effective means of reducing this overpopulation to a safe level in areas menaced by wildlife rabies. The public health veterinarian can assist the local health department in this activity by working closely with the federal and state wildlife agencies and utilizing predator-control specialists who can train locally hired trappers and hold practical short course demonstrations in trapping for farm groups.

Other important measures are restraint of dogs while the control campaign is under way, and pursuit of a continual and energetic publicity campaign. Essential to the success of the program is good organization under health department and veterinary medical auspices, with the fullest use of all technical resources in the community.

In the event of a human rabies fatality, complete epidemiologic investigation should be carried out for information which should include: age, sex, date of exposure, location, severity, and nature of exposure on body, where the episode occurred, date of onset, date of death, type of animal including species, breed, age, vaccination status including type of vaccine, whether diagnosis was established by clinical or laboratory methods or both, disposition of the animal, names of other exposed persons, whether the victim received local wound treatment, and vaccine history of treatment (type, including manufacturer and lot number).

(4) *Management of known exposed animals.* Whenever new cases of rabies appear in the community, it is important that information be secured regarding the exposure of other animals in an effort to check the spread of the disease. All dogs and cats bitten by a known rabid animal should be: (1) destroyed immediately; (2) if the owner is unwilling to destroy the exposed animal, it should be placed in

strict isolation in a kennel for six months; (3) if the animal has been vaccinated previously within one year with nervous tissue vaccine or three years with chicken-embryo vaccine, revaccinate and restrain (leashing, confinement) for thirty days.

State. Coordination of control activities is the keynote of a successful, state-wide rabies-control program. Experience has shown that this is best effected by delegating the administration of such a program to a qualified, public health trained veterinarian at the state or provincial level. The development of a state-wide program under the state public health veterinarian can insure effective uniformity of control practice among the local health jurisdictions. At the present time, there are thirty-three such state programs in the country. In his capacity to promote the state-wide program, the public health veterinarian stimulates the interest of private practicing veterinarians of the state and obtains their participation in local control programs. He also enlists the support of livestock organizations, animal protection societies, kennel and sportsmen's clubs. He acts in a liaison capacity between the public health, wildlife, and livestock disease control agencies of this state. He arranges for regular exchange of information on control with neighboring states and keeps abreast of the latest technical and administrative control procedures. By organizing a state-wide reporting system and working closely with the state diagnostic laboratories, he keeps apprised of the geographic movement of infection throughout the state and is in a position to alert counties of the presence of rabies in neighboring areas.

The health department veterinarian is responsible for collecting and evaluating epidemiologic data on human exposures and on infection in animals and man. In his role as coordinator, he improves methods for shipment of specimens to diagnostic laboratories, surveys facilities for the collection and impoundment of stray dogs, and prepares and distributes educational material throughout the state. By frequent visits and consultation, he assists local health units in the organization of sound programs, based on the latest technical information on effective control procedures.

National. Meyer (1954) has stated that no general measure has proved as effective as quarantine for preventing the establishment of the disease in rabies-free countries. Australia, New Zealand, the Hawaiian Islands and Great Britain have been successful in insuring their rabies-free status by imposing strict quarantine regulations on all dogs and cats entering the area. In the United Kingdom, where there is a six-month quarantine regulation rabies has occurred in twenty-two imported dogs while in quarantine since the regulations were put into effect in 1919. From time to time, pressures are brought on authorities in these countries to relax the regulations for the convenience of pet owners. In each case, thus far, the rabies control officials, after thorough investigation and evaluation of these procedures, have elected to continue rigid enforcement of quarantine. It is felt that lowering of safeguards would invite the added danger of introducing the disease into the wild fauna of the area. One of the most dramatic illustrations of this danger is the sad experience of Puerto Rico, where the disease became firmly established in the mongoose population of the island in 1950 (Tierkel *et al.*, 1952). Mongoose rabies continues to be a major and costly public health problem in Puerto Rico, which previously had been one of the world's rabies-free areas. The last report of the WHO Expert Committee on Rabies (1960) recommends that countries free of rabies prohibit the importation of dogs and cats or subject them to a prolonged period of quarantine, preferably 6 months at the port of entry.

ITEMS OF NOTE

1) Rabies is a disease to which all warm-blooded animals are susceptible.

2) Elimination of rabies in dogs usually serves to eradicate the infection in urban communities. In recent years, the number of cases in wild carnivorous species, such as skunks and foxes, has exceeded those in dogs. Bat rabies has become increasingly important.

3) The virus of rabies is an ultramicroscopic filtrable virus.

4) After symptoms of rabies appear, there is no known cure.

5) Not more than one person in six bitten by rabid animals develop the disease, even though no antirabic treatment is taken.

6) Bites on the exposed surfaces, as the face and hands, are most dangerous.

7) Rabies is an infection usually requiring a broken skin for entrance of the virus.

8) Ingestion of the virus is not dangerous unless lesions are present in the mouth or throat. The gastric juice of the stomach quickly destroys the virus.

9) Air-borne transmission of rabies to foxes and coyotes has been observed in a bat cave in Texas.

10) Rabies is an all the year round disease, occurring during every month. In temperate zones it is most prevalent during late winter and early spring.

11) Antirabic post-exposure vaccination is highly effective, in the vast percentage of cases, in preventing the disease in man when administered promptly. It should not be administered to persons who do not need it.

12) A reduced regimen of avian embryo rabies vaccine followed by a booster can serve as good pre-exposure prophylaxis in individuals in high risk occupations such as laboratory workers, veterinarians, rabies control personnel and wild predator control specialists.

13) The fluorescent antibody test has been developed as a practical, rapid, highly specific procedure in the laboratory diagnosis of rabies.

14) Living attenuated chicken embryo vaccines (Flury strain) for dogs have been shown to be superior in duration of immunity to the older type inactivated, nervous tissue vaccines.

15) The successful control of rabies in a community requires the vaccination of all owned dogs, elimination of all strays and reduction of wild vector animals such as foxes and skunks.

REFERENCES

APPELBAUM, E., GREENBERG, M., AND NELSON, J.: (1953) Neurological complications following antirabies vaccination. *J. A. M. A.,* *151:*188-191.

BALTAZARD, M., AND BAHMANYAR, M.: (1955) Essai pratique au serum antirabique chez les mordus par loups enrages. *Bull. World Health Organ.,* *13:*747-772.

BELL, J. F., BURGDORFER, W., AND MOORE, G. J.: (1957) The behavior of rabies virus in ticks. *J. Infect. Dis.,* *100:*278-283.

BELL, J. FREDERICK: (1959) Transmission of rabies to laboratory animals by bite of a naturally infected bat. *Science,* *129:*1490-1491.

BURNS, K. F., FARINACCI, C. F., MURNANE, T. G., AND SHELTON, D. F.: (1956) Insectivorous bats naturally infected with rabies in southwestern United States. *Am. J. Pub. Health,* *46:*1089-1097.

BURNS, K. F., SHELTON, D. F., AND GROGAN, E. W.: (1958) Bat rabies: Experimental host transmission studies. *Ann. New York Acad. Sc.,* *70:*452-466.

CAMARGO, F.: (1955) The derriengue problem in Mexico. *Proc. 59th Ann. Meeting U. S. Livestock Sanitary Assoc.,* pp. 313-318.

CARNEIRO, V., BLACK, J., AND KOPROWSKI, H.: (1955) Rabies in cattle, V. Immunization of cattle in Brazil against exposure to street virus of vampire bat origin. *J. Am. Vet. M. A.,* *127:*366-369.

CARSKI, T. R.: (1960) in manual by Cherry, W. B., Goldman, M. and Carski, T. R. Fluorescent antibody techniques, Communicable Disease Center Publication, *1*:64-67.

CONSTANTINE, D. G.: (1957) Bat rabies investigations. Unpublished Communicable Disease Center Report.

CONSTANTINE, D. G.: (1958) An automatic bat-collecting device. *J. Wildlife Management, 22*:17-22.

CONSTANTINE, D. G.: (1960) Bat rabies investigations. Unpublished Communicable Disease Center Report.

CONSTANTINE, D. G.: (1962) Rabies transmission by non-bite route. *Public Health Reports, 77*:287-289.

COOK, E. B. M., STEARNS, C., FIELD, J., AND IRONS, J. V.: (1955) Report on the use of phenolized vaccine in Texas from 1949 through 1953. *Texas Rep. Biol. & Med., 13*:234-250.

DAMON, S. R., AND SELLERS, T. F.: (1941) A note on the probability of error in the diagnosis of rabies by microscopic search for Negri bodies. *J. Lab. & Clin. Med., 27*:71-74.

DAWSON, J. R., JR.: (1941) A study of chick embryo adapted virus. *Am. J. Pathol., 17*:177-187.

DEAN, D. J.: (1956a) Vaccine recommendations for puppies. Working Document WHO/Rabies/57 September 14, 1956.

DEAN, D. J.: (1956b) Immunization of cats. Working Document WHO/Rabies/58, September 14, 1956.

DEAN, D. J.: (1956c) The epidemiology of bovine rabies in New York State. Working Document WHO/Rabies/56.

ENRIGHT, J. B., SADLER, W. W. MOULTON, J. E., AND CONSTANTINE, D. G.: (1955) Isolation of rabies virus from insectivorous bat *(Tadarida mexicana)* in California. *Proc. Soc. Exper. Biol. & Med., 89*:94-96.

ERZOGOVAC, D. T.: (1956) Ergebnisse experimenteller Arbeiten auf dem Gebiet der Tollwutprophylaxe. *Wien. tieraztl. Monataschr., 43*:288-306.

FERNANDES, M. V. AND POMERAT, C. M. (1961) Cytopathogenic effects of rabies virus in nervous tissue *in vitro. Zeitschr. f. Zellferschung, 53*:431-437.

FOX, J. P.: (1958) Prophylaxis against rabies in humans. *Ann. New York Acad. Sc., 70*:480-494.

FOX, J. P., CONWELL, D. P., AND GERHARDT, P.: (1955) Immunization of man with living avianized rabies virus (Flury strain). *Calif. Vet., 8*:20-24.

FOX, J. P., CONWELL, D. P., AND GERHARDT, P.: (1956) Antirabies vaccination of man with HEP Flury virus. *Bull. Tulane Univ. Med. Fac., 16*:108.

FOX, J. P., KOPROWSKI, H., CONWELL, D. P., BLACK, JR., AND GELFAND, H. M.: (1957) Study of antirabies immunization of man. Observations with HEP Flury and other vaccines, with and without hyperimmune serum in primary and recall immunization. *Bull. World Health Organ., 17*:869-904.

GOLDWASSER, R. A., AND KISSLING, R. E.: (1958) Fluorescent antibody staining of street and fixed rabies virus antigens. *Proc. Soc. Exper. Biol. & Med., 98*:219-223.

GOLDWASSER, R. A., KISSLING, R. E., CARSKI, T. R., AND HOSTY, T. S.: (1959) Fluorescent antibody staining of rabies virus antigens in the salivary glands of rabid animals. *Bull. World Health Organ., 20*:579-588.

GOMEZ, C., BLACK, J., AND KOPROWSKI, H.: (1955) Rabies in cattle. III. Comparative studies on vaccination of cattle in Colombia with Flury virus and chloroform inactivated vaccine. *J. Am. Vet. M. A., 127*:360-363.

GREENBERG, M. AND CHILDRESS, J.: (1960) Vaccination against rabies with duck embryo and Semple vaccines, *J.A.M.A.*, *173*:333-337.

HABEL, K.: (1940) Evaluation of a mouse test for the standardization of the immunizing power of antirabies vaccines. *Public Health Rep.* (U.S.), *55*:1473-1487.

HABEL, K.: (1957) Rabies prophylaxis in man. *Public Health Rep.* (U.S.), *72*:667-673.

HAUPT, H., AND REHAAG, H.: (1921) Durch Fledermause verbreitete seuchenhafte Tollwut unter Viehbestanden in Santa Catharina (Sud-Brasilien). Z. Infektions-krankh. parasit. *Krankh. u. Hyg. Haustiere*, *22*:104-127.

HELMBOLDT, C. F., AND JUNGHERR, E. L.: (1955) Distemper complex in wild carnivores simulating rabies. *Am. J. Vet. Res.*, *16*:463-469.

HEMPT, A.: (1925) *Ann. inst. Pasteur, 39*:632 from VAN ROOYEN, C. E., AND RHODES, A. J.: (1948) *Virus Diseases of Man*, pp. 792-906. Thomas Nelson, New York.

HOTTLE, G. A., MORGAN, C., PEERS, J. H., AND WYCKOFF, R. W. G.: (1951) The electron microscopy of rabies inclusion (Negri) bodies. *Proc. Soc. Exper. Biol. & Med.*, *77*:721-723.

HUMPHREY, G. L., KEMP, G. E. AND WOOD, E. G.: (1960) A fatal case of rabies in a woman bitten by an insectivorous bat, *Public Health Rep.* (U.S.), *75*:317-326.

HURST, E. W., AND PAWAN, J. L.: (1931) An outbreak of rabies in Trinidad without history of bites and with the symptoms of acute ascending myelitis. *Lancet, 221*:622-628.

HURST, E. W., AND PAWAN, J. L.: (1932) A further account of the Trinidad outbreak of acute rabic myelitis: Histology of the experimental disease. *J. Path. & Bact.*, *35*:301-321.

JOHNSON, H. N.: (1942) Significance of the Negri body in the diagnosis and epidemiology of rabies. *Illinois M. J.*, *81*:382-388.

JOHNSON, H. N.: (1945) Experimental and field studies of canine rabies vaccination. *Proc. 49th Ann. Meeting U. S. Livestock Sanitary Assoc.*, pp. 99-107.

JOHNSON, H. N.: (1948) Methods of rabies control. *Proc. 4th Intern. Congr. Trop. Med.*, Washington, *1*:587-594.

JOHNSTON, R. V., NEWBERNE, J. W., YORK, C. J., BURCH, G. R., AND BRUECKNER, A. H.: (1957) Studies with Flury rabies vaccine in pups. *J. Am. Vet. M. A.*, *130*:61-63.

KAEBERLE, M. L.: (1958) Newer tools for the prevention of rabies in domestic animals. *Ann. New York Acad. Sc.*, *70*:467-477.

KAPLAN, M. M., GOOR, Y., AND TIERKEL, E. S.: (1954) A field demonstration of rabies control using chicken-embryo vaccine in dogs. *Bull. World Health Organ.*, *10*:743-752.

KAPLAN, M. M., WECKER, E., FORSEK, Z., AND KOPROWSKI, H.: (1960) An indicator plaque-forming system for demonstration of interference by non-cytocidal strains of rabies virus. *Nature, 186*:821-822.

KISSLING, R. E.: (1957) Failure to isolate rabies virus from the blood of experimentally infected dogs. Unpublished Communicable Disease Center Report.

KISSLING, R. E.: (1958) Growth of rabies virus in non-nervous tissue culture. *Proc. Soc. Exper. Biol. & Med.*, *98*:223-225.

KISSLING, R. E. AND EIDSON, M.: (1955) Vaccination of puppies 2-4 months of age. Unpublished Communicable Disease Center Report.

KLECKNER, M.: (1958) Studies in wildlife rabies. Unpublished Communicable Disease Center Report.

KLIGLER, I. J., AND BERNKOPF, H.: (1938) Cultivation of rabies virus in the allantois of the developing chick embryo. *Proc. Soc. Exper. Biol. & Med.*, *39*:212-214.

KOPROWSKI, H.: (1949) Experimental studies on rabies virus. *Canad. J. Pub. Health*, *40*:60-67.

KOPROWSKI, H.: (1956) Inoculation of normal human subjects with HEP Flury vaccine. Working Document WHO/Rabies/67.

KOPROWSKI, H., AND BLACK, J.: (1950) Studies on chick-embryo-adapted rabies virus. II. Pathogenicity for dogs and use of egg-adapted strains for vaccination purposes. *J. Immunol., 64:*185-196.

KOPROWSKI, H., AND BLACK, J.: (1952) Studies on chick embryo adapted rabies virus. III. Duration of immunity in vaccinated dogs. *Proc. Soc. Exper. Biol. & Med., 80:*410-415.

KOPROWSKI, H., AND BLACK, J.: (1954) Studies on chick embryo-adapted rabies virus. V. Protection of animals with antiserum and living attenuated virus after exposure to street strain of rabies virus. *J. Immunol. 72:*85-93.

KOPROWSKI, H., AND COX, H. R.: (1948) Studies on chick-embryo-adapted virus. I. Cultural characteristics and pathogenecity. *J. Immunol., 60:*533-554.

KOPROWSKI, H., BLACK, J., AND JOHNSON, W. P.: (1955) Rabies in cattle. IV. Vaccination of cattle with high egg-passage chicken embryo-adapted rabies virus. *J. Am. Vet. M. A., 127:*363-366.

LEACH, C. N.: (1938) Comparative methods of diagnosis of rabies in animals. *Am. J. Pub. Health, 28:*162-166.

LEACH, C. N., AND JOHNSON, H. N.: (1940) Human rabies with special reference to virus distribution and titer. *Am. J. Trop. Med., 20:*335-340.

LENNETTE, E. H., LOWE, O. A., NAKAMURA, K. AND KELLOG, R. H.: (1960) A fatal human case of rabies following the bite of a rabid bat (Lasionycteris noctivagans), *J. Lab. & Clin. Med., 55:*89-93.

LEPINE, P., AND CROISSANT, O.: (1951) Microscopic electronique des corps de Negri dans la rage des rues. *Ann. Inst. Pasteur, 81:*1-8.

LILLIE, R. D.: (1948) *Histopathologic Technic*, p. 225. Lippincott, Philadelphia, Pennsylvania.

McKENDRICK, A. G.: (1940) A ninth analytical review of reports from Pasteur Institute on the results of anti-rabies treatment. *League Nations Bull. Health Organ., 9:*31-78.

MAGENDIE, F., AND BRESCHET, G.: (1821) *J. physiol. exptl., 1:*42 from STIMSON, A. M.: (1910) Facts and problems of rabies Hyg. Lab. Bull. U. S. Public Health Serv., No. 65, 1-90.

MALAGA-ALBA, A.: (1958) Tropical bat rabies as a public health and veterinary problem. Unpublished report. Pan American Sanitary Bureau.

MALAGA-ALBA, A., AND CAMPILLO SAENZ, C.: (1957) Rabia humana transmitida por murcielagos, confirmacion del primer casos en Mexico. *Bol. Ofic. san. pan-am., 42:*567-570.

McQUEEN, J. L., LEWIS, A. L. AND SCHNEIDER, N. J.: (1960) Rabies diagnosis by fluorescent antibody. *Am. J. Pub. Health, 50:*1743-1752.

MEYER, K. F.: (1954) Can man be protected against rabies? *Bull. World Health Organ., 10:*845-866.

NEGRI, A.: (1903) Beitrag zum Studium der Actiologie der Tollwuth. *Z. Hyg. Infektionskrankh., 43:*507-528.

NEHAUL, B. B. G.: (1955) Rabies transmitted by bats in British Guiana. *Am. J. Trop. M. Hyg., 4:*550-553.

PAIT, C. F., AND PEARSON, H. E.: (1949) Rabies vaccine encephalomyelitis in relation to the incidence of animal rabies in Los Angeles. *Am. J. Pub. Health, 39:*875-877.

PASTEUR, L., with collaboration of C. CHAMBERLAND, E. ROUX, AND L. THUILLER: (1882) Nouveaux faits pour servir a la connaisance de la rage. *Compt. rend., 95:*1187-1192.

PAWAN, J. L.: (1936a) The transmission of paralytic rabies in Trinidad by vampire bats (Desmodus rotundus murinus, Wagner, 1840). *Ann. Trop. Med. Parasitol., 30:*101-130.

PAWAN, J. L.: (1936b) Rabies in the vampire bat of Trinidad with special reference to the clinical course and the latency of infection. *Ann. Trop. Med. Parasitol., 30:*401-422.

PECK, F. B., JR., POWELL, H. M., AND CULBERTSON, C. G.: (1955) A new antirabies vaccine for human use. Clinical and laboratory results using rabies vaccine made from embryonated duck eggs. *J. Lab. & Clin. Med., 45:*679-683.

PECK, F. B., JR., POWELL, H. M., AND CULBERTSON, C. G.: (1956) Duck embryo rabies vaccine. Study of fixed virus vaccine grown in embryonated duck eggs and killed with beta-propiolactone (BPL). *J. A. M. A., 162:*1373-1376.

PEREZ-GALLARDO, F., ZARZUELO, E., AND KAPLAN, M. M.: (1957) Local treatment of wounds to prevent rabies. *Bull. World Health Organ., 17:*963-978.

POWELL, H. M., AND CULBERTSON, C. G.: (1950) Cultivation of fixed rabies virus in embryonated duck eggs. *Public Health Rep.* (U. S.), *65:*400-401.

REED, L. J., AND MUENCH, H.: (1938) A simple method of estimating fifty percent endpoints. *Am. J. Hyg., 27:*493-497.

SANDOZ, M.: (1954) *The Buffalo Hunters.* Hastings House, New York.

SCHLEIFSTEIN, J.: (1937) A rapid method for demonstrating Negri bodies in tissue sections. *Am. J. Pub. Health, 27:*1283-1285.

SCHROEDER, C. R., BLACK, J., BURKHART, R. L., and KOPROWSKI, H.: (1952) Rabies in cattle. I. Prevention of vampire bat paralytic rabies derriengue, by vaccination with chick-embryo-adapted rabies virus. *Vet. Med., 47:*502-506.

SELLERS, T. F.: (1954a) Rabies. In *Principles of Internal Medicine.* (T. R. Harrison, ed.), 2nd ed., pp. 1106-1109. McGraw-Hill, New York.

SELLERS, T. F.: (1954b) World Health Organization Monograph Ser. No. *23:*32-35.

SELLERS, T. F. (1948) Rabies, the physician's dilemma. *Am. J. Trop. Med., 28:*453-456.

SEMPLE, D.: (1919) On the nature of rabies and antirabies treatment. *Brit. M. J., II:*333-336.

SHARPLESS, G. R., BLACK, J., COX, H. R. and RUEGSEGGER, J. M.: (1957) Preliminary observations in antirabies immunization of man with different types of high-egg-passage Flury virus. *Bull. World Health Organ., 17:*905-910.

SHAUGHNESSY, H. J., and ZICHIS, J.: (1943) Prevention of experimental rabies. Treatment of wounds contaminated by rabies virus with fuming nitric acid, soap solution, sulfanilamide or tincture of iodine. *J.A.M.A., 123:*528-533.

SHAUGHNESSY, H. J., and ZICHIS, J.: (1954) Treatment of wounds inflicted by rabid animals. *Bull. World Health Organ., 10:*805-813.

SOAVE, O. A., JOHNSON, H. N. and NAKAMURA, K.: (1961) Reactivation of rabies virus infection with adenocorticotropic hormones. *Science, 133:*1360-1361.

STAMM, D. D., KISSLING, R. E., and EIDSON, M. E.: (1956) Experimental rabies infection in insectivorous bats. *J. Infect. Dis., 98:*10-14.

STARR, L. E., SELLERS, T. F., and SUNKES, E. J.: (1952) Apparent recovery of a dog from rabies. *J. Am. Vet. M. A., 121:*296.

STARR, L. E., CLOWER, T. B., BROMLEY, C. L., and ROUTH, C. F.: (1954) Antirabic immunization of cattle in Georgia using living virus vaccine of chick embryo origin. *Vet. Med., 49:*366-371.

STOVALL, W. D., and BLACK, C. E.: (1940) The influence of pH on the eosin methylene blue method for demonstrating Negri bodies. *Am. J. Clin. Pathol., 10:*1-8.

Sulkin, S. E., and Greve, M. J.: (1954) Human rabies caused by a bat bite. *Texas State M. J.,* 50:620.

Tierkel, E. S.: (1956) Effects of an intensified canine rabies vaccination campaign in Houston, Texas. Working Document WHO/Rabies/ 96 Nov. 26, 1956.

Tierkel, E. S.: (1958) Antibody response of human volunteers to HEP rabies vaccine. Unpublished Communicable Disease Center Report.

Tierkel, E. S., and Neff, H. D.: (1957) Rabies: Methods in Laboratory Diagnosis, p. 23. *Public Health Service Publication No. 568.* U. S. Government Printing Office.

Tierkel, E. S., Koprowski, H., Black, J., and Gorrie, R. H.: (1949) Preliminary observations in the comparative prophylactic vaccination of dogs against rabies with living virus vaccines and phenolized vaccine. *Am. J. Vet. Res.* 10:361-367.

Tierkel, E. S., Graves, L. M., Tuggle, H. G., and Wadley, S. L.: (1950) Effective control of an outbreak of rabies in Memphis and Shelby County, Tennessee, *Am. J. Pub. Health,* 40:1084-1088.

Tierkel, E. S., Arbona, G., Rivera, A., and de Juan, A.: (1952) Mongoose rabies in Puerto Rico. *Public Health Repts.* (U.S.) 67:274-278.

Tierkel, E. S., Kissling, R. E., Eidson, M. E., and Habel, K.: (1953) A brief survey and progress report of controlled comparative experiments in canine rabies immunization. *Proc. 90th Ann. Meeting Am. Vet. M. A.,* Toronto, Canada, pp. 443-445.

Tierkel, E. S.: (1961) Pre-exposure immunoprophylactic protection of laboratory personnel against rabies. *Proc. 65th Ann. Meeting, U.S. Livestock San. A.* 269-272.

Umeno, S., and Doi, Y.: (1921) A study in the antirabic inoculation of dogs. *Kitasato Arch. Exper. Med.,* 4:89-108.

Webster, L. T., and Dawson, J. R.: (1935) Early diagnosis of rabies by mouse inoculation. Measurement of humoral immunity to rabies by mouse protection test. *Proc. Soc. Exper. Biol. & Med.* 32:570-573.

Wells, C. W.: (1954) The control of rabies in Malaya through compulsory mass vaccination of dogs. *Bull. World Health Organ.,* 10:731-742.

Wilsnack, R. E.: (1960) Guest Editorial, The fluorescent antibody diagnosis of rabies. *J. A. Vet. M. A.,* 137:319-320.

Wolman, M., and Behar, A.: (1952) A cytochemical study of the nature of Negri bodies. *J. Infect. Dis.,* 91:69-71.

World Health Organization: (1954) Expert Committee on Rabies, Second Report. *World Health Organ. Tech. Rep. Ser. No. 82.*

World Health Organization: (1957) Expert Committee on Rabies. Third Report. *World Health Organ., Tech. Rep. Ser. No. 121.*

World Health Organization: (1960) Expert Committee on Rabies, Fourth Report. *World Health Organ. Tech. Rept. Series No. 201.*

World Health Organization: (1960) World Survey of Rabies, Mimeographed Report, Rabies/Inf./1.

Zinke, G. G.: (1804) Neue Ansichten der Hundswuth, ihrer Ursachen und Folgen, nebst einer sichern Behandlungsart der von tollen Tieren gebissenen Menschen. *Fur Arzte und Nichtarzte bestimmt.,* C. E. Gabler, Jehna, 16:212.

Chapter 10

PSITTACOSIS (ORNITHOSIS)

Howard J. Shaughnessy, Ph.D.

PSITTACOSIS is a natural disease of birds from which it is transmitted to man. The word, psittacosis, first suggested by Morange in 1895, was derived from the Greek word for parrot (psittacus) and referred to the virus disease contracted from psittacine birds. Since it is now known that not only fifty odd species within the parrot family but also many other non-psittacine birds may act as hosts, the name psittacosis should perhaps be dropped in favor of the broader designation, ornithosis. The latter term, however, has also been used in the narrower sense in reference only to the disease manifested in non-psittacine birds infected with psittacosis virus.

During the past few years the existence of a large group of viruses related to the virus of psittacosis has been demonstrated largely by immunologic reactions. These viruses are widely distributed and some cause human infections. Others isolated from laboratory animals inoculated with material from sick persons, are probably latent viruses carried by the former. Included in the group, usually designated as the psittacosis-lymphogranuloma group of viruses, are the avian viruses of psittacosis and ornithosis; the animal viruses of meningo-pneumonitis, mouse pneumonitis, enzoötic abortion of sheep, calf enteritis virus, and cat-scratch fever; and those certainly or probably of human origin such as the viruses of lymphogranuloma venereum, inclusion conjunctivitis, trachoma and human pneumonitis (SF, Illinois, and Louisiana types). There is increasing evidence that the mammalian pneumonitis viruses are transmitted from animal to animal or man to man.

HISTORY

Psittacosis was probably first described by Ritter in 1879 as "pneumotyphus," a disease occurring among the members of a household

who had received a shipment of sick exotic birds. Following an outbreak of highly fatal cases involving forty-nine persons in Paris in
1892 and another epidemic in 1893, also in Paris, it was decided that
it was a specific illness from contact with infected parrots. Nocard
cultured a Gram negative motile bacillus from infected parrots
which was believed to be the causative agent. Other investigators,
beginning with Nicolle in 1898, failed to support Nocard's conten-
tions. An outbreak with eight cases in Germany in 1893 demonstrated that parrakeets could cause the human infection.

From 1894 to 1929, individual cases and small outbreaks of psittacosis occurred in Italy, Germany, England and the United States.
The epidemic of 1917, reported by McClintock in Wilkes-Barre,
Pennsylvania, originated in the basement of a large department store
where many sick parrots were stored, has since had its counterparts
in outbreaks observed by Badger in New York (1930) and in Pitts-
burgh (1934).

From a rare and obscure disease psittacosis was suddenly raised
into a malady of worldwide interest when in July, 1929, Barros informed a number of prominent physicans and later the Medical
Society of Cordobas, Argentina, concerning the appearance of over
100 cases of a serious and peculiar pneumonia among the inhabitants
of Cordobas, Alta, Graciá and Tucuman. He diagnosed the disease
as psittacosis since the epidemiologic investigations showed that a
large consignment of psittacine birds had been imported into Argentina from Brazil; that there had been a great mortality among the
birds and that from this shipment the patients had purchased the
parrots which had fallen ill, and in a number of instances had died.
Local attention was directed to the strange disease in October when
in Buenos Aires a theatrical troupe of twelve persons, all of whom
fell ill and two succumbed following the use on the stage of a parrot
which died shortly before the human cases developed. The population was now warned and the trade in parrots stopped entirely in the
Argentine. However, the passengers of steamers calling at the Ar-
gentinian ports, ignorant of the existence of an epidemic disease of
parrots transmissible to man, bought many of the infected birds from
unscrupulous dealers. Thus the malady was conveyed to many countries. It reached the United States in November, 1929, while England reported cases in July and then in December. During the early
months of 1930, the newspapers gave accounts of outbreaks in at

least twelve countries (Austria, Italy, Switzerland, France, Denmark, Algeria, Holland, Egypt, Czechoslovakia, Germany, Sweden and United States of America). In many of the reports, it was stated that shipments of sick parrots had arrived in those countries. Later a perusal of the records of 1930 left no doubt that the South American parrots were not the only sources of infection. In England, in the United States and Switzerland psittacosis developed following the exposure to love-birds and canaries. The importance of the parrakeets was only appreciated when K. F. Meyer and B. Eddie in cooperation with the California State Department of Public Health recognized in 1931 and 1932 the wide distribution of latent psittacosis in the local breeding establishments and aviaries of California. Fortner and Pfaffenberg (1934, 1935) and Haagen and Krückeberg (1937) in extensive studies have fully confirmed the American findings for Germany, while Gerlach (1936) discovered endemic psittacosis in the bird stores and aviaries of locally bred and raised parrakeets, canaries and finches in Austria. The parrakeets raised in France were also infected (Aujaleu and Jude, 1936).

The pandemic of 1929-30 with approximately 750 to 800 cases and the subsequent endemic distribution of parrakeet psittacosis involving the United States and Germany with another 500 cases offered a splendid opportunity to many investigators for a thorough study of the disease from a clinical, etiologic and epidemiologic point of view. The reports from every country have converged in the same direction and it is now firmly established that psittacosis is an infection with a filtrable, corpuscular, microscopically demonstrable and cultivatable "virus." The hypothesis of a *Salmonella* infection has been entirely abandoned.

In 1942, Meyer and his associates called attention to the disease in pigeons, with reports of several human infections. Subsequent studies by a number of investigators have revealed the importance of chickens, ducks, turkeys, gulls, fulmars and other birds. The mammalian sources of infection emerged still later.

PREVALENCE AND DISTRIBUTION

Ornithosis is distributed throughout the World, wherever birds are found. It is probable that more human cases of this disease are contracted from non-psittacine birds than not. In the U.S.A., at least, most cases probably are now of non-psittacine origin. In the latter country the number of cases has risen sharply since 1951 when the Interstate Quarantine Regulations were changed to permit shipment of psittacine birds except into areas where state laws prohibited their entry. This change in previous restrictions apparently increased the demand for parrakeets and other birds and poorly operated aviaries sprang up all over the country. Birds were sold by the millions, many of them being carriers of psittacosis virus, and, consequently, infections occurred among aviary workers, store clerks, and purchasers of the birds.

TABLE 42

CASES AND DEATHS FROM PSITTACOSIS—UNITED STATES (PUBLIC HEALTH SERVICE)

	Cases	Deaths
1929–1930	170	33
1931–1934	133	32
1935–1939	25	7
1940–1944	51	10
1945–1949	147	3
1950–1954	918	13
1955–1959	1485	13
1960	113	—

The number of cases reported since 1929 is shown in Table 42. It is obvious that the actual number of cases is much higher. Single cases, even when severe, are often overlooked and many mild cases occurring in small epidemics never come to the attention of public health authorities. Thus, Dean (1956) found that among some 2,000 purchasers of birds there were ninety-five who had psittacosis-like illnesses; of forty-nine of these who were studied further six had complement-fixation titers of 1:64 or higher. Among fifty individuals who handled these birds in the course of their occupation four probably had had psittacosis. Of the ten or more probable cases found through this investigation it is doubtful if more than one or two would have come to attention through ordinary channels.

During the past few years it has been increasingly evident that the newly discovered sources of infection—pigeons, chickens, turkeys and probably other birds—may overshadow the reservoir of infection in psittacine birds. This fact probably explains in part the increased prevalence indicated in Table 42.

THE ETIOLOGIC AGENT

Independently, first by Bedson and Western (1930) in England, Levinthal (1935) in Germany, Armstrong and McCoy in the United States and Sacquépée in France, the virus character of the psittacosis disease agent was established. Of particular importance was the discovery by Krumwiede, McGrath and Oldenbusch (1930) that the virus was readily transmitted to white mice. It is now fully recognized that the elementary bodies measuring from 0.22 to 0.36 μ (Lazarus and Meyer, 1939) and generally described as the Levinthal-Cole-Lillie bodies or *Microbacterium multiform psittacosis*, independently discovered by the three investigators in the exudates, blood and organs of diseased birds, mammals and man represent the virus. They are readily demonstrated in the infective material by the Macchiavello (aqueous basic fuchsin pH 7.4 heated and differentiated with citric acid) or the Castaneda stain. The Giemsa and Heidenhain iron haematoxylin stain are sometimes useful. Bedson (1935), Bland and Canti (1935) have followed in detail in the spleen of mice and tissue cultures the morphologic changes incident to the intracellular growth of these bodies. In all psittacosis infections whether birds, rodents or man, the essential injury is the invasion and destruction of the reticulo-endothelial system. Virus bodies should be searched for in these cells (see Figure 76A).

Weiss (1949) who studied several mammalian viruses of the psittacosis-lymphogranuloma group came to the conclusion that all of them have a simple developmental pattern similar to that shown in Figure sixty-three. The elementary body (the infectious unit) produces in the infected tissue a larger body called the initial body. The initial body may produce either a cluster of granules smaller than itself or may grow and divide into a cluster or small plaques. Clusters and plaques develop into vesicles which may contain granules the size of elementary bodies or larger granules, plaques or vacuoles. The vesicles, which have a limiting membrane, rupture and release elementary bodies or plaques. The latter also break up and liberate elementary bodies.

The "virus" of ornithosis is actually an intermediate form of life, having some of the properties of viruses and bacteria, but being more closely related to the latter. Its relationship to the bacteria is shown by the presence of both deoxyribonucleic and ribonucleic acids, enzymes and co-enzymes, a cell wall of the bacterial type and sensitivity to antibiotics. Its obligate intracellular parasitism and developmental cycle are typical of the viruses.

On account of its size, the filtrability of the psittacosis virus is rather limited. Only the more porous types of filter candles or colloidal pads allow the virus to pass. Organ suspensions or sputum specimens, which are infectious to mice in high dilutions, frequently yield non-infectious filtrates when passed through Seitz pads or Berkefeld V filters. Through fractional sedimentation in angle cen-

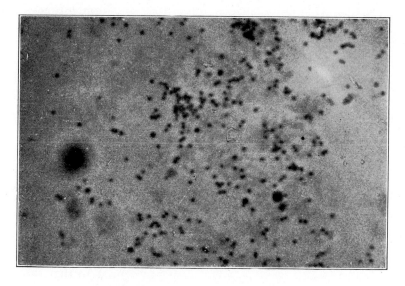

Fig. 76A. Levinthal-Cole-Lillie (L.C.L.) bodies of psittacosis in the peritoneal exudate of infected mouse. x3600.

trifuges the L.C.L. (Levinthal-Cole-Lillie) bodies may be secured in a high state of purity. The elementary bodies grow freely in the ectodermal cells of the chorion-allantoic membrane of the chick for several hundred passages without losing their infectiousness (Bland and Canti, 1935; Burnet and Rountree, 1935; Lazarus and Meyer, 1939; Fortner and Pfaffenberg, 1935). On lifeless media no growth is obtainable. However, in fluid tissue cultures consisting of Tyrode solution and chick embryo cells (Maitland method), excellent growth has been secured through forty passages (Yanamura and Meyer, 1941; Levinthal, 1935 and Haagen and Crodel, 1936). The infectiousness persists undiminished; 0.5 cc. of a dilution 10^{-9} is fatal to a mouse in fourteen days.

The virus may also be grown readily in roller tube tissue cultures containing a nutrient fluid consisting of serum ultrafiltrate and Simms' solution (Morgan and Wiseman, 1946). The elementary bodies are specifically agglutinated by antisera produced in guinea pigs or other animals. They act as excellent antigens in the complement fixation test (Bedson, 1933; Yanamura and Meyer, 1942). The psittacosis virus contains two antigens, one resistant to boiling and the other rapidly destroyed at this temperature (Bedson, 1936). The heat-stable component is the group-specific antigen and the heat-labile substance, probably a carbohydrate, is the strain-specific antigen.

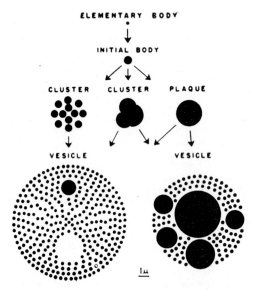

Fig. 76B. Stages in the development of viruses of the psittacosis-lymphogranuloma venereum group (Chlamydozoaceae). (From Weiss, Emilio: *J. Infectious Diseases, 84*:130, 142, March-April, 1949.)

The virus is not very resistant to glycerin but quite so to desiccation. Dried by the lyophile method, it remains active for over six months. When exposed to formaldehyde (0.2 per cent) at room temperature, the virus remains infectious for periods up to ten days; however, it is quite heat labile (15 minutes at 70° C.).

Experimentally the virus has been transmitted to a variety of psittacine birds (parrots, shell parrakeets, ricebirds, sparrows and canaries). It should be borne in mind that these birds may carry latent infections (psittacosis and salmonellosis) and that in the infected state they are dangerous sources for laboratory infections. The mouse as a universal and relatively safe experimental animal has displaced the birds. The gross anatomic lesions in form of an enlarged spleen, liver necrosis, a ballooned duodenum, peritoneal exudate and occasional patches of pneumonia with cells of the reticulo-endothelial system filled with L.C.L. bodies are very characteristic. The rodents may be infected by any route even by feeding and contact exposure. Mice inoculated with small doses of the virus survive the infection and may carry the virus for over 200 days or develop a sterile immunity. Gophers *(Thomomys bottae)* are readily infected by the subcutaneous route (Hoge, 1934). The intratracheal injection of guinea pigs, squirrels and monkeys leads to extensive and highly characteristic pneumonic lesions with an abundance of virus. Macacus monkeys infected with virus by the subcutaneous route may prove resistant to intratracheal re-infection. Virus passage through mice stabilizes the infectiousness and maintains the virulence through hundreds of transfers.

Usually intraperitoneal inoculation of guinea pigs with non-mammalian strains of virus fails to cause infection. On the other hand, guinea pigs are readily infected by the Louisiana and SF human pneumonitis strains when injected by this route.

Most, if not all of the viruses of the psittacosis-lymphogranuloma venereum group produce toxins. This was first shown in 1943 by Rake and Jones with the virus of lymphogranuloma venereum and later for the several pneumonitis viruses (Rake and Jones, 1944; Hamre and Rake, 1944; Hamre, Rake and Rake, 1947; and Manire and Meyer, 1950a). These toxins kill mice when injected intravenously. There is a great deal of variation in the potency of the toxins produced by different strains. In general, those which are most lethal for man, the Louisiana, Illinois and turkey viruses, produce the most potent toxins. A toxin neutralization test has been very useful in differentiating the psittacosis viruses into groups (Manire and Meyer, 1950b).

GENERAL EPIDEMIOLOGY

As a rule, the epidemiologic facts in household outbreaks are stereotype in nature; suddenly a patient with an atypical pneumonia is observed in a family in which recently a parrot or a pair of parrakeets, rarely canaries or finches, have been introduced as cage pets. Quite often in rapid succession, additional cases are seen among the relatives and even guests or visitors. The responsible pet birds may or may not be visibly sick. Usually two to three weeks elapse between the acquisition of the birds and the onset of the first case. A seasonal prevalence during the winer months (January-April) is probably due to the frequency with which human beings receiving birds as gifts are brought in contact with them through prolonged exposure in the closed rooms of a winter household. The majority of psittacosis infections have occurred in people of middle age (Elkeles —66 per cent for age group thirty to fifty; Sturdee and Scott—60 per cent over the age of forty). The disposition to clinical psittacosis is very low in children under ten years of age. However, young children do become infected, sometimes fatally, and it is probable that infections in this age group may be overlooked because of the general opinion that psittacosis does not occur among them.

A significant difference in the susceptibility of the sexes has only been noted in the outbreaks due to shell parrakeets. The greater frequency in women is in part due to the fact that they are either engaged in the breeding of the birds or as lovers of pets, come more closely in contact with the virus. The mortality rate is higher in the groups between 40 and sixty years of age. The case fatality rates from 25 to 40 per cent in the outbreaks preceding and during the pandemic have declined during the past few years due in part to the recognition of mild or missed infections but also because of the lower virulence of some of the viruses now reaching people and particularly because of antibiotic therapy.

The occurrence of this disease as an occupational liability among persons engaged in the breeding, raising, transportation and sale of parrots and parrakeets is well known. The personnel of pet and department stores has suffered greatly from psittacosis (Badger, Hegler and others). Seamen bringing home parrots to sell and baggage car employees shipping parrakeets contracted parrot fever. Physicians, veterinarians, health department officials and inspectors experienced several attacks of psittacosis (Leichtenstern, Hamel, Buchanan, Glage, Hegler, Elliot and Hatfield, Haagen and Krückeberg). During the experimental investigations of avian psittacosis in 1929 and 1930, at least thirty-eight laboratory infections were contracted. Sulkin and Pike (1949) reported seventeen more instances of psittacosis due to laboratory infections.

Human case to case infections are by no means infrequent (Meyer, 1942, Berman *et al.*, 1955). Professional nurses or persons who care for psittacosis patients are prominently represented. In the Louisiana bayou outbreak of 1942 (Olson and Trenting, 1944) infection of those attending the sick was a prominent feature. There were nineteen cases with eight deaths among those who nursed primary cases.

Milzer (1952) has described an interesting example of person to person infection. Because of overcrowding of the hospital, a patient ill with pneumonitis was placed in the same room with a surgical patient. The latter was "protected" with daily doses of penicillin the first ten days of contact and with a broad spectrum antibiotic from the fifth to tenth days of contact. However, after fifteen days of residence in the room with the pneumonitis patient the surgical patient contracted pneumonitis and he as well as the original patient was proved by laboratory tests to have had psittacosis.

The pathways of transmission from bird to man are twofold: (a) by the aerogenic route — the inhalation of dust contaminated with infective particles derived from desiccated fecal droppings, urine, feathers, cadavers, etc., and droplets from the nasal secretions, and (b) rarely by direct contact through bite wounds. The high infectivity of the psittacosis virus which resembles that of smallpox or measles is reflected in the histories in which short exposure occurred in a pet shop where diseased birds were kept. Contrary to general belief among the laity, actual contact or possession of diseased psittacine birds is not necessary since air currents may disseminate the virus particles.

Pigeons have been responsible for the disease in man on a number of occasions. Meyer, Eddie and Yanamura (1942) reported ten such cases in New York, Massachusetts, Minnesota and California. Other cases have been reported by Alicandri (1942) in New York, Levinson, Gibbs and Bearwood (1944) in Philadelphia, Favour (1943) in Boston and Turgasen (1944) in Wisconsin. The virus which is found in pigeons is less virulent for man than is the virus found in the psittacine birds. The droppings of pigeons probably contain the virus, with human infections occurring by inhalation.

Most of these cases resulted from contact with domesticated pigeons. An outbreak involving seven persons and apparently due to wild pigeons occurred in a railroad car shop in Decatur, Illinois in 1946 (Shaughnessy, 1955). Pigeons were so plentiful in the shop that 300 had been shot in the building about six weeks prior to the outbreak and metal screens had to be placed over the drinking water fountains to protect them from pigeon droppings. Six of the seven infected persons and five of thirteen pigeons tested were found to have complement-fixing antibodies against psittacosis.

Chickens are known to be infected with the ornithosis virus but apparently have not played an important part in human infections. Ward *et al.* (1954) described an interesting series of outbreaks in Northwestern Illinois in which mild cases of a psittacosis-like disease occurred during a period of several successive years in late winter and spring. Sick individuals were found to have positive complement fixation titers that were much higher than those in control groups. Because of the absence of psittacine birds in the area, they ascribed the source as being possibly in chickens. About one-third of the sera collected from chickens in the vicinity were positive in the indirect complement fixation test with lygranum antigen.

Ducks have been found to be infected in a number of areas in the U.S.A. and Europe. Human cases from this source have usually been mild, but it is possible that a more virulent virus may be introduced by wild birds.

A number of outbreaks of human ornithosis have occurred among persons working in turkey processing plants in Texas, New Jersey, Wisconsin, Oregon, Washington, and British Columbia (Graber and Pomeroy, 1958). These have involved some 500 persons with about a dozen deaths. Careful studies have shown that the processors who were engaged in jobs which caused them to come in contact with cloacal contents or aerosols containing dried cloacal contents were most likely to be infected. The strains of virus isolated from turkey flocks involved in these epidemics were of high virulence, resembling the egret strains implicated in the Louisiana bayou epidemics.

IMMUNITY

Recovery from an attack of psittacosis, or injection of living virus in monkeys (Rivers and Schwentker, 1934) may be followed by the appearance of neutralizing antibodies in varying amounts and a persistence of complement fixing antibodies. Persons constantly exposed to the virus may have a high neutralization index of their blood. The resistance to re-infection in mice is frequently an infection immunity associated with the latency of the virus in the viscera.

Active immunization of mice with antigens prepared by inactivating infected tissue, tissue culture or embryonated eggs with formalin, photodynamic action or by irradiation with ultraviolet light protects them against up to several million lethal doses of virus. Bedson (1938) stated that the immunity following vaccination was not complete and that the challenge inoculation appeared to set up inapparent infections lasting for several months. Later investigators (Morgan and Wiseman, 1946; Francis, Milzer and Gordon, 1947; and Wagner *et al.*, 1946) do not mention this phenomenon, possibly because they used what seem to be more potent vaccines.

A satisfactory method for immunizing man has not been developed. Rivers and Schwentker recommended the active immunization of laboratory workers with live virus but, in view of the tendency of psittacosis virus to remain latent, this method apparently has not had general acceptance.

LABORATORY DIAGNOSIS

The blood obtained during illness may contain the virus; it should be inoculated, either defibrinated or as serum, intraperitoneally into mice. Bedson and Meyer and Eddie found the blood virulent up to the fourth and tenth day, Gerlach even on the fifteenth and sixteenth. At any stage of the disease, the sputum is the most likely material to yield positive findings on inoculation of unfiltered, centrifuged or filtered sputum extracts into mice or ricebirds. The virus is not always present and repeated examinations are indicated. It has been found even up to the seventy-fifth day (Gerlach) after the onset of the disease. At post-mortem the infective agent has repeatedly been demonstrated in portions of the lung, spleen and liver in the order mentioned. Extreme precautions should be exercised since any material containing the psittacosis virus must be regarded as highly pathogenic and dangerous. Experimental inoculations should not be attempted except in especially equipped laboratories.

The complement fixation test with heated antigens prepared from spleens of infected mice or tissue cultures has proven of great value in the early diagnosis of the disease.

Cross-reactions occur in the complement-fixation test due to infection with other viruses of the group such as lymphogranuloma venereum, feline pneumonitis and cat-scratch fever. The necessity of showing an increase in titer by testing acute and convalescent phase sera should be emphasized. Early treatment of the disease with antibiotics may delay the production of complement-fixing antibodies for twenty to forty days. In diagnosing infection in the avian species, the indirect complement fixation test (Hilleman, Haig and Helmbold, 1951) has been found to be a useful tool.

THE SPONTANEOUS DISEASE IN TROPICAL BIRDS

The recognition that a variety of tropical birds and, in particular, shell parrakeets *(Melopsittacus undulatus)* may act as sources of infection is one of the important contributions resulting from the researches in psittacosis since 1931. Equally far-reaching is the discovery that visibly "healthy" birds may harbor the virus and as shedders disseminate the infective virus. The incidence of these inapparent latent infections in aviaries and breeding establishments may vary from 10 to 90 per cent. Although the importation embargoes against South American parrots, which were instituted by practically every country following the pandemic of 1929-30 throttled the exotic bird trade but disclosed the existence of endemic psittacosis in the domestic breeding establishments of California, Germany, Austria, France and England. With the aid of newer laboratory methods, the disease of the birds has been carefully studied. It is quite generally admitted that the clinical manifestations of parrots or parrakeets infected with psittacosis are by no means characteristic. Sick birds may be recognized by their behavior and appearance, sleepiness, motionless sitting on the perches, ruffled feathers, semiclosed or closed eyes, fits of shivering, loss of weight with atrophic breast muscles and labored breathing may be noted. Diarrhea with greenish stools or soiled tail feathers with grayish mortar-like concretions are occasionally observed. The mortality among parrots may be very high, while among parrakeets held in a fairly sanitary environment only five to 10 per cent actually succumb to psittacosis. Young birds are more susceptible than the older ones. Through contact experiments in the incubation time has been found to be from five to twenty days, and not infrequently much longer (100 days). Relapses are quite common in carefully observed cage birds and the disease may last for weeks. In order to prove the psittacosis nature of the parrot or parrakeet disease, autopsy and laboratory examinations are important. The gross anatomic changes, aside from emaciation and in the acute cases septic hemorrhages are not very extensive and are confined to the abdominal cavity. The liver may be enlarged, saffron-colored and studded with fresh or partially healed necroses and infarcts, and the catarrhal inflammation of air sacs and degenerative changes in the kidneys.

An enlargement of the spleen, variable as to size in the different stages of the disease, is rarely absent. Direct smears from these organs,

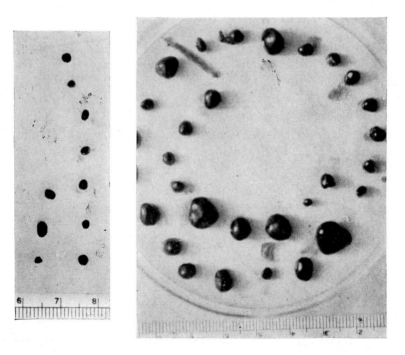

Fig. 76C. Spleens of parrakeets, showing normal spleen (left) and spleens from parrakeets infected with psittacosis (right) 2.5 mm. to 10.0 mm. in diameter.

when adequately stained, reveal the elementary L.C.L. bodies, while organ suspensions infect mice. The routine diagnosis of latent psittacosis in parrakeets segregates the non-infected from the infected birds by the size of the spleen (see Figure 76C). Spleens with a diameter of over 3 to 4 mm. yield on inoculation a high percentage of virus infections. The histopathologic altreations have been studied by Lillie (1933). Thus the parrot disease of psittacine birds is primarily a disease of the liver and spleen with no lesions in the lung and occasional latency up to 812 days in parrakeets.

The veterinary differential diagnosis must take into consideration the Salmonella infections which are by no means uncommon in South American tropical birds. Psittacosis and salmonellosis may exist in a carrier stage in the same parrotlet. The so-called Pacheco virus disease of parrots studied by Rivers and Schwentker must be considered in the examination of diseased parrots.

Spontaneous psittacosis infections responsible for human disease have been proven in the following species of the order *Psittaciformes:* Blue-fronted Amazon *(Amazona aestiva),* various Cuban, Mexican and Panama species *(Amazona barbadensis* Gmelin), macaw *(Ara ararauna)* short-tailed parrot *(Graydidasculus brachyurus* Temminck and Kuhl), shell parrakeets or budgerigars *(Melopsittacus undulatus),* sulphur-crested cockatoos *(Kakatoe galerita),* galah *(Kakatoe roseicapilla)* and Murrum bidgee smoker parrots *(Barnardius sp).* Enzootic, acute and latent psittacosis among wild parrots and parrotlets has been demonstrated by mouse tests in the following Australian species: Shell parrakeets, lorikeets *(Trichoglossus chlorolepidotus* and *moluccanus* 58 per cent), grass parrot *(Psephotus haematonotus* 41 per cent), cockateels *(Leptolophus hollandicus* 60 per cent), roseleas *(Platycercus sp);* African species: Mask *(Agapornis)* and ring-necked parrakeet *(Palaoernis torquatus);* and South American species: Spectacled parrotlet *(Psittacula conspicillata),* Spengel parrotlet *(Psittacula spengeli)* and brown-throated conures *(Eupsittula pertinax aeruginosus).* Experimentally a great many other species have been successfully infected with the psittacosis agent; for example, senegal parrots *(Poeocephalus senegalus),* conures *(Conurus solstialis, Eupsittula canicularis, E. cacurum),* orange-bellied grass parrakeet *(Neophenia chrysogastea),* Quaker parrakeet *(Myiopsitta monachus),* African love-birds or masks or peach faces *(Agapornis roseicollis, personata),* etc. Combining all these findings, the uniform disposition of the psittacine birds to psittacosis is fully established and further evidence strongly supports the belief that the infection is widely distributed among wild parrots and parrakeets, perhaps as a population regulator. The high incidence of prolonged latent infections in certain species, particularly those desired as cage birds, is important. Crowding, lack of sunlight and of cleanliness and malnutrition so prevalent in transit and in bird stores diminish the resistance of the birds to the infective agent lying dormant in the tissues. The active psittacosis which follows not only exposes other birds but becomes the main source of human infections.

THE SPONTANEOUS DISEASE IN FINCHES

Epidemiologic observations by Roubakine (1930), Sturdee and Scott (1930) have definitely incriminated the canary bird *(Serinus canaria),* while Meyer and Eddie and more recently Gerlach proved conclusively the role of this finch as a potent source for human psittacosis infections. In fact, various other finches, thrushes and sparrows [goldfinch *(Carduelis carduelis),* bullfinch *(Pyrrhula pyrrhula),* nonpareil *(Cyannospiza ciris),* Lady gould finch *(Poephilamirabilis),* blackbird *(Turdus meurla),* crossbill *(Loxia curvirostra),* titmouse *(Parus major),* siskin *(Spinus pinus),* yellow-crowned sparrow *(Zonotrichia),* Bengalese *(Uroloncha acutocauda),* pekin robin *(Liothrix luteus)*] exposed in bird shops or accidentally fed on contaminated seeds from infected stores (Gerlach) may contract the disease and spread it to other birds and even man (in Holland firefinch, *Lagonosticta senegala L).* Particularly susceptible are ricebirds *(Padda oryzivora);* they are used as sentinels in aviaries to detect the presence of the psittacosis virus among apparently healthy parrakeets (Meyer and Eddie). Chickens exposed in breeding pens with diseased budgerigars have contracted psittacosis (Meyer and Eddie).

THE SPONTANEOUS DISEASE IN PIGEONS

Ornithosis of pigeons is probably widespread in the United States. Meyer, Eddie and Yanamura (1942) studied flocks from many different areas of the country and found that 30 per cent to 75 per cent gave positive complement fixation reactions. The virus was isolated from many of the birds tested.

Eddie and Francis (1942) found that 61 per cent of loft and market pigeons in Michigan gave positive complement-fixation reactions. Virus was isolated from only two of thirty-six birds studied.

"Wild" pigeons have been examined by Zichis, Shaughnessy, and Lemke (1946) in Chicago, Labzoffsky (1947) in three Ontario cities, and Davis and Ewing (1947) in Baltimore, Maryland. Virus was isolated by the three groups of investigators from 22, 16 and 15 per cent respectively, of the birds. The relative importance of this vast reservoir of infection is not yet understood. There have been reports of infections from pigeons and one wonders how often cases of "atypical pneumonia" may be contracted from these birds without the source being known.

The virus possesses a highly adapted latent parasitism for pigeons, similar to psittacosis virus for parrots. Parrakeets and ricebirds are fatally infected by feeding or inhalation of the pigeon strain of virus. Pigeons (and an occasional dove) are clinically not affected by feeding or intramuscular injection, but continue to carry the virus for many weeks in their organs.

Infection seems to be acquired when the pigeons are young, in the nest, or soon after. Adverse conditions, such as crowding in unsanitary cages or improper feeding causes a flare-up of the disease.

THE DISEASE IN TURKEYS

In young poults, except for respiratory distress and diarrhea in a few birds, the first sign of disease may be depression, followed quickly by death. In older turkeys the disease is more marked with anorexia, respiratory distress, manifested by gasping and rales and diarrhea, followed by cyanosis, weakness and death. At postmortem pericarditis, peritonitis, perihepatitis, splenomegaly, pneumonia and tracheitis are commonly found. The air sacs are coated with caseous exudates in most instances. Since many other respiratory infections may produce similar symptoms and lesions, isolation of ornithosis virus is recommended for establishing the diagnosis.

THE SPONTANEOUS DISEASE IN OTHER BIRDS

The domestic fowl (*Gallus gallus*) is sometimes infected (Meyer and Eddie, 1942; Karrer, Eddie and Meyer, 1950; Mandel and Jordan, 1952) as is the domestic duck (*Anas platyrhynchos*). Evidence, direct or indirect, has been collected to indicate that the English sparrow *(Passer domesticus)*, fulmers or petrels, terns, gulls, turkeys, and pheasants, carry the virus to a greater or lesser degree. Many of these birds are in close contact with man and it is not strange that infections are believed to have been transmitted by most of those listed (Davis, 1947; Irons, Sullivan, and Rowen, 1951; Mandel and Jordan, 1952). The possibility of transmission to domestic fowl from birds like petrels, gulls or pigeons must also be kept in mind.

THE DISEASE IN MAN

The clinical manifestations listed in the numerous histories of severe cases are remarkably uniform (Adamy, Sturdee and Scott, Gorham, Calder and Vedder, Polayes, Maclachlan, Permar and Rogers, Rabinowitz and others). The incubation time, although difficult to establish in many instances, varies from seven to fifteen days after initial contact. Since an incubationary latency cannot be excluded, it is not surprising to observe occasionally an incubation time of from thirty to thirty-nine days. The onset of the disease may be abrupt or begins gradually and insidiously with indefinite influenza-like symptoms like malaise, anorexia, headache, backache, photophobia and chills. Restlessness, insomnia, delirium, typhoidal state, non-productive cough, constipation, occasionally diarrhea with abdominal distension and tenderness are, as a rule, present during the height of the infection. Epistaxis occurs in about 25 per cent of the cases. Rose spots may appear on the pale icteric skin. The temperature rises rapidly and assumes the character of a continuum which may begin to fall by lysis during the second or third week. One of the characteristic features of the disease is the relative slowness of the pulse compared with the temperature. In the fatal cases the pulse becomes rapid and feeble. The spleen is rarely palpable. Phlebitis with thrombosis are frequent complications. The lungs are involved in every case except the mild and ambulatory cases. Physical signs may develop slowly and have a peculiar migratory character; roentgen-ray examinations indicate that the parenchymatous consolidation begins early in the course of the disease. As a rule, the cough when present is not productive; despite extensive respiratory involvement, the sputum is scanty (sputumless pneumonia), mucoid and very rarely rusty or blood tinged. Due to secondary infections, the ensuing bronchitis produces a copious frankly purulent sputum. A remarkable feature of the disease is the frequent absence of rapid or deep breathing even when the physical signs in the lungs indicate extensive involvement. In the second week encephalitic manifestations in form of lethargy, stupor, etc., may make their appearance. In fact, the apathy and toxemia are entirely out of proportion to the clinical signs of exhaustion and organic involvement. White blood counts reveal a leucopenia or a slight leucocytosis.

Hepatitis and myocarditis are being increasingly recognized as complications or sequelae of psittacosis. Convalescence is very slow and tedious; relapses are by no means rare. Mild and ambulatory cases may last for one day to one week and are only recognized in the course of epidemiologic investigations. No effort should be spared to make an etiologic diagnosis by examination of nasal washings or sputum specimens in the mouse test or the complement fixation test of the serum.

Successful treatment of psittacosis with penicillin, aureomycin, or terramycin, has been reported by a number of investigators (Turgasen, 1944; Wolins, 1948). The impression that aureomycin is more effective than penicillin is borne out by the studies in animals. Penicillin merely prevents division of the virus particle but the abnormal virus continues to produce injury to the host cells (Weiss, 1950); aureomycin almost completely stops growth of the virus and thus prevents severe damage to the host cells (Gogolak and Weiss, 1950). Due in part to the use of antibiotics the case fatality rate has dropped from about 18 per cent in the pandemic years of 1929 and 1930 to less than 2 per cent at the present time. (Meyer and Eddie, 1951a.)

The morbid anatomy of fifty-two cases were admirably summarized by Lillie in 1933. Anatomically the focal or lobular pulmonary consolidation involves the alveolar epithelial cells which desquamate and become embedded in a serous exudate poor in polymorphonuclear leucocytes. Interstitial infiltration is usually lacking and the bronchioles may remain clear. In the hematopoietic system congestion and phagocytic activity prevail, while in the liver focal necrosis of the parenchyma and vacuolation of the Kupffer's cells are found.

Gerlach, by sputum examinations of two persons, exposed to clinical cases of psittacosis has indicated the probable existence of inapparent, silent human infections. According to Haagen, the virus may persist in the spleen for at least two weeks after recovery from acute psittacosis.

Meyer and Eddie (1951b) described in detail the history of a human carrier of psittacosis virus. Virus was isolated from this man for at least eight years after his original attack of the disease. During much of that time he had a history of paroxysmal coughing spasms which were productive of a moderate amount of thick tenacious sputum. Apparently he did not infect anyone during his long carrier condition. However, it would be well to look for a human carrier when cases occur which cannot be explained on the basis of contact with birds. The two fatal cases described by Zichis and Shaughnessy (1945) had no known contacts with birds or with one another but did have common human contacts and developed their infection at the same time.

PROTECTIVE AND PREVENTIVE MEASURES

Psittacosis of psittacine origin could be readily controlled, provided the public would appreciate the possible danger inherent to contact with birds, psittacine, varieties or finches, particularly of unknown origin. However, the love for pets, so deeply rooted in human nature, cannot be changed. Some degree of protection has been obtained by means of restrictive measures, such as embargo of exotic birds, quarantine, isolation, etc. During 1930 practically every country prohibited the importation of parrots including any bird of the group known as "Psittaciformes." However, gradually exceptions have been adopted.

The Interstate Quarantine Regulations adopted in 1932 required that no psittacine birds could be transported in interstate commerce without a certificate from the State health authority certifying that the birds were free from psittacosis. This regulation was unworkable because the respective states, except California, did not have the machinery for investigating the health of the birds.

The 1951 Act removed all Federal restrictions on interstate shipments of psittacine birds unless the Surgeon General has determined that birds from a certain area are dangerous to the public health.

The importation of tropical birds, except as individual pets (limit two per household per year) which have been in the owner's possession for four months prior to arrival, is prohibited by Federal Quarantine Regulations. However, Meyer and Eddie (1951a) indicate that smuggling of tropical parrots across the Mexican border is prevalent and probably cannot be halted by the present enforcement staff.

Since the commercial aviaries engaged in the breeding and raising of shell parrakeets are the principal spreaders of diseased birds, and the creators of epizootics among canaries and finches in pet shops, etc., every effort should be made to create a bird industry free from psittacosis.

California's experience in attempting to control the disease is illuminating. In 1933 all persons engaged in the parrakeet business were required to submit birds to laboratory tests before the breeders could obtain certificates permitting parrakeets to be sold. Laboratory tests showed that the incidence of the disease declined steadily to almost zero by 1937. There were subsequent small rises in incidence in the decade beginning in 1940. The number of human cases and deaths in California and elsewhere showed a similar decline.

Because of the cost and difficulty of enforcement California has permitted its controls to die. It will be of interest to see whether the infection rate will rise to its former heights.

Doubtless the many thousands of parrakeets bred and sold in this country are creating a huge potential reservoir of infection. It appears that there has been a recent increase in human infections which may be related to the increased sale of psittacine birds or may reflect the importance of other sources of infection.

Recently, it appears that infection of psittacine birds may be controlled by feeding them with one of the tetracycline antibiotics. (Meyer *et al.,* 1958). In larger birds (turkeys, for example) intramuscular injection of these drugs in oil may be used in place of feeding. These procedures seem to be indicated in aviaries and also among infected flocks of turkeys. Individual owners may also wish to use them to try to prevent excretion of virus by pet birds.

While psittacosis is not one of the important human diseases, it is largely preventable. The medical and veterinary professions and the public should realize the danger from close contact with psittacine birds. The role of other birds and fowl needs to be studied. Above all we need to know how much human psittacosis exists and what are its principal reservoirs.

ITEMS OF NOTE

1) Psittacosis (ornithosis) is a disease of the psittacine birds, pigeons, turkeys, domestic fowl, duck, and other birds.

2) The disease has appeared in endemic form in many bird breeding establishments and pet shops.

3) Psittacosis is caused by a virus.

4) Pigeons in the United States seem to be infected commonly with psittacosis virus.

5) Man is highly susceptible to the virus of psittacine origin, less so to the virus of pigeon origin.

6) The domestic fowl and duck apparently play a small role in the epidemiology of the disease.

7) Person to person infection occurs with considerable frequency.

8) Turkeys have become an important source of human infections.

9) Control of the disease calls for an appreciation of the dangers inherent to contact with pet birds, especially of unknown origin, together with the creation of a bird industry free from psittacosis.

REFERENCES

ALICANDRI, H.: *J.A.M.A., 118:*1214, 1942.

AUJALEU, E. and JUDE, A.: *Presse méd., 44:*1094, 1936.

BEDSON, S. P. and WESTERN, B. T.: *Brit. J. Exper. Path., 11:*502, 1930.

BEDSON, S. P.: *Brit. M. J., 1:*890, 1931; *13:*65, 1932; and *461:*14, 162 and 267; *15:*243, 1934; *17:*109, 1936; *Lancet, 2:*1277, 1935; *2:*1477, 1937.

BERMAN, S. *et al.: Pediatrics, 15:*752, 1955.

BLAND, J. O. W. and CANTI, R. G.: *J. Path. & Bact., 40:*231, 1935.

BURNET, F. M.: *J. Hyg., 35:*412, 1935.

BURNET, F. M. and ROUNTREE, P. M.: *J. Path. & Bact., 40:*471, 1935.

DAVIS, D. J. and EWING, C. L.: *Proc. Soc. Exper. Biol. & Med., 62:*1484, 1947.

DAVIS, D. J.: *Proc. Soc. Exper. Biol. & Med., 66:*77, 1947.

DEAN, D. J.: Discussion at *Second Symposium on Psittacosis.* Auspices Rutgers Univ., New York City, Feb. 16-17, 1956.

EDDIE, B. and FRANCIS, T. F.: *Proc. Soc. Exper. Biol. & Med., 50:*291, 1942.

ELKELES, G. and BARROW, E.: *Ergebn. Hyg. Bakt., Immunitatsforsch. Exper. Therap., 12:*529, 1931.

FAVOUR, C. B.: *Am. J. M. Sc., 205:*162, 1943.

FORTNER, J. and PFAFFENBERG, R.: *Ztschr. Hyg. u. Infectionskr., 116:*397, 1934a; *117:*286, 1935; *Deutsche tierarztl. Wchnschr., 2:*720, 1934b; *Berl. tierarztl. Wchnschr., 52:*405, 1936.

FRANCIS, R. D., MILZER, A. and GORDON, F. B.: *Proc. Soc. Exper. Biol. Med., 66:*184, 1947.

GERLACH, F.: *Ztschr. Hyg.*, *118:*574 and 709, 1936; *Wien. tierarztl. Monatschr.*, *23:*552, 1936.

GOGOLAK, F. M. and WEISS, E.: *J. Infect. Dis.*, *87:*264, 1950.

GRABER, R. E. and POMEROY, B. S.: *Am. J. Pub. Health*, *48:*1469, 1958.

HAAGEN, E. and CRODEL, B.: *Zento Bakt. Parasitenk*, *138:*20, 1936, Abt. 1, Orig.

HAAGEN, E. and KRUCKEBERG, E.: *Veroff a. d. Gebiete d. Volksgesundheits dienstes*, *48:* 1937; Heft 423, 384.

HAMRE, D., RAKE, H. and RAKE, G.: *J. Exper. Med.*, *86:*1, 1947.

HEGLER, C.: *Handb. Innern Med.*, 3rd Ed. 1934, Bd. 1, p. 1085; *Ergebn. d. ges. Med.*, *19:*423, 1934.

HILLEMAN, M. R., HAIG, D. A. and HELMHOLD, R. J.: *J. Immun.*, *66:*115, 1951.

HOGE, V. M.: *Pub. Health Rep.*, *49:*451, 1934.

IRONS, J. V., SULLIVAN, T. D. and ROWEN, J.: *Am. J. Pub. Health*, *41:*931, 1951.

KARRER, H., EDDIE, B. and MEYER, K. F.: *J. Infect. Dis.*, *87:*13, 1950.

KRUMWIEDE, C., MCGRATH, M. and OLDENBUSCH, C.: *Am. J. Path.*, *2:*585, 1930.

LABZOFFSKY, N. A.: *Canad. J. Pub. Health*, *38:*187, 1947.

LAZARUS, A. and MEYER, K. F.: *J. Bact.*, *38:*153, 1939.

LEVINSON, D. C., GIBBS, J. and BEARDWOOD, J. T.: *J.A.M.A.*, *126:*1079, 1944.

LEVINTHAL, W.: *Lancet*, *1:*1207, 1935.

LILLIE, R. D.: *Nat. Inst. Health Bull.* No. 161, Washington, 1933.

MANDELL, A. and JORDAN, W. S.: *Am. J. Hyg.*, *55:*230, 1952.

MANIRE, G. P. and MEYER, K. F.: *J. Infect. Dis.*, *86:*226, 1950a; *86:*241, 1950b.

MEYER, K. F. and EDDIE, B.: Proceedings of Twelfth International Veterinary Congress, *3:*182, 1935; *Klin. Wchnschr.*, *13:*865, 1934; *Am. J. Pub. Health*, *25:*571, 1935; *Arch. Gewerbepath. Gewerbehyg.*, *5:*501, 1934.

MEYER, K. F.: *Medicine*, *21:*175, 1942.

MEYER, K. F. and EDDIE, B.: *Proc. Soc. Exper. Miol. & Med.*, *49:*522, 1942.

MEYER, K. F., EDDIE, B. and YANAMURA, H. Y.: *Proc. Soc. Exper. Biol. & Med.*, *49:*609, 1942.

MEYER, K. F. and EDDIE, B.: *Bull. Hyg.*, *26:*1, 1951a; *J. Infect. Dis.*, *88:*109, 1951b.

MEYER, K. F., EDDIE, B., RICHARDSON, J. H., SHIPKOWITZ, N. L. and MUIR, R. J.: In *Progress in Psittacosis Research and Control*, Beaudette, F. R., (Ed.). Rutgers University Press, 1958.

MILZER, A.: 1952. Personal communication.

MORGAN, H. R. and WISEMAN, R. W.: *J. Infect. Dis.*, *79:*131, 1946.

OLSON, B. J. and TREUTING, W. L.: *Pub. Health Rep.*, *59:*1299, 1944.

PACHECO, G.: *Mem. Inst. Oswaldo Cruz*, *26:*169, 1932; *Compt. rend. Soc. biol.*, *105:*109, 1930.

PFAFFENBERG, R.: *Erg. Hygiene*, *18:*251, 1936.

RAKE, G. and JONES, H.: *Proc. Soc. Exper. Biol. & Med.*, *53:*86, 1943; *J. Exper. Med.*, *79:*463, 1944.

RIVERS, T. M. and ASSOCIATES: *J. Exper. Med.*, *54:*91, 105, 119, 129, 1931; *55:*911, 1932; *J. Immunol.* 26:328, 1934; *J.A.M.A.*, *96:*2061, 1931.

RIVERS, T. M. and SCHWENTKER, F. F.: *J. Exper. Med.*, *60:*211, 1934.

RIVERS, T. M. and BERRY, G. P.: *J. Exper. Med.*, *61:*205, 1935.

ROUBAKINE, A.: League of Nations Monthly Epidemiological Report, April 15, 1930, 9th Year, No 4, p. 141.

SHAUGHNESSY, H. J.: In *Psittacosis*, Beaudette, F. R. (Ed.). Rutgers Univ. Press, 1955.

STURDEE, E. L. and SCOTT, W. M.: Reports on Public Health and Medical Subjects. *61:* London, 1930.

SULKIN, S. E. and PIKE, R. M.: *New England J. Med., 241:*205, 1949.

TURGASEN, F. E.: *J.A.M.A., 126:*1150, 1944.

WAGNER, J. C., MEIKLEJOHN, G., KINGSLAND, L. C. and HICKISH, H. W.: *J. Immunol., 54:*35, 1946.

WARD, C. S., HILDINGER, A. L., MORRISSEY, R. A. and BIRGE, J. P.: *J.A.M.A., 155:*1146, 1954.

WEISS, E.: *J. Infect. Dis., 84:*125, 1949; *87:*249, 1950.

WOLINS, W.: *Am. J. Med. Sc., 216:*551, 1948.

YANAMURA, H. Y. and MEYER, K. F.: *J. Infect. Dis., 68:*1, 1941; *J. Immunol., 44:*195, 1942.

ZICHIS, J. and SHAUGHNESSY, H. J.: *Science, 102:*301, 1945.

ZICHIS, J., SHAUGHNESSY, H. J. and LEMKE, C.: *J. Bact., 51:*616, 1946.

Chapter 11

VESICULAR STOMATITIS

ROBERT P. HANSON, PH.D.

VESICULAR STOMATITIS is a virus disease affecting chiefly cattle, swine and horses. The disease is characterized by the successive appearance of macules, vesicles and erosions in the mucus membranes of the mouth, and sometimes in the skin of the foot and teat. Although affected cattle resemble animals with foot and mouth disease, vesicular stomatitis does not produce as great an economic loss, as recovery ordinarily occurs within a week or ten days. Man and seven other species of mammals may become infected.

HISTORY

Vesicular stomatitis has probably existed in the Americas for many years and may have arisen there. Perhaps the earliest account of sore mouth of horses was written by John Spenser of Maryland and published in 1826. In 1862, horses belonging to the Army of the Potomac suffered an epizootic of "hoof and mouth" disease that resembled vesicular stomatitis in all respects. Notable outbreaks of the disease have occurred in the United States in 1889, 1906, 1916, 1926, 1937, 1944 and 1949. Vesicular stomatitis is enzootic in such American countries as Columbia, Venezuela and Mexico.

However, it was in the eastern hemisphere that vesicular stomatitis was first recognized as a clinical entity. Theiler (1901) described the disease as a malady of South African horses. Years later, in 1916, after the French had reported vesicular stomatitis in horses shipped from the United States and Canada, it was belatedly recognized in America.

Cotton (1927) established the virus etiology of the disease in 1926, and in the following year demonstrated the existence of two serological types of the disease.

374

ETIOLOGICAL AGENT

The virus is one of the few rod shaped animal viruses. The particles are 60 to 69 mμ in diameter and 175 to 210 mμ in length (Chow *et al.,* 1954 and Bradish *et al.,* 1956). It is found in high titer in the vesicles fluids of affected animals and for a short time in the blood and saliva. The virus may be cultivated in tissue culture, in embryonating hen's eggs, and in the skin or the nervous system of a number of laboratory animals.

Virus introduced into the yolk sac or allantoic chamber of seven or eight day old embryos results in death of the embryos in about twenty-four hours. Titers of 10^4 to 10^7 embryo LD_{50} in 0.1 ml. are obtained in fluids and membranes. Incubation of eggs at temperatures of 38 to 39°C. renders them less susceptible to the virus than incubation at the lower temperatures of 35 to 36°C. (Sigurdsson, 1943). Embryos of seven to eight days are susceptible at both temperatures, although the titers of virus produced differ and older embryos of ten to eleven days are often completely refractory at the higher temperatures. Several kinds of tissue cultures, chicken fibroblasts, bovine kidney cells, human HeLa cells and guinea pig kidney cells are readily susceptible (Bachrach *et al.,* 1955; McClain and Hackett, 1958). In all instances the virus is cytopathic. Titers of 10^4 to 10^5 are obtained.

The physical stability of vesicular stomatitis virus has not been adequately defined (Hanson, 1952). At 56°C. some strains of the virus remain active from ten to fifteen minutes, others slightly longer. At the body temperatures of various mammals, i.e., 37 to 38°C. the virus may remain viable for three to four days. At 6-8°C. infectivity of the virus persists for six to eight weeks and when frozen it can be demonstrated much longer. Oxidizing compounds, weak acids and bases, and even isotonic sodium chloride are harmful to the virus. Sunlight and ultraviolet light rapidly destroy it; serum and tissue components are protective. The usual chemical disinfectants, cresol and chlorine compounds, are used in practical measures to destroy vesicular stomatitis virus.

Two immunologically distinct types of vesicular stomatitis virus are known: New Jersey and Indiana serotypes. Animals immune to one strain are still susceptible to the other. Humoral antibodies that develop following infection and which may be demonstrated by their ability to neutralize virus fail to reveal any cross reaction between the two serotypes. Complement fixing antibodies are likewise distinct. Partial identity can be shown by means of precipitin lines in gel.

Both virus types are distinguishable, on the basis of the serum neutralization or complement fixation tests, from the viruses of foot and mouth disease, vesicular exanthema, equine encephalomyelitis, pseudorabies, herpes and Colorado tick fever.

While only a few strains have been compared, it appears that the Indiana serotype of vesicular stomatitis virus differs from the New Jersey type in several ways. Most outbreaks of Indiana type virus have been in southwestern United States. It apparently occurs every year in Mexico (Camargo, 1954). New Jersey type virus is more widely distributed; and even in Mexico it is more frequently isolated than is Indiana. Reported cases of Indiana infection have been less severe than have some described cases of New Jersey infection. Indiana virus appears to be less pathogenic for cattle and horses. Experimental New Jersey virus had greater potential neuropathogenicity, as it induced death in cattle inoculated intracerebrally with the virus while the Indiana type stimulated nervous signs but did not cause death.

The viruses possess, to different degrees, the ability to vary or mutate. Intracerebral passage of New Jersey and Indiana types in mice led to the rapid development of neurotropism in the line from the New Jersey stock and to little change in Indiana type. Galloway (1933) observed that the virus particle grown in the chicken embryo appeared to be smaller when measured by filtration than virus obtained from guinea pig foot pads. He did not determine whether this change was transitory. Strains of a single serotype have been found to differ in pathogenicity. The Wisconsin isolant of the New Jersey serotype, while as pathogenic for cattle and embryonating eggs as the Missouri isolant, has often required six to ten days to produce foot pad lesions in guinea pigs rather than the usual one to two days required by the latter.

GEOGRAPHIC DISTRIBUTION

Vesicular stomatitis appears to be enzootic in the tropical and semitropical regions of America (Figure 77A). It is seen during most of the year in Colombia, Venezuela and Mexico, but the extent of the disease was never realized until facilities for its differential diagnosis from foot and mouth disease were established. More than a hundred isolations were made in Mexico during a two year period.

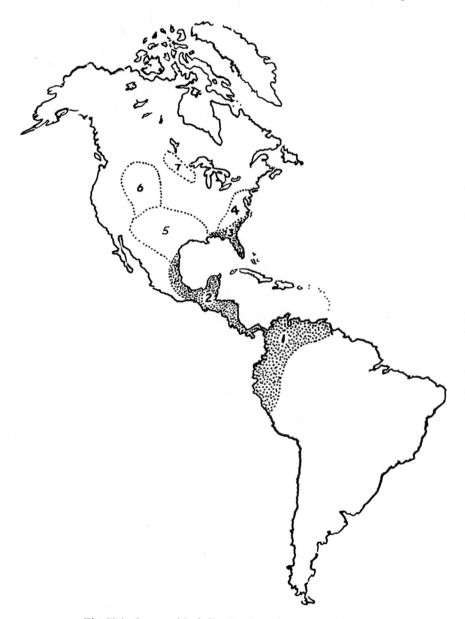

Fig. 77A. Geographical distribution of vesicular stomatitis

The disease tends to move north into the United States during the summer season appearing first in the gulf states in April or May and later in June, July or August as far north as Manitoba in Canada. Outbreaks have occurred with greater frequency in Texas and Colorado and with less frequency in Wisconsin or Montana. Three regions of the United States have suffered repeated epizootics. They are: 1) an area covering the states bordering on the Gulf of Mexico and extending up the Appalachian range to Maryland, 2) an area in the upper Mississippi Valley, and 3) an area in the Rocky Mountains.

Northeastern United States, northwestern United States, most of Canada and all of Alaska have never been known to have experienced the disease. In large areas of the United States, as the Great Plains, vesicular stomatitis has appeared as a sporadic disease generally traceable to importation of infected animals, particularly in stock yards, remount depots or serum plants. In all parts of the United States and Canada, vesicular stomatitis has been limited to the frostless season of the year.

South of Colombia and Venezuela in South America, vesicular stomatitis has been reported in Argentina and Peru. There the disease has resembled that in the United States, occurring as recurrent epizootics rather than as an enzootic.

In the eastern hemisphere vesicular stomatitis has occurred in both Africa and Europe. Theiler (1901) described two epizootics in South Africa in 1884 and 1897. There is no evidence that the disease has reappeared in South Africa since that time. Vesicular stomatitis was introduced into Europe during the 1915-1917 period by importation of American and Canadian horses for military purposes. While the disease spread to European horses and a few cattle, it failed to persist. The presence or absence of vesicular stomatitis in Asia cannot be established on present evidence.

SEASONAL PREVALENCE

Vesicular stomatitis in the temperate zones appears only during the frost-free seasons. The great majority of the cases in the United States have been reported in August and September. In tropical and semitropical regions, cases have been seen throughout the year.

ANIMAL SUSCEPTIBILITY

The virus of vesicular stomatitis has been isolated from diseased cattle, horses and hogs. Serological evidence of the natural infection of these species as well as of man and five species of wild animals has been obtained. The wild animals known to possess antibody in enzootic areas include white tailed deer, feral swine, raccoon, bobcat and skunk. The involvement of sheep and dogs cited upon isolated clinical and circumstantial evidence has not been confirmed. The experimental host range of vesicular stomatitis includes, in addition to the naturally infected species listed, six rodents—the mouse, rat, hamster, guinea pig, rabbit and chinchilla; one carnivore, the ferret; and two primates, the Cynomologus and Macacus monkeys, as well as the chicken. Two types of clinical disease are induced: first, epidermotropic following intradermal injection; or second, the neurotropic, typified by the fatal encephalitis of mice which follows intracerebral inoculation. Some animals have an inapparent infection. Infection can sometimes be induced by natural routes in these animals. Aerosols or nasal instillation produces disease of young mice, chinchillas and ferrets. Contact transmission has been observed among young pigs and between adult ferrets.

Transmission among the natural hosts, cattle, swine and horses, was once assumed to occur by contact. Theiler (1901) was the first to point out that the disease was transmitted with difficulty or not at all even when animals were in close contact, unless abrasions were present in or about the mouth. Cotton (1927) in his description of the 1926 New Jersey outbreak and Heiny (1945) in the report of Colorado outbreaks pointed out that it often is impossible to explain the spread of the disease by usual contact transmission. These observations, considered with several other lines of evidence such as: 1) the sharp seasonal prevalence, most cases occurring in August and September; 2) the disappearance of the disease during the winter months, 3) the rapidity of spread in such epizootic areas as the upper Mississippi Valley; and 4) the tendency of the disease to recur in certain geographical areas, particularly river valleys, suggest that a vector of some sort is instrumental in the transmission of the disease.

Ferris *et al.* demonstrated in 1954 that vesicular stomatitis could be transmitted in the laboratory by several species of biting Diptera. Transmission was mechanical and not biological. The biting parts, contaminated while feeding on an infected animal, were capable of transmitting the virus for a period of three or four days. The insects included mosquitoes, stable flies and horse flies.

THE DISEASE IN ANIMALS

Vesicular stomatitis is of economic consequence in cattle. The animals lose weight and, in most instances, there is a marked temporary loss in milk production which is aggravated by teat involvement.

The first and cardinal sign of the disease, salivation, develops within one to three days after infection and is found on close inspection to be associated with various degrees of maceration and exfoliation of the mucous membrane of the tongue, gums, hard palate and lips. The infective process progresses repaidly to ulceration and secondary necrosis of the partly denuded tissues, and the saliva and exudate often become quite viscid. Movement of the tongue, lips and jaws as a result of salivation and pain give rise to the smacking sounds of cattle and "grinding" of the teeth of horses.

Failure to observe vesiculation in infected animals is not unusual. The transient temperature rise which is concurrent with the vesicular stage of infection, likewise, is seldom detected in the field. Teat lesions are observed in many cattle, and often lesions of interdigital and coronary areas of the feet of otherwise affected cattle are seen.

THE DISEASE IN MAN

Burton (1918), while working with vesicular stomatitis in England during World War I, reported that he and two assistants developed the disease. Almost thirty years later three cases of vesicular stomatitis in men who had handled lesions on cows' teats were reported by Heiny (1943) in Colorado. These individuals had vesicular lesions and experienced general malaise. Neither Burton or Heiny had the opportunity to isolate the agent or obtain serological evidence of infection.

A series of five infections occurred among the laboratory personnel at the University of Wisconsin in 1950 (Hanson, *et al.*, 1950). Each individual was exposed to experimentally infected animals. The degree of response varied from a mild coryza to an illness severe enough to necessitate confinement in bed.

In a typical case (Figure 77B) the inset was repid, occurring forty-eight hours after exposure. Pain was experienced in the muscles of the legs, back and in the eyes. Mental dullness and headaches appeared early and increased in severity during the afternoon of the

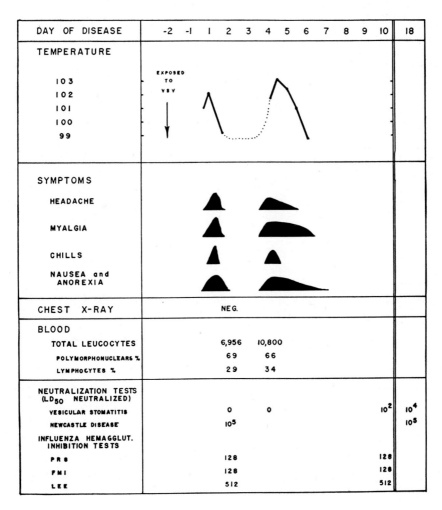

DAY OF DISEASE	-2	-I	I	2	3	4	5	6	7	8	9	10		18
TEMPERATURE														
103														
102			EXPOSED TO VSV											
101														
100														
99														
SYMPTOMS														
HEADACHE														
MYALGIA														
CHILLS														
NAUSEA and ANOREXIA														
CHEST X-RAY					NEG.									
BLOOD														
TOTAL LEUCOCYTES				6,956		10,800								
POLYMORPHONUCLEARS %				69		66								
LYMPHOCYTES %				29		34								
NEUTRALIZATION TESTS (LD$_{50}$ NEUTRALIZED)														
VESICULAR STOMATITIS				O		O						10^2		10^4
NEWCASTLE DISEASE				10^5										10^5
INFLUENZA HEMAGGLUT. INHIBITION TESTS														
P R 8				128								128		
F M I				128								128		
L E E				512								512		

Fig. 77B. Symptoms of vesicular stomatitis infection. (Courtesy of *J. Lab. & Clin. Med., 36:*1950.)

first day. The oral temperature was 102°F. at 4 P.M.; a frank chill occurred at 7 P.M. Generalized myalgia accompanied by repeated chills continued during the early evening. Between 9 and 10 P.M.

perspiration was profuse; the temperature decreased from 102 to 100°F., chills ceased, and there was symptomatical improvement. Twenty-four hours after onset, although weakness persisted, the patient considered himself recovered. At this time injection of the conjunctivae, slight oropharyngeal erythema, and a small red papule on the buccal surface of the lower lip were the only abnormalities observed. On the following day the patient continued to be subjectively well.

On the fourth day a sudden recurrence of symptoms occurred, characterized by malaise, myalgia, headache and anorexia, associated with chills and fever to 103°F. The symptoms were less severe than on the day of onset. However, the patient appeared to be acutely ill. The skin was hot and dry and the conjunctivae were injected. The papule on the buccal mucosa of the lower lip had developed into a small herpetiform ulcer about 2 mm. in diameter with punched-out edges and a clean grayish floor which was surrounded by an area of intense erythema. The tonsils were swollen. The anterior cervical and submental lymph nodes were swollen and tender, most marked on the right. Other lymphadenopathy was not evident and the spleen and liver were not palpable. The chest was clear. Fever of 101°F., malaise, anorexia and myalgia continued for the next two days. Thereafter recovery was prompt and complete except for residual weakness which persisted for a week. Specific therapy was not administered. Serum neutralizing antibodies developed within ten days from none to 10,000.

Laboratory infection with vesicular stomatitis has occurred in other laboratories. The prevalence of infection among the personnel working at the animal disease station at Beltsville, Maryland, as determined by the development of complement fixing titers is disclosed in Table 43 which was prepared by Dr. Mott of the Bureau of Animal Industry. Three types of contact are tabulated. The laboratory workers had had frequent exposures to both types of viruses and five possessed complement fixing antibodies to both types of virus. The animal caretakers tended infected cattle, swine and horses in the isolation barns. The trainees were a group of field men who spent two weeks studying the disease, handling infected animals and materials. Among those who had contact with the disease, 54 per cent developed specific titers and 35 per cent reported clinical symptoms.

Although the virus was not isolated in either Wisconsin or Maryland, virus was isolated from a cutaneous form of the disease in man. Dr. Schoening of the Bureau of Animal Industry and formerly with the Mexican-American Foot and Mouth Disease Commission described in a personal communication an accident occurring in the Palo Alto Laboratory in Mexico in which the finger of a worker was infected with New Jersey type vesicular stomatitis virus. In forty-eight hours a large vesicle 3 cm. long developed. Fluid from the vesicle caused food pad lesions in guinea pigs typical of vesicular stomatitis virus.

TABLE 43

PREVALENCE OF VESICULAR STOMATITIS AMONG A GROUP OF 55 MEN AT BELTSVILLE, MARYLAND, ON THE BASIS OF COMPLEMENT FIXING ANTIBODIES

Type of Exposure	*NJ-CF Antibodies*	*Ind-CF Antibodies*	*Non-Specific CF Reaction***	*Negative*	*Total*	*% Developed Positive Titers*	*% Developed Symptoms*
Lab workers	6* (6)	7* (6)	1	0	9	100	87
Animal caretakers	2 (1)	2 (1)	2	7	13	36	18
Trainees	0	8 (4)	7 (2)	10	25	44	22
No contact	0	0	0	8	8	0	0
Total	8 (7)	17 (11)	10 (2)	25	55		

*Five possessed both New Jersey (NJ) and Indiana (Ind) CF antibodies.
**Cases not included in percentage figures.
( )Number in bracket is the number which experienced clinical symptoms of disease.

In 1955, Fellowes *et al.* reported the isolation of virus from the blood of an individual who became infected in a laboratory. The virus was recovered in chicken embryos and shown by neutralization tests to be New Jersey serotype. It produced typical lesions in bovine tongue and guinea pig foot pads. Antibodies for vesicular stomatitis, New Jersey serotype, were found in the sera of the individual fourteen and eighty days after infection.

Reports from farmers and veterinarians living in northern Wisconsin in the area of the 1949 vesicular stomatitis epizootic suggest that human cases occurred during that outbreak (Brandley, *et al.,* 1951). The similarity of the disease which develops in man to many other mild febrile conditions, particularly influenza and herpangina, would make clinical diagnosis most difficult. Presumably, isolation of the virus or serological tests would have to be relied upon to distinguish the disease.

Vesicular stomatitis virus is a common human pathogen in regions in which the virus is enzootic in the livestock population (Hanson and Karstad, 1956). Approximately 30 per cent of a group of human serum samples obtained by the State Public Health Laboratory at Waycross in southeast Georgia contained neutralizing antibodies to New Jersey type vesicular stomatitis. All individuals possessing antibody lived in rural communities or spent part of their time in such areas. Many lived on farms where cattle and swine had neutralizing antibodies. The nature of the disease caused by vesicular stomatitis virus in rural human populations is yet unknown. Presumably it is similar to the disease described among laboratory workers. It may cause a portion of the febrile illnesses which are common among farmers in southern Georgia. Two instances are on record in which such individuals developed antibody to vesicular stomatitis virus following a febrile illness.

Serious sequelae, particularly orchitis, have been ascribed to vesicular stomatitis virus in man. Evidence to substantiate such claims has not been presented.

PREVENTION AND CONTROL

A practical method of preventing the spread of the disease among cattle has not been devised. Infection of livestock appears to be primarily dependent upon exposure to an effective vector. Since stabled animals and animals kept in open, upland pastures rarely have been infected, animals could be managed to avoid infection. A vaccine for swine has been studied. Whether a vaccine will eventually be marketed depends upon research and upon the economics of livestock production. Animals are usually given plenty of water and placed on soft feeds. If food intake can be maintained, weight losses will be minimized and recovery speeded. Available antibiotics have not been effective in treatment. Means by which man can avoid infection in an enzootic area are not known. By exercise of due precaution in handling the virus, laboratory workers should be able to avoid infection.

ITEMS OF NOTE

1. Vesicular stomatitis is a virus disease of cattle, swine and horses resembling foot and mouth disease clinically.

2. Vesicular stomatitis appears to be enzootic in tropical and subtropical America from where it moves northward during the sum-

mer and creates, in certain years, widespread epizootics in the United States.

3. The virus is readily cultivated in embryonating eggs, tissue cultures and mice. Many laboratory animals are susceptible.

4. Vesicular stomatitis in man resembles influenza, being characterized by a fever, general malaise and myalgia.

5. Diagnosis of vesicular stomatitis virus infection of man and other animals should be based on a history of exposure, clinical observations and demonstration of the development of specific antibodies or isolation of the virus.

REFERENCES

BACHRACH, H. L., CALLIS, J. J., and HESS, W. R.: The growth and cytopathogenicity of vesicular stomatitis virus in tissue culture. *J. Immunol., 75:*186-191, 1955.

BRADISH, C. J., BROOKSBY, J. B., and DILLON, J. F., JR.: Biophysical studies of the virus system of vesicular stomatitis. *J. Gen. Microbiol., 14:*290-314, 1956.

BRANDLY, C. A., HANSON, R. P., and CHOW, T. L.: Vesicular stomatitis with particular reference to the 1949 Wisconsin epizootic. *Proc. Book, Am. Vet. M.A.,* 61-69, 1951.

BURTON, A. C.: Stomatitis contagiosa in horses. *Vet. J., 73:*234-242, 1917.

CAMARGO, N. C.: A contribution to the study of vesicular stomatitis in Mexico. *U. S. Livestock San. A., 58:*379-389, 1954.

CHOW, T. L., CHOW, FU HO, and HANSON, R. P.: Morphology of vesicular stomatitis virus. *J. Bact., 68:*724-726, 1954.

COTTON, W. E.: Vesicular stomatitis. *Vet. Med., 22:*169-175, 1927.

FELLOWES, O. N., DIMOPOULLOS, G. T., and CALLIS, J. J.: Isolation of vesicular stomatitis virus from an infected laboratory worker. *Am. J. Vet. Res., 16:*623-626, 1955.

FERRIS, D., HANSON, R. P., DICKE, R. J., and ROBERTS, R. H.: Experimental transmission of vesicular stomatitis virus by Diptera. *J. Infect. Dis., 96:*184-192, 1955.

GALLOWAY, I. A., and ELFORD, W. J.: The differentiation of the virus of vesicular stomatitis from that of foot and mouth disease with particular reference to a rapid and certain method of resolving mixtures of the two viruses. *Brit. J. Exper. Path., 16:* 588-613, 1933.

HANSON, R. P., and KARSTAD, L.: Enzootic vesicular stomatitis. *Proc. U. S. Livestock San. A., 16:*288-292, 1956.

HANSON, R. P., RASMUSSEN, A. F., BRANDLY, C. A., and BROWN, J. W.: Human infection with the virus of vesicular stomatitis. *J. Lab. & Clin. Med., 36:*754-758, 1950.

HANSON, R. P.: The natural history of vesicular stomatitis virus. *Bact. Rev., 16:*179-204, 1952.

HEINY, F.: Vesicular stomatitis in cattle and horses in Colorado. *North Am. Vet., 26:* 726-730, 1945.

KARSTAD, L. H., ADAMS, E. V., HANSON, R. P., and FERRIS, D. H.: Evidence for the role of wildlife in epizootics of vesticular stomatitis. *J.A.V.M.A., 129:*95-96, 1956.

McCLAIN, M. E., and HACKETT, A. J.: A comparative study of the growth of vesicular stomatitis virus in the tissue culture systems. *J. Immunol., 80:*356-361, 1958.

SIGURDSSON, B.: The influence of host and temperature incubation on infection of the chick embryo with vesicular stomatitis virus. *J. Exper. Med., 78:*17-26, 1943.

THEILER, S.: Eine contagiöse Stomatitis des Pferdes in Süd-Afrika. *Deutsch tierarztl. Wochenschr., 9:*131-132, 1901.

Chapter 12

THE POX DISEASES OF MAN AND ANIMALS

D. W. Bruner, B.S., D.V.M., Ph.D.

Smallpox, or *variola,* is a disease primarily of man. It is ordinarily transmitted directly from man to man. It can, however, be transmitted by inoculation to a variety of animal species, in which it is generally quite mild and usually localized. Rarely the infection is transmitted from smallpox patients to animals by natural contacts. When smallpox virus becomes adapted to animals, it generally loses much of its virulence for man, and when carried back to man, by inoculation, the disease produced is mild and localized and is known as *vaccinia.* Vaccinia confers immunity in man to smallpox, and vaccination has long been used for protecting people against this dangerous and disfiguring malady.

Diseases with skin eruptions similar to those of smallpox in man occur in cattle, horses, swine, sheep, goats, rabbits, and other mammals. We also have pox diseases in birds but the manifestations are somewhat different from those in mammals. Generally the animal poxes are naturally restricted to their own host species but experimentally most of those affecting mammals can be inoculated successfully into rabbits, and some of them into other animal species. In experimental animals the character of the lesions is practically alike, irrespective of the original host species. These facts have led many to believe that the pox diseases of man and other mammals have originated from a common stem and that the host specificity seen today is the result of adaptations to different hosts. The relationship of the virus adapted to cattle (cowpox) to the one adapted to man (smallpox) is particularly interesting and important.

HISTORY OF SMALLPOX

The history of smallpox has been lost in prehistoric times. Its original home is not known but the earliest records show that it prevailed in the Orient. The first precise description of the disease was given by Rhazes, an Arabian physician, in the ninth century, A.D. It is certain, however, that it had existed for several centuries before the Christian era in China. The *pesta magna* described by Galen in the second century is believed to have been smallpox. The disease was prevalent in the sixth century and it existed among the crusaders who carried it from Asia Minor into the countries of western Europe. The disease was a scourge in Europe throughout the middle ages and later. During the 18th century it has been estimated that as many as 60,000,000 people died of it. Most children contracted it, and those who escaped it in childhood generally suffered from it later in life. Numerous references in English literature indicate the fear and terror which it inspired in the popular mind. Ben Jonson, about 1600, wrote:

> 'Envious and foule disease, could there not be,
> One beautie in an age and free from thee.'

Lord Macauley has given a powerful word picture of conditions about 1700:

> 'The small pox was always present, filling the churchyard with corpses, tormenting with constant fears all whom it had not stricken, leaving on those whose lives it spared the hideous traces of its power, turning the babe into a changeling at which the mother shuddered, and making the eyes and cheeks of the betrothed maiden objects of horror to the lover.'

Smallpox was introduced into the Western Hemisphere by the Spaniards shortly after the continent had been discovered by Columbus. There it proceeded to devastate the Indian population. Catlin has estimated that at least 6,000,000 of them died with the disease prior to the time that the continent was heavily colonized by the white men. Similar pictures of the disease have been presented from many other parts of the world.

It was under conditions such as these that Edward Jenner was reared. Jenner was a country doctor, practicing in western England. It was he who showed the way to change smallpox from the devastating disease that it had long been, to the much milder one that we know today. In 1798, Jenner published a pamphlet entitled *An Inquiry into the Causes and Effects of the Variolae Vaccinae, a Disease*

Discovered in Some of the Western Counties of England, Particularly Gloucestershire, and Known by the Name of the Cow Pox in which he showed that it was possible to protect people against smallpox by "vaccinating" them with lymph taken from the lesions of cowpox. It seemed that it was common gossip at the time among country folk that an infection with the mild cowpox would give them protection against the deadly smallpox. To determine whether this belief was correct, Jenner, on May 14, 1796, collected lymph from the hand of Sarah Nelms, a dairy maid affected with cowpox, and transferred it to the arms of James Phipps, an eight-year-old boy. A typical "take" followed. Six weeks later the boy was inoculated with smallpox. He proved to be immune to it. Such experiments were multipled with the same results. It was true that the mild cowpox would immunize to the virulent smallpox and the method soon was widely used for this purpose.

Probably the first vaccinations in America were done by Waterhouse who, in 1800, vaccinated his own son with cowpox lymph obtained from England, dried upon threads. In 1802 an experiment was conducted in Boston in which nineteen boys were vaccinated. Three months later, twelve of them were infected with smallpox without result. Two others, not previously vaccinated, developed the disease following inoculation with the same virulent material which had been used on the vaccinated boys. These experiments did much to develop faith in vaccination as a means of controlling smallpox in America.

THE ETIOLOGIC AGENTS

All of the pox diseases are caused by filtrable viruses. They are characterized, in mammals, by the appearance of skin eruptions which begin as papules and later become pustules with characteristic umbilications in their centers. Before the skin eruption appears, virus can be found in the blood and internal organs of persons suffering from either variola or vaccinia. In the cells of the deeper layers of the corium of the affected skin in all pox diseases, characteristic bodies may be found. Those of smallpox were first described by Guarnieri in 1892 and they were regarded by him as the cause of the disease. In his honor they are now known as Guarnieri bodies. They are relatively large and stain readily with tissue stains. They lie in the cytoplasm of the affected cells. The exact nature of these bodies is still uncertain but they belong to a group of such structures, found in many virus diseases, which are now known as *inclusion bodies*. They cannot of themselves be the causative agent of small-pox, because the virus is filtrable through Berkefeld filters whereas Guarnieri bodies are far too large to pass such filters.

Structures similar to Guarnieri bodies are found in the pox lesions of all animals. Some of them are given other names, e.g., the Bollenger bodies of fowlpox, but most of them are unnamed.

In 1906, Paschen described small bodies, much smaller than the Guarnieri bodies, in the lymph and infected epithelial cells of the lesions of vaccinia in children. Paul inoculated the cornea of the eye of rabbits with suspensions of these bodies, washed free of extraneous matter, and produced characteristic pox lesions that contained Guarnieri bodies. These findings have been corroborated by many others. The minute bodies are now known as Paschen bodies, or elementary bodies. Because purified suspensions readily produce pox, and because they agglutinate in immune serum, the bodies are now regarded as the virus elements. They measure about 0.2 microns in diameter, and readily pass through the coarser Berkefeld filters. They are among the largest of the viruses according to Elford and Andrews. Studies with the electron microscope show that these bodies are cuboidal in shape. Electron micrographs of films made from suspensions remind one of a large number of dice.

Similar elementary bodies have been found in the other pox diseases. Those of fowlpox are known as Borrel bodies. They have been thoroughly studied by Woodruff and Goodpasture who found that they were resistant to tryptic digestion and thus could be freed from tissue elements by digesting the suspensions with artificial pancreatic juice. Suspensions of such purified bodies readily produce fowlpox. When the bodies are centrifuged out of suspension the supernatant fluid becomes innocuous. These experiments strengthen the belief that the bodies actually constitute the virus of pox.

Pox virus is destroyed by heating at 100° C for three minutes. It is especially resistant to drying. According to Paschen, dried vaccine virus will remain viable for as long as 229 days. It is resistant to many common disinfectants. In 0.5 to 1.0 per cent phenol solution the virus remains alive for long periods. Commercial vaccine virus is commonly preserved in 50 per cent glycerol solution plus a dye, brilliant green, since these agents have little effect on the virus but tend to restrain multiplication and eventually destroy any bacteria which may be present.

Vaccine virus may be propagated indefinitely by serial passage through rabbits which have been inoculated either on the cornea of the eye or into the tissue of the testicle. Parker and Nye cultivated the virus, free of bacteria, in tissue cultures of cells taken from the testes of the rabbit. Rivers cultivated vaccine virus in pure culture in minced chick embryo suspended in Tyrode's solution. Goodpasture, Woodruff, and Buddingh used the chorioallantoic membrane of the developing chick embryo for the same purpose. By the use of these special technics, the elementary bodies of vaccinia have been collected in large amounts for study and for the making of vaccine.

THE ANIMAL POXES

Jenner believed that smallpox, cowpox, and an eruption occurring on the pasterns of horses which was known as "grease" were modified forms of the same disease. Early in the 19th century observations were made in both Europe and America which indicated that cowpox and smallpox were identical diseases except that one occurred in cattle and the other in man. The Lyons Commission in France about 1864 produced lesions in cows identical with those of cowpox by inoculating them with material from cases of human smallpox. Freyer not only produced typical vaccinia in cows by the use of smallpox material, but he used lymph from these animals for successful vaccination of people. These results have been confirmed by many and are now accepted facts. The virus of smallpox can readily be converted into the virus of vaccinia by animal passage. None has been able to change the virus of vaccinia into that of smallpox.

Methods of artificial culture of vaccinia virus have made it possible to collect large numbers of elementary bodies in a relatively pure state. With such suspensions it is possible to conduct most of the serological tests that are used for establishing the identity of strains of bacteria. Agglutinins, lysins, and complement-fixing bodies have been produced which react with the elementary bodies in the same way that such antibodies react with bacteria. These antibodies react with the elementary bodies of variola and vaccinia alike. The viruses of smallpox and cowpox are considered to be virtually identical immunologically.

Cowpox and PseudoCowpox (Paravaccinia). The literature on naturally-occurring cowpox is conflicting and confusing. It seems likely that there are at least two entities, perhaps more, that are included in the clinical syndrome. One of these is the true cowpox, already discussed, which is immunologically closely related to small-pox in man. This infection can be transmitted easily from cow to cow by inoculation, and recovered animals are thereafter highly resistant to inoculation with vaccine virus. This is the classical cow-

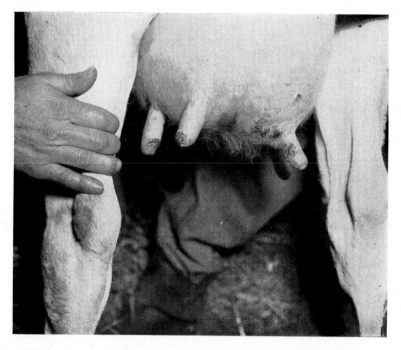

Fig. 78A. Pox lesions on the teats of a cow. (From Hagan and Bruner: *Infectious Diseases of Domestic Animals,* 4th Ed. Ithaca, New York, Comstock.)

pox of Jenner—the one that conveyed smallpox resistance to the milkers. This disease apparently was much more common in Europe and America a century ago than it is at present. Because smallpox was also more prevalent then than now, it seems likely that the bovine disease had its reservoir in the human family. In more recent times there have been a number of reports of cowpox outbreaks in dairy herds as a result of infection from recently vaccinated milkers. Boerner has reported such an outbreak in Pennsylvania in which the infection, introduced in this way, spread through an entire herd and a number of persons were infected secondarily. Another such outbreak was reported by Sayer and Amoss in New York in which two herds were infected by the same recently-vaccinated milker and in which additional milking personnel in both herds became infected. There have been other reports both from this country and abroad, and additional instances are known which have never been reported in the literature. These experiences teach the lesson that *recently vaccinated persons should never be permitted to work as milkers on dairy farms until their vaccine reactions are well healed.*

A disease which is universally known as cowpox is common in all dairy districts in this country and in Europe as well. The lesions occur for the most part on the teats but often on the skin surface of the udder itself. They begin as papules which change to vesicles and finally pustules. The vesicles often coalesce and those on the teats usually rupture through the friction of the milking process, leaving raw surfaces. These become covered with dry crusts. Healing is delayed in milking animals by the breaking off of the scabs in milking. When such lesions occur near the end of the teats, they often pave the way for bacterial invasion of the udder and the production of cases of suppurative mastitis. If mastitis does not result, the general health of the animals is not noticeably affected, but the soreness of the teats makes them difficult to milk. The disease usually spreads through the herd, obviously by the milking process since nonlactating animals usually escape infection.

This disease deserves more study than has been given it so far. For several reasons it seems obvious that it is not true cowpox. For one thing, infection of the people who handle and milk these animals very seldom occurs and when it does the clinical picture is not that described by Jenner and by others. More convincing perhaps is the fact, shown by Christen in Switzerland, and confirmed by Hester, Boley, and Graham and Gibbons in this country, that vaccine virus neither prevents this disease, nor does this disease render the animals insusceptible to subsequent vaccination. Also, Christen, and Hester, Boley, and Graham, were not successful in transmitting the disease by inoculation to normal cattle. This does not accord with the experience of many who worked with the genuine cowpox in past years. The commonly-occurring disease which we call cowpox today obviously is not cowpox, or it is a pox strain which has become more closely adapted to cattle and less adapted to man than those of earlier days. In the German literature the disease has been called para-vaccinia. English and American authors have referred to it as pseudo-cowpox. Its relation to an affliction of man will be discussed in the next chapter (see Chapter 13).

THE POXES OF ANIMALS OTHER THAN CATTLE

Horsepox. This disease, also known as contagious pustular stoma-titis of horses, now seems to be rare in Europe and there are no records of its occurrence in North America. According to Zwick, who investigated the disease thoroughly, the causative agent is the virus of vaccinia. The disease is characterized by papules, vesicles, and pustules which appear on the mucous membrane of the mouth and occasionally on the skin.

Sheeppox. According to reports this disease often is quite prev-alent and destructive in southeastern Europe. It has not been re-ported in North America. The virus can easily be transmitted to other sheep but is not readily transmitted to rabbits or other species. Inclusion bodies resembling those seen in vaccinia are found in the affected epithelial cells.

Similar in many respects to sheeppox, except that it is usually localized in the mucous membrane of the lips, is the disease known as "sore mouth" or contagious ecthyma. This is a very common dis-ease on the sheep ranges of our western states, and many farm flocks in other parts of the country frequently become infected (see Chap-ter 14).

Swinepox. This is a rather common disease in this country and abroad. In general it is not considered to be serious, but there are those who feel that its importance is greater than is generally thought. The lesions are usually found on the under parts of the body and it is known that the common hog louse plays an important role in the spread of the disease. As in cattle, it is obvious that there are two different diseases masquerading under the name of pox in swine. One of these is the true pox, associated with a virus that is closely related to vaccinia, and the other is caused by an unrelated virus. True swinepox is reported in Europe but there are no authen-tic reports of its existence in America. The so-called swinepox of this country cannot be transmitted to animals other than swine, according to McNutt, Murray, and Purwin; Schwarte and Biester; and Shope. There are no reports of the American disease having been transmitted to man.

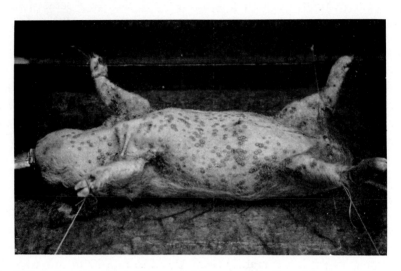

Fig. 78B. Swinepox. (From Hagan and Bruner: *Infectious Diseases of Domestic Animals,* 4th Ed., Ithaca, New York, Comstock.)

Fowlpox. The pox diseases of birds (chickens, pigeons, turkeys, canaries, etc.) are caused by viruses which are not closely related to vaccinia, immunologically. Neither do the lesions resemble those of true pox in mammals. They are seen most frequently around the head but also occur on the feathered portions of the body. They consist generally of epithelial thickenings, rather than of vesicles and pustules as in mammals. In the affected cells there are bodies which resemble the Guarnieri and Paschen bodies of vaccinia. The bird poxes usually affect only the species in which they originate, but a certain amount of cross immunity can be produced by inoculation, thus pigeonpox virus is used practically for immunizing laying hens against chickenpox. Vaccinia virus does not easily "take" on birds, and does not immunize against the bird viruses, and vice versa.

PREPARATION AND USE OF VACCINE VIRUS

Smallpox vaccine has been produced on a commercial scale longer than any other of the biologic products used for prophylaxis. For many years all vaccine was produced by propagating the virus on the scarified skins of calves, and much of it is still made in this way. Animals with white skins and weighing up to 250 pounds are preferred. They are carefully examined for any abnormalities before being purchased for vaccine manufacture. This includes tests for tuberculosis and brucellosis. They are then kept in quarantine for observation for a week or more. After the vaccine is harvested the animals are destroyed and subjected to a postmortem examination as a final check on their health before the pulp is processed for use.

It appears that most, if not all, vaccine made in this country is manufactured from the same strain of virus which probably originated from Jenner's stock. It is produced under license from the National Institutes of Health which, under law, has the responsibility of setting up regulations for all biological products intended for use on man and which go into interstate trade.

From time to time manufacturers pass their virus strain through rabbits or through man because it tends to lose its effectiveness as an immunizing agent. Except for this, the strain is maintained constantly by passage through calves. For vaccine production, the hair is clipped and the animal thoroughly washed. It is then fastened to an operating table which exposes the abdomen and the inner aspect of the thighs, and these areas are shaved and thoroughly scrubbed. Sterile water, soap, and brushes are used for this process. When the area is ready, inoculation is done with a metal scarifier which makes superficial, longitudinal scratches about 0.5 to 1.0 cm apart. No blood is drawn. The "seed pulp" which may have come from a rabbit or from another calf is then applied and rubbed in with a spreader. After the pulp has dried on the skin, the animal is released from the table and returned to its stall. No dressing is applied to the scarified area. The animal is fed as usual, and is allowed to lie down at will. The stall is kept scrupulously clean. Some manufacturers spray the scarified area daily with a 1:1,000 aqueous solution of brilliant green. This helps to restrain bacterial growth but does not affect development of the virus.

The vaccine pulp is collected about the sixth or seventh day. After the whole area has been carefully washed with sterile water and dried with sterile towels, the dried crusts are removed and discarded and the pulpy material lying underneath is collected with a curette and placed in sterile bottles. The calf is anaesthetized during this process, and destroyed immediately afterward. The vaccine "pulp" contains not only the vaccinia virus but a considerable number of bacteria, some of which may be pathogenic.

For many years the extraneous microorganisms in vaccine pulp have been reduced by mixing it with 50 per cent glycerol and 1.0 per cent phenol, and storing it for some time at a temperature of about 5° F. Investigations in the New York City Health Department have shown that the dye, brilliant green, in a final concentration of 1:10,000 does not affect the virus but greatly hastens the destruction of bacteria. It is frequently used for this purpose. Recent work has shown that the virus is not affected by concentrations of penicillin which will destroy streptococci and some of the noxious anaerobes.

Tests for purity and potency are made before the vaccine pulp suspension is placed in capillary tubes for clinical use. The vaccine must be free from tetanus bacilli and relatively free of all bacteria. Its virulence is tested on the shaved skin of rabbits. It is considered satisfactory in this respect when numerous typical pustules result from rubbing a 1:1,000 suspension of the finished product into the shaved area.

In years past vaccine virus was dried on bone "points" or used in bulk. Regulations now prohibit any distribution except in sealed capillary glass tubes.

The virus may also be grown for vaccine purposes on the chorioallantoic membrane of the chick embryo or in chick embryo tissue culture. Because the virus is grown under sterile conditions problems of bacterial contamination are avoided. Glycerol and other substance do not need to be added to destroy bacteria. However, these vaccines do not seem to be as effective immunizing agents as the calf lymph preparation, possibly because of adaptive changes to chicken tissue.

EFFICACY OF VACCINE VIRUS

The protective power of vaccine virus has been demonstrated on numerous instances. In Sweden during the twenty-eight years before vaccination (1774-1801) the annual death rate from smallpox per million population averaged 2,050; in the forty years following vaccination, smallpox deaths averaged only 158.

Wherever a determined effort has been made to vaccinate a large part of the population, smallpox has almost disappeared; when laxity begins to prevail smallpox again becomes prevalent. This was strikingly illustrated in England and in the Philippine Islands.

In England and Wales, smallpox vaccination was voluntary prior to 1871. In that year vaccination of infants became compulsory.

The reduction of the incidence of smallpox was spectacular. The deaths from this disease immediately before and after this legislation, reported by decades was as follows:

1867-1876	52,218
1877-1886	18,026
1887-1896	5,092
1897-1906	4,761
1907-1916	139
1917-1926	138

In 1898, a "conscience" clause was introduced into the English law which exempted from vaccination those who claimed conscientious scruples against this practice. This had no immediate effect on the incidence of the disease because the few unprotected individuals were relatively well protected from exposure because of the fact that most of their contacts were vaccinated persons. As the number of susceptibles increased, however, smallpox returned and the increase was notable after about 1930.

In the Philippine Islands, prior to the time of the American occupation, there were about 40,000 deaths annually from smallpox. Compulsory vaccination caused the disappearance of the disease in all areas where it was applied. The mortality in Manila and surrounding provinces fell from 6,000 annually to zero. For seven years prior to 1914 there was not a single death from smallpox in Manila. Then laxity occurred and the disease reappeared. In 93 per cent of the cases, the victims were unvaccinated. Resumption of enforcement of the compulsory vaccination law again caused the disease to disappear.

Formerly smallpox was widespread and deadly in the United States. After 1900 most of the numerous outbreaks were of the mild, nonfatal type of the disease, but often these outbreaks became malignant and fatal. As late as 1929, 42,282 cases of smallpox were reported to the United States Public Health Service. The enactment of compulsory vaccination laws by many of the states, and the general recognition of the desirability of childhood vaccination has resulted in the elimination of the disease in the United States. The number of cases reported in recent years in the United States are as follows:

1946	356	1949	48
1947	173	1950	37
1948	56	1960	0

Smallpox continues to take a heavy toll in many parts of the world where vaccination is not generally practiced. It is especially prevalent and virulent in many parts of Asia. As late as 1945, more than 100,000 cases were reported from India alone.

Certain criticisms have been advanced against vaccination. One is that it spreads syphilis. This was possible and probable under the old method of transferring scabs directly from arm to arm; under the present procedure of manufacturing vaccine virus it is impossible. Another is that it is responsible for tetanus. In 1903 Rosenau showed that some of the vaccine virus offered for sale in the United States contained tetanus spores. In 1917, McCoy and Bengston demonstrated the presence of tetanus organisms on bone-point scarifiers which were at that time in use for performing vaccinations. Regulations at the present time are sufficiently stringent to prevent the distribution of vaccine virus contaminated with tetanus spores. Armstrong has studied postvaccination tetanus occurring in thirty-two states in this country between 1914 and 1928. He found that dressings, bunion pads, shields, and the like were responsible for the few cases of tetanus that developed. Recent methods of vaccination recommended by the United States Public Health Service absolutely avoid all dangers of tetanus infection.

Another complication that is rarely observed is generalized vaccinia infection. This is seen most often in persons who suffer from eczema. Such persons should not be vaccinated while their disesase is active, or great precautions should be taken to see that the vaccination site is so protected that virus is not likely to reach the eczematous areas. It should be kept in mind also that persons suffering from eczema should be protected against accidental infection from other recently vaccinated persons (see Ellis; Graves and Dowman).

Still another complication is postvaccination encephalitis. This complication is rare. It appears to occur more often in Europe than in the United States for reasons that are not clear. It is probable that some vaccine virus strains have a greater predeliction for nerve tissue than others, and that greater incidences in some areas rather than others may be due to this factor. A study of a sixty-year-history of vaccination in Germany, made in 1935, showed that the complications of vaccination are not sufficiently serious to warrant the weakening of compulsory vaccination laws.

ITEMS OF NOTE

1) Smallpox of man and the pox diseases of several of the lower animals are definitely related. This is especially true of the disease in cattle.

2) Smallpox virus, passed through cattle by natural contact or artificial inoculation, becomes weakened for man and can be used for preventive inoculation. This is the vaccine (Latin, vacca = calf) virus used for vaccination.

3) Vaccine virus has been proved by more than a century of experience to be efficient in suppressing outbreaks of smallpox, and in preventing their occurrence.

4) Present governmental regulations insure that vaccine virus is a harmless product for use on man.*

REFERENCES

ARMSTRONG, CHAS.: *U.S. Pub. Health Rep., 40:*1351, 1925.
ARMSTRONG, CHAS.: *J.A.M.A., 90:*738, 1928.
BOERNER, F., JR.: *J.A.V.M.A., 64:*93, 123.
BUDDINGH, G. J.: *Am. J. Pub. Health,* 27:1135, 1937.
CHRISTEN: *Schweiz. Arch., 81:*53 and 108, 1939.
ELFORD, W. J. and ANDREWS, C. H.: *Brit. J. Exp., Path., 13:*36, 1932.
ELLIS, F. A.: *J.A.M.A., 104:*1891, 1935.
FREYER, *Zeitschr, Hyg., 23:*322, 1896.
GIBBONS, W. J.: *Cornell Vet., 34:*235, 1944.
GOODPASTURE, E. W., WOODRUFF, A. M. and BUDDINGH, G. J.: *Am. J. Path., 8:*271, 1932.
GRAVES, G. W. and DOWMAN, C.: *N. Y. State J. Med., 37:*1833, 1937.
GUARNIERI, G.: *Centrbl. Bakt.* 16:299, 1894.
HESTER, H. B., BOLEY, L. E. and GRAHAM, R.: *Cornell Vet., 31:*360, 1941.
KRUMWIEDE, C., FIELDER, F. S., and WATSON, T. A.: *J. Infect. Dis., 22:*118, 1918.
LYONS COMMISSION: *Report of Rev. gen. med. Vet.,* 1865.
McCOY, G. W. and BENGSTON, I. A.: *Hyg. Lab. Bull., 115:* (1918), U.S. Pub. Health Service.

---

*The author wishes to thank William A. Hagan, D.V.M. for his contributions to this chapter.

McNutt, S. H., Murray, C. and Purwin, P.: *J.A.V.M.A., 74:*752, 1929.

Newsom, I. E. and Cross, F.: *J.A.V.M.A., 84:*799, 1934.

Parker, F. and Nye, R. N.: *Am. J. Path., 1:*325 and 327, 1925.

Paschen, E.: *Arch. Kinderheilk., 47:*168, 1908.

Paul, G.: *Deutsch. med. Wchnschr., 39:*2136, 1913.

Rosenau, M. J.: *Hyg. Lab. Bull., 16:* (1903), U.S. Pub. Health Service.

Rivers, Thos. M.: *J. Exper. Med., 54:*453, 1931.

Sayer, S. W. and Amoss, F. B.: *N. Y. State J. Med., 36:*1163, 1936.

Schwarte, L. H. and Biester, H. E.: *A.J.V.R., 2:*136, 1941.

Shope, R. E.: *J. Bact., 39:*39, 1940.

Chapter 13

MILKER'S NODULES

D. W. Bruner, B.S., D.V.M., Ph.D.

Two kinds of lesions occur on persons who have a history of associating with cattle suffering from a skin affection that involves the udder and teats and is commonly diagnosed as cowpox. Both types usually infect the hands and forearms of milkers, suggesting that they are infections contracted by direct contact with the lesions of the cows. Frequently, if not always, the lesions appear where there have been abrasions of the skin.

One of these types develops in the form of discrete, usually multiple papules which progress through vesicular and pustular stages to crusts which finally fall off leaving a healed surface. These lesions are typical of vaccinia, and they induce immunity to variola or smallpox as was first shown by Edward Jenner. Such lesions are described and illustrated in many of the earlier textbooks, and it appears that they were not uncommon in early times. Such lesions have not been reported in this country in many years, and Taylor says that they are rare in England today although quite common many years ago.

The second syndrome in man associated with "cowpox" in cattle is known under the name of "milker's nodules" or "milker's warts." These lesions appear on the hands of milkers and usually are not numerous. In most instances only one or two occur, however Groth saw a case in a German milkmaid in which there were forty on one hand and twenty on the other. Milker's nodules begin as papules surrounded by erythematous areas in from five to seven days after exposure. They gradually enlarge into firm, elastic, bluish-red nodules from one to two centimeters in diameter. There is never any evidence of pustulation. Usually they are quite painless but frequently they induce an itching sensation. Sometimes there is slight swelling of the axillary lymph nodes. Having attained full development the nodules are semiglobular with a slight central depression in their centers. Gradually they tend to flatten as healing progresses. If the grayish epithelium is broken the substance of the lesion is observed to consist of highly vascular granulation tissue. From four to six weeks are required for complete involution of these nodules. Healing occurs without a break in the integument and usually no scars

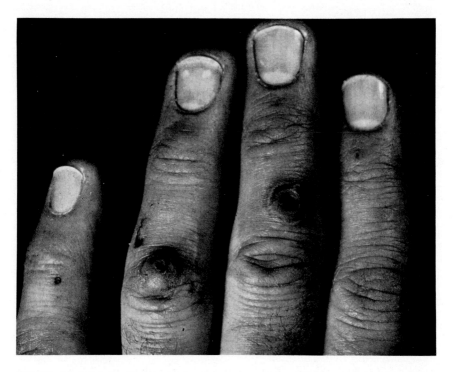

Fig. 79. Nodules on the hand of a dairyman. (From Hagan and Bruner: *Infectious Diseases of Domestic Animals,* 4th Ed. Ithaca, New York, Comstock.)

are left. Bonnevie, in Denmark, and Brants, in Latvia, describe secondary efflorescences on other parts of the body. Hagan states that he has seen one such case in New York State. When these occur, and they do not appear to be common, the rash develops well after the primary nodules and it usually disappears within one week, long before the nodules have become absorbed. It is believed that these rashes are of allergic or toxic origin.

PREVALENCE

Milker's nodules have been described by a number of European workers representing a number of different countries and indicate that the condition is wide-spread. The only description of them in the United States is that of Becker. Hagan has seen two cases, both associated with the same outbreak of pseudopox, and inquiry has shown that the condition has been observed by many veterinarians and dairymen. It seems that the disease is not nearly so frequent in man, however, as is the corresponding disease in cattle. Apparently man is not highly susceptible to infection, or perhaps peculiar conditions are required for its transmission from cattle to man.

THE CAUSE OF MILKER'S NODULES

The relationship of these lesion to pox or poxlike lesions in cattle is clear. It is not so clear, however, whether the nodules are the result of the virus of true cowpox, or of a pseudopox producing agent.

In Germany, Schultz, Seifried, and Schaaf produced poxlike lesions on a calf by inoculating it with material from what they considered to be a milker's nodule. From this calf they obtained a virus which caused infection when inoculated into other animal species including the rabbit. In the cornea of the rabbit Guarnieri bodies were produced. After recovery from the inoculations, the animals proved refractory to reinoculations with the same virus and with vaccinia virus as well. They thus proved that they were working with a virus identical with or at least very closely related to that of cowpox. They believed that this virus was the cause of the milker's nodules, which the Germans call "Steinpocken," "Warzenpocken," or "Spitzpocken." The question raised about the work of this group is whether the original material consisted of typical milker's nodules; several believe that they were not.

Bonnevie quotes the experiences of Dolgov and Morosov which are enlightening. These workers failed to infect rabbits but succeeded in reproducing the disease in cattle and sheep, using human material for inoculation. Of interest is an outbreak that was regarded to be milker's warts in a slaughter house in Odessa. Forty-seven of the 300 employes developed the disease. Only four of this group had milked cows, but all of them had handled cows, sheep, and swine on which "pox papules" occurred. In this case they were successful in infecting a number of animals and also several persons who had been recently vaccinated and were immune to vaccinia. As a result of this experience the authors concluded that the causative agent was a virus, but was not the virus of cowpox. They believed that it might be identical with the paravaccinia virus of Lipschutz. Stark and co-workers concluded that the infective agent in these cases of atypical animal pox and milker's warts was a variola virus which had been altered in its biological properties by continued parasitism in foreign hosts. Two of the patients described by Becker in the United States were vaccinated after recovery from an attack of milker's nodules with typical "takes," indicating that the nodules had not induced immunity to vaccine virus.

Additional evidence that this disease in man is not related to the virus of cowpox has been obtained through studies made on the associated condition in the cows. Christen in Switzerland, on the basis of extensive work, concludes that the common udder pox which prevails in that country is not true cowpox. This conclusion was based upon the fact that the disease did not respond to vaccination with vaccinia virus, and that recovered animals did not develop any immunity to vaccinia virus. By contrast he found that true cowpox, which he studied in one herd that had been accidentally infected by a recently vaccinated milker, did respond promptly to vaccination. Numerous attempts to transmit the common udder pox failed, a situation which he did not understand, inasmuch as the natural disease was clearly quite contagious.

Bonnevie had the opportunity to check the immunity to vaccine virus of one of the cows which had been the source of a nodule infection in a milker. The animal was supposed to have suffered from cowpox, yet he was able to obtain a typical "take" with vaccine virus. Hester, Boley, and Graham in the United States studied the disease in cattle. They were unable to produce the typical disease in other cattle, or to obtain infection in rabbits. Furthermore, they were able to show that animals that had recovered from so-called cowpox, gave typical reactions to vaccine virus. Animals that had recovered from vaccination with vaccine virus could not be successfully revaccinated. They were not able to stop natural outbreaks of the disease in cattle by vaccinating them with vaccine virus. Gibbons also found that vaccination was not effective in halting the bovine disease. Hardenbrook, continuing the work of the Illinois group, confirmed the earlier work that the cattle disease was not related to vaccinia. He has isolated an unidentified species of *Actinomyces* from early lesions of the disease with which he was successful in producing vesicular lesions on the udder of cattle. These lesions do not resemble the natural ones, hence further work is necessary to show the relationship, if any, between the fungus and this disease.

The situation with respect to the etiology of the so-called cowpox or udder pox of cattle which is a relatively common disease in this country and abroad, and the rather uncommon human disease known as milker's nodules which is associated with it is uncertain at present. The bulk of the evidence indicates that these conditions are not due to cowpox virus. The difficulty which most workers have experienced in transmitting these infections to other individuals suggests that they may not even be induced by a virus. Further work is necessary to clarify the situation.

ITEMS OF NOTE

1) Milker's nodules or milker's warts occur, in most instances, in persons who have milked cows suffering from a disease which is commonly called cowpox.

2) The condition in the cows associated with the human disease apparently is not true cowpox, and there is much evidence that the human disease, likewise, is not cowpox or vaccinia.

3) The causative agent of the cattle and human diseases is believed to be identical, but its nature at present is unknown.*

REFERENCES

1. BECKER, F. T.: *J.A.M.A., 115:*2140, 1940.
2. BONNEVIE, P.: *Brit. J. Dermat., 49:*164, 1937.
3. BRANTS: *Arch. Dermat. u. Syph., 178:*87, 1938.
4. CHRISTEN: *Schweiz. Arch., 81:*53 and 108, 1939.
5. DOLGOV, A. and MOROSOV, M.: *Sov. vestnik. Dermat., 9:*338, 1931.
6. GIBBONS, W. J.: *Cornell Vet., 34:*235, 1944.
7. GROTH, A.: *Munch. med. Wchnschr.,* 2128, 1929.
8. HARDENBROOK, E.: Master's thesis, University of Illinois. Personal communication from Dr. Robert Graham.

---

*The author wishes to thank William A. Hagan, D.V.M. for his contributions to this chapter.

9. HESTER, H. B., BOLEY, L. E. and GRAHAM, R.: *Cornell Vet., 31:*360, 1941.

10. JENNER, E.: An inquiry into the Causes and Effects of the Variolae Vaccinae, a Disease Discovered in Some of the Western Counties of England, Particularly Gloucestershire, and Known by the Name of the Cowpox., London, Sampson Low, 1798.

11. SCHULTZ, W., SEIFRIED, O., and SCHAAF, J.: *Zeitschr. Infectionskr., 31:*295, 1927.

12. STARK, A. M. *et al.: Arch. Dermatol, u. Syph., 170:*38, 1934.

13. TAYLOR, R. W.: *Brit. M. J., 1:*424, 1932.

Chapter 14

CONTAGIOUS ECTHYMA OF SHEEP AND GOATS

(Sore Mouth of Sheep and Goats)

W. T. HARDY, D.V.M.

CONTAGIOUS ECTHYMA of sheep and goats (sore mouth of sheep, contagious pustular dermatitis) is a communicable disease of sheep and goats, caused by a filtrable virus. Man is infected at rather infrequent intervals.

GEOGRAPHIC DISTRIBUTION

The disease is probably of worldwide distribution. In the United States it has been reported from many sheep-raising areas of the west; in the eastern states sporadic cases are encountered.

SEASONAL PREVALENCE

The disease in the United States is most prevalent during the spring and early summer months. This coincides with the period when young lambs and kids are susceptible. Later in the year, after an attack of the disease, they have attained an immunity and few cases appear.

THE ETIOLOGIC AGENT

The etiologic agent is a filtrable virus. It remains viable in scabs from lesions for many months when kept dry and cold and was infective after twenty-two years and eight months (Livingston and Hardy). It survives winter temperature in the soil of pasturelands and infects new lambs in the spring when they begin to graze.

ANIMALS SUSCEPTIBLE

Contagious ecthyma is a disease of sheep and goats. It has been reported in no other domestic or wild animals.

THE DISEASE IN SHEEP

Contagious ecthyma is a common disease of lambs and kids. While it may occur in very young animals, it is more prevalent in lambs four to six months old (Marsh and Tunnicliff). Older sheep have usually obtained immunity from an attack of the disease or vaccination. The infection makes itself apparent first as whitish spots on the buccal mucosa. These tend to grow and enlarge until they coalesce, forming a false membrane. If this is pulled off, it leaves a bleeding, eroded area; if it is allowed to stay on, it forms a heavy scab which eventually falls off, leaving no scar. During the course of the disease, which lasts about one month, lambs are unable to eat normally. Hence, there is malnutrition, stunting and sometimes death from starvation.

Fatalities are not great except in very young lambs complicated by other infections. Marsh and Tunnicliff in Montana found that lesions superimposed with infection by *Actinomyces necrophorus* were much more serious. Thorp reported serious losses by death from this cause. Boughton and Hardy in Texas reported cases of contagious ecthyma which were invaded by larvae of the flesh fly, *Cochliomyia americana,* resulting in many fatilities.

Animals which have recovered from the disease have a solid immunity.

THE DISEASE IN MAN

According to Schmidt and Hardy the possibility of transmision of sore mouth to man was suggested by Williams of Belgium. Transmission of the disease to shepherds with the "occurrence of stomatitis, with vesicles on the gums, tongue, cheek and lips" was reported by Hatbiolos of Greece. Schmidt and Hardy in Texas encountered two similar instances, but lacked proof of the relationship to the virus affecting sheep and goats.

Price successfully infected a lamb from a lesion from his wrist which became infected while preparing contagious ecthyma vaccine.

Brandenburg reported an outbreak of lip and leg ulcer in North Dakota, where two men who were treating the animals developed lesions on the hands and arms to the elbow and on the legs to the knees. Larger, lentil-like nodules appeared, which were slightly painful and which smarted and itched if they were pressed upon or irritated in any way. The neighboring lymph glands were swollen.

Newson and Cross relate the experience of a sheep feeder and his two helpers who treated a large band of sheep for sore mouth, requring three days to finish the task. In removing cockleburs from the wool, the workers irritated the skin on their hands. Four days later there appeared on the hands of the feeder several large vesicles, the larger ones being composed of several small compartments. They were surrounded with a reddened zone and moderate swelling. Lymph glands in the armpits were swollen, with considerable pain. The lesions when opened emitted a thin limpid fluid. Both helpers were afflicted with similar lesions.

Fluid from one of the lesions on the hand was rubbed into a scratch on the inside of the thigh of a lamb. Five days later there was considerable reddening around the scratch, then a pustule along its entire length, which attained its maximum development eleven days after inoculation. Another lamb inoculated in the same manner developed vesicles in four days.

The prevalence of human infections is probably small. The disease in lambs is very widespread and quite common, yet reports of man being infected are rare. Practically all workers preparing vaccine in the laboratory usually become infected through skin abrasions. Possibly the lesions produced by the cockleburs in the cases of Newson and Cross had some effect. The feeder in that instance had been associated fifteen years with infected animals, without contracting the trouble.

The duration of the disease in man is about three weeks, with uneventful recovery.

PREVENTION AND CONTROL

Pastures and premises once infected with the virus of contagious ecthyma remain in that condition for a long period of time, resulting in new infections that are difficult to control.

Boughton and Hardy have reported a vaccine that is used to immunize young lambs and kids. Dried scabs from lesions are ground and suspended in 50 per cent glycerin, one part scab to 100 parts solution. A drop of this is applied and rubbed into a scratch on the skin, inside the flank. A small vesicle appears, developing into a pustule and then a scab. The lamb develops a permanent immunity without the usual manifestations of the disease, unless the animal nibbles at the lesion and infects the lips. In the small percentage of such instances, the disease runs a much milder course than usual.

In man the disease is so rare and so mild that the ordinary precautions of hygiene are sufficient. Considerably less than one percent of ranch workers using the vaccine in the spring (usually carelessly) become infected.

ITEMS OF NOTE

1)   Contagious ecthyma of sheep and goats is probably widespread over the world.

2)   Sheep and goats are the only susceptible animals.

3)   The etiologic agent is a filtrable virus which may remain infective for years.

4)   Man is infected only at rare intervals and the course of the disease is mild.

5)   Lambs and kids may be protected by vaccination.*

REFERENCES

BOUGHTON, I. B. and HARDY, W. T.: *Texas Agri. Exper. Sta. Bull., 504*, 1935.
BRANDENBURG, T. O.: *J.A.V.M.A., 81*:818-820, 1932.
LIVINGSTON, C. W., JR. and HARDY, W. T.: *J.A.V.M.A., 137*:651, 1960.
MARSH, H. and TUNNICLIFF, E. A.: *J.A.V.M.A., 61*:600, 1937.
NEWSON, I. E. and CROSS, F.: *J.A.V.M.A., 84*:799-802, 1934.
PRICE, D. A.: *Southwestern Veterinarian, 5*:344, 1951-1952.
SCHMIDT, H. and HARDY, W. T.: *Texas Agri. Exper. Sta. Bull., 457*, 1932.
THORP, F., JR.: *Colo. Farm Bull., 4*, 1939.

----

*The author acknowledges the contribution of Thomas G. Hull to certain portions of this chapter.

Chapter 15

NEWCASTLE DISEASE

C. H. CUNNINGHAM, B.S., M.S., D.V.M., PH.D.

NEWCASTLE DISEASE is a highly contagious and fatal virus infection of domestic poultry and of wild birds characterized by pneumonic and neurologic disturbances. Certain animals are susceptible and human infection has been recognized.

Other names under which the disease has been known are avian pneumoencephalitis, respiratory-nervous disorder, fowl pest, pseudo-fowl pest and avian distemper. Numerous colloquial or indigenous names have been used to identify the disease such as Ranikhet disease, Philippine fowl pest, Madras fowl pest, Batavia disease and others. (Beach, 1942; Beaudette, 1943, 1949b, 1950; Brandly, 1950, Brandly, 1959, Brandly *et al.*, 1946a.)

HISTORY

Kraneveld first referred to the disease in 1926 as one prevalent in poultry in the Netherland East Indies. Later in the same year the disease appeared at Newcastle-on-Tyne in England where it was investigated by Doyle (1927) who clearly established the nature and cause of the disease and proposed the name of Newcastle disease. Since that time the disease has been encountered throughout the world. Due to the widespread distribution of the disease, the name Newcastle disease is obviously unsuited but has been retained to avoid confusion with the plurality of other names (Doyle, 1933).

Outbreaks in a previously free continent have been near seaport towns. It appears that the disease was spread largely along channels of trade through introduction of infected birds or their offal.

Newcastle disease is now considered to have been present in California as early as 1935, and perhaps earlier, but it was not until 1944 that the virus of the disease first called a "respiratory-nervous disorder" of chickens and later "avian pneumoencephalitis" (Beach,

411

1942; Stover, 1942a, 1942b) was recognized as being immunologically identical with the virus of Newcastle disease (Beach, 1944). Newcastle disease was diagnosed in the eastern United States in 1944 (Brandly, 1959, Brandly *et al.,* 1946b) and has since been identified in all States.

SEASONAL PREVALENCE

In the United States, Newcastle disease may be encountered at any time during the year. In typical farm flocks the incidence is usually higher in the spring, summer and fall than in the winter. In areas of concentrated poultry production such as broiler raising, the disease may be encountered at any time due to the rapid turnover of the flock and the introduction of new stock.

ETIOLOGIC AGENT

Evidence that the etiologic agent of Newcastle disease is a virus was first demonstrated by Doyle (1927) with a filtrate from a saline suspension of mouth exudate passed through Chamberland L3 and Berkefeld filters. The virus passes through all grades of Berkefeld, Mandler and Seitz filters and Chamberland L3 and L5 filters (Beaudette, 1943, 1949b, 1950; Beaudette *et al.,* 1949; Brandly, 1950; Brandly *et al.,* 1946b; Doyle, 1927).

On the basis of filtration through graded collodion filters the size of the virus has been estimated to be from 80 mμ to 120μ (Burnet and Ferry, 1934). Spherical as well as sperm-shaped particles have been observed by electron microscopy (Bang 1948c, 1949; Cunha *et al.,* 1947; Reagan *et al.,* 1948). The virus is spherical in solutions of physiologic concentration but increasing hypertonicity produces filamentous and sperm-shaped particles that are to be considered as artifacts (Bang, 1948c, 1949). The head piece of the sperm-shaped particles is about 70 mμ x 180 mμ (Cunha *et al.,* 1947), 83 mμ x 146 mμ (Bang, 1948c), and the tail piece about 500 mμ (Cunha *et al.,* 1947). The diameter is from 100 mμ to 125 mμ (Reagan *et al.,* 1948). There are no appreciable morphological differences among strains of the virus from various parts of the world (Macpherson, 1956).

On the basis of radiation data (Wilson and Pollard, 1958), Newcastle disease virus is considered to be about 56 mμ in diameter containing an outer radiation-resistant coat and an inner radiation-sensitive unit (the infectious unit). The outer structure of low absorbing power for electrons is thought to be a limiting membrane (Sharp *et al.*, 1952).

The hemagglutinins and hemolysins, which have separate entities (Wilson, 1958a, 1958b), are distributed over the surface of the virus (Wilson and Pollard, 1958). The virus is a complex of about 67 per cent protein, about 27 per cent lipid and a relatively small amount of nucleic acid, some of which is of the desoxypentose type (Cunha *et al.*, 1947). The virus contains trypsin-resistant rings of ribonucleo-protein consisting of a protein core stabilized by threads of ribo-nucleic acid along its surface (Valentine and Isaacs, 1957). The phospholipid fraction of Newcastle disease virus is essential. The virus contains little or no desoxynucleic acid (Franklin, *et al.*, 1957).

Newcastle disease virus has been classified as *Tortor furens* (van Rooyen, 1954) but it is included in the group of myxoviruses (Andrewes *et al.*, 1955; Gottschalk, 1957; Anderson, 1959) which possess an enzyme capable of splitting off neuraminic acids derivatives from some common mucoproteins.

Newcastle disease virus is rendered non-infective by 0.025 per cent beta propiolactone at 37°C. for two hours (Mack and Chotisen, 1955).

Certain mixtures of Newcastle disease, infectious bronchitis, fowl pox and laryngotracheitis viruses, and Crawley's agent can be re-solved by physical-chemical treatment (56 C., pH and chemical agents) of the inocula (Quiroz and Hanson, 1955).

The hemagglutinin of Newcastle disease virus is extremely re-sistant to radiation inactivation (McRea, 1960). The hemolysin is influenced by the physical treatment of the virus, is inhibited by calcium ions, and is dependent upon pH and the temperature of incubation (Wilson, 1958a).

On the basis of pathogenicity for embryonating chicken eggs, Newcastle disease virus strains may be differentiated into three types as determined by the difference in death time of a minimum lethal dose: lentogenic (more than 100 hours), mesogenic (60 to 90 hours) and velogenic (about 50 hours) (Hanson and Brandly, 1955; Methods, 1959). Among other criteria for typing of strains are the intra-cerebral pathogenicity and intravenous pathogenicity indices for susceptible chickens (Methods, 1959).

An embryo infective unit is about ten virus particles (Bang, 1948a, 1948b).

Some of the common chemical agents capable of inactivating the virus in from three minutes to one hour are phenol (3 per cent), ethyl alcohol (95 per cent, 70 per cent), mercuric chloride (0.1 per cent), Lysol (1 per cent), tincture of green soap, tincture of iodine (1 per cent), Lugol's solution (0.1 per cent), potassium permanganate (0.1 per cent), tincture of metaphen (0.5 per cent), tincture of zepharin (0.1 per cent), liquor cresolis saponatus (1 per cent), merthiolate (0.1 per cent), sodium orthophenylphenate (1 per cent), Phemerol (3 per cent), Disilyn (0.02 per cent), Clorox (5 per cent), formalin (2 per cent) and Roccal (1 per cent). Sodium hydroxide in 2 per cent concentration is effective according to some authors but ineffective according to others (Beamer and Prier, 1950; Cunningham, 1948a; Tilley and Anderson, 1948). Fumigation of egg incubators with formaldehyde and potassium permanganate inactivates the virus (Beamer *et al.*, 1949; Schmittle and Mansfield, 1950). Ultraviolet light (1600-1800Å) inactivates the virus (Brandly *et al.*, 1946b) but is not of practical value for control of the disease. Maximum stability of the virus occurs from pH 5 to pH 9 at one week (Moses *et al.*, 1947).

The heat stability of the hemagglutinative activity and embryo infectivity of certain strains of the virus at 56° C. for thirty minutes is variable. With some strains the hemagglutinative activity is more stable than the embryo infectivity and with others the opposite is found (Hanson *et al.*, 1949).

The virus may be preserved in 50 per cent glycerol for at least one year (Prier and Alberts, 1950), by freezing at —70° C. and by lyophilization and refrigeration for at least two years (Brandly *et al.*, 1946b) and by dehydration in vacuo over P_2O_5 and refrigeration for three years (Iyer, 1943).

Penicillin and streptomycin are without effect on the virus (Brandly *et al.*, 1946b).

The virus may remain infective in carcasses of chickens for as long as 196 days at 24-35° F. and for 300 days at —40° C. (Asplin, 1949; Gordon, *et al.*, 1948). The virus may remain infective for long periods of time on materials such as cloth, burlap, feces, mash and eggs subjected to various environmental conditions (Jungherr, 1950; Olesiuk, 1951) and in the soil (Boyd and Hanson, 1958).

Certain strains of virus can be obtained from the Newcastle Disease Virus Repository maintained at the Department of Veterinary Science, University of Wisconsin, Madison.

VECTORS

Arthropods have not been incriminated in the natural spread of Newcastle disease, although the virus has been isolated from ticks *(Argas persicus)* (Komarov, 1940), common chicken lice (Bolin, 1948), and feather mites *(Liponyssus sylviarum)* (Hofstad, 1949a). Arthropods may become infected during the viremic stage of the natural disease but no virus has been transferred by the bites of arthropods.

ANIMALS SUSCEPTIBLE

Other than chickens and turkeys, the following avian species are susceptible to Newcastle disease virus: pheasant, duck, goose, guinea fowl, pigeon, swan, parrot, osprey, parakeet, quail, partridge, sparrow, crow, mayas (martin), starling, dove, owl and gannet. It is believed that all avian species may be infected (Beaudette, 1943, 1949b, 1950; Brandly, 1959; Brandly *et al.,* 1946a; Ingalls *et al.,* 1951, Zuydam, 1952).

Experimental infection has been produced in the monkey, ferret, guinea pig, rabbit, hamster (Brueckner *et al.,* 1950) mouse, (Brandly *et al.,* 1946b; Brueckner *et al.,* 1950; Hanson *et al.,* 1951; Kilham *et al.,* 1952; Upton *et al.,* 1951) cave bat, (Reagan and Brueckner, 1951) pig and sheep (Hofstad, 1950). Natural infection has been reported in the calf (Yates *et al.,* 1952) and cat (Moses, 1951). The virus has been isolated from a case of shipping fever in cattle (Ozawa and Chow, 1958).

DISEASES IN ANIMALS

Pneumonic and neurologic signs dominate the disease produced by American strains of the virus. The mortality rate varies with the age group of chickens. Infection with strains of the virus from other parts of the world is accompanied by a 100 per cent mortality and pneumonic and gastro-intestinal involvement is more obvious. The incubation period is about five or six days with extremes of from two to fifteen days (Beaudette, 1943, 1949b, 1950; Brandly *et al.,* 1946b; Hofstad, 1949b).

In chicks the disease begins with respiratory signs of gasping and coughing. About four days later there is a general malaise, depression, stupor, ataxia, lateral recumbency, torticollis, opisthotonus and posterior or circular propulsion. The neurologic involvement may be transient or permanent. Respiratory signs may or may not be followed by nervous signs. The mortality rate is variable but it averages about 25 or 30 per cent and may be as high as 50 to 100 per cent.

In adult chickens the clinical picture is similar to that observed in chicks but in some instances the pneumonic signs, and especially the neurologic signs, may be so slight as to escape notice. The mortality rate is usually about 5 or 10 per cent. The most characteristic feature of the disease is a precipitous drop of egg production within four days to a week following the appearance of the disease. Production may cease completely and it is usually five or six weeks before it returns to normal. In some instances the pre-infection level is never attained. When the flock is returning to production, the first few eggs may be small, soft-shelled or even without shells, malformed, and of poor quality (Parnell, 1950) and with an abnormal color.

At necropsy the usual findings are cloudy air sac membranes which contain yellow, caseous material, dehydration of the carcass, excess mucus in the trachea and bronchi, and gastro-enteritis. The basic microscopic pathologic alterations are necrotizing in character in the abdominal viscera and proliferative in the lung and central nervous system (Jungherr *et al.*, 1946).

Virus is excreted from naturally infected chickens by the respiratory and gastro-intestinal tracts (Brandly *et al.*, 1946b) and has been detected in the yolk sac of four-day-old chicks, embryos and infertile eggs laid by hens during the active stages of the infection (DeLay, 1947). Contamination of commercial fowl pox and laryngotracheitis vaccines with Newcastle disease virus has been detected (Zargar and Pomeroy, 1950). Apparently virus is not present in eggs laid by hens during recovery from infection or vaccination and egg transmission does not seem to be a factor in spread of the disease from hen to chick (Bivins *et al.*, 1950; Hofstad, 1949b; Prier *et al.*, 1950). Virus has been recovered from the air in pens of infected chickens (DeLay *et al.*, 1948).

The virus of lymphomatosis may be a contaminant in chicken

embryos used for the production of Newcastle disease vaccine (Burmester *et al.*, 1956).

Chicks hatched from eggs produced by hens recovered from or vaccinated against Newcastle disease may have a naturally acquired passive immunity for three or four weeks. Antibodies may be detected in the yolk of such eggs and chicks (Brandly and Jungherr, 1946d; Schmittle, 1950; Schmittle and Millen, 1948).

In avian species other than chickens the signs and lesions are usually not as pronounced and may be overlooked due to only a mild or transient nature (Beaudette, 1943, 1949a, 1950; Brandly, 1950; Brandly *et al.*, 1946c).

DISEASE IN MAN

Newcastle disease may represent a potential occupational hazard to certain persons. Numerous literature references are available (Hanson and Brandly, 1958). One source of infection is the respiratory discharges and natural aerosols from chickens in the incubative stages of the disease (DeLay *et al.*, 1948). Artificial aerosols from sprayed or nebulized fluid virus or virus dust vaccines are a considerable hazard to those administering vaccines by these methods (Hitchner and Reising, 1952). Another important source for exposure of man to aerosols and to contact with the virus is the laboratory where the virus is studied and vaccines produced. Persons working in diagnostic laboratories or eviscerating plants are exposed when handling infected carcasses and infection may be by aerosol or contact (Hofstad, 1951). There is no evidence that the virus is transmitted from infected chickens to man through arthropods.

In general, the disease is characterized by a superficial, unilateral, acute granular conjunctivitis often with periauricular adenitis. Subcutaneous hemorrhage, edema of the eyelids, subconjunctival hemorrhage, hyperemia of the scleral and conjunctival vessels, secondary infiltration of the corneal epithelium and a mucopurulent discharge may be observed (Anderson, 1946; Burnet, 1943; Gustafson and Moses, 1951; Hunter *et al.*, 1951; Ingalls and Mahoney, 1949; Keeney and Hunter, 1950; Thompson, 1950). A systemic syndrome of fever, chills, headache, general malaise, mild leucopenia and relative lymphocytosis indicates that the virus is not always limited to the conjunctiva. Virus has been recovered from blood serum seven hours after the onset of chills and fever on the second day after infection and from conjunctival washings as late as the sixth day (Hunter *et al.*, 1951). Nasal and lachrymal secretion and saliva have been proved to be infectious. The significance of inclusion body-like particles in the epithelial cells of the conjunctiva during the early stages of the infection has not been fully established (Keeney and Hunter, 1950). Inclusion bodies have not been conclusively demonstrated in the natural host (Jungherr *et al.*, 1946). Recovery is complete in one or two weeks without sequelae. Medication is without effect.

DIAGNOSIS

In addition to clinical history, signs and lesions, laboratory diagnosis of Newcastle diesase in birds may involve one or more of the following procedures: 1) isolation of virus in embryonating chicken eggs; 2) hemagglutination (HA) test of virus-infected allantoic fluid; 3) hemagglutination-inhibition (HI) test of serum and of egg yolk; and 4) serum neutralization (SN) test.

Brain, spleen, lung and trachea are collected during the respiratory stage of the disease in birds as virus is less readily isolated from specimens collected during the nervous stage of the disease (Brandly *et al.*, 1946b; Cunningham, 1960; Hofstad, 1951). The specimens are ground and suspended in either broth or phosphate-buffered saline. Penicillin and streptomycin (10,000 units and 100 mgm., respectively, per ml. of suspension) are added (Brandly *et al.*, 1946b; Cunningham, 1960; Methods, 1959). Portions of the suspension are inoculated into the allantoic cavity of nine to twelve day embryonating chicken eggs. With typical Newcastle disease virus infection, the embryos are killed by the virus by the third or fourth postinoculation day. All embryos might not die from primary inoculation. In this case, allantoic fluid should be collected from the dead embryos and used to inoculate additional eggs. Usually on the second or third passage all embryos die. Allantoic fluid should be collected from dead embryos for use in HA, HI and SN tests. Dermal petechiation and congestion and hemorrhage of the yolk sac may be observed in the dead embryos (Jungherr *et al.*, 1946) but there are no characteristic pathologic alterations that can be used for diagnosis.

Newcastle disease virus possesses the ability to agglutinate red blood cells of chickens and other avian species as well as those of certain mammals (Brandly *et al.*, 1946b; Hanson *et al.*, 1950; Winslow *et al.,* 1950). This property of the virus can be assayed by titration and expressed as hemagglutinative units (HA units) (Brandly, 1959; Cunningham, 1960; Methods, 1959).

The ability of Newcastle disease virus antibodies to inhibit hemagglutination by the virus can be measured quantitatively by the HI test using either the alpha (decreasing virus-constant serum) procedure or the beta (constant HA units of virus-decreasing serum) procedure (Brandly, 1959; Cunningham, 1960; Methods, 1959). Using the alpha procedure for chicken serum, an HI titer of 80 or more is considered positive for Newcastle disease virus antibodies, 40 is suspicious, and 5 or 10 are considered as within a normal range (Brandly *et al.,* 1946b; Brandly *et al.,* 1947).

According to the beta procedure using 10 HA units, an HI value of 10 has been considered as of questionable diagnostic significance. A value of 20 or higher indicates prior infection of the chicken. (Brandly *et al.,* 1947; Doll *et al.,* 1950c; Schmittle, 1950; Schmittle and Millen, 1948).

Egg yolk extracted with ethylene dichloride and ether may be used in the HI test in place of serum. It is essential that no egg albumen be included (Schmittle, 1950; Schmittle and Millen, 1948).

Modifications of the HI test to use plates instead of tubes have been described (Luginbuhl and Jungherr, 1949; Zargar and Pomeroy, 1949).

For the SN test serial 10-fold dilutions of virus-infected allantoic fluid and equal parts of serum and diluted virus are mixed. At least four, preferably five, nine to twelve day embryonating chicken eggs are used per dilution and inoculated via the allantoic cavity. (Brandly *et al.,* 1946b; Cunningham, 1960c; Doll *et al.,* 1950c, 1951a; Methods, 1959).

The endpoints of infectivity of the virus and of the virus-serum mixtures are expressed as the LD_{50} and the difference as the LD_{50} Neutralization Index (NI). The $LD_{50}NI$ of serum from normal chickens would not be expected to exceed 10^1 (Doll *et al.,* 1950c, 1951a), $10^{1.001} \pm 10^{0.0262}$ (Cunningham, 1951). An $LD_{50}NI$ of 10^2 or higher is considered as positive for Newcastle disease virus antibodies (Doll *et al.,* 1950c).

An indirect complement-fixation test for Newcastle disease in chickens has been described (Wolfe *et al.,* 1949).

Newcastle disease virus antibodies can be detected in human

serum by HI, SN and complement-fixation tests (Howitt, 1950; Hunter *et al.,* 1951; Luginbuhl and Jungherr, 1949; Wenner *et al.,* 1950). The serum should be heated at 56° C. for thirty minutes before use. Serologic diagnosis of Newcastle disease in man should be done with paired serum from the acute and convalescent stages of the disease. Only significant increases in titer should be considered as criteria for diagnosis of the disease. A 4-fold increase in the HI titer has been detected on the sixth and eleventh days after infection and a thirty-two fold increase on the fourteenth through the 110th days (Hunter *et al.,* 1951). A serologic relationship of mumps and Newcastle disease has been observed but it is suggested that a diagnosis of Newcastle disease in humans be made with caution, especially in the absence of virus isolation (Jungherr *et al.,* 1949).

The affinity of Newcastle disease virus to the influenza group, (Anderson, 1947; Burnet, 1942; Florman, 1948) receptor destruction by viruses of the mumps-Newcastle disease-influenza group, (Hirst, 1950a, 1950b) modification of red blood cells by Newcastle disease virus and use of these cells in serologic studies of infectious mononucleosis and viral hepatitis (Evans, 1950; Kilham, 1950) and Newcastle disease hemolysin (Kilham, 1949) have been reported. While these reports indicate certain serologic relationships of the viruses studied and their possible adaptation to diagnosis of human infections, evaluation of the specificity of the reactions must await further investigation.

PREVENTION AND CONTROL

Vaccines of avian embryo origin are used for immunization of birds against Newcastle disease. Two major types of vaccines, inactivated virus and live virus, are in general use. The virus in the inactivated virus vaccine is treated with chemical agents such as formalin or crystal violet. Adjuvants such as alumina gel are added. The vaccine is inoculated intramuscularly (Hofstad, 1953, 1954, 1955).

Modified or attenuated virus is used for the live virus vaccines which are administered by several routes including the "stick" or wing web puncture, intramuscular injection, "drop" intranasal or conjunctival sac installation, spraying or nebulizing, dusting for inhalation, and adding the virus to the drinking water (Beaudette, 1948, 1949a, 1950; Clancy *et al.*, 1949; Doll *et al.*, 1950a, 1950b, 1951b; Hanson and Brandly, 1955; Hitchner and Johnson, 1948; Hitchner *et al.*, 1950, 1951; Luginbuhl *et al.*, 1955; Markham *et al.*, 1949, 1954, 1955, 1956).

Advantages and limitations of each vaccine are generally recognized (Beaudette, 1948, 1949a, 1950; Brandly, 1950; Brandly, 1959). All the vaccines are capable of producing a measurable degree of immunity. Killed virus vaccine does not introduce the living agent in a flock and does not produce a systemic reaction or mortality. Living modified virus vaccines introduce the living agent in a flock and may produce a systemic reaction and some mortality. The mortality is not as heavy as experienced with natural infection.

In practice it is not expected that any one kind or type of vaccine is universally suitable for all circumstances. In some instances revaccination is desirable to augment or prolong immunity. With all vaccines it is not considered good practice to vaccinate chicks during the period in which naturally acquired passive immunity is expected to be present (Doll *et al.*, 1950b). Critical evaluation and standardization of vaccines is necessary to characterize strains of virus capable of production of an effective immunity response.

Control of Newcastle disease embraces a program of good management and sanitation in the flock and in the hatchery. Traffic in infected birds, crates and other equipment, as well as visitors to an affected flock, are among the common means of dissemination of the disease. Such factors as a previous outbreak of the disease, amount of poultry traffic, and incidence of the disease in the locality need to be considered before initiating a vaccination program. Prophylactic vaccination is recommended in flocks in which the disease has previously occurred or in which survivors of a past outbreak remain; in flocks in an enzootic area; and as emergency vaccination at the beginning of an outbreak. In the latter case, birds in the noninfected pens should be vaccinated first. Vaccination is not a substitute for good management and sanitation. Vaccination is not recommended in a flock where there is little or no poultry traffic, where the disease is not present in the locality, or if the flock is affected with other diseases.

ITEMS OF NOTE

1) Newcastle disease is encountered throughout the world.

2) Newcastle disease virus is capable of infecting birds, animals and man.

3) Pneumonic and neurologic symptoms characterize the disease in birds.

4) In man, the disease is characterized by a conjunctivitis and a syndrome of fever, chills, headache and general malaise.

5) Laboratory diagnosis is based on isolation of the virus and serologic tests such as hemagglutination-inhibition and serum neutralization.

6) Killed virus vaccine and living modified virus vaccines are capable of stimulating immunity.

7) Control of the disease in poultry embraces good management and sanitation complemented by vaccination where indicated.

REFERENCES

ANDERSON, S. G.: A note on two laboratory infections with the virus of Newcastle disease of fowls. *Med. J. Australia, 1:*371, 1946.

—— The reaction between red cells and viruses of the influenza group. Studies with Newcastle disease virus. Austral. *J. Exper. Biol. & Med. Sc., 25:*163-174, 1947.

—— Hemagglutination by animal viruses. *The Viruses,* Vol. 3, Edited by F. M. Burnet and W. M. Stanley. New York, Acad. Press, 1959.

ANDREWES, C. H., BANG, F. B., and BURNET, F. M.: A short description of the myxovirus group (influenza and related viruses). *Virology, 1:*176-184, 1955.

ASPLIN, F. D.: Observations on the viability of Newcastle disease virus. *Vet. Rec., 65:*159-160, 1949.

BANG, F. B.: Studies on Newcastle disease virus. I. An evaluation of the method of titration. *J. Exper. Med., 88:*233-240, 1948a.

—— Studies on Newcastle disease virus. II. Behavior of the virus in the embryo. *J. Exper. Med., 88:*241-249, 1948b.

—— Studies on Newcastle disease virus. III. Characters of the virus itself with particular reference to electron microscopy. *J. Exper. Med., 88:*251-266, 1948c.

—— Formation of filamentous forms of Newcastle disease virus in hypertonic concentration of sodium chloride. *Proc. Soc. Exper. Biol. & Med., 71:*50-52, 1949.

BEACH, J. R.: Avian pneumoencephalitis. Proc. 46th. An. Meet. U. S. Livestock San. Assn. 202-223, 1942.

—— The neutralization *in vitro* of avian pneumoencephalitis virus by Newcastle disease immune serum. *Science, 100:*361-362, 1944.

BEAMER, P. D., SUTHERLAND, A. K., and SCHMITTLE, S. C.: Studies on Newcastle disease. II. The resistance of Newcastle disease virus to formaldehyde fumigation. *Am. J. Vet. Res., 10:*384-387, 1949.

——, and PRIER, J. E.: Studies on Newcastle disease. III. Resistance of Newcastle disease virus to certain chemical agents. *Cornell Vet., 40:*57-60, 1950.

BEAUDETTE, F. R.: A review of the literature on Newcastle disease. Proc. 47th An. Meet. U. S. Livestock San. Assn. 122-177, 1943.

—— The immunization of birds against Newcastle disease. Proc. 52nd An. Meet. U. S. Livestock San. Assn. 254-265, 1948.

—— Twenty years of progress in immunization against virus diseases of birds, *J.A.V.M.A., 115:*367-377, 1949a.

—— An addendum to a review of the literature on Newcastle disease. Proc. 53rd An. Meet. U. S. Livestock San. Assn. 202-220, 1949b.

—— Recent literature on Newcastle disease. Proc. 54th An. Meet. U. S. Livestock San. Assn. 132-153, 1950.

BIVINS, J. A., MILLER, B. R., and BEAUDETTE, F. R.: Search for virus in eggs laid during recovery postinoculation with Newcastle disease virus. *Am. J. Vet. Res., 11:*426-427, 1950.

BOLIN, F. M.: Isolation of Newcastle disease virus from feces of the domestic cat and the common chicken louse. *Proc. 48th An. Meet. Soc. Am. Bact.,* 43, 1948.

BOYD, R. J., and HANSON, R. P.: Survival of Newcastle disease virus in nature. *Avian Dis., 2:*82-93, 1958.

BRANDLY, C. A.: Newcastle disease. *J.A.V.M.A., 116:*139-146, 1950.

—— Newcastle Disease. *Diseases of Poultry,* 4th edition. Edited by H. E. Biester and L. H. Schwarte. Ames, The Iowa State Univ. Press, 1959.

——, MOSES, H. E., JUNGHERR, E. L., and JONES, E. E.: Epizootology of Newcastle disease of poultry. *Am. J. Vet. Res., 7:*243-249, 1946a.

—— Isolation and identification of Newcastle disease virus. *Am. J. Vet. Res., 7:*289-306, 1946b.

——, JONES, E. E., and JUNGHERR, E. L.: Immunization of chickens against Newcastle disease. *Am. J. Vet. Res., 7:*307-332, 1946c.

——, and JUNGHERR, E. L.: Transmission of antiviral activity via the egg and the role of congenital passive immunity to Newcastle disease in chickens. *Am. J. Vet. Res., 7:*333-342, 1946d.

——, HANSON, R. P., LEWIS, S. H. and WINSLOW, N. S.: Variables and correlations in laboratory procedures for Newcastle disease diagnosis. *Cornell Vet., 37:*324-336, 1947.

BRUECKNER, A. L., REAGAN, R. L., SCHENCK, D. M., WERNER, H. O., and HICKMAN, J. W.: Mammalian adaptations of Newcastle disease virus. Proc. 87th An. Meet. A.V.M.A. 163-166, 1950.

BURMESTER, B. R., CUNNINGHAM, C. H., COTTRAL, G. E., BELDING, R. C., and GENTRY, R. F.: The transmission of visceral lymphomatosis with live virus Newcastle disease vaccines. *Am. J. Vet. Res., 17:*283-289, 1956.

BURNET, F. M., and FERRY, J. D.: The differentiation of the viruses of fowl plague and Newcastle disease: Experiments using the technique of chorioallantoic membrane inoculation of the developing egg. *Brit. J. Exper. Path., 15:*56-64, 1934.

—— The affinity of Newcastle disease virus to the influenza group. *Australian J. Exper. Biol. & Med. Sc., 20:*81-88, 1942.

—— "Human infection" with the virus of Newcastle disease of fowls. *Med. J. Australia, 2:*313-314, 1943.

CLANCY, C. F., COX, H. R., and BOTTORFF, C. A.: Laboratory experiments with living Newcastle disease vaccine. *Poul. Sci., 28:*58-62, 1949.

CUNHA, R., WEIL, M. L., BEARD, D., TAYLOR, A. R., SHARP, D. G., and BEARD, J. W.: Purification and characters of the Newcastle disease virus. *J. Immunol., 55:*69-89, 1947.

CUNNINGHAM, C. H.: The effect of certain chemical agents on the virus of Newcastle disease of chickens. *Am. J. Vet. Res., 9:*195-197, 1948a.

—— Newcastle disease and infectious bronchitis neutralizing antibody indexes of normal chicken serum. *Am. J. Vet. Res., 12:*129-133, 1951.

—— A Laboratory Guide in Virology. 4th ed. Minneapolis, Burgess Publishing Co., 1960.

DeLay, P. D.: Isolation of avian pneumoencephalitis (Newcastle disease) virus from the yolk sac of four-day-old chicks, embryos, and infertile eggs. *Science, 106:*546, 1947.

——, De Ome, K. B., and Bankowski, R. A.: Recovery of pneumoencephalitis (Newcastle) virus from the air of poultry houses containing infected birds. *Science, 107:*474-475, 1948.

Doll, E. R., McCollum, W. H., and Wallace, M. E.: Immunization against Newcastle diesase with a virus of low virulence. *Vet. Med., 45:*231-236, 1950a.

—— Immunization of chicks hatched from hens immunized against Newcastle disease. *Vet. Med., 45:*365-369, 1950b.

——, Wallace, M. E., and McCollum, W. H.: Interpretation of serologic procedures for the diagnosis of Newcastle disease. *Am. J. Vet. Res., 11:*265-271, 1950c.

—— Newcastle disease virus-neutralizing indexes of normal chicken serums. *Am. J. Vet. Res., 12:*345-346, 1951a.

—— Susceptibility to Newcastle disease infection of chickens vaccinated with a killed virus vaccine. *Am. J. Vet. Res., 12:*368-371, 1951b.

Doyle, T. M.: A hitherto unrecorded disease of fowls due to a filter-passing virus. *J. Comp. Path. Therap., 40:*144-169, 1927.

—— Newcastle disease. (In: The virus diseases of animals with special reference to those of poultry). *J. Comp. Path. Therapy., 46:*90-107, 1933.

Evans, A. S.: Serological studies on infectious mononucleosis and viral hepatitis with human erythrocytes modified by different strains of Newcastle disease virus. *J. Immunol., 64:*411-420, 1950.

Florman, A. L.: Some alterations in chicken erythrocytes which follow treatment with influenza and Newcastle disease virus. *J. Bact., 55:*183-196, 1948.

Franklin, R. M., Rubin, H., and Davis, C. A.: The production, purification and properties of Newcastle disease virus labeled with radiophosphorus. *Virology, 3:*96-114, 1957.

Gordon, R. F., and Reid, J., and Asplin, F. D.: Newcastle disease in England and Wales. Proc. 8th World's Poul. Cong., 642-650, 1948. Copenhagen, Denmark.

Gottschalk, A.: Virus enzymes and virus templates. *Physiol. Rev., 37:*66-83, 1957.

Gustafson, D. P., and Moses, H. E.: Isolation of Newcastle disease virus from the eye of a human being. *J.A.V.M.A., 118:*1-2, 1951.

Hanson, R. P., and Brandly, C. A.: Identification of vaccine strains of Newcastle disease virus. *Science, 122:*156-157, 1955.

——, and Brandly, C. A.: Newcastle disease. *Ann. N. Y. Acad. Sc., 70:*585-597, 1958.

——, Upton, E., Brandly, C. A., and Winslow, N. S.: Heat stability of hemagglutinin of various strains of Newcastle disease virus. *Proc. Soc. Exper. Biol. & Med., 70:*283-287, 1949.

——, Winslow, N. S., Brandly, C. A., and Upton, E.: The antiviral activity of Newcastle disease immune sera. *J. Bact. 60:*557-560, 1950.

——, Upton, E., and Brandly, C. A.: Pneumopathogenicity of Newcastle disease virus for adult white mice. *J. Bact., 62:*545-547, 1951.

Hirst, G. K.: Receptor destruction by viruses of the mumps-NDV-influenza group. *J. Exper. Med., 91:*161-175, 1950a.

—— The relationship of the receptors of a new strain of virus to those of the mumps-NDV-influenza group. *J. Exper. Med., 91:*177-184, 1950b.

HITCHNER, S. B., and JOHNSON, E. P.: A virus of low virulence for immunizing fowls against Newcastle disease (avian pneumoencephalitis). *Vet. Med., 43:*525-530, 1948.

——, REISING, G., and VAN ROEKEL, H.: The intranasal vaccine—Its role in a Newcastle disease program. Proc. 54th An. Meet. U. S. Livestock San. Assn. 154-160, 1950.

—— Characteristics of the B1 strain of Newcastle disease virus. *Am. J. Vet. Res.,* 12:246-249, 1951.

——, and REISING, G.: Flock vaccination for Newcastle disease by atomization of the B₁ strain of virus. *Proc. 89th An. Meet. A.V.M.A.* 258-264, 1952.

HOFSTAD, M. S.: Recovery of Newcastle disease (pneumoencephalitis) virus from mites, *Liponypsus Sylviarum,* after feeding upon Newcastle-infected chickens. *Am. J. Vet. Res., 10:*370-371, 1949a.

—— A study on the epizootology of Newcastle disease (pneumoencephalitis). *Poul. Sc., 28:*530-533, 1949b.

—— Experimental inoculation of swine and sheep with Newcastle disease virus. *Cornell Vet., 40:*191-198, 1950.

—— A quantitative study of Newcastle disease virus in tissues of infected chickens. *Am. J. Vet. Res., 12:*334-339, 1951.

—— Immunization of chickens against Newcastle disease by formalin-inactivated virus. *Am. J. Vet. Res., 14:*586-589, 1953.

—— The secondary immune response in chickens revaccinated with inactivated Newcastle disease virus vaccine. *Am. J. Vet. Res., 15:*604-606, 1954.

—— The immune response in chickens following the use of three different types of inactivated Newcastle disease vaccine. *Am. J. Vet. Res., 16:*608-612, 1955.

HOWITT, B.: A nonspecific heat-labile factor in the serum neutralization test for Newcastle disease virus. *J. Immunol., 64:*73-84, 1950.

HUNTER, M. C., KEENEY, A. H., and SIGEL, M. M.: Laboratory aspects of an infection with Newcastle disease virus in man. *J. Infect. Dis., 88:*272-277, 1951.

INGALLS, W. L., and MAHONEY, A.: Isolation of the virus of Newcastle disease from human beings. *Am. J. Pub. Health, 39:*737-740, 1949.

——, VESPER, R. W., and MAHONEY, A.: Isolation of Newcastle disease virus from the great horned owl. *J.A.V.M.A., 119:*71, 1951.

IYER, S. G.: Studies on Newcastle (Ranikhet) disease virus. *Indian J. Vet. Sc. & Anim. Husb., 13:*1-26, 1943.

JUNGHERR, E.: Studies on sanitizing used feed bags. *J.A.V.M.A., 117:*324-328, 1950.

——, TYZZER, E. E., BRANDLY, C. A., and MOSES, H. E.: The comparative pathology of fowl plague and Newcastle disease. *Am. J. Vet. Res., 7:*250-288, 1946.

——, LUGINBUHL, R. E., and KILHAM, L.: Serologic relationship of mumps and Newcastle disease, *Science, 110:*333-334, 1949.

KEENEY,(A. H., and HUNTER, M. C.: Human infection with the Newcastle virus of fowls. *Arch. Ophtham., 44:*573-580, 1950.

KILHAM, L.: A Newcastle disease virus (NDV) hemolysin. *Proc. Soc. Exper. Biol. & Med., 71:*63-66, 1949.

—— Evaluation of the agglutination of erythrocytes sensitized by Newcastle disease virus (NDV) as a serologic test in infectious mononucleosis. *J. Immunol., 65:*245-253, 1950.

——, LOOMIS, L. N., and PEERS, J. H.: Variations in behavior of Newcastle disease virus on passage through brains of adult mice. *Am. J. Vet. Res., 13:*95-98, 1952.

KOMAROV, A.: Newcastle disease in Palestine. *Palestine Vet. Bul., 6:*107-111, 1940.

KRANEVELD, F. C.: Over een in Ned.-Indie heerschende Ziekte onder het Pluimvee. *Nederl-Indische Bladen voor Diergeneesk., 38:*448-450, 1926. Cited by BEAUDETTE, 1943.

LUGINBUHL, R. E., and JUNGHERR, E.: A plate hemagglutination-inhibition test for Newcastle disease antibodies in avian and human serums. *Poul. Sc., 28:*622-624, 1949.

——, JUNGHERR, E. L., and CHOMIAK, T. W.: Administration of Newcastle disease and infectious bronchitis vaccines through the drinking water. *Poul. Sc., 34:*1399-1403, 1955.

McCREA, J. F.: Ionizing radiation and its effects on animal viruses. *Ann. N. Y. Acad. Sc., 83:*692-705, 1960.

MACK, W. N., and CHOTISEN, A.: Beta-propiolactone as a virus altering agent for a Newcastle disease vaccine. *Poul. Sc., 34:*1010-1013, 1955.

MACPHERSON, L. W.: Electron-microscope studies of the virus of Newcastle disease. *Canad. J. Comp. Med., 20:*72-78, 1956.

MARKHAM, F. S., COX, H. R., and BOTTORFF, C. A.: Field trials with living virus vaccine for Newcastle disease. *Poul. Sc., 28:*52-57, 1949.

——, COX, H. R., and BOTTORFF, C. A.: Newcastle disease: a serologic study in vaccination and revaccination. *Cornell Vet., 44:*324-345, 1954.

——, HAMMAR, A. H., GINGHER, P., and COX, H. R.: Vaccination against Newcastle disease and infectious bronchitis. 1. Preliminary studies in mass vaccination with live virus dust vaccines. *Poul. Sc., 34:*442-448, 1955.

——, HAMMAR, A. H., PERRY, E. B., and TESAR, W. C.: Combined Newcastle disease-infectious bronchitis vaccines and the absence of interference phenomena. *Cornell Vet., 46:*538-547, 1956.

Methods for the Examination of Poultry Biologics. Publication 705, Washington, D. C., National Academy of Sciences—National Research Council, 1959.

MOSES, H. E.: Cats and Newcastle disease virus. *J.A.V.M.A., 119:*213, 1951.

——, BRANDLY, C. A., and JONES, E. E.: The pH stability of viruses of Newcastle disease and fowl plague. *Science, 105:*477-479, 1947.

OLESIUK, O. M.: Influence of environmental factors on viability of Newcastle disease virus. *Am. J. Vet. Res., 12:*152-155, 1951.

OZAWA, Y., and CHOW, T. C.: A study and identification of Newcastle disease virus (NDV) from ranch cattle infected with shipping fever. *Poul. Sc., 37:*802-809, 1958.

PARNELL, E. D.: The keeping quality of shell eggs in storage as affected by Newcastle disease. *Poul. Sc., 29:*153-155, 1950.

PRIER, J. E., and ALBERTS, J. O.: Studies on Newcastle disease. VII. Viability of live embryo Newcastle disease virus in buffered glycerol. *Cornell Vet., 40:*300-303, 1950.

——, MILLEN, T. W., and ALBERTS, J. O.: Studies on Newcastle disease. IV. The presence of Newcastle disease virus in eggs of hens vaccinated with live vaccine. *J.A.V.M.A., 116:*54-55, 1950.

QUIROZ, C. A., and HANSON, R. P.: Physical-chemical treatment of inocula as a means of separating and identifying avian viruses. *Avian Dis., 2:*94-98, 1958.

REAGAN, R. L., LILLIE, M. G., HAUSER, J. E., and BRUECKNER, A. L.: Electron micrographs of the hamster-adapted Newcastle virus. *Cornell Vet., 38:*418-420, 1948.

——, and BRUECKNER, A. L.: Effects of nasal installation of virus strains of Newcastle disease virus into the cave bat *(Myotis Lucifugus)*. *Am. J. Vet. Res., 12:*347-348, 1951.

SCHMITTLE, S. C.: Studies on Newcastle disease. V. A comparison of Newcastle disease antibody titers in blood and egg as measured by the hemagglutination-inhibition test, *Am. J. Vet. Res., 11:*226-230, 1950.

——, and MILLEN, T. W.: Studies on Newcastle disease. I. Detection of hemagglutination-inhibition antibodies in unincubated eggs. *Cornell Vet., 38:*306-309, 1948.

——, and MANSFIELD, M. E.: Studies on Newcastle disease. VI. A field test on hatchery fumigation with formaldehyde against Newcastle disease virus. *Cornell Vet., 40:*90-92, 1950.

SHARP, D. G., ECKERT, E. A., BEARD, D., and BEARD, J. W.: Morphology of the virus of avian erythromyeloblastic leucosis and a comparison with the agent of Newcastle disease. *J. Bact., 63:*151-161, 1952.

STOVER, D. E.: A filterable virus, the cause of a respiratory-nervous disorder of chickens. *Am. J. Vet. Res., 3:*207-213, 1942a.

—— Respiratory-nervous disorder in eight-months old pullets. *Am. J. Vet. Res., 3:*239-241, 1942b.

THOMPSON, JR., C. H.: Newcastle disease infection in man. *Mil. Surgeon, 106:*276-281, 1950.

TILLEY, F. W., and ANDERSON, W. A.: Germicidal action of certain chemicals on the virus of Newcastle disease (avian pneumoencephalitis). *Vet. Med., 42:*229-230, 1947.

UPTON, E., HANSON, R. P., TEPLEY, N. W. and BRANDLY, C. A.: Neurotoxicity of Newcastle disease virus for hamsters and mice. Proc. 51st Gen. Meet. Soc. Am. Bact. 87, 1951.

VALENTINE, R. C., and ISAACS, A.: The structure of viruses of the Newcastle disease-mumps-influenza (myxovirus) group. *J. Gen. Microbiol., 16:*680-685, 1957.

VAN ROOYEN, C. E.: A revision of Holmes's classification of animal viruses, Suborder III (Zoophagineae). *Canad. J. Microbiol., 1:*227-284, 1954.

WENNER, H. A., MONLEY, A., and TODD, R. N.: Studies on compliment fixation with Newcastle disease virus. *J. Immunol., 64:*323-333, 1950.

WILSON, D.: Radiation studies on the hemolysin of Newcastle disease virus. *Radiation Res., 8:*142-149, 1958a.

WILSON, D. E.: The inactivation of Newcastle disease virus hemolysin by antiserum and high -energy electrons. *Proc. Soc. Exper. Biol. & Med., 99:*205-208, 1958b.

——, and POLLARD, E. C.: Radiation studies on the infective property of Newcastle disease virus. *Radiation Res., 8:*131-141, 1958.

WINSLOW, N. S., HANSON, R. P. UPTON, E., and BRANDLY, C. A.: Agglutination of mammalian erythrocytes by Newcastle disease virus. *Proc. Soc. Exper. Biol. & Med., 74:*174-178, 1950.

WOLFE, D. M., KORNFELD, L., and MARKHAM, F. S.: Simplified indirect complement-fixation test applied to Newcastle disease immune avian serum. *Proc. Soc. Exper. Biol. & Med., 70:*490-494, 1949.

YATES, V. J., FRY, D. B. and HENDERSON, JR., B. W.: Isolation of Newcastle disease virus from a calf. *J.A.V.M.A., 120:*149-150, 1952.

ZARGAR, S. L., and POMEROY, B. S.: A rapid whole blood plate test for the diagnosis of Newcastle disease. *J.A.V.M.A., 115:*354, 1949.

—— Isolation of Newcastle disease virus from commercial fowlpox and laryngo-tracheitis vaccines. *J.A.V.M.A., 116:*304-305, 1950.

ZUYDAM, D. M.: Isolation of Newcastle disease virus from the osprey and the parakeet. *J.A.V.M.A., 120:*88-89, 1952.

Chapter 16

CAT SCRATCH DISEASE
(Cat Fever; Benign Inoculation Lymphoreticulosis)

Warren J. Warwick, M.D.

CAT SCRATCH DISEASE is usually a mild infection confined to a regional group of lymph nodes. As far as is known, it is strictly a disease of man, but it is included here because the majority of cases occur following a cat scratch or bite.

HISTORY

The establishment of cat scratch disease as a specific entity by Debré, in 1950,[2] is a good example of international cooperation. In 1947, Drs. L. Foshay of Cincinnati and R. Debré of Paris compared notes on a disease entity each had observed and studied for twenty years. Using a skin test antigen, prepared from heated pus of a suppurative lymph node by Drs. F. M. Hanger and H. M. Rose of New York, Debré and Foshay established the presumptive identity of the cases in the three cities.

GEOGRAPHIC DISTRIBUTION

Cat scratch disease has been recognized on all continents and in all climates, but the majority of published cases have been in Europe and North America.

SEASONAL PREVALENCE

Three epidemics of cat scratch disease have been recognized and reported,[3,4,8] each of which occurred during the winter months from October to March. About 90 per cent of the cases observed in North America have occurred in the six months from September through

February, with a peak in November and December.[6,8] This seasonal occurrence supports the thesis that cat scratch disease is an infectious disease.

VECTORS

Cats are unquestionably important in the transmission of this disease, even though they do not acquire the infection or demonstrate reactivity to the skin test antigen. There has been a cat contact in almost 90 per cent of the recorded cases, and all reported family epidemics have occurred in families with a pet cat.[6] The offending cat, almost always a kitten, may merely be a mechanical transmitter of the infectious virus acquired from an unknown source.

ETIOLOGY

The absence of microorganisms in pathologic specimens, and failure to isolate the causative agent on bacteriologic culture media, in tissue cultures of cells, in embryonated eggs, and in laboratory animals, are presumptive evidence that the causative agent is a virus. A few workers have had limited success in their search for the causative agent. In France, Mollaret and co-workers[5] produced the disease in a human volunteer after four inoculations, and in the Old World monkeys, *Cercopithecus aethiops sabaeus* and *Macaca mulatta*. In Germany, Zwissler[12] also used aspirated pus to produce the disease in four human beings, and by passage of the material through rat testes and chick embryo yolk sacs he produced both a skin test and a precipitation test antigen. In the United States, another group[7] isolated a virus, antigenically related to herpes simplex, from the node of a patient with cat scratch disease, and found that this virus produced hemagglutination of rabbit and rat erythrocytes. Some convalescent patients have had hemagglutination-inhibiting antibody. So far no one has reported duplication of the work of any of these investigators.

A high incidence of elevated titers against lymphogranuloma-psittacosis antigens suggests that the virus belongs to that group.

MECHANISM OF TRANSMISSION

The virus gains entrance to the body through puncture wounds of the skin. Cat scratches and bites cause most cases, although any penetrating injury to the skin by thorns, splinters of wood, fish hooks, porcupine quills, biting insects, and superficial cuts may be sufficient if there is cat contact and, rarely, even without cat contact.

THE DISEASE IN ANIMALS

Natural infection is unknown in animals. No animal, including man, is readily susceptible to this infection, and this fact has seriously hampered both clinical and laboratory investigations of the disease. The disease produced experimentally in the monkey *Ceropithecus* is clinically and histologically like that in human beings.

THE DISEASE IN MAN

The principal characteristic of cat scratch disease is a regional lymphadenitis, usually involving the axillary, cervical, or the femoral and inguinal nodes, although any lymph node may be affected. The nodes are often tender or painful. They remain enlarged for periods of a few weeks to several months, and about one-third of them suppurate. Only rarely is there generalized lymphadenopathy or hepatosplenomegaly. In about one-third of the cases a primary lesion, an erythematous, scaly papule, is found at the site of inoculation.

Constitutional symptoms are usually mild and of short duration. Two-thirds of the patients have a mild fever, 100 to 102° F., but occasionally temperatures of 104° or more occur. Less frequent symptoms include chills, malaise, anorexia, generalized aching, nausea, stomach ache, and pallor. Skin rashes, infrequent and evanescent, have also been reported, including those of the scarlatiniform, morbilliform, pleomorphic, macular and papulovesicular types, and occasionally erythema nodosum.

Parinaud's oculoglandular syndrome is commonly caused by cat scratch disease. Other complications, which are rare, include encephalitis, osteolytic bone lesions, and thrombocytopenic purpura.

Of the routine laboratory studies, hemoglobin determinations and urinalyses are characteristically normal. Normal or slightly elevated white blood counts and erythrocyte sedimentation rates are usual; marked elevation is uncommon.

DIAGNOSIS

The following criteria are helpful in establishing that a case of *regional lymphadenopathy* is cat scratch disease.[10] With a typical case history,[1] any three are sufficient, but with an atypical case all four should be established.

1. History of cat contact.
2. Laboratory studies negative for the other etiologic possibilities: tuberculosis, brucellosis, infectious mononucleosis, tularemia, lymphogranuloma venereum, Hodgkin's disease, lymphosarcoma and lymphoma.
3. Biopsy of nodes, and findings consistent with cat scratch disease histopathology.[11]
4. A positive skin test to 0.1 cc. of cat scratch disease antigen. The positive skin test has a diagnostic reliability of 95 per cent. Rare false-negative tests do occur, however, so that when the other criteria are positive the patient should be tested with a second antigen from another source.

TREATMENT

Treatment is seldom required after the diagnosis is made. Antibiotics are ineffectual. Suppurative nodes should be aspirated. Surgical draining is contraindicated. Excision is indicated to abort a severe, complicated, or prolonged illness.

PREVENTION

Because of inadequate knowledge of the causative agent and its natural hosts, effective preventive measures are unknown. However, avoidance of cat scratches will obviously prevent many infections.

ITEMS OF NOTE

1) Cat scratch disease has been established as a specific entity.
2) It is world-wide in distribution.
3) The etiology is unknown, but probably a virus.
4) Natural infection in animals is unknown.
5) Infection in man is usually, but not always, caused by the bite or scratch of a cat.
6) Symptoms in man are usually mild and of short duration.

REFERENCES

1. DANIELS, W. R., and MACMURRAY, F. G.: *J.A.M.A., 154:*1247, 1954.
2. DEBRÉ, R., LAMY, M., JAMMET, M. L., COSTIL, L., and MOZZICONACCI, P.: *Bull. et mém. Soc. méd. hôp. Paris, 66:*76, 1950.

3. HÖRING, F. O., and ZWISSLER, T.: *Verhandl. Deutsch. Ges. inn. Med., 60:*624, 1954.

4. MARSHALL, C. E.: *Canad. M.A.J., 75:*724, 1956.

5. MOLLARET, P., REILLY, J., BASTIN, R., and TOURNIER, P.: *Presse méd., 59:*701, 1951.

6. SPAULDING, W. B., and HENNESSY, J. N.: *Am. J. Med., 28:*504, 1960.

7. TURNER, W., BIGLEY, N. J., DODD, M. C., and ANDERSON, G.: *J. Bact., 80:*430, 1960.

8. WARWICK, W. J., and GOOD, R. A.: *A.M.A. J. Dis. Child., 100:*228, 1960.

9. WARWICK, W. J., and GOOD, R. A.: *A.M.A. J. Dis. Child., 100:*236, 1960.

10. WARWICK, W. J., and GOOD, R. A.: *A.M.A. J. Dis. Child., 100:*241, 1960.

11. WINSHIP, T.: *Am. J. Clin. Path. 23:*1012, 1953.

12. ZWISSLER, T.: *Ztschr. klin. Med., 154:*227, 1956.

Chapter 17

INFECTIONS PRODUCED BY
ANIMAL PARASITES

Ernest Carroll Faust, Ph.D.

THE ANIMAL parasites of man are closely related to those which cause infection in domestic and wild animals, and a few parasite species are identical (*viz.*, the "trichina worm," the hydatid cysts and the sheep liver fluke). In many instances the parasites are morphologically identical but have developed strain differences in different host species, so that cross infection is rare or not demonstrated (*viz.*, *Ascaris lumbricoides* of man and the hog, *Hymenolepis nana* of man and domestic rodents). In other instances, for example *Ascaris* of man and the horse, and hookworms of man and the dog, they are specifically different. Again, man may be susceptible to parasites of the reservoir host but is not commonly exposed to these infections; conversely domestic or wild animals may only occasionally be exposed to infection with parasites which are common in the human host. Thus, susceptibility or refractoriness, as well as frequent or only occasional opportunity for exposure are often determining factors in the epidemiology of these animal parasitoses. Yet viewing the broad spectrum of the parasite species common to both types of hosts, one becomes impressed with the importance of the species of animal parasites of wild and domestic animals hosts which from time to time infect man.

The methods by which man is exposed to infections with parasites commonly or incidentally infecting domestic or wild animal hosts may be grouped for the most part in the following categories:

1. Passive introduction of the parasite into the body by the oral route.
   a. When the infective-stage cysts, eggs or larvae have been voided in the feces of the reservoir host and have entered the mouth in polluted food, drink or from contaminated

fingers. Examples: Cysts of *Balantidium coli* from hogs or monkeys; eggs of the hydatid tapeworms *Echinococcus granulosus* and *E. multilocularis* from canine hosts, larvae of *Trichostrongylus* from sheep, goats and other herbivorous animals.

    b. When larvae of the parasite are introduced in supposedly clean food which is eaten in an uncooked state. Examples: *Trichinella* in pork; *Clonorchis sinensis* and *Diphyllobothrium latum* in fresh-water fish; *Taenia saginata* in beef.

    c. When the larval stage in its appropriate insect host accidentally gets into the mouth and is swallowed. Examples: *Dracunculus medinensis* in Cyclops; *Hymenolepis diminuta* in rat fleas and *Dipylidium caninum* in dog fleas.

2. Active penetration of the infective-stage of the parasite into the skin.

    a. From moist soil. Examples: Hookworm and *Strongyloides* larvae.

    b. From water. Example: Blood flukes, *Schistosoma* spp.

    c. Following deposition of the organism onto the skin by a biological or mechanical vector. Examples: *Trypanosoma cruzi* by triatomid-bug intermediate hosts; *Dermatobia hominis* eggs by mosquito carriers; filarial worms by blood-sucking flies.

3. Introduction of the parasite into the skin by an obligatory alternate host. Example: Malaria parasites, by mosquitoes, African trypanosomes, by tsetse flies.

4. Skin contamination by infective stage of the parasite.

    a. Direct contagium from the animal reservoir. Example: *Sarcoptes scabiei* from horses and possibly other domestic animals.

    b. Eggs or larvae deposited on skin by a myiasis-producing fly. Examples: *Oestrus ovis* (sheep bot) *Hypoderma bovis* (cattle bot).

It must be understood that the problem of human infection with animal parasites involving animal hosts is a serious one only when the parasite is a relatively common invader of both the reservoir host and man and when the strains of these parasites in the two types of hosts are physiologically adapted to invasion and infection of the reciprocal host. Hundreds of species of animal parasites which commonly infect domestic and wild animals are only incidental or "rare" parasites of man, but comparatively few species commonly occur in both types of hosts. Special emphasis will be placed on this smaller group.

PROTOZOAN PARASITES

Among the large numbers of species of Protozoa described from vertebrate hosts, very few, indeed, are known to infect man. *Entamoeba histolytica,* (Subphylum *Sarcodina*) the only pathogenic ameba able to invade the intestinal wall of the human host, is a natural parasite of monkeys and less frequently of dogs and rats, but the opportunities for transfer of the cysts (which are the infective stage) from these animals to man, are very few compared with the daily chances of human carriers producing contamination of food, drink and soiled clothing. In a few instances the hog ameba, *Entamoeba polecki,* has been diagnosed as a human infection.

No intestinal flagellates (Subphylum *Mastigophora*) of domestic or wild animals are known to be commonly infective for man.

With respect to members of the Subphylum Sporozoa, two species of coccidia (Subclass Coccidia), *viz., Isospora belli* and *I. hominis,* which are occasionally diagnosed from human feces, have also been found in the excreta of dogs and cats. Among the species of the Subclass Haemosporidea, those belonging to the genus *Plasmodium* which are regarded as exclusively human parasites, *viz., P. vivax, P. malariae, P. falciparum* and *P. ovale,* have identical or closely related counterparts in higher simian hosts, while a few species of *Plasmodium* considered to be exclusively simian parasites are capable of infecting man. A third major group of the Sporozoa (Class Sarcosporidea) contains the genus *Sarcocystis,* which has infrequently been diagnosed from human tissues, usually at autopsy. This infection is relatively common in the muscles of cattle, sheep, horses, hogs, rabbits and other mammals. Infection is probably acquired from food or drink contaminated with feces containing spores of the parasite. Human infection is of subclinical grade.

One intestinal protozoon of the Subphylum *Ciliophora,* class *Ciliatea, Balantidium coli,* is often found in the large bowel of monkeys and the domestic pig; it is a dangerous parasite of man in warm climates. This organism burrows into the wall of the large bowel, producing basally enlarged, deeply excavated lesions, comparable to those of *Entamoeba histolytica* on a somewhat larger scale. Human infection is most probably acquired from the reservoir host as a result of contamination of food or drink with pig droppings which contain the encysted organisms. Patients with balantidiasis often give a history of close association with pigs. The relatively low incidence in man compared with the amount of exposure suggests a considerable degree of refractoriness to the infection. The infection in the porcine host is apparently harmless. However, once the infection has been established in man, it may be either chronic or acute and at times developes in epidemic form. Furthermore, there is no satisfactory drug for the eradication of the infection in the human host.

Some species of hemoflagellates (i.e., those flagellate *Protozoa* which have become adapted to the blood stream, the cells of the reticulo-endothelial system and at times other tissues of the body of vertebrates) are common parasites of both wild or domesticated mammals and man. *Leishmania donovani,* the agent of visceral, leishmaniasis (kala-azar), *L. tropica,* the agent of cutaneous leishmaniasis (Oriental sore, Delhi boil, Aleppo button, etc.), and *L. braziliensis,* causing human muco-cutaneous leishmaniasis in tropical America, have reservoirs in canine hosts (China, Iraq, Iran, Mediterranean countries, tropical America) and in wild rodents (southern U.S.S.R.), and constitute important sources for infection of the sandfly which is the insect vector of these diseases. The human trypanosomes are also related to reservoir infections in wild and domestic mammals. *Trypanosoma gambiense* and *T. rhodesiense* are species of organisms causing African sleeping sickness in man. Clinically and possibly biologically, these organisms are specifically different from one another, as well as from *T. brucei* of big game animals and domestic cattle. Morphologically, however, these three species are identical and are transmissible to the next mammalian host by the same species of tsetse flies.

Nevertheless, *T. gambiense* and *T. rhodesiense* have become so specifically adapted to the human host that they are not readily infective for the large game animals and, similarly, *T. brucei* is apparently not adapted for residence in man. A much closer association is found in *Trypanosoma cruzi,* which has an extensive distribution in mammalian reservoirs and in man from Central Chile and Northern Argentina to the Southwestern United States. This parasite utilizes various species of blood-sucking bugs (Family *Triatomidae*) as intermediate hosts and transmitting agents. The many reservoir hosts include armadillos, opossums, squirrels, bats, numerous species of rodents, monkeys, dogs, and cats. From the reservoir hosts the disease is readily picked up by the blood-sucking bugs and after an incubation period the organisms are inoculated into unsuspecting human beings.

Parasitologists regard toxoplasmosis, produced by *Toxoplasma gondii* as a protozoan infection. This disease is cosmopolitan in distribution; in infants and at times in older children it is highly disabling, at times fatal. This organism not uncommonly parasitizes certain rodents and birds.

HELMINTHIC PARASITES

The Helminths, or parasitic worms, belong primarily to two large Phyla of the Animal Kingdom, the roundworms and the flatworms. In addition, there are two minor groups which parasitize domestic animals and occasionally man, *viz.,* Acanthocephala (thorny-headed worms) and Hirudinea (leeches). The roundworms (Phylum Nematoda) are the most common helminthic parasites of vertebrates. Some species of roundworms parasitize invertebrates, others invade healthy plant tissues and by far the largest number of species is free-living. Forms of human importance include *Trichinella spiralis,* the hookworms and their allies, *Strongyloides stercoralis, Ascaris lumbricoides, Trichuris trichiura,* the filarial worms and *Dracunculus medinensis.* The flatworms (Phylum Platyhelminthes) consist of two parasitic groups, the tapeworms (Class Cestoidea) and the flukes (Class Trematoda), and, in addition, two nonparasitic groups, the turbellarians and the nemerteans. Common tapeworms of man include beef and pork tapeworms, the broad (fish) tapeworm and the dwarf tapeworm.

THE "TRICHINA" WORM, TRICHINELLA SPIRALIS

This nematode, which has a cosmopolitan distribution, is most common as a human parasite under conditions where raw or inadequately cooked pork is consumed by man. The worm was first discovered by Peacock at a human autopsy in London, in 1828, and was first obtained from hog's flesh by Joseph Leidy of Philadephia in 1846. Leuckart (1855) and Virchow (1859) first demonstrated the life cycle and Zenker (1860), the clinical importance of the infection. Except in the Balkan states and Poland the disease is much less important in Europe than it was a century ago, but in the United States (especially in New York, Massachusetts, Connecticut, Minnesota, Missouri and California) a marked increase in incidence of the infection in man has been reported since 1929. This may be due to more careful laboratory and postmortem diagnosis or to an actual increase in cases.

TABLE 44

INCIDENCE OF TRICHINOSIS AND CONDITION OF TRICHINAE BY AGE AT DEATH IN 855 POSITIVE CASES (WRIGHT, JACOBS AND WALTON, 1944)

Age at Death	Total Number Cases	Positive Cases		Condition of Larvae		
		Number	Per Cent	Live	Mixed	Dead
1–44	1,967	248	12.6	102	65	81
45 and over	3,304	603	18.3	143	77	383
1–4	85	1	1.2	1	—	—
5–9	63	4	6.3	—	1	3
10–14	65	8	12.3	4	3	1
15–19	122	7	5.7	4	2	1
20–24	195	21	10.8	10	7	4
25–29	228	27	11.8	14	8	5
30–34	251	37	14.7	19	8	10
35–44	958	143	14.9	50	36	57
45–54	1,050	190	18.1	68	35	87
55–64	1,031	186	18.0	40	22	124
65–74	817	156	19.1	27	18	111
75 and over	406	71	17.5	8	2	61
Unknown	42	4	9.5	—	—	4
Total	5,313	855	16.1	245	142	468

Man has also acquired trichinosis from consumption of bear meat (Northwestern U.S., Alaska and Canada) and walrus meat (Greenland). Rats become infected from eating infected rats or discarded hog trimmings in country slaughter houses; dogs, cats and many other mammals, develop infection from infected rats or other primary reservoirs.

Infected meat contains the encysted *Trichinella* larvae. When this meat is eaten raw or inadequately processed, the larvae are digested out of the flesh in the patient's stomach, become excysted in the duodenum and invade the duodenal and jejunal mucosa, where

TABLE 45

INCIDENCE OF TRICHINELLA SPIRALIS IN VARIOUS POPULATION GROUPS AS FOUND IN
5,313 POST-MORTEM EXAMINATIONS (WRIGHT, JACOBS AND WALTON, 1944)

	Total Number in Group	Number Infected	Per Cent Injected
Males..	3,736	623	16.7
White.......................................	2,757	465	16.9
Colored.....................................	915	152	16.6
North American Indians......................	8	1	—
Chinese....	9	0	—
Japanese....................................	4	1	—
Filipinos....................................	10	0	—
Mexican....................................	25	3	—
Race unknown..............................	8	1	—
Females..	1,575	232	14.7
White.......................................	942	140	14.9
Colored.....................................	608	86	14.1
North American Indians.....	8	0	—
Japanese....................................	1	0	—
Mexican....................................	10	4	—
Race unknown..............................	6	2	—
Sex unknown....................................	2	0	—
Whites...	3,699	605	16.4
Negroes..	1,523	238	15.6
Other races....................................	75	9	—
Race unknown..................................	16	3	—
Military (Army-Navy)........................	324[1]	41	12.7
Officers (commissioned and warrant)...........	117	19	16.2
Enlisted men................................	207[1]	22	10.6
Army.......................................	203[2]	27	13.3
Navy.......................................	121[2]	14	11.6
Families and relatives of military men.........	64	11	—
Civil..	4,984	813	16.3
Civilian Conservation Corps....................	54[3]	5	—
Farmers....................................	289	48	16.6
Villagers...................................	147	16	10.9
Veterans, mostly World War I................	765[3]	157	20.5
Military—Civil status unknown.................	5	1	—
Sea (Navy-Merchant Marine)..................	300	36	12.0
Merchant Marine...........................	179	22	11.3
Land..	5,013	819	16.3
Mentally deranged under hospitalization.........	684	115	16.8
Mentally sound or not under hospitalization......	5,629	740	16.0
High economic-social status....................	1,189	179	15.1
Low economic-social status....................	3,788	630	16.6
Economic-social status unknown................	336	46	13.7
Total cases...............................	5,313	855	16.1

[1]One case, both soldier and sailor, counted only once.
[2]One case, both soldier and sailor, counted in both groups.
[3]Two cases, both CCC and veteran, counted in both groups.

in three to five days they develop into adult males (1.4-1.6) mm. by 40-60 microns) and females (somewhat larger than the males). After fertilization the females invade the tissues of the intestinal wall more deeply and begin to deposit living young, many of which burrow into the mesenteric vessels and are carried to skeletal muscles, where they are filtered out and soon become encysted. Larviposition by the female worm covers a period of about six weeks. The heaviest infection occurs in muscles poor in glycogen.

The pathology and symptomatology of trichinosis is divided into three periods: 1) that of *invasion* of the intestinal wall, with symptoms resembling acute food poisoning; 2) that of *larval migration*, with severe myositis and edema; and 3) the toxic stage, following encystation of the larvae, with a variety of symptoms of toxic origin. The disease is usually accompanied by a hypereosinophilia. Although the above picture is typical of the severe cases, and death or prolonged invalidism may be a sequela, unquestionably a preponderant number of cases in the United States, exhibit mild symptoms or are without apparent symptoms.

Diagnosis of trichinosis may be suggested by the patient's history and a high eosinophilia, and is confirmed by recovery of the larvae from centrifugalized specimens of blood or from digests of biopsied samples of biceps muscle, as well as by the Bachman intradermal reaction, using antigen in dilution of 1 to 5,000—10,000. No specific therapeutic is known; only symptomatic treatment is available.

While many ideas have been advanced for the prevention of trichinosis in the human population, the majority of these are impracticable. In the United States infected pork from country slaughter houses provides the largest number of serious clinical cases, but the larger government-inspected slaughter houses provide little guarantee of trichina-free meat unless it has been subjected to refrigeration at 5° F. for twenty days or at 2° F. for twenty-four hours. Smoking, salting and drying do not necessarily kill the larvae. If no garbage slops containing infected pork trimmings or viscera were fed to hogs on the farm or in the slaughter pens, the incidence and amount of infection in the hogs would soon be reduced to the vanishing point. Until this protection is provided, the only simple safeguard is the thorough heating or deep freezing of all pork to be consumed. The same precaution applies to bear meat, which is not infrequently infected with this parasite. The rat, while often harboring the parasite, is of less importance than was formerly thought in spreading trichinosis to man or hogs.

TABLE 46

SUMMARY OF 4,864 AUTOPSY EXAMINATIONS MADE FOR TRICHINAE IN MAN IN THE UNITED STATES

Year	Author	Locality	Method	Number of Exams.	Infected Number	Infected Per Cent
1901	Williams	Buffalo, N. Y.	Pressed Muscle	505	26	5.3
1910	Simonds: Indianapolis	St. Louis	Pressed Muscle	100	2	2
1931	Queen	Rochester, N. Y., Boston	Digestion	402	75	18.6
1934	Riley and Scheifley	Minneapolis	Pressed Muscle	117	20	17.1
1936	Hinman: New Orleans	New Orleans	Digestion	200	7	3.5
1936	McNaught and Anderson	San Francisco	Digestion	200	48	24
1937	Hall and Collins	Washington, D. C.	Digestion and Pressed Muscle	300	41	13.6
1937	Queen	Denver, Colo.	Digestion	431	70	16.3
1937	Magath	Rochester, Minn.	Pressed Muscle	220	17	8
1937	Scheifley	Minneapolis and St. Paul	Pressed Muscle	118	15	12.7
1938	Walker and Breckenridge	Alabama	Digestion and Compression	100	33	33.0
1939	Sawitz	New Orleans, La.	Digestion	400	24	6.0
1939	Butt and Lapeyre	Los Angeles, Cal.	Digestion	170	31	18.2
1939	Harrell and Johnson	Durham, N. C.	Digestion and Compression	105	3	2.8
1940	Oosting	Dayton, O.	Digestion	134	27	20.1
1940	Catron	Ann Arbor, Mich.	Digestion	300	44	14.7
1940	Gould	Detroit, Mich.	Digestion and Compression	500	93	18.6
1941	Merrill	Northern Utah		47	0	0
1941	Meleney	Nashville, Tenn.	Digestion and Compression	209	21	10.0
1944	Broders and Porter	Richmond, Va.	Digestion and Compression	100	6	6
1948	Brooks, Ward and Holder	Mississippi	Digestion and Compression	50	3	6
1951	Beard	San Francisco	Digestion	161	13	8

HOOKWORMS AND THEIR ALLIES

The two common human hookworms, *Nectaor americanus* and *Ancylostoma duodenale,* are rarely found in reservoir hosts, and the common dog hookworm, *Ancylostoma caninum,* seldom, if ever, parasitizes man. On the other hand, a hookworm of dogs and cats in warm climates, *Ancylostoma ceylanicum,* is an occasional intestinal parasite of man in Brazil, Ceylon and the Philippines. Another species commonly parasitizing the dog, *A. braziliense,* is present along the south Atlantic and the Gulf coastal areas of the United States, in coastal southern Brazil and in isolated foci elsewhere. This worm produces only a cutaneous manifestation in man, referred to as "larva migrans" or "creeping eruption." This is due to the fact that the infective-stage larvae of this worm, on penetrating the skin, appear to be incapable of reaching the peripheral blood vessels, but continue to live for weeks or months in serpiginous tunnels which they produce in the skin. *Bunostomum phlebotomum,* a hookworm of cattle, has also incidentally produced "creeping eruption" in man.

Other roundworms, more or less akin to the hookworms, which are relatively common in domestic mammals and occasionally parasitize man, include the following: 1) *Haemonchus contortus,* the sheep wireworm; 2) *Metastrongylus elongatus,* which parasitizes the respiratory tract of hogs, sheep and cattle; 3) *Ternidens deminutus* and species of *Oesophagostomum,* which commonly infect simian hosts. On the other hand, *Strongyloides stercoralis,* which is not uncommon in the human host and the chimpanzee in certain warm areas of the world, is occasionally found in dogs, which possibly obtain their infection from human sources. Larvae of other nematodes commonly found in domestic animals may produce granulomatous lesions in the human eye (ophthalmic nematodiasis of Wilder), or hepatic lesions (visceral larva migrans of Beaver *et al.*) due to migration of the dog Ascarid, *Toxocara canis,* in the viscera of the human host.

One of the most interesting, and historically the most important, roundworms is the dragon worm *(Dracunculus medinensis),* commonly found as a parasite of man in parts of India, Arabia, Iran, Iraq, and Africa. Upon becoming mature, the meter-long female worm crawls from the patient's viscera to the skin layers and produces a little cutaneous blister at the point where its head nears the surface of the skin. On contact with fresh water the blister ruptures and a swarm of active larvae is discharged. These larvae may be picked up by little water "fleas" (Cyclops), in the body cavity of which the larvae mature. When human beings accidentally ingest the Cyclops in raw drinking water, they acquire the infection. In China dogs are reservoirs of this worm and in the United States it parasitizes fur-bearing mammals, although in neither of these countries is the parasite known to infect man.

INCIDENTAL ROUNDWORM INFECTIONS OF MAN

From time to time clinicians and medical parasitologists have reported cases of "rare" infections of man due to roundworms. Almost without exception these worms are relatively common parasites of domestic or wild animals, which accidentally or incidentally occur in the human subject. Mention may be made of *Syngamus laryngeus,* a relatively common parasite of the upper respiratory tract of cattle, water buffaloes and goats, with at least twenty-two reported infections from man; several species of *Trichostrongylus* and *Ostertagia,* commonly parasitizing the intestinal tract of many species of herbivorous mammals and reported from time to time in man, particularly in Asia and Africa; *Gongylonema pulchrum,* a relatively common esophageal parasite of ruminants, monkeys, hedgehogs, bears and pigs, with at least eighteen reported instances from man (buccal mucosa); *Gnathostoma spinigerum* of feline, canine and other reservoir hosts, and *G. hispidum* of the pig, producing subcutaneous abscesses and at times tunnels (so-called "creeping eruption") in man, and *Thelazia callipaeda,* the conjunctival worm of the dog, as well as *T. californiensis* of the dog and cat, both of which have on rare occasions been recovered from the human conjunctiva.

Increasing interest has developed in recent years in immature (and occasionally the adult) stages of filarial worms not well adapted to the human host, discovered in the tissues of man. Cases were reported in earlier years from the Mediterranean countries, the Near and Middle East and once each in Argentina, Brazil and Louisiana. More recently several larval filarial infections have been reported from Southeastern United States, of which a majority have acquired the infection in Florida. Most, if not all of these larval filariae, and the three or four cases of adult worms, have been diagnosed as belonging to the genus *Dirofilaria* and classified as *Dirofilaria conjunctivae.* The most likely natural host is the dog, and the transmitter a domestic mosquito, although wild mammalian hosts may possibly serve in the same capacity as definitive hosts. In the Western Hemisphere the cosmopolitan canine filaria is *D. immitis.* In man, a large majority of the human infections involve the subcutaneous tissues, on the head, trunk and forearms. In view of the migrating propensity of these larval filariae, the clinical entity in the human host has been referred to as "filarial larva migrans."

Only a few years ago the species of filariae found in man were all considered to be specific for the human host. Now at least three of these species are known to have wild mammalian hosts, *viz., Acanthocheilonema streptocerca* and *Loa loa,* both of Tropical Africa, parasitizing the chimpanzee, and *Brugia malayi,* in the Malayan Federation, commonly infecting domestic cats and their wild relatives. In contrast, there is no evidence that man, whose species of *Onchocerca (O. volvulus)* produces serious disability in the human subject, is a susceptible host of other species of this genus which are common parasites of horses and cattle.

The ascaris of the hog, *Ascaris lumbricoides* var. *suum,* is morphologically indistinguishable from that of man but is biologically different. Man may occasionally become infected from ingesting infective-stage *Ascaris* eggs from porcine sources. The adult cat ascarid *Toxocara cati,* has at times been reported from the human intestine.

THE TAPEWORMS

Domestic animals play an important role in most of the tapeworm infections of man, serving either as reservoir or intermediate hosts. The rat and mouse are reservoirs of the dwarf tapeworm (*Hymenolepis nana*) and the rat tapeworm, (*H. diminuta*), while the dog and cat serve as reservoir hosts of the double-pored tapeworm (*Dipylidium caninum*). *H. diminuta* and *D. caninum* are relatively uncommon human parasites and are acquired from accidentally swallowing infected insects which are ectoparasites of the reservoir host. *H. nana* requires no intermediate host. It is relatively common as a human infection. Although rats and mice are commonly infected with this worm, they are infrequently the source of human infection, since the human and rodent strains of this tapeworm are not readily infective for the reciprocal hosts. Dogs serve as reservoir hosts of the broad fish tapeworm, *Diphyllobothrium latum,* but man is usually the indirect source of his own infection, which necessarily is carried though: 1) a water "flea" (*Diaptomus* or *Cyclops*), and 2) a fresh-water fish, before becoming infective for a mammalian host.

Rarely man has become accidentally infected with tapeworms normally parasitic in simian hosts, as, for example, *Bertiella studeri,* or in birds, as for example, *Drepanidotaenia lanceolata,* a common parasite of ducks.

The most important relationship of domestic mammals as reservoirs or intermediate hosts of human tapeworm infections is illustrated by the species of Taenia *(T. saginata* and *T. solium)* and the related hydatid worm *(Echinococcus granulosus).* In the case of the beef tapeworm *(Taenia saginata),* man is the only known host of the mature worm, while the ox is the necessary host of the larval or *cysticercus* stage. Similarly man harbors the mature pork tapeworm *(T. solium),* while the hog is the usual host of the larval stage. However, man is also a very acceptable host for the cysticercus stage of *T. solium (C. cellulosae),* which commonly lodges in the brain, producing epilepsy and paralysis. Human cysticercosis is rare in the United States and Canada, but rather frequent in Latin America and India. The larvae (cysticerci or bladder worms) develop respectively in the striped muscles of the ox or hog, after these animals have ingested the eggs which have been evacuated in stools of infected persons. When man eats inadequately heated or inadequately processed beef or pork that is infected, he acquires the infection. Pork tapeworm infection is rarely encountered in the United States, but beef tapeworm infection is widely distributed in this country and elsewhere, and, furthermore, shows no evidence of diminishing in the human population. In endemic foci cattle should not be allowed to pasture on ground contaminated with polluted sewage. All beef and pork should be thoroughly cooked or frozen as a simple safeguard against infection. The hydatid worm *(E. granulosus)* reaches maturity in the intestine of the dog and its wild relatives. Eggs are discharged in dog's feces and are the source of infection in the larval stage *(hytadid cyst)* of sheep, hogs, cattle, other herbivorous mammals and man. Sporadic human infection with hytadid cyst is reported from the United States. This infection in man is prevalent in Southern Brazil, Uruguay, Argentina, Chile, the Middle East and Southern Australia. Control of this serious infection requires deep burying of the carcasses of sheep, hogs and cattle which have died of the disease and meticulous care on the part of human beings not to allow dog's feces to contamniate food, drink, play objects, or mess kits.

The related hydatid worm, E. *multilocularis,* is common as an adult in foxes, and its hydatid larval stage in mice of the tundra of the northern boreal regions and other mice of woodlands in Central

Europe. In these areas human infection with the larva (alveolar hydatid) is not infrequent.

THE TREMATODES OR FLUKES

Man and the higher vertebrate animals are parasitized by only those trematodes which require some mollusc as an intermediate host (i.e., the digenetic trematodes). In the mollusc two or more generations of the life cycle are developed. There emerge from the mollusc (usually a snail) swarms of tailed larvae, called cercariae, which either invade the definitive host directly via the skin route, or first encyst in the tissues, or on the surface of a second inter-mediate host. When the infected tissues of this latter host are con-sumed by the appropriate final host, the trematode is enabled to proceed with its life cycle.

The blood flukes or schistosomes produce cercariae which directly penetrate the skin of the definitive host. The adults live in the portal blood stream and caval tributaries and their eggs are evacuated from the host's body either in the feces or urine. Of the several blood flukes living in mammals, three species are relatively common and produce very serious symptoms in large portions of the human popu-lation in endemic areas, namely *Schistosoma haematobium* (Africa and Western Asia), *S. mansoni* (Africa and parts of Tropical Amer-ica), and *S. japonicum* (Oriental area). *S. haematobium* and *S. mansoni* almost exclusively parasitize man, rarely infecting wild mammals. *S. japonicum,* which is distributed through extensive areas in Central and South China, and occurs in a few foci in Japan, Formosa and five islands of the Philippines, has been recorded from dogs, cats, rodents, cattle, water buffaloes and other mammals suf-ficiently often to indicate the importance of these animals as res-ervoirs of this infection. In addition, *S. bovis,* a common parasite of domestic animals in portions of the Eastern Hemisphere, has, on a few occasions, been diagnosed as a human infection.

In contrast to the blood flukes, many of those trematodes which encyst in second intermediate hosts and infect man by the buccal route, are parasites common to both man and other vertebrate hosts. Attention may be directed to a few typical examples. From eating raw or inadequately cooked fresh-water fish, man and other fish-eating mammals acquire infection with the Chinese liver fluke

(Clonorchis sinensis) and its close relatives *(Opisthorchis felineus and O. viverrini)*. Canines and felines are especially prone to infection with these worms. Other flukes acquired from consuming raw fish include minute heterophyoid species, as *Metagonimus* and *Heterophyes*. Some of these small flukes, as well as species of echinostomes, are more commonly parasitic in birds than they are in mammals. The sheep liver fluke *(Fasciola hepatica)* is common in sheep, less frequent in other mammals and man. It gains entrance to the hosts' body through consumption of raw vegetation on which the cercariae have encysted. At least one human case of fascioliasis has been reported from the Continental United States; it is endemic in Cuba, Puerto Rico, Mexico, South America, Hawaii and in the Mediterranean countries, where man acquires the disease from eating watercress salad. Occasional human infection has been reported with the giant cattle liver fluke, *Fasciola gigantica*. The giant intestinal fluke *(Fasciolopsis buski)* which is prevalent in certain areas in the Far East, is a common parasite of both pigs and man in these localities. The Oriental lung fluke *(Paragonimus westermani),* which mammals acquire from eating the soft parts of crabs and crayfishes, parasitizes man, felines and canines. In the United States, a closely related species, *P. kellicotti,* is known as a parasite of several species of fur-bearing mammals, but only one probable human infection is on record. Potentially amphistomate flukes of the hog, cattle and certain wild ruminants may infect man but reported human infections are very few. Echinostomate flukes of the dog *(Echinochasmus perfoliatus)* and even of the duck *(Echinostoma revolutum)* are occasional human parasites.

ARTHROPOD PARASITES AND VECTORS

Many insects and other arthropods are parasitic on man and other animals. A few actually invade the tissues of their victims but most of them are only ectoparasites, visiting the host to obtain a blood meal.

A few species of mites enter the human skin. Most notorious of these is the mange mite, *Sarcoptes scabiei,* but it is doubtful if the variety which infests man has an animal host. On the other hand, the variety of this mite which infests horses, possibly also the bovine and ovine varieties, occasionally produce dermatitis in man. Likewise, *Demodex folliculorum* of the dog may produce follicular dermatitis in man.

The rat mite, *Bdellonyssus bacoti,* causes an itchy dermatitis affecting mainly the legs but also other parts of the body. The parasite ordinarily inhabits dark crevises where it lays its eggs. Hence, the semidarkness of motion picture theaters and also parts of hospitals, office buildings and department stores are favorable sources of infestation. In cold weather the mites even turn to warmer rooms, like the bathroom and kitchen. They remain on the brown rat only a few hours during feeding and a lesser time on human beings. It is thus only a temporary parasite of the skin, like the bed bug. The disease has been recognized, particularly in Texas (Shelmire); since many cases are observed in Texas and Louisiana this dermatitis runs a close second to scabies in frequency of parasitic dermatoses. The incidence rises during anti-rat campaigns, when the parasite deserts its favorite host and turns to man. Children are affected the more extensively, with lesions on the face and hands, but the ankles, beltline, upper parts of shoulders and neck may be involved. Vesicles are present in addition to the wheals and papules observed in adults.

The fowl mite, *Dermanyssus gallinae,* is an ubiquitous parasite that deserts sick and dead fowls, whereupon the attendants of such fowls receive their attention. The skin of the hands becomes scaly, dry and covered diffusely by papules. In severe cases pustules and crusts may form. Experimental and epidemiological evidence suggests that this mite is a vector of St. Louis encephalitis and Western equine encephalomyelitis from fowl to fowl reservoir of the virus. The mouse mite, *Allodermanyssus sanguineus,* is a vector of rickettsialpox to man (New York City and Boston). Chiggers in the southwest Pacific and East Asia transmit scrub typhus to man. Tongue worms *(Linguatula)* occasionally infest man.

The chigoe *(Tunga penetrans)* and many species of fly maggots infest both man and a variety of mammalian species.

THE PROBLEM OF PREVENTION OF ANIMAL PARASITES INFECTING MAN

Where man is the sole or only important host of an infection, public health measures directed against the dispersal of unsterilized human excreta, together with specific therapeutic procedures, if available, should ultimately wipe out the disease. But where reservoir hosts are involved, the situation is more complicated, since the parasite may be propagated in spite of these control measures. In such instances, as well as those in which animal or plant tissue serves as a medium for transfer of the organisms to man, mankind must be taught the sources of the infection and the means for protecting his food and drink, as well as his skin, from the invader. The successful completion of this latter type of protection cannot be carried out solely by police powers of a government but requires cooperation of all individuals in the community. It pressupposes, therefore, a higher type of civilization than is found in primitive peoples, in whom diseases of animal etiology are most prevalent. Yet the incidence of trichinosis and beef tapeworm infection in our supposedly civilized communities indicates that much remains to be accomplished along these lines.

In the case of arthropods which serve as biological or mechanical vectors of parasitic infections DDT has proven to be of inestimable aid in eradicating the vector, hence the transmission of the disease. However, strains of filth flies, such as *Musca domestica*, of several culicid mosquitoes and at least one strain of the body louse, *Pediculus corporis*, have developed resistance to DDT and will require other potent insecticides for purposes of disease control.

ITEMS OF NOTE

1) Numerous parasites classified in the Animal Kingdom infect or infest other animals; comparatively few such parasites are common to animal hosts and man.

2) Protozoan parasites of animals cause the following diseases in man:

Amebic dysentery, caused by *Entamoeba histolytica,* a natural parasite of monkeys and sometimes of dogs and rats. Dysentery caused by *Balantidium coli* from monkeys and domestic pigs. *Kala-azar,* Oriental sore and allied conditions caused by *Leishmania donovani* and *L. tropica* from canine and rodent hosts. African sleeping sickness caused by *Trypanosoma gambiense* and *T. rhodesiense* closely akin to trypanosomes of wild game in Africa, as well as Chagas' disease caused by *T. cruzi,* common in domestic and wild mammals in Latin America.

3) Parasitic roundworms of animals are responsible for the following ailments of man:

Trichinosis caused by *Trichinella spiralis,* a parasite of hogs, bears, the walrus and rats.

Creeping eruption (cutaneous larva migrans) caused by the hookworm *Ancylostoma braziliense,* an intestinal parasite of dogs and cats in warm climates, and visceral larva migrans caused by the dog ascarid, *Toxocara canis,* a parasite of the dog in warm climates.

Dracontiasis caused by the dragon worm, *Dracunculus medinesis,* a parasite of dogs in China and of fur-bearing animals in the United States (although the disease does not occur in man in either of these countries).

Other roundworm infections include *Trichostrongylus* from herbivorous animals, the sheep wireworm *Haemonchus contortus* from sheep and cattle, *Metastrongylus elongatus* from the respiratory tracts of hogs, sheep and cattle, *Ternidens deminutus* from monkeys and *Syngamus laryngeus* from cattle. The thread-worm *Strongyloides stercoralis* is found in dogs. Various other roundworms are occasionally acquired by man from animals. Some of these in their larval state may migrate into ectopic sites in the human body, as the eye, brain and liver, where they cause serious tissue damage.

4) Tapeworm infections are rather commonly transmitted from animals to man:

The dwarf tapeworms, *Hymenolepis nana,* is found in rats and mice, but man is probably rarely infected from rodent sources. The rat tapeworm, *Hymenolepis diminuta,* is found in rats and mice, but human infection is acquired from swallowing an infected insect which serves as intermediate host.

The double-pored tapeworm (dog tapeworm) *Dipylidium caninum,* is acquired from dogs and cats by swallowing an infected flea.

The broad fish tapeworm, *Diphyllobothrium latum,* finds the dog as a host, but man is infected by eating fish.

The beef tapeworm, *Taenia saginata,* and the pork tapeworm, *Taenia solium,* are acquired from insufficiently cooked beef and pork. Cerebral disease frequently develops in man when he becomes infected with the cysticercus stage of *T. solium,* which typically develops in the hog.

Hydatid disease, caused by *Echinococcus granulosus,* is acquired from the dog, but sheep, hogs, cattle and other herbivorous animals are the usual hosts of the hydatid larva.

5) The trematodes—flukes—which parasitize man all require some mollusc, usually a snail, as an intermediate host:

Several liver flukes find a host in the dog or the cat among other animals. Infection with *Clonorchis sinensis, Opisthorchis felineus* and *Heterophyes* or *Metagonimus* is contacted by these animals from eating raw fresh water fish.

The sheep liver fluke *Fasciola hepatica,* which is common in sheep, is acquired from eating raw plants which carry the encysted metacercariae.

The giant intestinal fluke *Fasciolopsis buski* is carried by the hog, which acquires it from ingesting infested plants.

The Oriental lung fluke *Paragonimus westermani* is contracted by dogs and cats from eating crabs and crayfish. The closely related *P. kellicotti* is found among fur-bearing animals in the United States.

The blood flukes, *Schistosoma haematobium* and *S. mansoni* occasional parasites of wild mammals, *S. japonicum* of dogs, cats, cattle and rodents, and *S. bovis* of cattle penetrate the skin directly.

6) Arthropods from animals hosts cause the following afflictions in man:

(a) Dermatitis, caused by *Sarcoptes scabiei* from horses, *Bdellonyssus bacoti* from rats, *Demodex folliculorum* from dogs, *Dermanyssus gallinae* from birds.

(b) Rickettsial, bacterial and spirochetal diseases, *viz.,* rodent fleas transmit plague and murine typhus; trombiculid mites transmit scrub typhus; ticks transmit spotted fever, relapsing fever and tularemia; and the mouse mite transmits rickettsialpox.

7) Prevention consists in education and a better appreciation of the sources of infection. In case of arthropods, DDT and benzene hexachloride (for bugs) constitute valuable weapons of control.

REFERENCES

ALICATA, J. E.: *Hawaiian M. J., 12:*196-201, 1953.
BEARD, R. R.: *J.A.M.A., 146:*331-334, 1951.
BEAVER, P. C. *et al.: Pediatrics, 9:*7-19, 1952.
BEAVER, P. C.: *Exp. Parasit., 5:*587-621, 1956.
BIOCCA, E.: *J. Helminth., 25:*1-10, 1951.
CHANDLER, A. C.: *J.A.M.A., 78:*636-639, 1922.
CHANDLER, A. C.: *Introduction to Parasitology,* 8th Ed., New York and London, 1949.

CRAIG, C. F. and FAUST, E. C.: *Clinical Parasitology*, 6th Ed., Philadelphia, 1957.

DEANE, L. M. and DEANE, M. P.: *O Hospital* (Brazil), *45:*703-707, 1954.

DESPORTES, C.: *Ann. de Parasit., 20:*160-190, 1944-1945.

EYLES, D. E., COATNEY, G. R. and GETZ, M. E.: *Science, 131:*1812-1813, 1960.

EYLES, D. E. and FRENKEL, J. K.: *U.S.P.H.S. Monogr.* No. 247, Washington, D.C. 1952.

FAUST, E. C. and KHAW, O. K.: *Am. J. Hyg. Monogr. Ser.* 3: 1927.

FAUST, E. C.: *Human Helminthology*, 3rd Ed., Philadelphia, 1949.

FAUST, E. C., AGOSIN, M., *et al.: Am. J. Trop. Med. & Hyg.*, 1:239-249, 1952.

FAUST, E. C.: *Amebiasis.* Springfield, Thomas, 1954, 154 pp.

FAUST, E. C., GIRALDO, L. E., CAICEDO, G. and BONFANTE, R.: *Am. J. Trop. Med. & Hyg., 10:*343-349, 1961.

FRYE, W. W. and MELENEY, H. E.: *Am. J. Hyg., 16:*729-749, 1932.

GOULD, S. E.: *Trichinosis.* Springfield, Thomas, 1945, 365 pp.

HALL, M. C.: *Control of Animal Parasites,* Evanston, Ill., 1936.

HEGNER, R. and CHU, H. G.: *Am. J. Hyg., 12:*62-108, 1930.

HIRST, L. F.: *Indian J. M. Res., 10:*789-820, 1923.

HUTCHINSON, M. P.: *Ann. Trop. Med. & Parasit., 47:*156-168, 169-182, 1953; *48:*75-94, 1954.

KERSHAW, W. E.: *Trans. R. Soc. Trop. Med. & Hyg., 49:*143-150, 1955.

KESSEL, J. F. and JOHNSTONE, H. G.: *Am. J. Trop. Med., 29:*311-315, 1949.

KIRBY-SMITH, J. L., DOVE, W. E. and WHITE, G. F.: *Arch. Dermat. & Syph., 13:*137-173, 1926.

KNOX, J. M.: *J. Louisiana State Med. Soc., 105:*69-72, 1953.

KUNTZ, R. E. and MALAKATIS, G. M.: *J. Parasit., 41:*467-475, 1955.

LAING, A. B. G., EDESON, J. F. B., and WHARTON, R. H.: *Ann. Trop. Med. & Parasit.,* 92-99, 1960.

MAGATH, T. B.: *Am. J. Trop. Med., 9:*17-48, 1929.

MATHESON, R.: *Medical Entomology,* 2nd Ed., Ithaca, N. Y., 1950.

MOORTHY, V. N. and SWEET, W. C.: *Indian M. Gaz., 71:*437-442, 1936.

MORISHITA, K. O. R.: *Ann. Trop. Med., 18:*23-26, 1924.

PEEL, E. and CHARDOME, M.: *Ann. Soc. belge de Med. Trop., 26:*117-156, 1946.

PROMMAS, C. and DAENGSVANG, S.: *J. Parasitol., 19:*287-292, 1933; *22:*180-186, 1936.

RAUSCH, R.: *Pub. Health Repts., 68:*533, 1953.

RAUSCH, R.: *Am. J. Trop. Med. & Hyg., 5:*1086-1092, 1956.

TOBIE, J. E.: *Proc. Soc. Exper. Biol. & Med., 45:*691-693, 1940.

VAN HOOF, L., HENRARD, C. and PEEL, E.: *Rec. trav. sci. med. Congo-Belge, 1:*53-68, 1942.

VOGEL, H.: *Deutsch. med. Wochenschrift, 80:*931-932, 1955.

WARDLE, R. A.: *Bull.* No. 45, *The Biol. Board of Canada,* Ottawa, 1935.

WILDER, H. C.: *Tr. Am. Acad. Ophth.,* Nov.-Dec., 1950.

WOOD, S. F.: *Am. J. Trop. Med., 29:*43-55, 1949.

WOODY, N. C. and WOODY, H. B.: *J.A.M.A., 159:*476-477, 1955.

WRIGHT, W. H., KERR, K. B. and WALTON, A. C.: *U. S. Pub. Health Reports, 59:*669-681, 1944.

Chapter 18

FUNGOUS DISEASES

CHARLES H. BRIDGES, D.V.M., PH.D.

BIOLOGY OF THE PATHOGENIC FUNGI

THE FUNGOUS DISEASES may be conveniently divided into two main groups: the superficial or dermatomycoses and the localized or systemic granulomatous mycoses. This division is based on a fundamental difference in the parasitic habitat of the fungi in each group, and it also largely reflects the biological adaptability of the infecting organism.

The fungi causing most superficial mycoses are parasites, perhaps not strictly obligate ones, but most commonly identified when living on animal tissue. However, a minority of them are common in soil and only occasionally are found in the parasitic state. All of these fungi have the special ability to grow within the keratin of the skin and its appendages. The actual substrate on which the organisms maintain their population in the soil is not known. However, they may be baited with hair or wool and subsequently isolated on selective artificial media.[11] Evidence for obligatory parasitism in the case of many dermatophytes is the fact that they have become adapted to animal hosts and are seldom found as free-living forms in nature. A few, however, have been found capable of reproducing in soil in the laboratory, but they have not been isolated from the soil of the environment of infected individuals. Furthermore, the dermatomycoses are seldom if ever fatal. Many of them are contagious, and transmission may occur readily from contaminated premises to animals to man. Control and prevention of most infections of this type are relatively simple, being based on the detection and treatment of infected hosts and the prevention of contact between healthy subjects, infected carriers, and contaminated premises or fomites.

The biology of the fungi causing the systemic mycoses is somewhat complex also. However, clinical evidence from both human and animal cases indicates that seldom are these fungi transmitted directly from infected to normal subjects. During recent years it has been found that most of these organisms live in the soil, sharing this habitat with plant pathogens and with hundreds of other fungi which lack pathogenic properties. There are increasing indications, however, that some of these pathogenic fungi are found in greater concentrations around areas containing relatively large amounts of organic matter such as that of decaying wood, about the roosts of birds, and dens of animals. Although some have a world-wide distribution, others have a rather restricted geographic distribution because of climatic conditions, soil types, adaptability of the organism, and unknown factors.

Infection appears to depend on incidental contact with the organism in its natural environment. In most cases this is through inhalation of contaminated dust or inoculation into wounds. Rather large inoculums of some fungi causing deep or systemic mycoses are necessary to establish progressive disease. According to Henrici,[7] progressive infection with some of these fungi frequently depends on repeated contact with the organism and does not occur until previous contact has rendered an animal hypersensitive. However, with others, pulmonary infection can be established in experimental animals quite regularly with a single inoculation of a large number of spores. The indications for host-susceptibility as a factor is indicated by the fact that age, hormonal balance and general individual peculiarities of the host appear to play a greater role in susceptibility or resistence than does variation in pathogenicity of the infecting fungus from time to time. There are, however, some strains within species of certain pathogenic fungi which are slightly more pathogenic than others. Scarification of inoculated skin greatly favors experimental infection with many dermatophytes and more obvious factors favoring systemic mycoses are certain debilitating diseases such as diabetes, advanced neoplastic diseases and changes in microbial flora of the mucous membranes caused by prolonged use of antibiotics. Epidemiological studies have revealed considerable evidence of the greater susceptibility of some species of animals and races of people to certain mycoses.

Many of the organisms producing systemic mycoses exhibit the phenomenon of dimorphism, i.e., they grow as yeastlike fungi in the host's tissues and as molds in the soil or on special artificial media. However, they may also grow as yeast forms on certain artificial media and at certain temperatures *in vitro*. They usually grow slowly in tissue, and the resulting inflammation is chronic and granulomatous in nature. Thus mycotic granulomas may superficially resemble

TABLE 47

VALID DERMATOPHYTE SPECIES
(AFTER AJELLO)

Epidermophyton floccosum	*T. gourvilii*
*Keratinomyces ajelloi**	*T. megninii**
*Microsporum audouinii**	*T. mentagrophytes**
*M. canis**	*T. rubrum**
*M. distortum**	*T. schoenleinii**
M. ferrugineum	*T. soudanense*
*M. gypseum**	*T. tonsurans*
*M. nanum**	*T. verrucosum**
Trichophyton concentricum	*T. violaceum*
*T. equinum**	*T. yaoundei*
*T. gallinae**	

*Those which also have been reported to infect animals. (This data was added by C.H.B.)

TABLE 48

HUMAN PATHOGENIC FUNGI OTHER THAN THE DERMATOPHYTES
(AFTER AJELLO)

ACTINOMYCETES	*Cephalosporium falciforme*
*Actinomyces israelii**	*Cladosporium carrionii*
*Nocardia asteroides**	*C. compactum*
*N. brasiliensis**	*C. pedrosoi*
Streptomyces madurae	*C. trichoides*
S. pelletierii	*C. werneckii*
S. somaliensis	*Coccidioides immitis**
	*Cryptococcus neoformans**
PHYCOMYCETES	*Geotrichum candidum*
*Absidia corymbifera**	*Histoplasma capsulatum**
*Basidiobolus ranarum**	*Madurella grisea**
Rhizopus arrhizus	*M. mycetomii*
R. oryzae	*Malasezzia furfur*
	Paracoccidioides brasiliensis
ASCOMYCETES	*P. loboi*
Allescheria boydii	*Phialophora jeanselmei*
Leptosphaeria senegalensis	*P. verrucosa*
*Piedraia hortai**	*Pyrenochaeta romeroi*
	*Rhinosporidium seeberii**
DEUTEROMYCETES	*Sporotrichum schenckii**
(Fungi Imperfecti)	*Trichosporon cutaneum**
*Aspergillus fumigatus**	
*Blastomyces dermatitidis**	
*Candida albicans**	

*Those which also have been reported to infect animals. (This data was added by C.H.B.)

tuberculosis although in many of them a purulent inflammation accompanies the granulomatous reaction. In instances where there is fast multiplication of the organism in the host's tissues due to lowered resistance or massive inoculation, the reaction may be necrotizing and basically purulent. Skin sensitivity, agglutinins, precipitins and complement-fixing antibodies may develop in the course of the host's immune reaction to a fungous infection.

Ajello[3] has listed the valid dermatophyte species and the human pathogenic fungi other than the dermatophytes (Table 47 and 48).

ACTINOMYCOSIS

Actinomycosis is a chronic infectious disease caused by the anaerobic to microaerophilic actinomycetes *Actinomyces bovis, Actinomyces israeli* and *Actinomyces baudetii*.[4] It is characterized by granulomatous inflammation which eventually suppurates, discharging the white to yellow granular bodies (sulfur granules or rosettes) measuring 0.25 to 1 mm. in diameter which are characteristic of the infection. These sulfur granules are composed of radiating refractile club-shaped structures with their larger end at the periphery of the granules. The shape of the "clubs" becomes more obvious when the granules are crushed and examined microscopically. At one time, actinomycosis and the sulfur granule were linked inseparably, and it was thought that the fungous hyphae actually formed all of the sulfur granule, thus the term "ray fungus" by which it was known for some time. Subsequent studies revealed that the clubs were composed of an acidophilic material which is deposited about the organism and is found deposited about other fungi, bacteria including staphylococci, and nonviable plant materials which are present in granulomatous lesions of similar nature.[21] Occasionally one may find a colony of the organism in the tissue without the rosette with its clubs.

In 1845, Langenbeck first recognized the white to yellow granules ("clumps") produced in the lesions. In 1857, Lebert published one of the earliest reports of a human case. In 1877, Bolinger demonstrated that bovine cases were caused by a fungus, and in the following year, Harz named this organism *Actinomyces bovis*. However, it was not until 1890 that it was cultured. Since that time it has been controversial whether the usual human isolates and the usual bovine iso-

lates were the same organism. Definite differences in colonial morphology and biochemical behavior have been found in the majority
of organisms isolated from each source. A rough colonial type *(A.
israeli)* is most often isolated from lesions in man and a smooth
colonial type *(A. bovis)* usually is associated with bovine lesions.[16,20,22]
However, rough as well as smooth types have been isolated from
cattle and pigs as well as man.[16,17,22] The recognition of the frequent
biological variation in fungi by many people apparently has prevented unanimous acceptance of their classification as two totally
different organisms. This is reflected by the variation in usage in present day medical literature where one may find either one or both of
the names used in publication, even in the same book having multiple authors. *A. bovis* and *A. baudettii,* the latter name given to some
canine isolates, also has been considered to be almost identical if not
the same as *A. israeli* by Vanbreuseghem who considers the latter to
be the only valid name for the etiologic agent of actinomycosis.[12]

Emmons[15] concluded that the early reports on both Actinomycosis
and Nocardiosis constituted an unsatisfactory chapter in the literature of veterinary mycology because of the lack of laboratory data,
particularly cultures.

Studies of human tonsils in Puerto Rico indicate that *A. bovis
(israeli)* may occur in the crypts simply as hyphae, i.e., without the
clubs which characterize the sulfur granule.[14] Significantly, at a
subsequent examination of the same patient colonies with clubs
have been found.

Inasmuch as the common clinical complexes of actinobacillosis of
cattle and actinomycosis are similar, care should be taken to distinguish between these and other sulfur granule or rosette forming
diseases in animals by cultural means or Gram stains.

The above considerations have an important bearing on animal
pathology, now that *A. bovis (israeli)* has been found in human
tonsils extirpated in Puerto Rico and *A. bovis* has been found in the
tonsils of hogs[13] and in the mouths of apparently normal cattle.[18]
It would appear, therefore, that the tonsils of both hogs, cattle, and
men may contain pathogenic Actinomyces which, living saprophytically, may not produce disease. Since such organisms escape readily
into the mouth, it can be understood how they might initiate actinomycotic lesions in the tissues here and in the gastrointestinal tract,
if, as and when the proper conditions for infection arise.

Geographic Distribution

Actinomycosis probably occurs in most parts of the world, although figures are lacking. In the United States, Sanford and Voelker collected reports on about 570 human cases from every state in the Union. However, the Mississippi Valley and the Northwest showed the greatest number of cases.

Transmission

The mode of transfer of the organism from one animal to another, from man to man, or from other environment to animal or man is not known. No consistent source has been found outside of animals or man, and because the organisms are more frequently found in the mouth of man and animals, the source of infection is believed to be endogenous. The transfer in this case must be by contact with carriers of the organisms and with fomites. Infected individuals no doubt also act as passive carriers at least, continuously distributing the fungus about the environment through contaminated saliva or through feces,—whether used as fertilizer or not. Attempts at substantiating direct infection of man from animals have failed, but people working with and about farm animals have a higher incidence of the disease. However, experimental reproduction of several of the granulomatous mycoses including actinomycosis have been unsatisfactory. This may well be a reflection on the necessity of host susceptibility or other contributing factors which have not been present in the experimental animals.

Animals Susceptible

Cattle are outstandingly affected, followed by man, horse, and swine. More rarely the dog, cat, sheep, goat, deer, guinea pig, rabbit, and goose have been concerned. The cultural identity of the infection has not been proven in many of the cases in these animals. Among wild animals, the monkey, lizard, grizzly bear, tapir, deer, llama, elephant, antelope and muskrat have been reported affected. Some of the latter were in captivity, but specimens shot in the wild, including stone sheep in British Columbia, prove that the disease can be acquired apart from human environment. Evidence of the disease was found in a fossil rhinoceros in northwestern Nebraska.

Actinomycosis in Man

Farmers and cattlemen are the classes most commonly diseased. As a result, males in the prime of life are the most common subjects. In Sanford's statistics, 670 cases in the United States revealed 80 per cent in males. The majority were young adults but no age group was immune.

The mode of infection is usually in doubt. Ewing collected records of 100 cases in the United States and could find no evidence of an infection from animal to man either through milk or meat or by accidental inoculation. One cannot help but compare this disease with other mycetomas in which there usually is a history of wounds caused by penetrating objects or other lesions with considerable depth. Therefore, it is not surprising that the lesions are found frequently in the area of an infected or recently extracted tooth.

There are three major clinical forms: cervicofacial, thoracic, and abdominal. One subcutaneous infection has been reported to have followed a human bite. As in cattle, the jaw of man is the most common location; the soft tissues being affected initially. In the late stages the adjacent bone and its periosteum may be invaded to form a true osteomyelitis such as that seen in cattle. The lesion is diffuse, comparing with cancer in its wooden hardness, and is comparatively painless. The surrounding skin is dusky red to violaceous. Progress is slow, the enlargement occurring by fits and starts. The multiple granulomas in the depths of the lesion coalesce, suppurate and discharge their exudates upon the surface by sinuses. However, the abscesses in the deeper parts are not adequately drained. The pus which escapes contains the well known sulfur granules, easily visible to the naked eye. Regional lymph nodes, although they may become swollen, do not contain granulomas and discharge pus.

The pulmonary and intestinal forms of the disease are often secondary to aspiration of exudate from discharging sinuses of the cervicofacial form. Generalization (approximately 2 per cent of cases) is delayed for many years but eventually may become widespread,—both by direct continuity of tissue and by the blood stream. Secondary to intestinal and particularly appendiceal involvement, the skin over the abdomen may become involved by direct extension. The same is true of pulmonary lesions which extend to the skin of the thorax. Primary actinomycosis of the skin is exceedingly rare.

The symptoms may thus simulate syphilis, tuberculosis, sarcoma, carcinoma or another mycetoma. The prognosis is bad in the pulmonary and intestinal forms unless actively treated in the earliest stages; generalized cases are invariably fatal but only after a long drawn-out course, i.e., up to fifteen years. The older treatment with iodides has recently been replaced or supplemented with penicillin and other antibiotics which must be given for long periods of time and accompanied by appropriate surgical intervention when indicated.

Prevention of Actinomycosis

Inasmuch as *A. israeli* and *A. bovis* have been found in lesions as well as the tonsils and carious teeth of some otherwise normal animals and man, but never free in nature except in exudate from lesions, prevention should be directed to good oral hygiene and prevention of spread of exudates from draining lesions.

Actinomycosis in Animals

Cattle are the animals most often affected. The earliest lesions are ulcers in the mouth, and it is presumable that the underlying bone is usually invaded from these initial areas of infection. True actinomycosis of cattle usually affects the bones as well as the soft tissues, most often in the lower jaw. Because of this, it usually can be distinguished clinically from actinobacillosis which instead has a predilection for the soft tissues.

The organisms invade the bone and surrounding tissues where they set up a granulomatous reaction. In cattle this is often complicated by secondary invasion with *Corynbacterium pyogenes* and other pyogenic bacteria. The large tumor-like growths which result may be either hard or soft, depending on whether granuloma formation or suppuration predominate in the tissue. The organism concurrently destroys bony tissue and stimulates production of new bone, thus forming the proliferative osteitis called "lumpy jaw." This osseous hyperplasia has been mistaken for osteogenic sarcoma, particularly before the suppuration has broken through to the surface. Once it does so, the presence of "sulfur granules" should lead one to suspect actinomycosis and to identify the infecting organism by cultural means. The incidence of the infection has been found to be high where cattle are fed on very rough forage, especially on barley straw in which sharp awns are found.[19] On the other hand it should be recalled that *A. bovis* has never been isolated from soil or animal foodstuffs. In other words, there is only presumptive evidence for any postulated mode of infection except for the possible contamination of wounds or other lesions about diseased teeth or tonsils by organisms which are already in the mouth.

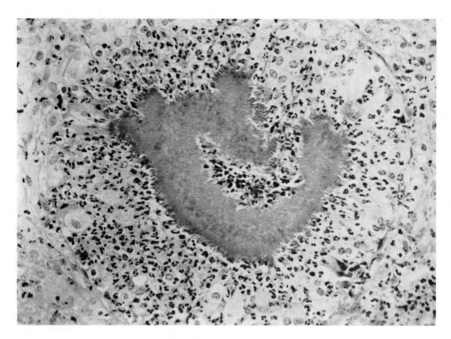

Fig. 80. Actinomycosis.

A. bovis is considerably less important in other animals than it is in cattle, and a number of reports of supposed infections are really those of actinobacillosis or of nocardiosis (z.v., page 463). In horses, *A. bovis* is reported to have been isolated along with *Brucella abortus* from the lesions of the atlantal and supraspinous bursae of the diseases called "poll-evil" and "fistulous withers." Similar lesions have been produced by injection of mixed cultures of these organisms into bursae. However, Emmons[15] has stated that these data among others could not be critically evaluated without bearing in mind that several types of aerobic to microaerophilic organisms resembling *A. bovis,* but probably including other poorly characterized species of *Actinomyces, Corynebacterium* and possibly *Lactobacillus* which have been encountered in a variety of lesions as contaminats.

In swine *A. bovis* has been cultured from the normal oral cavity and from infected tonsils. It has also been found in their lungs. Actinomycosis of the udder occurs in nursing sows: the infection is thought to enter from the mouths of the suckling pigs through wounds made by their sharp teeth. The so-called "scirrhous cord", a chronic funiculitis which follows castration, is often an actinomycotic infection in swine. The organism there presumably enters through the castration incision.

NOCARDIA INFECTIONS

The etiologic agent of *farcin du boeuf*, a chronic lymphangitis of cattle in the Republic of Guadeloupe, was first isolated and described by Nocard in 1888.[27] Subsequently a large number of similar organisms have been isolated from a wide variety of animals and given various names. With the change of nomenclature of the *Actinomycetaceae* in the sixth edition of Bergey's Manual,[4] a number of infections caused by obligate aerobic members of this family and which previously were termed "actinomycosis" were classified as nocardiosis and their etiologic agents listed in the genus *Nocardia*. Even in this classification one found a bewildering array of species of *Nocardia*. However, at the present time only two members of this genus, *Nocardia asteroides* and *Nocardia brasiliensis,* are considered to be pathogens affecting lower animals and man. *N. asteroides* appears to be the major pathogen for man and for animals, only one case of infection with *N. brasiliensis* having been reported in animals.[23] There is some evidence to indicate that *N. farcinica,* the reported etiologic agent of *farcin du boeuf* or bovine farcy, is identical to *N. asteroides*.[25] Reports concerning the cultural identification of *N. farcinica* and its differentiation from *N. asteroides* have not appeared in recent years.

Pathogenic Nocardia are commonly isolated from the soil and infection usually is considered to be derived from this source. *N. asteroides* appears to have a world wide distribution whereas reports on *N. brasiliensis* have come only from North and South America and Africa.[23]

Nocardiosis in Man

As presently defined nocardiosis is a chronic suppurative and granulomatous disease having two basic clinical and pathological forms, those of mycetoma and those of pulmonary and systemic infection.

Nocardial mycetoma is characterized by a chronic progressive infection with occasional temporary remissions usually affecting the extremities and especially the foot and leg. Clinical histories reveal that some time after an injury to the extremity a small painless nodule may develop, rupture and discharge a seropurulent exudate. This is followed by alternate remissions of and active progression of chronic suppurative inflammation which spreads to the adjacent tissues. Fistulous tracts containing the colonies of *Nocardia* surrounded by pus permeat the granulomatous tissue. The infective process is progressive and eventually erodes bone and destroys other junctional tissue. Colonies of *Nocardia* of varying colors are discharged to the surface in the seropurulent exudate. The disease takes a course of many months or years but remains localized. Clubs about the colonies are not seen frequently and then only in very chronic cases. Pulmonary and systemic nocardiosis usually arises in the lungs, apparently from inhalation of the pathogenic organism. Here the infection often does not remain localized and metatasis to a wide variety of organs is usual. Multiple abscesses in the skin are found and these rupture to form a chronic lesion similar to that seen in mycetoma. The usual causative agent is *N. asteroides*.

Nocardiosis in Animals

Nocardiosis in animals is no longer considered to be a rarity. The organism isolated from infections reported to date and in which the nomenclature can be correlated with present interpretations are largely *N. asteroides*. The one case of *N. brasiliensis* infection which has been reported was in a cat.[23] Nocardiosis has been reported in cattle, goats, dogs, cats, horses, rabbits, kangaroos, wallabies and a pig.[1] In the United States of America bovine infections are found most frequently in the mammary gland as a chronic progressive granulomatous inflammation with associated purulent exudate.[26,28,29] Metastasis to the lymph nodes, lungs, and liver has been observed in some infections arising in the mammary gland but usually it is limited to the affected glands.[29] *Farcin du bouef* is reported to occur as a chronic cutaneous form involving lymph nodes with occasional pulmonary lesions. A single etiologic agent for this clinical entity is not accepted,[1] but no doubt *Nocardia* are present in the lesions of some of the cases and certainly can be considered to be the cause of the pathologic change in such cases. Infection in dogs and cats may develop in the skin or mucous membranes with metastasis to internal organs or as a primary pulmonary infection. Metastasis to the other tissues is common. However, it is most difficult to identify which is first in most cases, pulmonary or cutaneous infection. Infections have occurred in the lung[1] and mammary gland of goats,[24] and leg joints and subcutaneously in horses.[1]

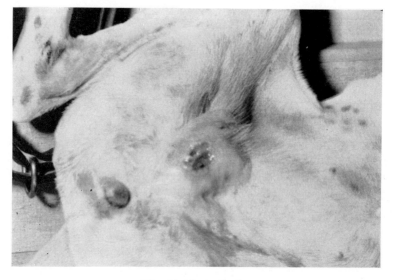

Fig. 81. Nocardiosis.

Prevention of Nocardiosis

Inasmuch as the Nocardia infecting man and animals are considered to be derived from their environment and infection is frequently known to be associated with trauma, good hygiene appears to be of paramount importance. Naturally, infected milk must be discarded.

SPOROTRICHOSIS

This is an infectious granulomatous disease caused by *Sporotrichum schenckii,* an organism which grows as cigar-shaped yeast forms in lesions and as a mycelial form with spores in nature as well as in artificial media. Like tuberculosis, actinomycosis and syphilis it follows a subacute, indolent course characterized by gumma-like lesions and ulceration,—naturally with variations.

S. schenckii has been isolated from several forms of vegetation (beech, oat grains and shave grass), as well as from the timbers in gold mines. Ample clinical evidence incriminates punctures by rose and barberry thorns, and the fungus which had caused several cases in florists has been isolated from sphagnum moss. Carnation and rose buds reportedly have been infected and retrocultures from them have produced sporotrichosis in experimental animals.[30] However, the interpretation concerning the infection of the plants has been questioned.[10] It is clear that the organism is widely distributed upon vegetation, thus affording the opportunity for direct infection of both man and lower animals. Man has been infected following the bite of various animals,[32,33] but since similar infection has followed injuries by splinters and contact with rotten sticks during the clearing of land, it would appear that animals act only as mechanical vectors. In a South African outbreak which involved 2,825 gold miners between 1941 and 1944, the fungus was found to be growing on the mine timbers. The epidemic was brought to a halt by impregnating the timbers with fungicides.[34]

S. schenckii is extremely difficult to demonstrate in pus or other tissue; cultural methods are mandatory. The fact that it produces agglutinins that are highly specific is almost unique in mycology. Spores from young colonies filtered through cotton serve as the antigen. They may be agglutinated in dilutions of 1:1500 up to 1:4000.

Sporotrichosis in Man

This begins as a solitary, granulomatous lesion in the skin on some exposed part of the body—usually on the hand or forearm, but occasionally on the lower extremities or face. The eyelids may become diffusely involved, leading to the mistaken diagnosis of trachoma, and lesions on the side of the nose have been erroneously regarded as due to dacrocystitis.

The lesion grows rather rapidly, attaining the size of a small marble in two or three weeks. It is firm, purplish red and painless. At about the fourth week it ruptures and develops into an ulcer. It thus suggests a furuncle, but one which is not violently inflammatory and which does not heal after rupture. Lesions of this sort should always prompt thoughts of sporotrichosis.

At times such a lesion may remain solitary, but in America secondary lesions generally develop and are distributed along the perivenous lymphatic channels. This leads to a tract of older and younger granulomas numbering up to twenty or thirty. While they may extend quite to the regional lymph nodes, the latter are themselves involved with the utmost rarity. Such a picture is almost pathognomonic. The patient remains in good general health and solitary lesions have been known to heal spontaneously, but usually the course of the disease is indefinite unless treated. Fortunately iodides are specific. Blood stream invasion occurs late and uncommonly, but once generalization occurs, any or all viscera are liable to involvement. When tuberculosis is associated with sporotrichosis, the two diseases appear mutually to aggravate each other.

Sporotrichosis in Animals

Sporotrichosis affects animals only sporadically, — rats, horses, mules, and dogs. The disease has also been seen in a camel, a cow and the domestic fowl.[9] Of these, Norway rats are more frequently concerned, cheesy nodules appearing on the tail and paws and producing a swelling of joints with deformity.[31] At times granulomas also appear in the viscera. In dogs, the features are similar to those of man, with emphasis upon the bones and joints; peritonitis secondary to hepatic involvement may be associated.

Watson,[35] who studied many cases in horses, described the disease in that species as taking two forms: 1) An ulcerating form, which is localized and involves the lymphatics; and 2) A nonulcerating form, which is usually disseminated. In this form the nodules are held loosely in the skin without lymphatic involvement. Although multiple nodules may form there is no tendency for them to coalesce. The disease has been mistaken for epizootic lymphangitis, but runs a much milder coarse and shows little or no tendency to spread in a herd. Whereas the organisms in epizootic lymphangitis usually are easy to see in the exudates from lesions, *S. schenckii* is not. *S. schenckii* is best identified by culturing exudates or by inoculation of mice intraperitoneally with them. The characteristic cigar shaped organism is abundant in the exudates from these latter animals (Fig. 82).

Transplantation from one arm to the other by direct contact has been reported and accidental infections of man in the laboratory have been recognized.[10] Although extremely unusual, direct transmission from man to man has been reported. Prevention requires avoiding injuries by vegetable matter and exposure either directly or indirectly through the bites of animals. The ubiquity of rats involving the soiling of splinters and other sharp materials incriminates these pests in one more connection as disease vectors.

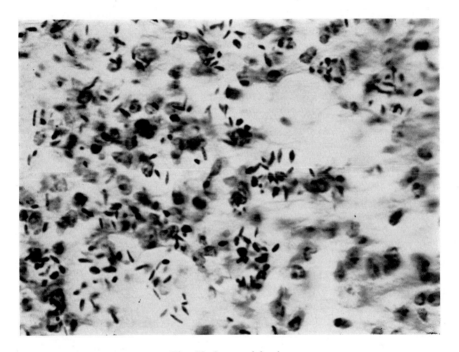

Fig. 82. Sporotrichosis.

CRYPTOCOCCOSIS

Cryptococcosis is a chronic infection of world-wide distribution caused by the yeastlike organism *Cryptococcus neoformans (Torula histolytica)*. The fungus was first found by Busse in human visceral lesions in 1895.[38] Mosberg and Arnold were able to find 167 cases in the literature up to 1950 and added five of their own.[48] Numerous others have been added since. The disease has been reported from most parts of the world.

The Disease in Man

The most common form is chronic cerebrospinal meningitis which must be distinguished particularly from tuberculous meningitis. Many cases have remained undiagnosed during life because cryptococcosis was not suspected. A specific diagnosis usually cannot be made unless the organism is demonstrated in the spinal fluid either by direct examination or by culture. The meningitis may run a chronic course of months and even years before terminating fatally.[37] In the cutaneous form the lesions are small granulomas which develop so rapidly as to simulate abscesses. The more superficial skin lesions may ulcerate, the subcutaneous ones do not do so. Enlargement of the lymph nodes may occur. The cutaneous form of cryptococcosis sooner or later is followed by the cerebrospinal form.[40]

Primary infections of the lungs occur and may simulate tuberculosis or neoplasia clinically. These two eventually terminate as cerebrospinal infections. Lung lesions have been found at autopsy of patients dying of meningitis who had shown no symptoms referable to the pulmonary system. This suggests that the lungs are often the portal of infection. However, the organism has been isolated from many parts of the body, including the pharynx and gastrointestinal tract. Generalized cryptococcosis in which all of the organs including bones and joints are affected occurs rarely.

Cryptococcosis occurs frequently in association with other diseases such as leukemia, malignant lymphoma and sarcoidosis.[53,54] In all but the cutaneous form the prognosis is very grave.

The Disease in Animals

C. neoformans has been identified as the cause of cryptococcosis in the horse, cow, cheetah, domestic cat, pig, monkey, small-toothed palm civet,[36] ferret,[51] guinea pig,[41] and goat.[52] The abundant capsular material of the cryptococci imparted a myxoma-like consistency to some lesions. Of particular public-health interest are outbreaks of cryptococcal mastitis in dairy herds in Maryland[46] and Wisconsin.[50] In the Maryland outbreak the organism caused severe and extensive damage to the glandular tissue of the udders (Fig. 83), which was followed by granulomatous inflammation in the later stages. One hundred and six of 235 cows were infected. Metastasis to the lung of one was found. Ulcerative endocarditis in a bull has been reported also.

Generalized cases of cryptococcosis have been found in the horse and the cheetah. In the latter animal the affected organs included the brain and meninges. Holzworth reported the first case of generalized infection in a cat, and since then has studied others.[44,45] Generalized infection as well as meningioencephalitis due to this organism has been seen in dogs.[36] Emmons found in mice inoculated intraperitoneally with *C. neoformans* that the fungi always invaded the meninges.[42] This has given experimental support to a predilection for the meninges that had long been observed by clinicians.

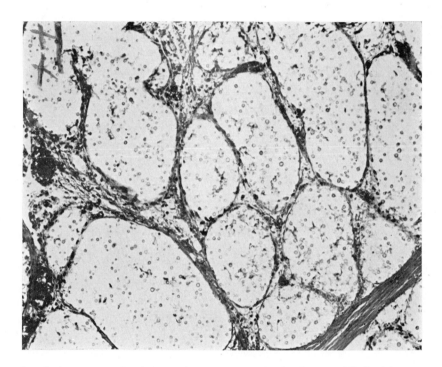

Fig. 83. Cryptococcosis of the udder in a cow. The lumina are filled with organisms, the fibrinous stroma is almost intact and there is an absence of inflammatory reaction. (J. R. M. Innes *et al.: Amer. Jour. Vet. Res., 13,* 1952.)

C. neoformans has been isolated from milk,[39] fruit and healthy human skin,[49] as well as from the soil,[42] pigeons nests and droppings[43,47] and from areas inhabited by chickens.[2] These are important indications of the potential sources of infection for both animals and man. Isolations were made from pigeon excreta from 16 of the 19 premises in one investigation.[43] These observations have since been confirmed by others. Infection of the pigeons was not found although the organism was present in the digestive tract of some of them. One can see a suggestion that a local concentration of the organism can be increased by the presence of a large amount of organic matter or other favorable conditions created by it and that it can be widely disseminated by transient birds. There is no report of transmission from animals to man, but in the case of this disease there is presumptive evidence that this may occur. Since *C. neoformans* occasionally invades the bovine udder, the possibility of it getting into a commercial milk supply is far from remote. It has in fact been isolated from a commercial bulk sample, although no disease could subsequently be found in the herd where the milk originated.[39] No infections were traced to the cryptococcal mastitis mentioned above.

COCCIDIOIDOMYCOSIS

Coccidioidomycosis is an infection caused by *Coccidioides immitis,* a fungus which grows as a mold in culture but as an endosporulating spherical organism in tissue (Figs. 84 and 85). It was first found in a human skin lesion in Argentina in 1892 by Posados and Wernicke. The vast majority of subsequent cases, however, have been found in certain arid and semiarid areas of southwestern United States, predominantly in the San Joaquin Valley of California. The endemic area also includes parts of Texas, Arizona and New Mexico. But, as one might expect, the adjoining states of Mexico (Sonora, Chihuahua, Baja California, and Choahuila) contain endemic areas associated with similar climatic and geographic characteristics. In addition, clinical cases have occurred in the Comayuga Valley of Honduras, in Venezuela (State of Lara and in the Grand Chaco-Pampa region), much of Paraguay and Argentina as well as a small area in Bolivia. Although a few cases have been reported in other parts of the world, there is suggestion in most cases that these are not endemic areas but that infection occurred through fomites or when the individuals were visiting endemic areas.[58]

The endemic areas in the United States has been described by Maddy[63] as coinciding with the portions of the Lower Sonoran Life Zone which have an arid to semiarid climate (Fig. 86). Mean summer temperatures (July) varying between 80 to 90° F. and the mean

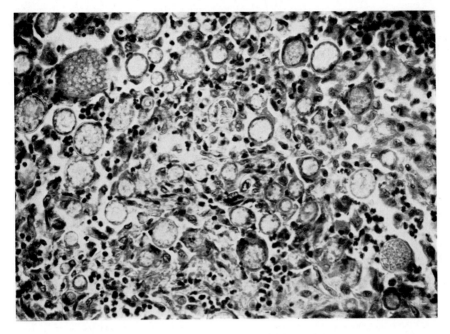

Fig. 84. Coccidioidmycosis.

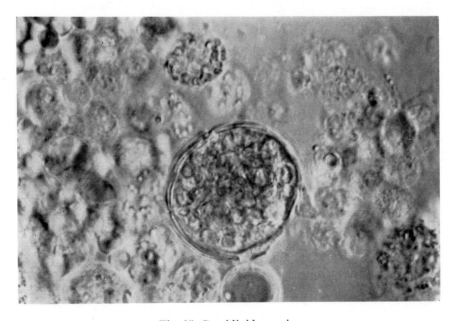

Fig. 85. Coccidioidmycosis.

winter (January) temperatures varying between 39 to 53° F. and the annual rainfall of about five to twenty inches as well as the presence of an alkaline soil are considered to be most favorable for the fungus. The organism is reported to survive in small areas six to eight inches beneath the earth's surface during the hotter and dryer months but to repopulate the upper soil a short time after rains. Cultivated soil has not been found to harbor the organism. Emmons[57] noticed that the organism appeared to be found most often in the soil about the burrows of desert rodents. Ajello *et al.*[55] found in their investi-

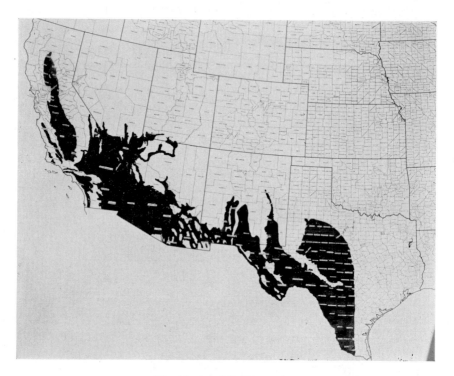

Fig. 86. Coccidioidmycosis.

gations that only one of twenty-four soil collection sites had *C. immitis,* and it was taken from a rodent burrow. Egeberg and Ely[56] found that of 120 soil samples taken at the end of the rainy season in April, 1955, in the San Joaquin Valley, forty animal burrows yielded 33½ per cent positives whereas samples elsewhere yielded 6.1 per cent positives. The endemic areas are characterized by frequent high winds and a soil which favors dust formation. This factor, of course, greatly favors pulmonary infection by inhalation.

The Disease in Man

There are two basic clinical forms. The first and most common form is an acute pulmonary inflammation which is usually benign because it is self-limiting. Some cases resemble a mild influenza, others are asymptomatic and are detectable only by immunologic tests. Infection results in an immune response which may be demonstrated by a skin test or by a complement fixation test. The antigen used in either test is coccidioidin, a filtrate of old broth cultures of the fungus.

A very few of the acute cases may lapse into the second form. This is a chronic generalized infection that involves the skin and subcutis, thoracic and abdominal viscera, testes, meninges, bones and joints. The generalized infection is progressive and is very resistant to treatment. The prognosis appears to be more favorable in those individuals developing hypersensitivity. The skin lesions resemble those of blastomycosis; the visceral lesions those of tuberculosis.[59] It is necessary to establish the presence of the fungus either histologically or by direct examination and culture of exudates in order to establish a diagnosis.

The Disease in Animals

The symptoms described in the dog are extremely inconsistent because the disease varies from inapparent to disseminate infection with progressive granulomatous inflammation leading to death.[61,64] Involvement of bone leads to a proliferative osteitis rather than a lysis as is seen in man. In cattle the disease has been recognized many times by meat inspectors in the Southwest.[65] It has been demonstrated that almost 100 per cent of the cattle in highly endemic areas of Arizona become infected within their first two years of residence.[64] The disease in this animal is benign and clinically asymptomatic. The lesions are granulomatous inflammation of the bronchial and mediastinal lymph nodes. Only rarely have small granulomas been concurrently found in the lungs. In abbatoirs where veterinary inspection is not provided it is almost certain that these minimal lesions would attract no attention. In view of this it probably is fortunate that bovine lungs and their adjacent lymph nodes are seldom used for human food. Interestingly enough, there is a report of a man who presumably contracted the infection by handling chicken food made from condemned cattle. The primary lesion occurred on the finger.[68] Apart from rodents, dogs and cattle, coccidioidomycosis has been reported in sheep, a chinchilla,[60] a pig,[64] coyotes,[67] a horse,[66] a mountain gorilla,[62] a llama, and a monkey.[64]

Various desert dwelling rodents have been found to harbor pulmonary coccidioidomycosis. However, there is considerable evidence that the organism can perpetuate itself in a saprophytic existence in the soil. Transmission from animals to man has not been found to occur, both animals and man apparently being infected through the inhalation of dust containing the organism. This hypothesis is supported by the observation that the incidence of the disease is high during the dusty season and low during the wet season. Based on this observation the U.S. Air Force instituted dust control measures (planting of lawns, paving and oiling of roads and runways) at air fields in the endemic areas which were successful in greatly reducing the rate of infection. It has been suggested that the habit of the dog of investigating rodent burrows may explain the great incidence of canine coccidioidomycosis.[58] Prchal[65] found that the disease in cattle was most common in those which were fed in dusty feed lots for two to three months. Infection is primarily by the arthrospores which are easily carried in the air currents. The infecting spherule is usually restricted to lesions or exudates.

RHINOSPORIDIOSIS

Rhinosporidiosis is a chronic local infection caused by the fungus *Rhinosporidium seeberi*. In man, the lesions occur in the form of granulomas in the mucosae of the nose, pharynx, conjunctiva, skin, the genitalia and the rectum. The nose is the most common seat of infection, and the granulomas occur in it as single polypoid masses which tend to coalesce as the disease progresses. Regardless of its site, rhinosporidiosis remains as a localized lesion and is seldom fatal; the chief clinical symptom is respiratory obstruction caused by the polyps. Cattle, horses, and mules are affected as well as man, but nasal lesions are the only ones that have been seen in animals.

In a review of the world literature up to 1949, de Mello[70] recorded 442 human cases and thirty-nine in animals. Sixteen of the human cases were from the United States, thirty-four from South America, nine from Africa, two from Italy, and one each from the Philippines, Malay and Israel. In contrast to this rather sporadic occurrence, there were thirty-one cases from Iran, 108 from Ceylon and 233 from India, in which countries the disease is apparently endemic. This incidence was somewhat paralleled by the animal cases, of which twenty-five had been reported from India, eleven from South America and three from South Africa. Smith and Frankson[73] have described the first case of rhinosporidiosis in an animal (a horse) in the United States (Fig. 87).

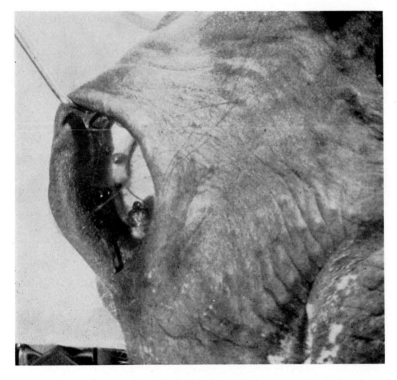

Fig. 87. Rhinosporidiosis.

Seeber first described the infection in man in 1900 and named the organism he found *Coccidium seeberi*. Still in the belief it was a protozoan, he renamed it *Rhinosporidium seeberi* in 1912, and it remained for Ashworth[69] to place it among the fungi some twelve years later. Ashworth also postulated that portion of the life cycle of the organism that could be deduced from the study of tissue sections. The infecting spore, a small round body six to seven microns in diameter, undergoes nuclear division until it becomes about 100 microns in diameter, when it forms a sporangium. A thick layer of cellulose is deposited inside the outer chitinous layer, except at one point where a "pore" is left. Further division results in a sporangium about 200 to 300 microns in diameter containing approximately 16,000 spores. When the spores have matured, they are liberated by the rupture of the thin walled pore. They can be found in the nasal discharge but apparently are not infective at this stage.

Many workers have attempted to culture the spores on a wide variety of media without success. Attempts to produce artificial infection with fresh material from nasal polyps have likewise been unavailing. Particular resourcefulness was shown by de Mello with respect to technics and the variety of organs and species he inoculated, but the organism could not be grown even in fetal tissue. Thus the complete life cycle of *R. seeberi,* particularly its source in nature and the mode of infection remain unknown.

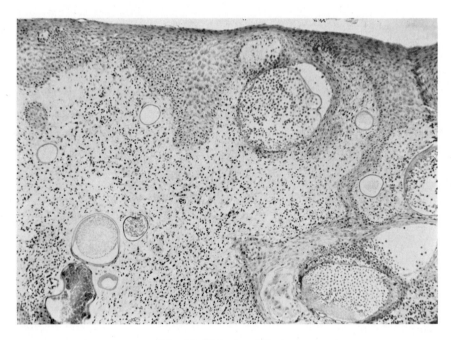

Fig. 88. Rhinosporidiosis.

The mode by which the disease is contracted is not known with certainty. Studies in India have revealed that infection of man was as high as 20 per cent in a group of individuals removing sand from the bed of stagnant river.[71] Only those who were exposed through diving or swimming became infected. Rao[72] suggested that the incidence is much higher in bullocks because they have their noses pierced whereas the cows do not, thus intimating that trauma may have a role.

The diagnosis of the disease is made by finding the large sporangia in the polyps, either in wet amounts of the fresh tissue or in histologic sections (Fig. 88). Treatment consists of surgical excision of the granulomas.

BLASTOMYCOSIS

The disease is caused by *Blastomyces dermatitidis,* a dimorphic fungus which occurs in the tissues as a budding yeast but grows as a mycelial form on artificial media at 25° F. and in the yeast phase at 37° F. on blood agar. The disease is found only in North America and with few exceptions, all of the human cases have been found in the United States and Canada; no animal cases have been reported outside this country. Menges[77] has reviewed 116 cases of the disease in animals. The cases came from nineteen states of the eastern half of the United States and Canada. The majority were hunting type dogs (Fig. 89).

Blastomycosis was first observed by Gilchrist in its cutaneous form in 1894; he and Stokes isolated the causative fungus from a human case in 1896.[76] They were able to infect a sheep, a horse, and two dogs by intravenous inoculation of the organism; all the animals developed chronic inflammatory foci in the lungs. They were unable to produce any infection in these animals by subcutaneous inoculation. The first case in animals were described by Meyer in 1912, and involved two dogs.[9]

Blastomycosis in Man

Laboring males are predominently infected, and there are three clinical forms: cutaneous, pulmonary and generalized. The pulmonary form usually terminates in the generalized form. The cutaneous form is seen on the exposed parts of the body as a localized papule which soon suppurates and ulcerates. This is followed by a chronic inflammatory hyperplasia of the skin around the margin of the ulcer. The lesions have a tendency to spread and involve an increasing area of skin with spontaneous healing of the center of the lesion.[5] Cutaneous blastomycosis comprises the bulk of the clinical cases, and the prognosis is good if it is treated before systemic involvement occurs. Iodides and roentgen irradiation are used in treatment, the former having been introduced by Gilchrist. Pulmonary blastomycosis may begin as an isolated pneumonic lesion anywhere in the lung. The

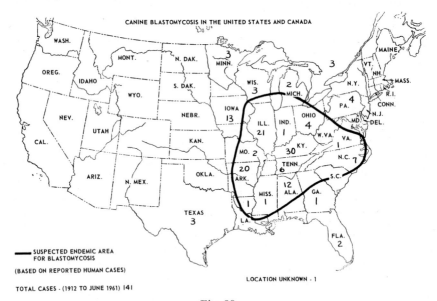

Fig. 89.

lesions have been mistaken for tuberculosis or neoplasm on x-ray examination. Histologically the lung lesion may be chiefly purulent, chiefly granulomatous or a mixture of both. Examination of the sputum is a diagnostic aid, since the fungus cells are often present in it. Most of the generalized cases include either lung or skin lesions so that the systemic involvement is traceable to spread from these organs. Unlike tuberculosis, the spleen, liver and intestines are seldom involved.

Patients with pulmonary or generalized blastomycosis should first be tested for hypersensitivity by skin testing with blastomycin. If sensitive, the patient should then be desensitized by subcutaneous injections of blastomyces vaccine. Unless this is done there is danger that the iodide therapy will promote the spread of the disease. The prognosis in generalized blastomycosis has been poor to date, a wide variety of therapeutic agents having been tried unsuccessfully. Stilbamidine and Amphotericin B also appear to have considerable therapeutic value.[77,80]

Blastomycosis in Animals

All but two of the infections in animals have been seen in dogs and the majority were those of fatal pulmonary infection or of generalized infection including the lungs.[79] There were lesions in the skin in approximately one-third of them. The lesions of granuloma-

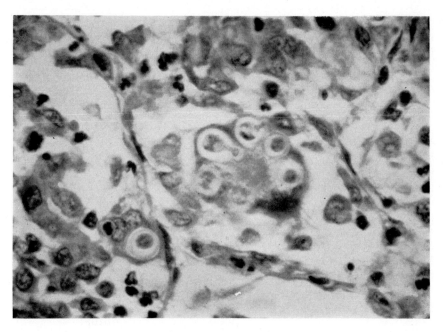

Fig. 90. Blastomycosis.

tous and suppurative pneumonia are similar to those in man (Fig. 90). The lymph nodes at or near the bifurcation of the bronchi were most frequently involved and frequently enlarged sufficiently to be seen roentgenographically. The disease in the captive Northern (Stellar) sea lion was generalized.[78] The single case in the mare was that of udder infection.[74] A complete autopsy was not performed on the latter animal, and it is likely that she too represented a case of generalized infection. Some of the dogs were subjected to treatment with a variety of chemotherapeutic and antibiotic agents, none of which were of value in arresting the disease.

Since *B. dermatitidis* has not been isolated from the soil, or from any source other than human or animal infection, its natural habitat is unknown. The cases of pulmonary infection are probably indicative of infection by inhalation and it is generally accepted that animals and man acquire it from the same source. A history of trauma preceding the infectious lesion is available in many of the cases of human skin infection. There are no well-authenticated instances of transmission from animal to man, but transmission from man to man by accidental self inoculation is reported.[75] No cases have developed in the personnel who handled the mare or a number of the canine cases even though these animals were presumably discharging the organism through accessible cutaneous lesions.

ASPERGILLOSIS

Aspergillosis has been recognized as an important infection of birds and mammals for over a century. Aspergilli are of world wide distribution. The species usually considered pathogenic for animals are *A. fumigatus, A. nidulans, A. niger,* and *A. flavus.*[1] The pathogenicity of the first species is well established, and that of *A. nidulans* has been recently demonstrated by Drake,[85] who found that intravenous inoculation produced death with typical lesions in rabbits. Henrici obtained a hemolytic toxin from a strain of *A. fumigatus* which had antigenic properties, eliciting the formation of antitoxin in rabbits.

The disease in Animals

Pneumomycosis due to *Aspergillus* infection often assumes epizootic proportions in domestic birds. Young squabs, chicks, ducklings and poults are particularly susceptible. Although the lesions appear chronic, the disease runs an acute clinical course in young birds and the mortality is high. In zoo and in pet birds, as well as in mammals, or older birds, cases are usually sporadic.[81] It is a major cause of death of penguins in zoos. Horses, cattle, lambs, cats (Fig. 91) and swine are also affected with pneumomycosis.[1,82,90] *Aspergillus* may invade the brain and meninges, and has been found there in turkey poults, horses and deer. It may localize in the fetal membranes of cattle and skin of fetuses, producing abortion. It has caused granulomatous lesions in the scrotum and inner aspects of the thighs of goats.[86] The fungus has been incriminated in a specific purulent conjunctivitis of chicks, and it has been found in the eyes of turkeys, where it causes a panophthalmia.[87,88] It grows in the tissues as a mycelial form and may have characteristic conidophores when it grows out into aeriated cavities such as bronchi or avian air sacs.

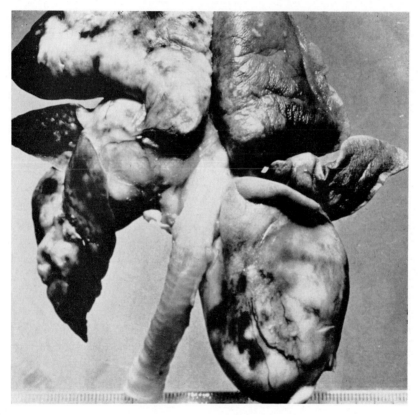

Fig. 91. Pneumomycosis due to Apergillus infection.

Aspergillosis in Man

Three of the forms of animal aspergillosis also occur in man: pneumomycosis,[89] meningoencephalitis and ophthalmitis;[83,84] in addition man is affected with otomycosis. The pulmonary form was once an occupational disease in France amongst those who chewed up grain for fattening squabs ("gaveurs des pigeons") or who worked with dry corn meal in the manufacture of wigs ("Peigneurs des cheveux"). Both occupations exposed workers to the *Aspergillus* spores, which are plentiful in moldy grain.[4] The exact origin of most of the sporadic cases is not known, but since the fungus is ubiquitous and extremely plentiful, animals and man probably acquire the infection through inhalation of spores. Of course, in the case of moldy hay, grain or bedding the number of spores which are inhaled is greater than in a normal environment. Since cases have occurred in ducklings as early as two days after hatching, the possibility of egg-borne infection is raised. Generally speaking, however, prevention depends upon avoiding contact with moldy grain or bedding. It is usually recognized that aspergilli are an important cause of destructive lesions when superimposed upon a previously debilitating disease such as pulmonary tuberculosis. One must consider this factor in interpreting the basic disease process. *A. fumigatus* is considered the main pathogen in human aspergillosis.

HISTOPLASMOSIS

The disease is caused by *Histoplasma capsulatum,* a fungus which usually occurs as a small budding yeast in infected tissues and as hyphae with spores when growing saprophytically in the soil or artificial media. Only occasionally are hyphae produced in tissues. Darling first reported it as a new disease in 1906 while studying human tissue sections in the Canal Zone in a search for kala-azar. He named the organism *H. capsulata* believing it to be a protozoan related to *Leishmania.* Subsequent study by Da Rocha-Lima indicated that it was really a fungus, but this was not conclusively proved until De Monbreun[95] isolated it from a human case in 1934. De Monbreun was able to infect puppies with a subculture from this case, and five years later he discovered the first natural case in a dog.[96]

The disease appears to be world wide in distribution. However, there are definite geographical areas in which it is more common. This is exemplified by the high percentage of histoplasmin reactions and clinical disease along the river valleys of Eastern United States. (Fig. 92) *H. capsulatum* has been isolated from the soil in many areas, the higher percentages being found in those frequented by birds, bats, and chickens such as chicken houses, coops, and the soil about farm homes,[6] as well as from caves inhabited by bats and birds.[91,103]

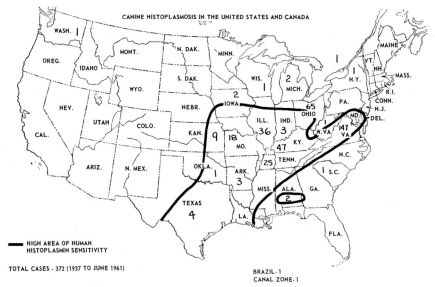

CANINE HISTOPLASMOSIS IN THE UNITED STATES AND CANADA

▬ HIGH AREA OF HUMAN
HISTOPLASMIN SENSITIVITY

TOTAL CASES - 372 (1937 TO JUNE 1961)

BRAZIL-1
CANAL ZONE-1

Fig. 92.

Histoplasmosis in Man

Most of the early cases were diagnosed at autopsy, hence the disease was known only as a highly fatal generalized infection. A series of brilliant epidemiological studies commencing with the work of Christie and Peterson have shown that histoplasmosis also occurs in a benign and self-limiting form. Infection is generally considered to begin in the lung following inhalation of the spores of the organism produced in its external habitat.

Many of the systemic cases first become manifest by ulcerative lesions on the tongue and in the mouth and pharynx. As the disease progresses, there follows ulceration and granulomatous inflammation of the intestinal tract with enlargement of the mesenteric lymph nodes, hepato- and splenomegaly and enlargement of various body lymph nodes suggestive of Hodgkin's disease. The clinical course is characterized by irregular fever, leucopenia, anemia and emaciation. The yeast cells can be found in sternal marrow and occasionally in the peripheral blood on smear or culture. When seen in smears or sections, they are characteristically found growing in large mononuclear phagocytes. Occasionally, extensive lung involvement is found at autopsy. The prognosis for generalized histoplasmosis usually is not favorable, but the development of some of the antibiotics such as Amphotericin B which has a suppressive action suggests a brighter future.

In a number of states in the Mississippi Valley, a high percentage of persons had been found in whom calcified focal pulmonary lesions could be detected roentgenographically, but who gave a negative tuberculin reaction. Such lesions had always been interpreted as tuberculous by radiologists, but when no correlation could be obtained with tuberculin reaction, it became evident that some other explanation must be sought. Christie and Peterson[92] showed in 1945 that there was an association between focal lesions in chest roentgenograms and histoplasmin sensitivity in tuberculin-negative children. Subsequent work by others has turned up many thousands of individuals in the Mississippi Valley who give a positive histoplasmin skin test. It is now apparent that the most common form of histoplasmosis is a benign self-limiting pulmonary infection with circumscribed lesions. These begin as small areas of cellular infiltration in the lungs which do not give rise to any symptoms and become calcified in the course of three or four years. The pathogenesis has been followed in consecutive x-ray pictures, and the organisms have actually been found in patients with such early lesions who came to autopsy after dying from some other cause. One of these was a three-month-old infant in which the lungs and spleen showed many chronic granulomatous lesions in which there was already evidence of healing.[93] There appears to be a second form of subclinical histoplasmosis, since the organisms have been found in a number of surgically removed appendices in children.

Histoplasmosis in Animals

Cole and associates[94] tested 2,867 dogs with histoplasmin and found thirty-eight reactors among them. The clinical signs were lung nodules in x-ray pictures, dysentery, chronic cough, ascites, emaciation, anorexia and vomiting. The clinical course of these dogs was acute progressive in three cases and chronic progressive in twenty cases, all with fatal termination. In three of the dogs the disease followed a benign course, and two dogs recovered after showing symptoms that had been classified as chronic progressive. The diagnosis was confirmed by biopsy of the visceral lymph nodes, liver, spleen, or lung and demonstration of the fungus in the tissue by microscopy or culture. Prominent autopsy findings in Cole's and other cases[9,101] include enteritis, enlargement of mesenteric lymph nodes, granulomatous lung nodules, spleno- and hepatomegaly and ulceration of the gastric and buccal mucosa. In one study forty-four

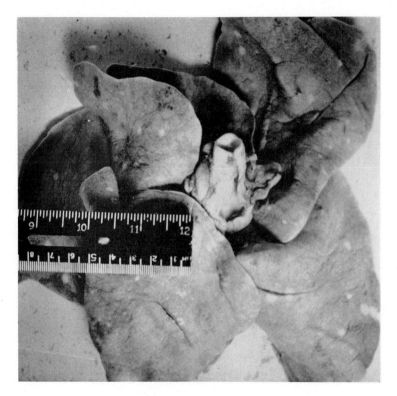

Fig. 93. Histoplasmosis.

percent of the apparently healthy dogs and cats examined had *Histoplasma* in their thoracic lymph nodes[104] (Figs. 93 and 94).

In addition to the canine cases, a number of histoplasmin reactors have been found in cattle, horses, sheep and swine in the Mississippi Valley, and the organism has been demonstrated in the cow.[102] Emmons and associates[98] have isolated *H. capsulatum* from domestic cats, the brown rat, roof rat, spotted skunk, striped skunk, house mouse, opossum, fox, and marmot. Having isolated the organism from rats, Emmons succeeded in isolating it from the soil of the farm where the animals had been caught.[97] Following these demonstrations that the fungus lived saprophytically in the soil, others have succeeded in isolating it from the environment in which human cases had originated.[99,100] There are one or two presumptive but no proved instances of animal to man transmission. The evidence at the present indicates that both man and dogs acquire the infection from the soil, probably by inhalation.

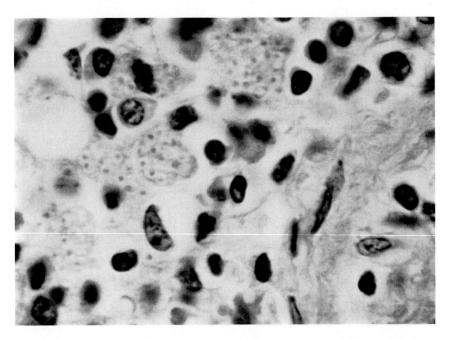

Fig. 94. Histoplasmosis.

Epizootic lymphangitis is a chronic suppurative infection of horses, mules, and donkeys caused by the fungus *Histoplasma farciminosum.* Infection is thought to occur through skin wounds, by direct contact between animals and by the use of contaminated grooming equipment. Insects also have been incriminated as mechanical vectors. Since there are no effective therapeutic agents, the disease often presents a formidable control problem in military units or other places where large numbers of horses are stabled.

The disease is enzootic in continental Europe, North Africa and various parts of Asia. It has been reported in the United States and in the Dominican Republic, but the cases were apparently those of sporotrichosis. No case reports have been found of the disease on this continent that will stand up to critical analysis with respect to the mycologic diagnosis.

Although large numbers of infected animals have been handled in the enzootic areas, reports of infection of human beings are strikingly rare. In none of the reported cases has the identity of the infection been confirmed by cultural means. In one instance, a pathologist attempted to infect himself by rubbing equine pus into the scarified skin. The attempt was unsuccessful, as have been all attempts to infect animals other than Equidae.[9] Indeed *H. farciminosum* shows a degree of host specificity indicative of adaptation to an obligate parasitic existence in Equidae: a specificity unique amongst the fungi causing systemic mycoses.

Diagnosis is made by microscopic examination of pus from the lesions or of tissue sections. The small yeastlike organisms are numerous, and many are present within swollen leucocytes. The mycelial phase occasionally has been observed in tissue, but usually is seen only in cultures.

ADIASPIROMYCOSIS (=Haplomycosis)*

Adiaspiromycosis is an infection in mammals caused by the fungus *Emmonsia* of which two species are recognized, *E. parva* (Emmons and Ashburn) 1942 and *E. crescens* Emmons and Jellison 1960. The organism grows readily as a sporulating mold on a variety of culture media at room temperature, 20-26° C., and has a yeast like phase in animal tissue or when cultured at 37° C. on blood agar or in blood broth. *E. parva* was first found in wild rodents in Arizona. *E. crescens* was described from an isolate made from a rodent in Norway but had been reported from Canada, United States, Japan, Korea, Sweden, and England as *Haplosporangium parvum* or *Haplosporangium* sp. It is now known from Finland, France, Yugoslavia, Germany, Italy, Africa, and South America. Natural infection has

*Prepared by William L. Jellison, Ph.D., U. S. Department of Health, Education, and Welfare, Public Health Service, National Institutes of Health, National Institute of Allergy and Infectious Diseases, Rocky Mountain Laboratory, Hamilton, Montana.

been observed in rabbits, carnivores, insectivores, and in a great many species of rodents. It is found in animals on mountain tops, hillsides, valleys, prairies, forests, rivers, swamps, and deserts, and from near the Equator to near the Arctic Circle.

Infection in Animals

The infection in animals appears to be extremely benign in most instances. However, McDiarmid and Austwick in England found dead moles, *Talpa,* heavily infected. Jellison, Vinson, and Borg reported pneumonic lesions and *E. crescens* in an otter, *Lutra,* which was found dead in Sweden.

Hundreds of apparently healthy wild animals have been trapped or shot and found to be infected with a few or many spherules. Histological study usually shows very little tissue reaction to the organism.

Laboratory animals, including mice, cavies, rabbits, sheep, and monkeys, succumb in twenty to sixty days after inocluation, but only if large doses of spores are used for inoculum.

Infection in Man

Evidence of human infection is based on passive cutaneous anaphylaxis tests only (Jellison, Owen, and Glesne, Rocky Mountain Laboratory, unpublished data). By testing a large number of stored human sera, two samples were found that gave a strong positive reaction to *Emmonsia* antigen and not to other fungal antigens. Fresh serum samples from both individuals repeatedly and consistently gave positive results. One probable case was a woman at Chiloquin, Oregon, who worked many years trapping and skinning muskrats. The other, a man, was a biologist with the Tennessee Fish and Game Department at Nashville. Both have been contacted, but do not have an account of previous or present illness than can be attributed to this infection.

It is difficult to conceive of a mycotic pathogen as widespread and abundant as *Emmonsia* that does not occasionally infect man. Other primates are readily infected in the laboratory.

In natural infections, the spherules are restricted to the lungs and it is obvious that infection is by inhalation. In the laboratory, mammals can be infected by intravenous, intramuscular, intraperitoneal, or subcutaneous inoculation or by nasal instillation. The organism has not been found in birds and several attempts to infect domestic chickens have failed.

Emmonsia has the following unusual or unique features:

1. *Emmonsia* grows, i.e., the tissue spherules, adiaspores, increase in size from $\pm 4 \mu$ to $\pm 500 \mu$ or approximately 1,000,000 volumes, but does not multiply in the living mammalian host.

2. The adiaspore can become one of the largest, if not the largest, pathogenic microbial cells known, as it often exceeds 400 μ in diameter. Cell walls 50 to 70 μ thick have been observed.

3. Nonparasitic growth at temperatures below 37° C. with development of mycelia and sporulation is essential before *Emmonsia* is infectious. Culture of conidiaspores at 37° C. produces spherules or adiaspores comparable to the parasitic stage.

4. Culture and production of conidia are essential for laboratory transmission. It could not possibly be transmitted in nature from rodent to rodent, rodent to man, or man to man except by death and decomposition of the host. However, the life cycle and perpetuation of the fungus in nature may occur entirely without the parasitic phase.

5. It is one of the few fungal parasites of rodents that has not been reported for man.

6. *Emmonsia* is restricted to the pulmonary tissues in naturally infected animals. Several other mycotic agents are usually systemic even though the lung may be the primary focus of infection. Other fungi are limited to cutaneous surfaces, mouth, mucosa, ears or gastrointestinal tract.

7. After a short initial incubation period, the organisms would probably not be found in the sputum even in massive infections as they become surrounded by lung tissue.

8. *Emmonsia* is the only "deep" mycotic agent of rodents known from the northern part of the temperate zone; its distribution approaches the Arctic Circle in Norway and Finland.

Emmonsia, as found in animals, has been a deceptive and cryptic organism, even though heavy infections in small rodents are often very conspicuous on autopsy. The tissue spherules are large in size and as a result have been misidentified as parasite eggs and cross sections of nematodes or set aside as nonidentified organisms. The adiaspore size is just below x-ray resolution.

Emmonsia shows a close relationship to *Histoplasma capsulatum* Darling in its mycelial stage and exhibits some resemblance to *Coccidioides immitis* Rixford and Gilchrist in its tissue phase. Both of these are important human pathogens.

SUPERFICIAL FUNGOUS DISEASES

The superficial fungus diseases or dermatomycoses of animals and man are caused by several genera and species of fungi commonly called dermatophytes which form a well defined group having a special affinity for growth in keratin. Therefore, in the parasitic form they are found growing only in the keratinized layer of the epidermis or hair follicles and the keratinized portions of the hair itself. Rare cases of deep infection have been reported.[115]

The dermatophytes have been divided into geophilic, zoophilic and anthropophilic groups on the basis of what appears to be their natural or usual habitats and their host preferences[3] which also reflect in their epidermiological behavior. The anthropophilic organisms are considered to be primary parasites of man which may affect animals also under unusual circumstances. The zoophilic organisms are primarily parasites of animals, many having definite species affinities but not limitations. The geophilic fungi which parasitize the skin are those which are found commonly in the soil of many localities and at present do not appear to necessitate an animal host for their perpetuation.

Of the twenty-one commonly recognized dermatophytes affecting man only the following five species are primarily zoophilic: *Microsporum canis, M. distortum, Trichophyton gallinae, T. verrucosum* and *T. equinum. T. mentagrophytes* which has two forms (var. *interdigitale* and var. *granulare*) cannot be classed as either zoophilic or anthropophilic because it affects both hosts about equally.[130] *M. gypseum* and *Keratinomyces ajello,* both geophilic organisms, are common to the soil but occasionally affect animals. Even so most of the anthropophilic dermatophytes have been found to cause dermatomycosis in animals and the zoophilic dermatophytes to affect man.

The anthropophilic fungi which affect animals on rare occasions are *M. audouinii,*[149] *T. rubrum,*[136] *T. schoenleinii,*[145] *T. nanum,*[3] and *T. megninii.*[145] *T. mentagrophytes* (var. *interdigitale*), which is the usual cause of chronic dermatitis pedis, is seldom isolated from animals.[130]

There are numerous reports which document the transmission of zoophilic dermatophytes from animals to man and a few of anthropophilic dermatophytes from man to animals and back to man. Both man[113] and animals[117,133,145] are infected by the geophilic organism *M. gypseum* through exposure to the soil and *K. ajello* has been found associated with lesions of animals.[129]

The mode of transmission of the dermatophytes is by direct contact of susceptible individuals with contaminated premises, fomites or infected hosts. Those infections of man which are derived from contact with infected animals usually involve those parts of the body which are not covered with clothes whereas the anatomic location of most infections with anthropophilic organisms except tinea capitis and tinea barbae are well covered with wearing apparel. It has been estimated that 70 to 80 per cent of the human infections which involve exposed parts of the body in rural areas are acquired from animals.[137] *T. mentagrophytes* (var. *granulare)* and *T. verrucosum* are the predominant etiologic agents in such cases.[126] Urban dermatomycosis usually involves the anthropophilic fungi *M. audouinii, T. tonsurans, T. rubrum,* the zoophilic *M. canis,*[126] the geophilic *M. gypseum* and *T. mentagrophytes* (var. *interdigitale).*

The Disease in Man

The dermatomycoses of man usually are classified according to the portions of the body which are affected because many of the various organisms involved produce similar lesions. However, some genera and species have a significant predeliction for specific areas of the body and some produce characteristic lesions and clinical behaviors. The common designations under this classification are tinea corporis, tinea barbae, tinea capitis, tinea cruris and tinea unguium. In addition, tinea imbricata and tinea favosa designate forms with particularly characteristic lesions.

Dermatomycoses of man which are derived from animals most frequently take the forms of tinea capitis, tinea barbae, tinea favosa, or tinea corporis, the latter usually involving the portions of the skin not covered by clothing, such as that of the neck, arms and hands.

The characteristic lesion of tinea corporis is the annular form of ringworm with a scaly, usually less active center and an active periphery which contains pustules and crusting vesicles. However, it may vary from focal scaliness of the epidermis to granulomatous inflammation. Most infections acquired from animals produce a more marked reaction on the part of the individual than do those caused by anthropophilic organisms.

Tinea barbae varies from simple focal ringworm to boggy kerion-type lesions and tinea capitis is similar with the addition of alopecia. Tinea favosa, usually involving the scalp, is characterized by the scutulum, a cup-shaped yellow mass of fungus and tissue debris with a mousy odor. This lesion frequently leads to scarring and to perm-anent focal alopecia.

M. canis does not cause epidemics of dermatomycosis in man but usually affects one or more members of a family or others living in close association. The organism may be transferred from one person to another but soon appears to loose its infectivity.[137] Dogs and cats have been proven as sources of human infection numerous times.[138,143,144,151,152] In several countries it is the major cause of tinea capitis. *M. canis* usually creates a greater reaction on the part of the human host than *M. audouinii,* the anthropophilic organism which is the primary cause of tinea capitis in children in the United States. Infection with the former frequently leads to self-limitation when assisted by simple scrubbing with soap,[139] whereas the latter tends to heal only after intensive treatment or when the individual has reached puberty.

Georg *et al.*[126] found in one series of cases that *T. verrucosum* caused approximately half of the rural ringworm, the other organism being *T. mentagrophytes* (var. *granulare).* The lesions were pri-marily around the neck and beard and most cases were traceable to cattle, either directly or indirectly. *T. equinum* also affects the beard of man primarily.

Trichophyton mentagrophytes (var. *granulare*), a variant of *T. mentagrophytes* (var. *interdigitale)* which is the most common cause of tinea pedis of man,[123] is an important cause of dermatomycosis of both animals and man. Infection of man with the *T. mentagrophytes* (var. *granulare)* contracted from animals causes a severe suppurative ringworm, usually affecting the scalp and beard and is most common in rural communities. Ajello[113] isolated *M. gypseum* from thirty-seven of 117 samples of soil from Tennessee and Georgia but it has been found in one analysis to cause only 2.1 per cent of the cases of human dermatomycosis.[137]

The Disease in Animals

Microsporum canis appears to be associated primarily with dermatomycoses in dogs and cats.[128,137,145] The clinical manifestations, especially in cats, frequently are missed on a casual inspection. There are indications that dietary deficiencies of cats favor increased clinical signs.[120] The disease occasionally is suspected in the pet by association when a child exposed to an animal develops lesions, the pet subsequently being submitted to laboratory examination for confirmation. (Fig. 97) The organism fluoresces in the lesion or hair

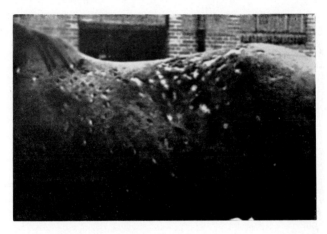

Fig. 95. Horse showing favus caused by *Microsporum gypseum*. (K. Bergner: *Ztschr. f. Infekt. d. Haustiere, 58,* 1942.)

when exposed to the Woods light (an ultra violet light shining through a nickel oxide or cobalt glass filter). The lesions in animals vary from the inconspicuous infection described above to focal or diffuse alopecia with breaking of the hair and occasionally to inflammation of such a degree that scabs and pustules are formed. The organism grows as a typical ectothrix with small spores forming a mosaic pattern about the hair. The head, ears, and legs or feet are most frequently affected but a generalized distribution of the lesion is not uncommon in dogs. *M. canis* infections appear to affect younger animals more frequently but it may affect the older ones also. Infections have been recognized also in the horse,[132,137] monkey,[137] chinchilla,[137] and sheep.[1]

M. distortum has been isolated from four monkeys and a dog which had contact with them.[135] The lesions on the monkeys varied from simple alopecia and scaliness of the skin to kerions, usually about the tail and extremities. Dermatomycoses developed in six people who had contact with the monkeys.

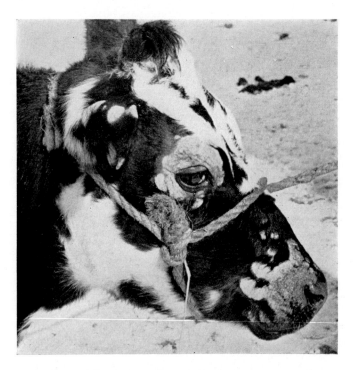

Fig. 96. Cow with *Trichophyton album* infection over eye and nose. (A. B. Hoerlein: *Cornell Vet., 35,* 1945.)

T. verrucosum is primarily a pathogen of cattle which is transmissible to man as well as to the goat, sheep, horse, donkey, burro[124] and camel.[119] The lesions, usually about the head and neck of cattle, but occasionally elsewhere, vary from a slight alopecia and scaliness of the epidermis to thick dense white to yellow-brown crusts (Fig. 96). The typhae invade the keratin of the hair and skin while sheaths of large spores of variable size (5-10 μ) form chains along the base of the hair. There is considerable inflammation in the dermis and epidermis. The organism has not been found growing in the soil or bovine dung as has *T. mentagrophytes*[8] but the spores may remain viable for four and one-half years in skin scrapings.[142]

T. equinum is considered to be the primary cause of dermatomycosis in horses in the United States, Europe and South America, approximately half of the isolates in one study being of this species.[127] Georg *et al.*[127] found the organism to have a complete requirement for nicotinic acid which is furnished in adequate quantities by the hair of the horse, donkey and mule but not by other animals. This

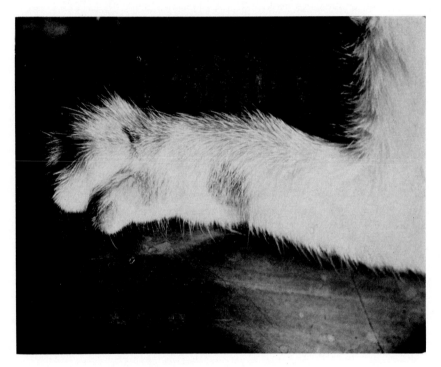

Fig. 97. Infection with microsporum canis.

may be the basic reason for the low incidence of human infection by this organism.

T. gallinae is the cause of favus in the fowl which is also called "white comb" because of the white crusty debris that forms on the normally glabrous wattles and comb. It is only an occasional parasite on man[153] and dog.[116]

T. mentagrophytes (var. *granulare*) is not an uncommon cause of dermatomycosis in many animals, both domestic and wild, including horses, cattle,[145] dogs, cats,[128] sheep,[125] pig,[141] chinchilla,[118,131] guinea pig,[146] muskrat,[122] squirrel,[121] silver fox,[145] and rabbit.[1] Evidence has been presented that it is abundant in areas frequented by domestic animals and is found most often on the hair of burrowing rodents which usually have no lesions attributable to it.[140] It has been suggested that the organism survives on the skin and fur where it obtains nutrition and grows so slow that no lesions develop.[126]

The geophilic dermatophyte *M. gypseum* is intermediate in parasitic behavior between *M. canis* and *M. cookii* inasmuch as it is quite commonly found as a saprophyte in the soil and occasionally found as a dermatophyte on man and animals. Considerations that infected animals might transmit it to human contacts must be tempered with the knowledge that both can become infected from the same source. Epidemics of infection have been reported to occur in horses[117,134] (Fig. 85) and infection is not uncommon in dogs.[148] Infection has been reported also in cats,[133] monkeys, a tiger, and a chicken.[113] It has been isolated from wild animals but none have had lesions.[140,147]

Keratinomyces ajello is a dermatophyte which is fairly common in some soils of many parts of the world from which it may be isolated using filaments of hair as a bait.[129,154] During the early years following its first recognition, it was isolated from lesions on the leg of an agricultural laborer,[11] four dogs, a calf[129] and a horse[150] but the organism was not demonstrated in the hairs or the epidermal debris of many of them. Its isolation from and demonstration in lesions on a Malabar squirrel with subsequent experimental reproduction of lesions in guinea pigs was the first proof that it truly could be classed as a dermatophyte.[129] Other isolates of this organism from lesions and the soil have failed to produce lesions experimentally[11,129]

Possibly completing the taxomonic scale from the obligate parasitic dermatophyte to the esesntially nonpathogenic keratinophilic fungus is *M. cookii* which has been isolated from the soil but more frequently from the hair of many animals.[114] Only one of the animals, a dog, had lesions but no fungus was found in them. Attempts to produce experimental infection in animals and man have failed. However, Ajello[114] has drawn attention to the fact that none of the wild animals from which *T. mentagrophytes, M. canis* and *M. gypseum* had been isolated in two studies[140,147] had lesions either.

CUTANEOUS STREPTOTHRICOSIS

Dermatophilus congolensis is the cause of a disease of animals known as cutaneous streptothricosis (not to be confused with nocardiosis or actinomycosis) which has been recognized for many years as an important enzootic dermatomycosis, especially of cattle, in Nyasaland,[166] Northern Rhodesia,[162] Nigeria,[163] British West Africa,[160] Kenya[163] and Belgian Congo,[165] as well as in occasional herds in Australia[155] and Great Britain.[164] It has been diagnosed in the United States more recently.[158] It is also known to affect the goat, horse, eland,[1] deer and man.[161] In the United States it has been diagnosed in horses in New York State[157] and Texas,[159] in cattle in Florida, Georgia and Texas[159] and in deer in New York.[161] Bridges[159] has identified a morphologically similar organism as a cause of extensive chronic pleuritis in a dog. The related species *D. dermatonomus* and *D. pedis* cause mycotic dermatitis and strawberry foot rot respectively in sheep.

The Disease in Animals

Dermatophilus spp. are characterized by narrow branching hyphae which divide by septae into three planes as they mature so that they become two to eight cells wide. Gram stain reveals that each cell contains a Gram positive coccoid spore. The latter, under appropriate conditions, may become motile. Grams stains of such maturing hyphae reveal parallel "chains of cocci." This organism has not been integrated into most classifications of fungi, the most thorough review of this phase being that of Austwick.[156]

The fungus invades the keratin of the epidermis and hair follicles, producing a focal hyperkeratosis with intraepidermal vesiculation and secondary purulent folliculitis. The hair is not invaded, a unique feature for a dermatophyte affecting animals. (*E. flocculosum* has a similar behavior in man.)

The lesions in animals varies from a small tuft of hair bound together by exudate and keratin, to focal raised white to gray or brown scabs sometimes resembling the scutula of favus. Persisting hairs protrude through the mass. The lesions are more common on the legs, back, neck and head.

Infection in Man

Soon after Bridges and Romane[158] reported the disease in cattle in Texas, Dean *et al.*[161] described the isolation of a species of *Dermatophilus* from two of four persons who developed furunculosis following handling an affected deer in the state of New York. The lesions consisted of multiple painless white "pimples" 2 to 5 mm. in diameter on the dorsal surface of one or both hands. One person who dressed the deer also developed lesions on the forearms as well as the hands. The lesions healed spontaneously in three to fourteen days.

There is considerable experimental evidence that the epidermis and hair follicles of animals must be damaged by scratches, excessive moisture or other debilitating factors before infection will become progressive. Such is true of some of the more usual dermatophytes also as illustrated by the higher incidence of experimental infections when the hair of the experimental animal is shaved before the dermatophytes are applied.

ITEMS OF NOTE

1) Actinomycosis occurs in many parts of the world in cattle, horses, swine and other animals. In man, farmers and cattlemen are the principal sufferers.

2) Nocardia infections, closely related to actinomycosis, are found in cattle, dogs and other animals. Man may be infected by contact.

3) Sporotrichosis is a disease of rats, horses, mules and dogs, with a few cases reported from other animals and the domestic fowl. Man is infected by animal bites and by puncture wounds from other sources.

4) Cryptococcosis has been found in horses, cattle, swine, cats, dogs, and man. There have been no reports of transmission of the disease directly from animals to man, but there is presumptive evidence that this may occur.

5) Coccidioidomycosis occurs in cattle and dogs, with a few cases reported from other animals. Man is infected apparently from inhalation of the spores of the organism in dust, in the same manner as animals are infected.

6) Rhinosporidiosis is a somewhat rare disease of cattle, horses and mules. Man is infected through some obscure source.

7) Blastomycosis is a disease of dogs, with a single case reported in the horse. The method of human infections is obscure.

8) Aspergillosis is an important infection of birds and poultry, as well as horses, cattle and swine. Man is probably infected by inhalation of Aspergillus spores.

9) Histoplasmosis occurs in dogs, with cases reported from the cat, horse, cow, sheep, hog, rat, mouse, skunk, opossum and marmot. It would seem that the bat, wild birds and domestic fowls are factors. Man is probably infected by inhalation of spore laden dust.

10) Epizootic lymphangitis, due to *Histoplasma farciminosum,* is an infection of horses, mules and donkeys. Infection occurs through skin wounds, by contact and possibly by insects serving as mechanical vectors.

11) Adiaspiromycosis is a natural infection of rabbits, carnivores, insectivores and rodents. The method of human infection is probably by contact.

12) Ringworm in its different forms is caused by various species of *Microsporum* and *Trichophyton.* Animals infected include the dog, cat, cow, horse, donkey, burro, camel, sheep, goat, hen and wild animals which suffer from one or another species of these organisms. Human infection is by direct contact.

13) Cutaneous streptothricosis is found in the goat, horse, cow, dog, deer and eland. Man is infected by contact.

REFERENCES

GENERAL REFERENCES

1. AINSWORTH, G. C. and AUSTWICK, P. K. C.: *Fungal Diseases of Animals.* Commonwealth Agricultural Bureaux, Farnham Royal, Bucks, England, 1959.
2. AJELLO, LIBERO: Soil as natural reservoir for human pathogenic fungi. *Science, 123:*876-879, 1956.
3. AJELLO, LIBERO: Geographic distribution and prevalence of the dermatophytes. *Ann. N. Y. Acad. Sc., 89:*30-38, 1960.
4. BREED, R. S., *et al.: Bergey's Manual of Determinative Bacteriology,* 6th Ed. Baltimore, Williams and Wilkins, 1948.
5. CONANT, N. F., SMITH, D. T., BAKER, R. D., CALLAWAY, J. L. and MARTIN, D. S.: *Manual of Clinical Mycology,* Ed. 2. Philadelphia, W. B. Saunders Co., 1954.
6. EMMONS, C. W.: Significance of saprophytism in the epidemiology of the mycoses. *Tr. New York Acad. Sc., Ser. II, 17:*157-166, 1954.
7. HENRICI, A. T.: Characteristics of fungous diseases. *J. Bact., 39:*113-138, 1940.
8. MUENDE, I., and WEBB, P.: Ringworm fungus growing as a saprophyte under natural conditions. *Arch. Derm. and Syph., 36:*987-990, 1937.

9. SAUNDERS, L. Z.: Systemic fungous infections in animals. A review. *Cornell Vet.,* *38:*213-238, 1948.

10. SKINNER, C. E., EMMONS, C. W. and TSUCHIYA, H. M.: *Henrici's Molds, Yeasts and Actinomycetes.* New York, Wiley, 1947.

11. VANBREUSEGHEM, R., GHISLAIN, E., and WELLENS, W.: Signification de l'isolement d'une souche de Keratinomyces ajello Vanbreuseghem 1952 a partier de l'homme. *Arch. belges Dermat, et Syph., 12:*130-134, 1956.

12. VANBREUSEGHEM, R. and WILKINSON, J.: *Mycoses of Man and Animals.* Springfield, Thomas, 1958.

ACTINOMYCOSIS

13. DAVIS, D. T.: Comparative study of crypt content of tonsils of man, pig, and cow, with special reference to actinomyces-like granules. *J.A.M.A., 81:*1172-1174, 1923.

14. EMMONS, C. W.: The isolation of Actinomyces bovis from tonsillar granules. *Pub. Health Rep., 53:*1967-1975, 1938.

15. EMMONS, C. W.: Mycoses of Animals, *Advances in Vet. Sci., 2:*47-63, 1955.

16. ERIKSON, D.: Pathogenic anaerobic organism of the Actinomyces group. *Med. Research Council Brit. Spec. Rept. Ser. No. 240,* p. 63.

17. ERIKSON, D. and PROTEUS, J. W.: *Commensalism in pathogenic anaerobic Actinomyces cultures. J. Gen. Microbiol., 13:*261-272, 1955.

18. FROST, B. M.: *A Study of the Actinomyces in the Mouths of Normal Cattle.* Thesis, Cornell, 1940.

19. HAGAN, W. A. and BRUNER, D. W.: *The Infectious Diseases of Domestic Animals,* 4th Ed. Ithaca, Comstock, 1961.

20. HOWELL, A. and PINE, L.: Studies on the growth of species of Actinomyces. I. Cultivation in a synthetic medium with starch. *J. Bact., 71:*47, 1956.

21. SMITH, H. A., and JONES, T. C.: *Veterinary Pathology,* Ed. 2. Philadelphia, Lea and Febiger, 1961.

22. THOMPSON, L.: Isolation and comparison of Actinomyces from human and bovine infections. *Proc. Staff Meetings Mayo Clinic, 25:*81-86, 1950.

NOCARDIA INFECTIONS

23. AJELLO, LIBERO, WALKER, W. W., DUNGWORTH, D. L., BRUMFIELD, G. L.: Isolation of *Nocardia brasiliensis* from a cat with a review of its prevalence and geographic distribution. *J.A.V.M.A., 138:*370-376, 1961.

24. DEFALLA, E. N. and GHARIB, H. M.: A study of mastitis in a goat caused by *Nocardia asteroides. Brit. Vet. J., 114:*143-145, 1958.

25. GORDON, R. E. and MIHM, J. M.: A comparative study of some strains received as Nocardia. *J. Bact., 73:*15-27, 1957.

26. JUNGERMAN, PAUL: Fungus mastitis: A case report. Vet. Med., 53:53, 1958.

27. NOCARD, M. E.: Note sur la maladie des boeufs de la Guadeloupe. *Ann. Inst. Pasteur, 2:*293-302, 1888.

28. PIER, A. C., GRAY, D. M., FOSSATI, M. J.: *Nocardia asteroides.* A newly recognized pathogen of the mastitis complex. *Am. J. Vet. Res., 19:*319-331, 1958.

29. PIER, A. C., MEJIA, M. J. and WILLERS, E. H.: *Nocardia asteroides* as a mammary pathogen of cattle. I. The Disease in cattle and the comparative virulence of 5 isolates. *Am. J. Vet. Res., 22:*502-517, 1961.

SPOROTRICHOSIS

30. BENHAM, R. W. and KESTEN, B.: Sporotrichosis: its transmission to plants and animals. *J. Infect. Dis., 50:*437-458, 1932.
31. LUTZ, A. and SPLENDORE, A.: Ueber eine bei Menschen and Raten beobachtete Mykose, *Centralbl. Bakt., 45:*631-637, 1907.
32. MOORE, J. J. and DAVIS, D. J.: Sporotrichosis following a field mouse bite, with immunological data. *J. Infect. Dis., 23:*252-265, 1918.
33. NORDEN, A.: Sporotrichosis, *Acta, Path. Microb. Scandinav., Suppl. 89:*1-119, 1951.
34. Proc. Transvaal Mine Medical Officers Assn. *Sporotrichosis Infection on Mines of the Witwatersrand.* Johannesburg, Transvaal Chamber of Mines, 1947.
35. WATSON, E. A.: A Note on equine sporotrichosis. *Canad. Vet. Res., 1:*18-19, 1920.

CRYPTOCOCCOSIS

36. BARRON, C. N.: Cryptococcosis in Animals *J.A.V.M.A., 127:*125-132, 1955.
37. BEESON, P. B.: Cryptococcic meningitis of nearly 16 years duration. *Arch. Int. Med., 89:*797-801, 1952.
38. BUSSE, O.: Ueber Saccharomycosis hominis. *Virchows Arch. f. Path Anat. 140:*23-46, 1895.
39. CARTER, H. S. and YOUNG, J. L.: A note on the isolation of *Cryptococcus neoformans* from a sample of milk. *J. Path. & Bact., 62:*271-274, 1950.
40. COWLEY, E. P., GREKIN, R. H. and CURTIS, A. C.: Turulosis. A review of the cutaneous and adjoining mucous membrane manifestations. *J. Invest. Dermat., 14:*327-344, 1950.
41. DEZEST, G.: Torulose spontanée chez le cobaye, *Ann. Inst. Pasteur, 85:*131-133, 1953.
42. EMMONS, C. W.: Isolation of *Cryptococcus neoformans* from soil. *J. Bact., 62:*685-690, 1951.
43. EMMONS, CHESTER W.: Prevalence of *Cryptococcus neoformans* in pigeon habitats. *Public Health Reports, 75:*362-365, 1960.
44. HOLZWORTH, J.: Cryptococcosis in a cat. *Cornell Vet., 42:*12-15, 1952.
45. HOLZWORTH, J. and COFFIN, D. L.: Cryptococcosis in the cat: a second case. *Cornell Vet., 43:*546-550, 1953.
46. INNES, J. R. M., SEIBOLD, H. R. and ARENTZEN, W. P.: The pathology of bovine mastitis caused by *Cryptococcus neoformans. Am. J. Vet. Res., 13:*469-475, 1952.
47. LITTMAN, M. L., SCHNEIERSON, S. S.: *Cryptococcus neoformans* in pigeon excreta in New York City. *Am. J. Hyg., 69:*49-59, 1959.
48. MOSBERG, W. H. and ARNOLD, J. G.: Torulosis of the central nervous system: Review of literature and report of five cases. *Ann. Int. Med., 32:*1153-1183, 1950.
49. RAVITZ, H. G.: Cutaneous cryptococcosis. A survey of cryptococci on normal and pathologic skin. *J. Invest. Dermat., 12:*271-284, 1948.
50. SIMON, J., NICHOLS, R. E., MORSE, E. V.: An outbreak of bovine cryptococcosis. *J.A.V.M.A., 122:*31-35, 1953.
51. SKULSKI, G. and SYMMERS, W. ST. C.: Actinomycosis and torulosis in the ferret *(Mustela furo). J. Comp. Path. and Therap., 64:*306-311, 1954.
52. SUTMÖLLER, P. and POELMA, F. G.: *Cryptococcus neoformans* infection (torulosis) of goats in the Leeward Islands region. *W. Ind. Med. J., 6:*225-228, 1957.
53. ZIMMERMAN, L. E., and RAPPAPORT, H.: Occurrence of cryptococcosis in patients with malignant disease of the reticuloendothelial system. *Am. J. Clin. Path., 24:*1050-1072, (1954).

54. ZIMMERMAN, L. E.: Fatal fungus infections complicating other diseases. *Am. J. Clin. Path., 25:*46-65, 1955.

COCCIDIOIDOMYCOSIS

55. AJELLO, L., REED, R. E., MADDY, K. T., BUDURIN, A. A., and MOORE, J. C.: Ecology and epizootiological studies on canine coccidioidomycosis. *J.A.V.M.A., 129:*485-490, 1956.

56. EGEBERG, R. O. and ELY, A. F.: *Coccidioides immitis* in the soil of the southern San Joaquin Valley. *Am. J. M. Sc., 231:*151-154, 1956.

57. EMMONS, C. W.: Isolation of Coccidioides from soil and rodents. *Pub. Health Rep., 57:*109-111, 1942.

58. FIESE, MARSHALL J.: *Coccidioidomycosis.* Springfield, Thomas, 1958.

59. FORBUS, W. D. and BESTEBREURTJE, A. D.: Coccidioidomycosis: A study of ninety-five cases of the disseminated type with special reference to the pathogenesis of the disease. *Mil. Surg., 99:*653-719, 1946.

60. JASPER, D. C.: Coccidioidomycosis in a chinchilla. *North Am. Vet., 34:*570-571, 1953.

61. LEVAN, N. E. and BURGER, C. H.: Coccidioidomycosis in dogs, a report of three cases. *California Med., 83:*379-380, 1955.

62. MCKENNEY, F. D., TRAUM, J., and BONESTELL, A. E.: Acute coccidioidomycosis in a mountain gorilla *(Gorilla beringeri)* with anatomical notes. *J.A.V.M.A., 104:*136-140, 1944.

63. MADDY, KEITH T.: Ecological factors possibly relating to the geographic distribution of *Coccidioides immitis. Proceedings of Symposium on Coccidioidomycosis, Public Health Service Publication,* No. 575, Dec. 1957.

64. MADDY, KEITH T.: A study of one hundred cases of disseminated coccidioidomycosis in the dog. *Proc. Symposium on Coccidioidomycosis, U.S. Public Health Service Publication,* No. 575, 1957.

65. PRCHAL, C. J.: Coccidioidomycosis of cattle in Arizona, *J.A.V.M.A., 113:*461-465, 1948.

66. REHKEMPER, J. A.: Coccidioidomycosis in the horse. A pathologic study. *Cornell Vet. 49:*198-211, 1959.

67. STRAUB, M., TRAUTMAN, R. J., and GREENE, J. W.: Coccidioidomycosis in 3 coyotes-*Am. J. Vet. Res., 22:*811-813, 1961.

68. VAN CLEVE, J. V.: Coccidioidal granuloma. *J. Kansas M. Soc., 37:*54-55, 1936.

RHINOSPORIDIOSIS

69. ASHWORTH, J. H.: On *Rhinosporidium seeberi,* with special reference to its sporulation and affinities. *Tr. Royal Soc. Edinburgh, 53:* (pt. 2) 301-342, 1923.

70. DE MELLO, M. T.: Rhinosporidiosis. *Mycopathologia, 4:*342-349, 1949.

71. MANDLICK, G. S.: A record of rhinosporidial polypi, with some observations in the mode of infection. *Indian med. Gaz., 72:*143-147, 1937.

72. RAO, M. A. N.: Rhinosporidiosis in bovines in the Madras Presidency with a discussion on the probable modes of infection. *Indian. J. Vet. Sci., 8:*187-108, 1938.

73. SMITH, H. A. and FRANKSON, M. C.: Rhinosporidiosis in a Texas horse, *Southwestern Vet., 15:*22, 1962.

BLASTOMYCOSIS

74. BENBROOK, E. A., BRYANT, J. B., and SAUNDERS, L. Z.: A case of blastomycosis in the horse, *J.A.V.M.A., 112:*475-478, 1948.

75. Evans, N. A.: Clinical report of a case of blastomycosis of the skin from accidental inoculation. *J.A.M.A., 40:*1172-1175, 1903.

76. Gilchrist, T. C. and Stokes, W. R.: A case of pseudo-lupus vulgaria caused by a blastomycete. *J. Exper. Med., 3:*53-78, 1898.

77. Menges, R. W.: Blastomycosis in animals. A review of an analysis of 116 canine cases. *Vet. Med., 55:*45-54, 1960.

78. Williamson, W. M., Lombard, L. S., and Getty, R. E.: North American blastomycosis in a Northern sea lion. *J.A.V.M.A., 135:*513, 1959.

79. Ramsey, F. K. and Carter, G. R.: Canine blastomycosis in the United States. *J.A.V.M.A., 120:*93-98, 1952.

80. Schoenback, E. B., Miller, J. M. and Long, P. H.: The treatment of systemic blastomycosis with stilbamidine. *Ann. Int. Med., 37:*31-47, 1952.

ASPERGILLOSIS

81. Ainsworth, G. C. and Rewell, R. E.: The incidence of aspergillosis in captive wild birds, *J. Comp. Path. and Therap., 59:*213-224, 1949.

82. Austwick, P. K. C., Gitter, M. and Watkins, C. V.: Pulmonary aspergillosis in lambs. *Vet. Rec., 72:*19-21, 1960.

83. Cogan, D. G.: Endogenous intraocular fungous infection. *Arch. Ophth., 42:*666-682, 1949.

84. Donahue, H. C.: Unusual mycotic infection of the lacrimal canaliculi and conjunctiva. *Am. J. Ophth., 32:*207-210, 1949.

85. Drake, C. H.: The pathogenicity of *Aspergillus nidulans. Mycopathologia, 4:*103-119, 1948.

86. Guha, A. N.: *Aspergillus fumigatus* infection in goats. *Indian vet. J., 36:*252-254, 1959.

87. Moore, E. N.: Miscellaneous diseases of turkeys. *Proc. 88th Annual Meeting, Am. Vet. M.A.,* 206-209, 1951.

88. Reis, J.: Queratomicose aspergilica epizootica em pintos. *Arq. Inst. Biol. (Sao Paulo), 11:*437-461, 1940.

89. Ross, C. F.: A case of pulmonary aspergillosis. *J. Path. and Bact., 63:*409-416, 1951.

90. Tscherniak, W. S.: Zur Lehre von den Broncho-und Pneumonomykosen der Pferde. *Arch. Tierheilk., 57:*417-444, 1928.

HISTOPLASMOSIS

91. Ajello, L., Briceño-Maaz, T., Campins, H., and Moore, J. C.: Isolation of *Histoplasma capsulatum* from an oil bird *(Steatornis caripensis)* cave in Venezuela. *Mycopathologia et Mycologia Applicata, 12:*199-206, 1960.

92. Christie, A. and Peterson, J. C.: Pulmonary calcification in negative reactors to tuberculin. *Am. J. Pub. Health, 35:*1131-1147, 1945.

93. Christie, A.: Histoplasmosis and pulmonary calcification. *Ann. New York Acad. Sc., 50:*1283-1298, 1950.

94. Cole, C. R., Chamberlain, D. M. and Prior, J. A.: Incidence, symptomatology and diagnosis of canine histoplasmosis. *Proc. 88th Annual Meeting Am. Vet. M. A.,* 179-181, 1951.

95. De Monbreun, W. A.: The cultivation and cultural characteristics of Darling's *Histoplasma capsulatum. Am. J. Trop. Med., 14:*93-125, 1934.

96. De Monbreun, W. A.: The dog as a natural host for *Histoplasma capsulatum. Am. J. Trop. Med., 19:*565-587, 1939.

97. EMMONS, C. W.: Isolation of *Histoplasma capsulatum* from soil. *Pub. Health Rep.,* *64*:892-896, 1949.
98. EMMONS, C. W., ROWLEY, D. A., OLSON, B. J., MATTERN, C. F. T., BELL, J. A., POWELL, E., and MARCEY, E. A.: Histoplasmosis: proved occurrence of inapparent infection in dogs, cats and other animals. *Am. J. Hyg., 61*:40-44, 1955.
99. FURCULOW, M. L. and LARSH, H. W.: Direct isolation of *Histoplasma capsulatum* from soil: Probable etiologic relationship to Camp Gruber pneumonitis. *Proc. Soc. Exper. Biol. & Med., 80*:246-248, 1952.
100. GRAYSTON, J. T., LOOSLI, C. G. and ALEXANDER, E. R.: The isolation of *Histoplasma capsulatum* from an unused silo. *Science, 114*:323-324, 1951.
101. MENGES, R. W.: Canine histoplasmosis. *J.A.V.M.A., 119*:411-415, 1951.
102. MENGES, R. W. and KINTNER, L. D.: Bovine histoplasmosis. Case report. *North Am. Vet. 32*:692-695, 1951.
103. MURRAY, J. F., LURIE, H. I., KAYE, J., KOMINS, C., BOROK, R., and WAY, M.: Benign pulmonary histoplasmosis (Cave Disease) in South Africa. *South African M.J., 31*:245-253, 1957.
104. ROWLEY, D. A., HABERMAN, R. T., and EMMONS, C. W.: Histoplasmosis: pathologic studies of fifty cats and fifty dogs from Loudoun County Virginia. *J. Infect. Dis., 95*:98-108, 1954.

ADIASPIROMYCOSIS

105. DOWDING, E. S.: Haplosporangium in Canadian rodents. *Mycologia, 39*:372-373, 1947.
106. EMMONS, C. W. and ASHBURN, L. L.: Isolation of *Haplosporangium parvum n. sp.* and *Coccidioides immitis* from wild rodents. Their relationship to coccidioidomycosis. *Public Health Rep., 57*:1715-1727, 1942.
107. EMMONS, C. W.: Coccidioidomycosis and haplomycosis. *Proc. 4th Internat. Cong. Trop. Med. and Malaria,* pp. 1278-1286, 1948.
108. EMMONS, C. W. and JELLISON, W. L.: *Emmonsia crescens. Ann. New York Acad. Sc., 89*:91, 1960.
109. JELLISON, W. L.: Haplomycosis in Montana rabbits, rodents, and carnivores. *Public Health Rept. 65*:1057-1063, 1950.
110. JELLISON, W. L., VINSON, J. W. and BORG, K.: Adiaspiromycosis (Haplomycosis) in Sweden. *Acta Vet. Scand., 2*:178, 1961.
111. McDIARMID, A. and AUSTWICK, P. K. C.: Occurrence of *Haplosporangium parvum* in the lungs of the mole *(Talpa europaea). Nature, 174*:843, 1954.
112. PEZENBURG, E.: Haplomykose beim Hasen. *Zeit. für Bakt., Parasiten, Infekt., und Hygiene, 178*:140, 1960.

SUPERFICIAL FUNGOUS DISEASES

113. AJELLO, L.: The dermatophyte, *Microsporum gypseum,* as a saprophyte and parasite. *J. Invest. Dermat., 21*:157-171, 1953.
114. AJELLO, L.: A new Microsporum and its occurrence in soil and on animals. *Mycologia, 51*:69-76, 1959.
115. ARAVIJSKY, A. N.: Rare findings in pathological material. *Mycopathologia, 11*:143-154, 1959.
116. BAUDET, E. A. R. F.: Sur une dermatomycose du chien produite par *Microsporum (Achorion) gallinae. Ann. Parasit. hum. Comp., 17*:443-446, 1940.
117. BERGNER, K.: Mikrosporon equinum und Achorion gypseum als Erreger von Flechtenerkrankungen bei Pferden. *Zeitschr. Infekt. Haustiere, 58*:121-142, 1942.

118. BLANK, F., BYRNE, J. L., PLUMMER, P. J. G., and AVERY, R. J., Isolation of *Trichophyton granulosum* Sabouraud, 1919, from chinchillas showing fur slipping. *Canad. J. Comp. Med. and Vet. Sci.*, *17:*396-402, 1953.

119. BLANK, F.: Dermatophytes of animal origin transmissible to man. *Am. J. M. Sc.*, *229:*302-316, 1955.

120. DE ALMEIDA, F., DA SILVA, A. C., BRANDÃO, C. H., MONTEIRO, E. L., MOURA, R. A.: Saprofitismo do *Microsporum canis* em gatos. *Rev. inst. Adolfo Lutz*, *10:*49-52, 1950.

121. DELAMATER, E. D.: The squirrel as a new host to a ringworm fungus. *Mycologia*, *31:*519-526, 1939.

122. ERRINGTON, P. L.: Observations on a fungus skin disease of Iowa muskrats. *Am. J. Vet. Res.*, *3:*195-201, 1942.

123. GEORG, L. K.: The relationship between the downy and granular forms of *Trichophyton mentagrophytes*. *J. Invest. Dermat.*, *23:*123-141, 1954.

124. GEORG, L. K.: The diagnosis of ringworm in animals. *Vet. Med.*, *49:*157-166, 1954.

125. GUILHON, J., CHARTON, A. and DURIEUX, J.: Teigne du mouton. *Bull. Acad. Vét. Fr.*, *28:*465-468, 1955.

126. GEORG, L. K., HAND, E. A., and MENGES, R. A.: Observations on rural and urban ringworm. *J. Invest. Dermat.*, *27:*335-353, 1956.

127. GEORG, L. K., KAPLAN, W., and CAMP, L. B.: Equine ringworm with special reference to *Trichophyton equinum*. *Am. J. Vet. Res.*, *18:*798-810, 1957.

128. GEORG, L. K., ROBERTS, C. S., MENGES, R. W. and KAPLAN, W.: *Trichophyton mentagrophytes* infections in dogs and cats. *J.A.V.M.A.*, *130:*427-432, 1957.

129. GEORG, L. K., KAPLAN, W., AJELLO, L., WILLIAMSON, W. M., and TILDEN, E. B.: The parasitic nature of the soil fungus *Keratinomyces ajello*. *J. Invest. Dermat.*, *32:*539-544, 1959.

130. GEORG, L. K.: Epidemiology of the dermatophytoses, sources of infection, modes of transmission and epidemicity. *Ann. N. Y. Acad. Sc.*, *89:*69-77, 1960.

131. HAYES, F. A.: Treatment of ringworm in chinchillas. *J.A.V.M.A.*, *128:*193-195, 1956.

132. HOERLEIN, A. B.: Studies on animal dermatomycosis. *Cornell Vet.*, *35:*287-307, 1945.

133. KAPLAN, W., GEORG, L. K., and BROMLEY, C. L., JR.: Ringworm in cats caused by *Microsporum gypseum*. *Vet. Med.*, *52:*347-349, 1957.

134. KAPLAN, W., HOPPING, J. L., and GEORG, L. K.: Ringworm in horses caused by the dermatophyte *Microsporum gypseum*. *J.A.V.M.A.*, *131:*329-332, 1957.

135. KAPLAN, W., GEORG, L. K., KENDRICKS, S. L., and LEEPER, R. A.: Isolation of *Microsporum distortum* from animals in the United States. *J. Invest. Dermat.*, *28:*449-453, 1957.

136. KAPLAN, W. and GUMP, R. H.: Ringworm in a dog caused by *Trichophyton rubrum*. *Vet. Med.*, *53:*139-142, 1958.

137. KAPLAN, W., GEORG, L. K. and AJELLO, L.: Recent developments in animal ringworm and their public health implications. *Ann. N.Y. Acad. Sc.*, *70:*636-649, 1958.

138. LATOUCHE, C. J.: The Leeds campaign against microsporosis in children and domestic animals. *Vet. Rec.*, *64:*398-399, 1952.

139. LEWIS, G. M., and HOPPER, M. E.: *An Introduction to Medical Mycology*. Chicago, Yearbook Pub. Co., 1943.

140. MCKEEVER, S., MENGES, R. W., KAPLAN, W., and AJELLO, L.: Ringworm fungi of feral rodents in southwestern Georgia. *Am. J. Vet. Res.*, *19:*969-972, 1958.

141. McPherson, E. A.: *Trichophyton mentagrophytes:* natural infection in pigs. *Vet. Rec., 68:*710-711, 1956.

142. McPherson, E. A.: The influence of physical factors on dermatomycosis in domestic animals. *Vet. Rec., 69:*1010-1013, 1957.

143. Marples, M. J.: Some observations on the occurrence and clinical course of tinea capitis and corporis in Otago. *New Zealand M.J., 50:*460-479, 1951.

144. Menges, R. W., and Georg, L. K.: Observations on feline ringworm caused by *Microsporum canis,* and its public health importance. *Proc. Am. Vet. M. A., Aug. 15-18:*471-474, 1955.

145. Menges, R. W. and Georg, L. K.: Animal ringworm study. *Vet. Med., 50:*293, 1955.

146. Menges, R. W., and Georg, L. K.: An epizootic of ringworm among guinea pigs caused by *Trichophyton mentagrophytes. J.A.V.M.A., 128:*395-398, 1956.

147. Menges, R. W., Love, G. J., Smith, W. W., and Georg, L. K.: Ringworm in wild animals in southwestern Georgia. *Am. J. Vet. Res., 18:*672-677, 1957.

148. Menges, R. W., and Georg, L. K.: Canine ringworm caused by *Microsporum gypseum. Cornell Vet., 47:*90-100, 1957.

149. Murrell, T. W., Jr.: *Microsporum audouini* isolated from a dog. *Arch. Dermat & Syph., 63:*638, 1951.

150. Pier, A. C. and Huges, J. P.: Isolation of *Keratinomyces ajello* from skin lesions of a horse. *J.A.V.M.A., 138:*484-486, 1961.

151. Roberts, L.: Note on a specimen of Tinea microsporon in the cat. *Brit. J. Dermat., 14:*327-332, 1902.

152. Saunders, W.: Small scale epidemic of ringworm caused by a pet. *New York State J. Med., 52:*1673, 1952.

153. Torres, G. and Georg, L. K.: A human case of *Trichophyton gallinae* infection. *A.M.A. Arch. Dermat., 74:*191-197, 1956.

154. Vanbrueseghem, R.: Interet théorique et practique d'un nouveau dermatophyte isolé du sol: *Keratinomyces ajello* gen. nov. sp. nov. *Bull. Classe des Sciences, 5th Series, 38:*1068-1077, 1952.

CUTANEOUS STREPTOTHRICOSIS (Dermatophilus Spp.)

155. Albiston, H. E.: Mycotic dermatitis in a calf. *Australian V. J., 9:*107, 1933.

156. Austwick, P. K. C.: Cutaneous streptothricosis, mycotic dermatitis and strawberry foot rot and the genus Dermatophilus Van Saceghem. *Vet. Rev. & Annot., 4:*33-48, 1958.

157. Bentinck-Smith, J., Fox, F. H., and Baker, D. H.: Equine dermatitis (cutaneous streptothricosis). Infection with Dermatophilus in the United States. *Cornell Vet., 51:*334-349, 1961.

158. Bridges, C. H. and Romane, W. M.: Cutanoeus streptothricosis in cattle. *J.A.V. M.A., 138:*153-157, 1961.

159. Bridges, C. H. and Schroeder, W. F.: Unpublished data. 1961.

160. Chodnik, K. S.: Mycotic dermatitis of cattle in British West Africa. *J. Comp. Path., 66:*179-186, 1956.

161. Dean, D. J., Gordon, M. A., Severinghaus, C. W., Kroll, E. T., and Reily, J. R.: Streptothricosis: a new zoonotic disease. *New York State J. Med., 61:*1283-1287, 1961.

162. Hudson, J. R.: Cutaneous streptothricosis. *Proc. Royal Soc. Med., 30:*1457-1460, 1937.

163. PLOWRIGHT, W.: Cutaneous streptothricosis in cattle. I. Introduction and epizootiological features in Nigeria. *Vet. Rec., 68:*350-355, 1956.
164. STABLEFORTH, A. W.: Cutaneous streptothricosis. A case in Great Britain. *Proc. Royal Soc. Med., 30:*1455, 1937.
165. VAN SACEGHEM, R.: Dermatose contagieuse (impétigo contagieux). *Bull. Soc. Pat. exot., 8:*354-359, 1915.
166. ZLOTNIK, I.: Cutaneous streptothricosis in cattle. *Vet. Rec., 67:*613-614, 1955.

Chapter 19

CHEMICALS IN ANIMAL PRODUCTS

R. D. RADELEFF, D.V.M.

THE NATURE OF THE PROBLEM

It is likely that every person who has cared for an animal producing milk for human consumption is aware that chemicals are readily absorbed and excreted with milk, producing bitterness, undesirable odors or colors. The sources of the commonly recognized undesirable changes have been various plants. More recently, organoleptic changes have been observed in milk following antiparasitic therapy with phenothiazine. Earlier in the history of the United States the excretion of tremetol by cows impeded the settlement of certain areas, notably Illinois and Kentucky and was a frequent cause of death. (See Chapter 20.) It is not surprising, then, to discover that synthetic organic compounds may be excreted in the milk of animals consuming them. It is probable that organic compounds of many kinds have always been stored in small quantities in the tissues of animals. In the absence of organoleptic evidence of such substances and the lack of immediate readily recognizable illness resulting from their consumption, most have gone unnoticed.

Effects isolated by time from their causes have always plagued scientists and the solution of such problems requires the most ingenious thought of persistent scientists. Binns, of the Animal Disease and Parasite Research Division of the United States Department of Agriculture, has described a cyclopian deformity of lambs occurring in the Rocky Mountain area for many years. Ranchers considered the condition to be a genetic problem and many were reluctant to have the condition studied. Although this condition is not transmissable to man, it is cited because of the significance it indicates must be attached to the presence of small quantities of an organic compound at a critical time and indicates the exquisite difficulty attendant upon demonstrating a cause when the effect is observed only after a relatively long period of time.

Observers in France found that fenugreek produces, in meat, an odor resembling that of hog manure and that calves may develop the odor from milk when their dams are fed the plant. Many chemicals are known to induce their own odors, hence are present, in meat after ingestion, absorption or injection. These common substances include, but are not limited to, ether, anise, asafoetida, valerian, benzene, camphor, carbolic acid, chloroform, tar and fennel. Some, such as ether, chloroform, phenol or chlorine, produce odors in tissues after being inhaled as vapors by the animal.

THE SIGNIFICANCE OF THE PROBLEM

It is neither amazing nor new knowledge, that chemicals applied to livestock or introduced into their feed will appear in their milk, or be stored in their tissues. The sulfonamides, antibiotics, anthelmintics, insecticides, and other agricultural chemicals have brought a series of problems. A very large proportion of these materials are stored in tissues, or secreted in milk. Their presence in food is considered by medical authorities to be potentially dangerous to the health of people. The primary worry in this regard is a concern over the effects of consumption for prolonged periods of time, possibly a lifetime. There is particular concern for the infants who must consume large quantities of milk and for the aged who may require large quantities of dairy products. It is generally thought, and usually true, that the young and the infirm are particularly susceptible to the effects of poisons.

Millions of pounds of the various agricultural chemicals and drugs are used in the United States each year. The use of antibiotics in the treatment of mastitis in cattle alone, required in 1958 more than seventy-five tons of the compounds. Pesticides are used in terms of millions of pounds. Considering the wide use of the chemicals, the many circumstances under which they may be applied, and the various species of livestock which might contact them, one is able to gain some idea of the immensity of the problem. Strong emphasis should be placed upon the fact that until the present writing (1961) there have been no confirmed instances in which people were frankly poisoned by agricultural chemicals in food as a result of

TABLE 49

RESULTS OF FEEDING VARIOUS LEVELS OF INSECTICIDES TO CATTLE AND SHEEP FOR VARIOUS TIMES, AND THE MAXIMUM FAT RESIDUES RESULTING FROM SUCH FEEDING. IN EACH CASE THE QUANTITY FED WAS HARMLESS TO THE ANIMALS. (FROM ARS 20-9, AGRICULTURAL RESEARCH SERVICE, U. S. DEPARTMENT OF AGRICULTURE, PAGE 138, SEPTEMBER, 1960.)

Chemical	Animals	Levels Fed in Total Diet (P.p.m.)	Period Fed (Weeks)	Maximum Fat Content (P.p.m.)
Aldrin	Cattle	5	16	8
		10	16	49
		25	8	78
	Sheep	5	16	17
		10	16	55
		25	8	78
BHC, all isomers	Cattle	100	16	250
	Sheep	100	16	119
BHC, Lindane	Cattle	1	12	1.5
		10	12	8
		100	12	98
Chlordane	Cattle	10	16	13
	Sheep	10	16	16
	Cattle	25	8	18
	Sheep	25	8	12
DDT	Cattle	10	4	6.8
	Sheep	10	4	3.1
	Cattle	25	16	40
	Sheep	25	16	15
Dieldrin	Cattle	1	16	5.5
	Sheep	1	16	3.9
	Cattle	2.5	16	14.3
	Sheep	2.5	16	10.5
	Cattle	10	16	44
	Sheep	10	16	48
	Cattle	25	8	75
	Sheep	25	8	69
Endrin	Cattle	2.5	16	1.6
	Sheep	2.5	16	3.2
	Cattle	5.0	16	2.4
	Sheep	5.0	16	2.2
Heptachlor	Cattle	1.0	8	4
	Cattle	2.5	16	1.5
	Sheep	2.5	16	2.1
	Cattle	10	16	7.5
	Sheep	10	16	8.5
	Cattle	60	16	62
Methoxychlor	Cattle	25	16	0
	Sheep	25	16	0
Toxaphene	Cattle	10	8	Less than 4
	Cattle	25	16	12
	Sheep	25	16	8
	Cattle	100	16	38
	Sheep	100	16	25

farm practices. There has been evidence that some persons consuming milk from cows treated with antibiotics have become allergic to the antibiotics involved, and that this has substantially restricted the number of drugs which might be used to treat these persons during various illnesses. At one time antibiotic levels in milk substances reached such an intensity that the processing of cheese and other dairy products was seriously interfered with.

Equal emphasis should be placed upon the fact that the careless use or management of agricultural chemicals, particularly insecticides, has resulted in the deaths of livestock, pets, and people. The total number of human poisonings in any year due to pesticides, however, has been far less than the number of deaths due to such common household items as aspirin or kerosene. Children, especially those under 5 years of age, account for a very high percentage of these poisonings. In livestock production, losses are still far greater from poisonous plants, toxic minerals, and industrial wastes than from agricultural chemicals.

Certain hormone-like substances and certain organic compounds that might have had some value in agriculture have been demonstrated to be carcinogenic under certain special laboratory conditions, usually involving tumor-susceptible laboratory animals and rather high dosages of the materials. Because of these findings, the food laws in the United States have been amended to prohibit, essentially, the presence in any quantity of any substance known to produce cancer when applied in any manner to any animal. The cattle disease, hyperkeratosis was never known to involve a transmission of the effect to humans, nor were its etiological agents, the highly chlorinated naphthalenes, shown to have a similar effect on people. This costly disease of cattle illustrates the fact that minute quantities of chemicals can have profound effects. In some tests the disease was induced in cattle exposed only to the vapors of the compound and not to direct contact. This disease also illustrates the fact that one can never be certain that a study in one animal, or even a series of animals, will completely answer the question of hazard to people. Toxicologists and pharmacologists are familiar with these deviations between species, and because they are aware of the deviation, those responsible for the safety of our foods in the United States conscientiously introduce a very high safety factor before permitting a chemical in foods.

PREVENTION, LEGISLATION AND INVESTIGATION

Under federal statutes, in the United States, chemicals may be present in food only if they are essential in the production of the food, and then only if toxicological studies have adequately demonstrated that the amounts present would not be harmful. In the United States milk is considered such a sensitive food that foreign chemicals are not permitted in any quantity.

Before a chemical can be properly evaluated there must be a thorough series of investigations. These begin with the characterization of the chemical, including a knowledge of the impurities that might be expected in routine manufacturing. There must then be an investigation of acute and chronic toxicity of the chemical to livestock and to laboratory animals, such as the rats, mice, guinea pigs, dogs and monkeys. These tests usually involve the application of the material by several routes. Feeding trials are conducted with laboratory animals and are usually designed to cover the lifetime of at least one species, preferably more. During the course of such toxicological studies, the absorption, excretion and storage of the material is investigated. An important part of this phase is the determination of the metabolites which the animal may produce from the original compound, for it is well established that animals readily convert such substances. The metabolites may be more toxic, equally toxic or less toxic than the parent compound. Indeed the body may be able to manufacture a nutrient from the metabolic products. Additional studies are required to determine the carcinogenic potential. Effects upon reproduction and longevity must be conducted.

During these studies a material is often recognized as having additional uses. In some cases the toxic effect of the chemical can be utilized. This was true of pival, which has a systemic effect against certain insects feeding on livestock, but unfortunately is an anticoagulent and in dosages sufficient for parasite control causes the death of the host by massive hemorrhages. This quality made it an excellent rodenticide.

Chemicals have specific behaviors. Some are readily absorbed and as readily eliminated, and their presence in the animal body is ephemeral. Others are poorly absorbed, therefore the total amount reaching the general circulation is very small. If the rate of excretion is not exceeded this small quantity disappears and creates no problems. In some instances such minute quantities persist for many months. There are other materials that are rapidly absorbed, stored in large amounts and excreted very slowly. Some require as much as a year for complete elimination.

BIOLOGICAL CYCLES

Biological cycles exist (see figure 98) with those materials that are readily stored but poorly eliminated. A treated cow will pass these substances to her calf in her milk. The calf in turn has difficulty in eliminating its accumulated residues and will retain that residue until it is marketed for beef. The same cycle can be observed if a farmer treats hay with these materials then sells it to a rancher.

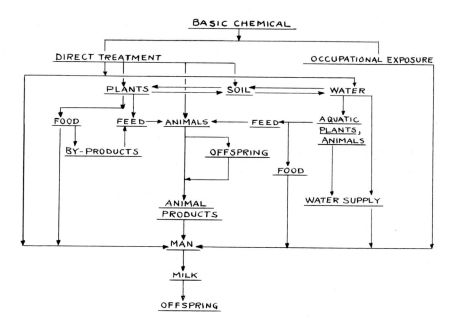

Fig. 98.

This cycle creates problems that are not easily solved because it is quite possible for the second man, that is, the owner of the calves to introduce into interstate commerce, meat of animals containing excessive amounts of the chemical. He has not personally contributed, nor did he, in all probability, have knowledge of the exposure when he put the animals on the market. Likewise, a farmer who fed

his cows the contaminated hay may not have been aware of the contamination. The farmer who treated his hay may not have treated
with the intention that the hay would be used for livestock to be
slaughtered. Establishing responsibility for the ultimate effect in
such a cycle is virtually impossible. This sort of cycle has caused
losses to some dairymen when milk was found to be contaminated,
although these men had not treated their animals nor used the
chemical on their premises. It is not practical to demand an analyses
to be provided with each lot of feed sold because of the tedious
technique required, nor does there appear to be a practical method
of coloring or otherwise identifying treated feeds. The only satisfactory solution is to restrict the usage or recommendation of chemicals, no matter how effective they may be, when the danger of starting a biological cycle is known.

Radioactive Isotopes

The development of nuclear explosives has introduced a special
form of hazard for man, animals and plants. Radioactive isotopes
are finding their way into the food chain from two sources other
than the naturally occurring minerals. Both sources are connected
with the production and use of atomic energy.

The explosion of nuclear devices creates showers of radioisotopes
from the casing and parts of the device and from solids and liquids
in the immediate vicinity of the point of explosion. Depending upon
the nature, size and point of explosion of such devices, radioisotopes
enter the atmosphere and may circulate above the earth for long
periods before settling to earth.

The purification of isotopes for use in explosive devices or for
atomic power involves the creation of sizable amounts of "waste"
products that are radioactive, and consequently, the problem of safe
disposition to avoid generally contaminating our environment.

Scientists are definitely not in full agreement concerning some of
the hazards said to exist. Scientists agree, however, on a number of
points:

1) Long lived isotopes are being concentrated or produced in the
development and use of atomic energy.

2) Radiation from these isotopes can alter the genetic material
of all living things.

3) A number of the isotopes are entering the food chain through plants and animals.

4) Certain isotopes have predilections for certain tissues and may be concentrated there even when the dietary level of intake is extremely small.

5) The radiation being received from the various sources would be best reduced.

6) Methods must be developed to minimize the contamination of our atmosphere, soil, water and food.

The greatest single problem is, of course, the control of this world wide contamination. The international nature of the use of atomic energy, both for peace and war, precludes simple legislative procedures. International agreements seem only a dream at this time.

The level of radioactivity from "fall-out" and wastes is presently detectable with the more sensitive radiometric equipment in much of the world. In the immediate area of the scenes of nuclear detonations there is usually a far higher level.

The careful, continuous, monitoring being carried on by various public health and research laboratories should provide us with ample warning of dangerous levels of the radioisotopes in our food and environment. The public press, radio and television services will undoubtedly convey the message. The real problem here is that they may sound unnecessary alarms so frequently as to dull our consciousness for the real warning.

Procedures for action in the event of atomic attack have been developed by the various responsible governmental agencies and will be activated when required.

ITEMS OF NOTE

1) Chemicals useful to man in controlling pests and diseases are essential in our modern economy, but have created problems with their residues in foods of animal origin as well as other foods.

2) The presence of chemical residues in foods of animal origin was recognized early enough in most cases to allow extensive studies that have lead to reasonable controls.

3) Frank poisoning of people by chemicals in foods of animal origin has not been observed, but sensitivities (allergies) have been developed by people, particularly to antibiotics.

4) The modern pesticides are not usually detectable organoleptically, therefore it is very difficult to recognize contaminated products.

5) Biological cycles may be instituted that lead to ultimate legal involvements and difficulty in determining the person at fault.

6) Radioactive isotopes are entering our animal foods, primarily from the testing of nuclear explosives and the preparation of materials for nuclear reactors for power production.

7) Chemicals in foods of animal origin are subject to reasonable control but the international scope of nuclear activities is not.

Chapter 20

MILK SICKNESS

Thomas G. Hull, Ph.D.

Milk sickness in man and trembles in animals results from poisoning with the white snake root or the rayless goldenrod. The disease is primarily one of animals transmitted to man through the milk, or milk products, of affected cattle. Other names by which milk sickness has been known are white snake root poisoning, slows, and puking fever in the East, and milk sick or alkali disease in the West.

HISTORY

Milk sickness was recognized as early as 1776 in North Carolina. It was a serious affliction of the early settlements of the Middle West, taking many lives in Tennessee, Ohio, Indiana, Illinois, Missouri, and other Mississippi River states.

Mather, in the *Making of Illinois,* mentions it in connection with the settling of the "New Design" in 1797, stating that it attacked many newcomers. It was one of the diseases which gave Illinois the reputation of being unhealthful and so retarded immigration to this territory for awhile.

Herndon, in his *Life of Abraham Lincoln,* describes the ravages of milk sickness in Kentucky, telling how whole settlements were abandoned to get rid of the peculiar malady. "In the fall of 1818, the scantily settled region in the vicinity of Pigeon Creek—where the Lincolns were then living—suffered a visitation of that dread disease common in the West in early days, and known in the vernacular of the frontier as the milksick! It hovered like a spectre over the Pigeon Creek settlement for over ten years and its fatal visitations and inroads among the Lincolns, Hanks, and Sparrows finally drove that contingent into Illinois. . . . It not only took off the people but it made sad havoc among the cattle. One man testifies that he lost four milk cows and eleven calves in one week. This, in addition to the risk of losing his own life, was enough, he declared, to ruin him, and prompted him to leave for points further west! . . . Early in October of the year 1818, Thomas and Betsy Sparrow fell ill of the disease and died within a few days of each other. Thomas Lincoln performed the services of undertaker. . . . Meanwhile Abe's mother had fallen a victim of the insidious disease. Her sufferings, however, were destined to be of brief duration. Within a week she, too, rested from her labors."

At the fifth annual meeting of the American Medical Association in 1852 Daniel Drake was appointed chairman of a "Committee on Milk Sickness, So Called." In his report to the Association in 1858 he "elaborated very extensively the theory that eating the *Rhus toxicodendron* produced the disease in cattle. In 1861, evidence was produced which tended to confirm the relation of white snake root to the disease in cattle. In 1907, Brown called attention to the sweetish odor of the breath and Walsh diagnosed the human disease as an acidosis.

"Alkali disease" had been known in the Pecos Valley of New Mexico and Texas since its earliest settlement.

The poisonous properties of the rayless goldenrod were first brought to the attention of the United States Department of Agriculture, when E. O. Wooten of Mesilla Park, New Mexico, submitted a specimen of the plant together with a history of losses in horses and cattle. Since that time a considerable number of reports have been recorded of alkali disease and milk sickness in New Mexico and Texas. The exact nature of the poison responsible for the disease was unknown. In 1909, Moseley published a report in which he ascribed the cause to aluminum salts in the plant. The work of Jordan and Harris indicated that it was of bacterial nature —*Bacillus lactimorbi*—but these findings were not confirmed by other investigators.

In 1926, Couch of the United States Department of Agriculture, isolated from white snake root and the rayless goldenrod the chemical substance responsible for the trouble. It has been named tremetol.

THE POISONOUS PLANTS

Two plants are responsible for milk sickness; white snake root and the rayless goldenrod.

White snake root *(Eupatorium ageratoides* or *urticaefolium),* also called richweed, boneset, polewort, or squaw weed, grows from Minnesota to Louisiana and east to North Carolina. There are over forty species of white snake root in the United States, but this is the only one that has given serious trouble. One other member *Eupatorium serotinum,* has been suspected of causing death in animals, but evidence has not been confirmed. The common thoroughwort belongs to the same family and grows in the same locality.

Eupatorium ageratoides grows in densely wooded areas. When the trees and underbrush are removed sufficiently to permit the growth of bluegrass the white snake root disappears almost completely. The plants do not thrive in the bright sunlight. It has been known to grow in pastures, however, and is found sparingly over a wide area in urban and rural communities.

In the more highly cultivated agricultural sections it has been found in orchard pastures.

The plant is a slender erect perennial herb which grows from one to four feet high. The leaves are opposite each other, three to five inches long, broadly ovate with sharply toothed or serrated edges. The leaf stalks are about one-fourth to one-half as long as the leaf. Each leaf has three main veins which extend from the base of the leaf and which give off many branches. In the late summer the white flowers of the plant appear as compound clusters having eight to thirty flowers, giving to pastures in heavily infested woodlands an attractive appearance. Other members of the family, including *Eupatorium serotinum,* grow more abundantly in open pastures.

The rayless goldenrod, or jimmy weed *(Aplopappus heterophyllus),* is distributed over a wide territory from southern Colorado to the Texas Panhandle and south to Arizona, Sonora, and Chihuahua. It is especially abundant in the irrigated portions of the Pecos Valley in Texas and New Mexico.

Aplopappus frutsiosus causes poisoning in some instances but it is less widely distributed.

The rayless goldenrod belongs to the composite family, bearing the flowers in compact heads as does the sunflower. It is a stout, erect, tufted perennial herb of one or two feet in height, except on the banks of irrigated ditches where it grows four feet or more high. The leaves are alternate, line-like or broader, one-eighth to one-fourth inch wide, and three-fourths to two and one-half inches long. The heads are numerous, with or without stems in terminal, flat-topped bunches, each head having seven to fifteen tubular flowers.

TREMETOL

Tremetol is the name given by James F. Couch of the Bureau of Animal Industry of the United States Department of Agriculture to the poisonous principle found in white snake root responsible for trembles in cattle and milk sickness in man.

White snake root contains three poisonous substances, a complex alcohol, a resinous acid, and a volatile oil. The latter two are only slightly poisonous and do not produce trembles. The complex alcohol is the substance that has been named tremetol. It is an optically active alcohol of the formular $C_{16}H_{22}O_3$ and is soluble in alcohol, ether, chloroform, benzene, and other organic solvents. It is insoluble in water, acids, or alkalis.

Tremetol may be altered by heat or by chemical reagents and when so changed it loses its poisonous properties. The temperature required for the pasteurization of milk, however, does not affect it. Couch devised a test for tremetol in plants, in milk, butter, cheese or meat. He described it as follows:

> "The suspected material is extracted with petroleum ether. Ordinary gasoline may be used if it does not give a red color with sulphuric acid. The solution is poured on the surface of 2 cc. of concentrated sulphuric acid in a dry test tube, when if tremetol is present, a red color appears at the junction of the two layers. Upon shaking the tube the petroleum ether layer is colored a transient red and on allowing the layers to separate the lower layer of acid is colored a fine cherry red while the upper layer is colorless. If the solution is very dilute only an orange color will result."

Milk or butter that respond to the color reaction are dangerous to health and should not be used as food. A few substances other than tremetol give a red color with sulphuric acid, but they are not likely to be present when tremetol is suspected.

Tremetol is rapidly destroyed by drying so that completely dried snake root is incapable of producing trembles. The poison of the rayless goldenrod, on the other hand, is not destroyed by drying and this plant is dangerous to cattle either green or dry.

THE DISEASE IN ANIMALS

Trembles appears in pastured animals—horses, cattle, and sheep being the ones naturally affected. During the autumn when pastures are dry, white snake root is green and cattle often turn to it as a last resort. Sometimes cattle will eat it even though pasture grass is abundant. The course of the disease is practically the same whether due to white snake root or the rayless goldenrod.

The first symptoms in cattle are drooping of head and ears, dull appearance, loss in weight, abnormal thirst, obstinate constipation, and general inactivity. A characteristic trembling of the voluntary muscles is responsible for the name trembles.

Marked muscular debility is noted in advanced stages when the animal lies prostrate on the ground unable to rise. The breath has a marked pungent odor. The pulse and respiration become irregular and slow as coma appears, followed by death. Not all cattle in a herd, develop the disease, while the severity of symptoms of those infected varies in different animals.

Milk cows exposed to white snake root may transmit the poison through the milk without showing any symptoms of the disease. It would appear that the milk absorbs the poison thus protecting the animal in lactation. When the animal goes dry the system at once becomes susceptible and the disease runs its usual course described above. Sometimes animals in lactation show symptoms however.

The disease runs a more rapid course in horses than in cattle. The usual symptoms seen in cattle are observed. Paralysis of the throat results in slobbering which is an early symptom. Death follows in two or three days.

Sheep exhibit symptoms similar to those seen in cattle. A drowsy, sleepy condition, bordering on coma usually precedes death.

No animal probably is immune from trembles, for in addition to horses, cattle and sheep, it has been observed in mules, swine, chickens, rabbits, dogs, cats and guinea pigs (Couch, 1933).

Prevention of trembles is better than attempts at cure. Each case that arises may be treated separately under the care of veterinarian but cure is not always certain.

THE DISEASE IN MAN

Milk sickness in man is the result of ingesting the poison tremetol from milk, butter, or cheese, from cattle which have partaken of white snake root or the rayless goldenrod. The poison is cumulative, causing a restless, weak, exhausted, languid feeling during the early stages of the disease. Later abdominal pains develop, with nausea, vomiting, constipation, thirst, loss of appetite, weak pulse, labored breathing, and subnormal temperature. The throat and intestinal tract apparently become paralyzed and in fatal cases death is often preceded by a prolonged coma. The incubation period is two to twelve days. Acetone breath is a characteristic symptom. The fatigue may last a long time with characteristic recurrences. Walsh describes a case poisoned in 1924 and repoisoned again in August, 1925. Three months after the poisoning, strenuous exercise brought on a marked attack of the disease. Relapses are common and the mortality is high in such instances.

Milk sick patients often find difficulty in retaining solid food and for this reason are put on a milk diet. If the milk was taken from the same source as the milk which caused the sickness in the first place, the condition of the patient is rendered much worse. In milk sickness an immediate change of milk and butter is imperative.

Meat from animals suffering from trembles probably does not contain tremetol. When dogs and cats were fed experimentally upon such meat, they developed no symptoms.

Couch believes that poisoned animals or man suffer from a ketosis which is a subsequent symptom to the toxic factor responsible for the onset of the disease. Acetone has been demonstrated both in the urine and expired air of the lungs.

The mortality from milk sickness is about 25 per cent. Wolff collected records of 320 cases of which seventy-seven died.

Milk sickness in man has been largely a rural problem. City milk supplies have been rendered safe by the dilution of any poisoned milk with milk from other sources. Pasteurization does not affect the poison.

The disease is rapidly becoming a medical curiosity, with fewer and fewer cases being reported.

PREVENTION

The prevention of trembles in cattle has been accomplished by the elimination of white snake root from pastures through the use of 2,4-D spray.

ITEMS OF NOTE

1) Milk sickness is due to a chemical poison found in the white snake root plant or the rayless goldenrod. This is in distinction to the other animal diseases which are bacterial in nature.

2) Tremetol, a complex alcohol, is the responsible agent in white snake root. The toxic agent in the rayless goldenrod is somewhat different in nature.

3) The poison is of danger chiefly to cattle, horses, and sheep.

4) Man is poisoned from ingesting milk or milk products from affected cattle.

5) Tremetol in milk is not destroyed by pasteurization temperatures.

6) Market milk is ordinarily rendered safe by dilution of the poisoned milk with milk from other sources.

7) Milk sickness in man has been largely a rural problem. The disease is becoming a medical curiosity.

REFERENCES

BROWN, T. R.: *Osler's Modern Medicine.* Philadelphia, 1907, *3:*547.

COUCH, J. F.: U. S. Department Agriculture, Bureau of Animal Industry, Circular Letter on Milk Sickness, Oct. 1926.

COUCH, J. F.: U. S. Department of Agriculture, Circ. 306, 1933.

DOYLE, J. T.: *North Carolina M. J., 8:*404-410, 1947.

DRAKE, DANIEL: *Tr. A. M. A., 11:*1858.

JORDAN, E. O. and HARRIS, N. M.: *J. Infect. Dis., 6:*401-404, 1909.

MARSH, C. W., ROE, G. C. and CLAWSON, A. B.: U. S. Department of Agriculture, Bull. 1391, 1926.

MOSEBY, E. L.: *Med. Rec., 75:*839-844, 1909.

UNIVERSITY OF ILLINOIS. Div. Animal Path. Exchange, Aug. 1927.

WALSH, W. E.: *Illinois M. J., 15:*422, 1909.

WOLFF, F. A., CURTIS, R. S. and KAUP, B. F.: *North Carolina Agri. Exper. Sta. Tech. Bull., 15:*1918.

SECTION TWO

DISEASES OF RODENTS
AND WILD ANIMALS
AND OCCASIONALLY OF
DOMESTIC ANIMALS

Chapter 21

PLAGUE

K. F. Meyer, D.V.M., Ph.D., M.D., D.Sc., LL.D.

Plague is an acute infectious disease caused by *Pasteurella pestis,* or preferably *Yersinia pestis,* affecting primarily wild rodents and commensal rats. It is maintained in many regions of the world as a continuous infection chain through a rodent reservoir and an insect vector. Man becomes the victim of bubonic plague accidentally by intervention in the rodent (usually rat)—flea—rodent sequence or by handling infected wild rodents. If the bubonic form becomes generalized and the lungs are secondarily affected, man to man infection ensues without the intervention by the flea.

HISTORY

During the 1,500 years before the Christian era there were forty-one major outbreaks designated as plague (Haeser, 1882; Sticker, 1908, 1910; Lloyd, 1925). One of the early records of its ravages is recounted in the *Bible* (I Samuel, Chapters 5 and 6). The Philistines made golden images of the "mice" that over-ran the land, in order to stay the pestilence. The outbreak began at the seaport town of Ashdad and moved inland. The mortality at Beth-shemesh has been given as 50,070.

Epidemics broke out from time to time during the ensuing centuries, but records were not sufficiently accurate to allow a certain diagnosis. Papon, however, stated that there were 109 epidemics of plague during the first 1,500 years of the Christian era and 45 from 1500 to 1720 (Lloyd, 1925).

The first authentic epidemic of plague began in 542 A.D. at Pelusium in Egypt, a leading center for trade between the East and the West. The main trade routes at that time between Europe and the East were along the Mediterranean Sea and overland through Turkey, Germany and France. The infection slowly spread till every country along these routes was afflicted, from Asia to Ireland. At the height of the epidemic the mortality was 5,000 persons daily and at times reached 10,000. According to Procopius "it spared neither island nor cave nor mountaintop where man dwelt. . . . Many houses were left empty and it came to pass that many from want of relatives or servants were unburied for several days. At that time it was hard to find anyone at business in Byzantium. Most people met in the streets were carrying a corpse. All business had ceased. All craftsmen had deserted their crafts." After about 200 years that epidemic subsided.

The second pandemic of plague, known then as the "Black Death," originated in Mesopotamia about the middle of the 11th century, attained its height in the 14th century and did not disappear till the close of the 17th century. It is thought that the Crusaders, returning from the Holy Land in the 12th and 13th centuries, were instrumental in hastening the spread of the disease. Again the land along trade routes was primarily involved and from them the infection spread east, west and north. During the course of the disease, 25,000,000 people perished, a fourth of the population of the world.

It was during this period that the system of quarantine and the issuing of official decrees establishing it came into use.

Though it is generally accepted that the plague pandemic of the 14th century originated in Central Asia and spread to Europe, to India and to China, only relatively recently has there been any documentary proof for this assumption. The Russian archeologist D. A. Chwolson discovered two old Nestorian graveyards near the Issyk-kul Lake, an area long thought to form part of the central Asia plague focus (Stewart, 1928). Inscriptions on three headstones made in 1338 and 1339 stated that the persons interred had died of plague. Chwolson also noted that the number of graves dating back to these years was exceptionally high. This is good evidence that plague existed in central Asia before Europe, India and China were ravaged by the Black Death.

Shortly after the plague of London in 1664 and 1665, the disease disappeared from the whole of western Europe. The last of these epidemics were in Ireland in 1650, Denmark in 1654, Italy in 1657, Spain in 1677-1681 and in eastern and southern Germany in 1679 and 1681. It is remarkable epidemiologically that in such a short time plague should totally disappear. Various explanations have been offered for this retrogression. The progress of civilization, in particular the control of epidemic diseases by sanitation, housing and cleanliness, and the supervision of the infectious sick were considered important factors. Liston (1924) related the disappearance of plague to a change in the rat population. In particular, the agrarian revolution led to the exclusion of rats from human dwellings and this favored the substitution of one species of rat for another. Another factor in the decline may be that, with the abandonment of the old trade routes, commercial activity became concentrated in Amsterdam and London, and the new connections with the Far East were by sea, not by land; this reduced the distribution of the disease (Simpson, 1905). These explanations are not fully satisfactory, but they doubtless cover important auxiliary factors even in recent years. Knowledge acquired since 1900 leads to the conclusion that the decline of plague at the end of the 17th century represents the operation of the great natural law of the rise and decline of epidemics. The seeming disappearance in the middle of the 19th century is merely a phase in the natural history of the disease itself, no more remarkable than the similar prolonged quiescence that followed the epidemics in the 8th century (Meyer, 1947).

During the 18th and the early part of the 19th century plague continued to prevail in Turkey, the Near East, Syria, Egypt and Greece. Then an outbreak near Vetlianka on the Volga in 1878-1879 marked the last appearance of plague in Europe for seventeen years.

The third great expansive pandemic is supposed to have originated in Yunnan Province in China where the rebellion of the Mohammedans beginning 1855 and possibly the movements of refugees propagated the disease. Progressing in slow stages, it reached the provincial capital of Yunnan-fu (now Kumming) in 1866, and not until twenty-eight years later did it extend to Canton and Hong-kong (in May, 1894). The number of deaths due to plague in Canton in that outbreak has been estimated at between 80,000 and 100,000. During the epidemic in Hongkong the cause of plague, *Pasteurella pestis,* was identified by Alexander Yersin on June 20, 1894 (Podach, 1952). Ports in south China became plague distribution centers. Between 1894 and 1922 it spread throughout the whole world, more widespread than during any great foregoing epidemics. Except in India and a few other Asiatic areas, the number of lives lost was relatively fewer than in the epidemics of old. Its expansion across the world was as vigorous as at any time in history and the prevailing disease types were as severe as they had been. Among the points infected were Bombay in 1896, Calcutta in 1898, Japan and the Philippines in 1897, Australasia in 1899, Hawaii, Central and South America in 1899, Cape Town and San Francisco in 1900, Egypt and Singapore in 1901, Bangkok in 1904, Guayaquil in 1908, Java in 1910 (Swellengrebel, 1950), New Orleans and Colombo in 1914, Galveston and Beaumont, Texas, and Pensacola, Florida in 1922, Macassar in 1944. Being at that time a seafaring disease, it struck nearly all European ports, causing local epidemics in Oporto, Odessa, Naples and Marseilles. The population of India suffered most and the country was the scene of appalling epidemics. The reported number of plague deaths between 1896 and 1917 was 9,841,396; the maximum, reached in 1907, was 1,315,892—a rate of 5.16 per thousand in population. Fortunately during the last twenty-five years the incidence curve has turned downward toward greatly diminished prevalence. In 1923, there were not over 250,000 deaths, in 1942 only 10,577; the figure rose in 1947 to 41,745, dropped to 9,757 in 1948 (Kaul, 1949) and to less than 200 in 1954-58 (W.H.O. 1961).

When this—the third—pandemic increased in magnitude, commissions appointed by several European governments proceeded to India to work on the problem, especially in Bombay. Of importance are the reports by the Austrians (1898-1900), the Germans (1899) and the Russians (1897). The Advisory Committee, appointed in 1905 by the Secretary of State for India, the Royal Society and the Lister Institute, published a long and very valuable series of reports (1906-1917), which greatly advanced the knowledge of plague.

The usual statements that nothing definite was known about the transmission of plague during the early epidemics is not entirely correct. Himalayan villagers long ago believed that unusual death among the rats preceded outbreaks of plague, and centuries earlier in the Israel-Philistine controversies mice were suspected of being in some way concerned in the outbreaks. Avicenna mentions plague in animals and according to Nicèphorus in 1348 mice died during the Black Death in Constantinople. This is probably true, for the black rat *(Rattus rattus)* came to the shores of Europe in the Crusaders' ships from the East. In China, the great scholar Hung-Liang-Chi (1736-1806) wrote of a great epidemic involving first the rats and then human beings. Plague in Canton and Hongkong was heralded by the death of rats. The opinion that the association of rats and human plague was not recognized during the Middle Ages is not supported by recently discovered evidence. For example, the Munich collection of copper plate prints contains a 15th century etching by the Dutch monogramist "W." It shows the plague saint, St. Quirin, with a rat-like animal in the foreground (Figure 99). The relationship of rat mortality to plague was again brought up in the Pali plague in India in 1837. Ogata (1897) described the

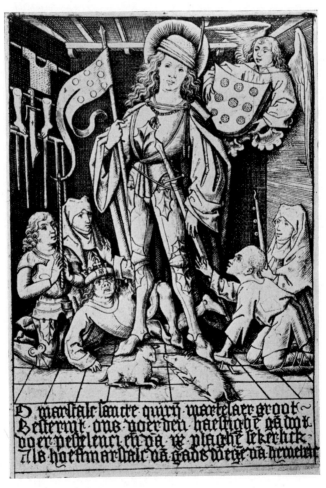

Fig. 99. Copy of a 15th century etching of the plague saint, St. Quirin. Note the rodent-like animals in the foreground.

Formosa epidemic as "rat pest." Paul Louis Simond noted the frequency of disease among those who had recently handled rats and the major part of the rat in the spread of the disease, later fully established by the Plague Research Commission in Bombay in 1905 and 1906.

The theory of transmission by the flea was specially developed by W. G. Liston (1905). The actual means by which certain fleas take the bacillus from host to host was elucidated by Bacot and Martin (1914).

Ever since Clemow in 1900 reviewed descriptions by the Russian workers Bieliavski and Riemshetmk of an epizootic disease affecting tarabagans (marmots) in Transbaikalia in Asia, east of Lake Baikal, it has become increasingly evident that wild rodents are prime carriers and reservoirs of the plague bacillus. The infection now smoulders and flares among wild rodents of the brush, deserts and mountains of China, the Buryat-Mongol Republic, Transcaucasia, southeast Russia, South and Central Africa, Argentina, Peru and the United States of America (Meyer, 1942; Davis, 1948; Link, 1951a; Pollitzer, 1954, 1960; Pollitzer and Meyer, 1961).

Recording valuable observations on plague manifestations in Iranian Kurdistan, Baltazard and co-workers (1960) postulated, in accordance with views already expressed by McCoy and by Meyer (1942, 1947)) that in general the slightly susceptible, rather than the highly sensitive, species were instrumental in perpetuating wild rodent plague. An exterminated rodent species can obviously not act as a true reservoir. Heisch and his co-workers in Kenya (1953) and Kartman and his colleagues (1958) in California agreed with Baltazard, but Pollitzer and Meyer (1961) in discussing the comparative importance of the wild rodent species state that vague mechanisms are at work that tend to limit the progress and consequently to favor the persistence of plague even in susceptible species. Emphasis is shifting from the large colonial rodents such as ground squirrels to the small, inconspicuous native field voles and mice such as *Microtus* and *Peromyscus*. Thus the ecology of plague, today less prominent among infections, is more complex than half a century ago.

A valuable history of plague may be found in *The Conquest of Plague* by L. Fabian Hirst (1953).

THE ETIOLOGIC AGENT

Pasteurella pestis, known also as *Bacillus pestis* or *Yersinia pestis,* is a member of the group of bacteria which cause hemorrhagic septicemias (pasteurelloses) in various animals. It is a rod, 0.5 to 0.7 μ wide by 1.5 to 2 μ long. It is gram-negative; the stain appears at both ends of the rod in a safety-pin pattern. It is seen singly or in pairs. In tissues it may be quite pleomorphic, globular and club-shaped; poorly stained forms are by no means uncommon. The bacillus is non-motile and does not form spores. Virulent strains have a readily demonstrable soluble slimy layer (Crocker *et al.,* 1956). *P. pestis* grows readily on ordinary culture media, slightly more abundantly at 30° than at 37° C. Colony formation is slow to appear but may be enhanced by the addition of cystine, blood or sodium sulfite to the medium. Colonies become distinctly visible after twenty- four hours; the growth of virulent strains proves quite stringy when touched with the loop. Milk is never coagulated by activity of the plague bacillus, acid is produced in glucose, maltose and mannite but indol is not formed. Action on glycerol is used for race differentiation of plague strains (Pollitzer, 1960). *P. pestis* has very little resistance to desiccation, sunlight or disinfectants. It may be readily agglutinated by specific antisera or lyzed by specific bacteriophage and thus differentiated from other organisms with which it might otherwise be confused.

Further evidence of plague in tissue material, sputum or ectoparasites may be obtained by subcutaneous inoculation or by rubbing such material on the freshly shaven, scarified skin of guinea pigs. The anatomical lesions produced are quite characteristic, and therefore this animal is most useful in the diagnosis of plague. Experimental work on plague also makes use of the high susceptibility of certain strains of white mice or sometimes black rats and rabbits.

The methods recommended for the experimental study of plague are detailed in a manual prepared by plague experts under the auspices of the World Health Organization (Baltazard *et al.,* 1956).

The existence of plague strains in different geographical areas distinguishable by their biochemical characteristics, such as action on glycerol and nitrates has been repeatedly demonstrated. Devignat (1951) defined three varieties of *P. pestis:* Variety I: *Pasteurella* (or *Yersinia*) *pestis* var. *orientalis* does not ferment glycerol, but

534 Diseases Transmitted from Animals to Man

does produce nitrous acid. It is the prevalent type in India, Burma
and China, is the pathogenic agent of Oriental plague responsible
for the 1894 pandemic and is present in the sylvatic plague foci
of North America, South Africa and rural plague in South America. Variety II: *P. pestis* var. *antiqua* ferments glycerol and produces nitrous acid. It is perhaps the oldest and came from central
Asia and, according to Devignat, may have provoked the famous
Justinian plague which spread through the Roman Empire. Since
then it has disappeared from Europe and has remained isolated in
Africa. Variety III: *P. pestis* var. *mediavalis* ferments glycerol, but
does not produce nitrous acid. It seems to have spread, in the 14th
century, from the Caspian Sea throughout the whole of Europe
where it caused the Black Death, and through the black rat established itself endemically during four centuries.

In subsequent contributions, Devignat drew attention to the tendency of his medieval strains to produce lung involvement in white
mice and also in white rats, adding that, if confirmed, these observations would throw light on the epidemiology of the plague manifestations at the time of the Black Death. However, considering that
by far the most violent pneumonic outbreaks of modern times, in
Manchuria and North China, have been caused by the "antiqua"
variety and that pneumonic plague manifestations were caused in
California by the "orientalis" variety one cannot share Devignat's
belief.

Pollitzer (1954, 1960) has recently reviewed the present knowledge
of the virulence, toxin and antigenic structure of the plague bacillus,
the mechanism of immunization, serodiagnostic methods and bacteriophage investigations.

GEOGRAPHIC DISTRIBUTION AND PREVALENCE

In two classical comprehensive accounts, Pollitzer (1954, 1960)
summarized the present distribution of plague and showed the intensity of the active foci in a map (Figs. 100, 101, 102A, 102B).

Plague maintains its patchy world-wide distribution of active endemic foci largely through epizootics among rats. Murine plague
still enhances the danger that maritime exchange along the lines of
travel and trade may introduce the infection into new territories.
Fortunately recent findings suggest that this spread by sea and even
land routes has been greatly diminished: 1) Plague, during the past

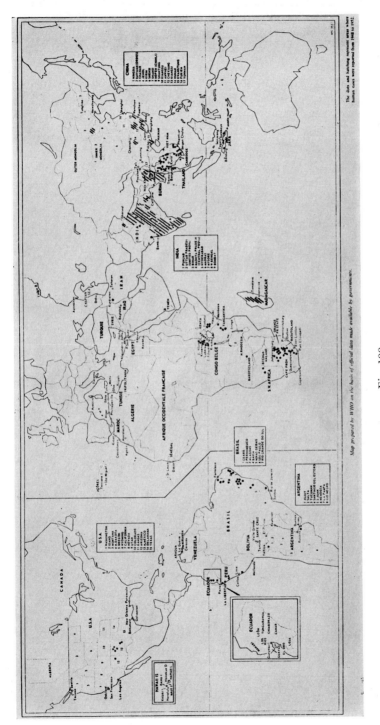

Map prepared by WHO on the basis of official data made available by governments.

The dots and hatching represent areas where human cases were reported from 1948 to 1952.

Fig. 100.

ten or fifteen years, has tended to establish its endemic home in
the cooler hinterland, rather than in the ports of warm countries.
2) Since 1929 the number of plague-infected vessels arriving on the
European, American and African continents from ports continuously infected, such as Rangoon, Colombo and Bombay, is quite
negligible; in fact, the only reported instance was on board the S.S.
Ville de Tamative in April, 1938 at Beirut. Today, the world is free
of shipborne plague (Link, 1951b). 3) Rat populations on ships have

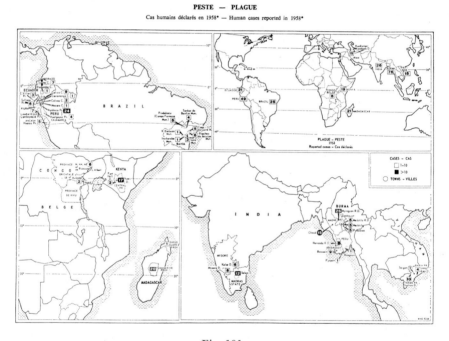

Fig. 101.

been considerably reduced through rat-proofing on a world-wide
basis. 4) Improved procedures adopted in ports exclude the transport
of rats in cargo, and fumigation with cyanide or other insecticides
of all grain and suspect cargoes, eliminates the infected fleas.

The accounts tell that in many countries dealt with, the incidence
of plague has markedly decreased within recent years and in some,
the disease has ceased to be manifest for the present. The decline
of plague throughout the world over the past fifteen years has been
large scale and rapid, though this in no way means that plague can

PESTE — PLAGUE

Cas humains déclarés en 1959 — Human cases reported in 1959

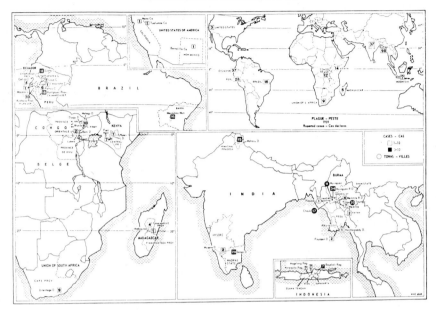

Fig. 102A.

PESTE — PLAGUE

Cas humains déclarés en 1960 — Human cases reported in 1960

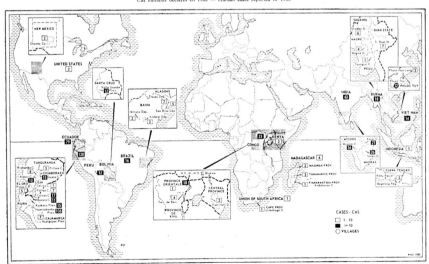

Fig. 102B.

be written off. The world incidence in 1959 was as low as in 1958; less than 300 cases of human plague were officially reported in ten countries of Africa, America and Asia (outside continental China). However, "accidental" single cases (in the United States, in California 1959, in New Mexico 1960 and 1961 and in Madagascar) and small foci in areas apparently free from human cases for one or more years (in northern India and the Union of South Africa), indicate that the infection is still maintained among rodents in wide areas of the three continents. No cases of plague were reported in ports and the disease was present in towns only in Burma. Today's situation reflects the success of a gigantic attempt—the first that could really be called "international" to correct one of the most tragic consequences of human "progress." From the beginning of the century, the successive sanitary conventions imposed increasingly heavy protective measures, including the search for and systematic examination of rats in ports and on vessels, the destruction of refuse, the separation of drains in ports, attempts to prevent the embarkation and debarkation of rats, in particular the employment of rat poison and the periodic fumigation of ships. The decline of plague marks the close of a unique period in the history of the 1894 pandemic in which the invention and wide use of the steamship enabled the disease to spread throughout the world. "Rat proofing" has gradually eliminated the rat from shipping. The value of this method, conceived and applied in the U.S.A. as early as 1907, was only officially recognized in 1926, when the Paris Conference introduced deratting exemption for rat-proof vessels. It became general only just before the Second World War. Rat proofing eliminates *R. rattus* from vessels at sea but its application to new buildings likewise gradually eliminates the species from the large ports as they become modernized. At the same time, the resistant species *R. norvegicus,* unaffected by the measures taken at the ports, is multiplying. The antagonism between the two species is encouraging the complete disappearance of *R. rattus.* One after the other the firmly established foci are dying out. The latest and most spectacular decline in plague has occurred in India and Java. Nevertheless, plague still clings to localities where conditions have favored its permanent establishment. During half a century, plague has more than doubled its area of distribution—now world-wide as a result of its territorial gains such as those in South Africa and the Americas. If control is continued it can safely be affirmed that the disease will never again assume pandemic proportions.

Oceanic plague has disappeared but maritime plague remains. Small boats, junks, sampans, neither rat-proofed nor deratted, plying in coastal waters between ports without facilities or supervision may create localized outbreaks. However, it seems certain that murine infection can be introduced into plague free areas only where *R. rattus* exists, and that the ensuing epizootic would be brief if *R. rattus* alone were present and could be prolonged only if *R. norvegicus* were also there. A permanent focus can become established only in wild and field rodents, and a balanced infection is maintained between resistant and susceptible species. (Baltazard *et al.,* 1960; Baltazard and Bahmanyar, 1960).

Asia: The active plague centers are in India, China and Burma. In systematic studies on the epidemiology of plague in Bombay province (Sharif, 1951) three endemic centers were designated near the foot of the Himalayas, one in central India comprising the water sheds of the Vindhya, Bhanier and Maikal Ranges and the Mahadeo Hills, and three centers in the water sheds of the western Ghats in Bombay and Hyderabad State and Mysore and the districts of Salem, Nilgiri and Madura. These foci have been very active. Wild rodents neither perpetuate nor transmit the infection there, only domestic rats do so. During the off-season the infection runs a slow subterranean enzootic course in some suitable place. When the rains begin, the rats move indoors. The temperature falls and humidity rises— conditions favoring an increase in the flea population. The fleas leave the rat burrow with the rats and then have opportunity to attack human beings.

Plague is both a rural and an urban problem; it moves from the commercial towns out to villages and flares up where it finds a highly susceptible rat population. Two types of plague epizootics have been recognized in India: On the warm tablelands the infections are severe and the heavy mortality among the rats causes the disease to ebb within a short time. In cooler regions, like the water sheds, the infection spreads slowly, but persists for a long time because of the light mortality among the rats. Areas with moderately moist and cool climates throughout most of the year constitute the endemic plague centers.

At the invitation of the Indian Government, the World Health

Organization entrusted the Institut Pasteur of Iran to determine the reasons for the persistence of plague and its spread in Uttar Pradesh—these being the only problems still requiring solution after fifty years of study. According to the results (Baltazard *et al.,* 1960), the infection in rural areas is spread by field rodents—*Millardia* and *Bandicota,* very susceptible species. Among them epizootics flare up, spreading from burrow to burrow and infecting village rats in passing. The persistence of rural plague is due to the relatively high resistance to the disease of the most plentiful field species, the Indian gerbil *(Tatera indica).* The principal role played by the domestic rat is to act as a liaison rodent between man the field rodents.

There are no permanent foci as there are in other parts of Asia, Africa and the Americas: the infection is constantly on the move, as Sharif had shown, affecting the villages on a serpentine course through the fields. Owing to widespread inundations during the monsoon, most rodents living in the low-lying parts of the area are drowned, those inhabiting higher ground survive. These rodents multiply rapidly after the floods have subsided, and their progeny becomes infected from the fleas *(Nosopsyllus, Xenopsylla)* carrying over the infection while subsisting on the resistant rodent species *(Tatera)* residing in the deep, closed burrows. The fact that "endemic" areas in north India are mostly situated in districts least liable to inundations supports this concept. There is also a marked predominance of *Tatera indica* in the "endemic" areas. However, this rodent is neither resistant nor sedentary enough to ensure the existence of true pockets of infection.

According to reports to the W.H.O. Expert Committee on Plague (1959), in urban centers, particularly Bombay and Calcutta, the steadily declining incidence of the commensal rat species is compensated by an increased frequency of *Bandicota bengalensis.* But epidemiological observations in Calcutta showed that proximity of plague-infected rats was essential for the appearance of human infection. Of considerable interest is the observation that the rats are sedentary; the range of their movement rarely exceeded 200 yards.

In China outbreaks varying in intensity were perennial in Hongkong until 1923. Canton has been free since the end of the First World War, but Pak-hoi was seriously involved (627 cases) from January to September, 1950. From Kwang-tung the infection has spread to other coastal provinces, and outbreaks due to dispersion along inland routes from Manchuria were proponderantly bubonic, but occasionally were pneumonic. Plague has also reappeared in Yunnan Province. The great epidemics of pneumonic plague of 1910-11 which cost 60,000 lives seems to have begun in Transbaikalia in tarabagan or marmot country.

A smaller epidemic (9,300 deaths) originated in Manchuria where marmot hunters contracted bubonic plague complicated by pneumonia and dispersed microbe-laden droplets of moisture into the foul atmosphere of overcrowded inns. All who inhaled the infected air would develop primary pneumonic plague and speedily spread it to the large Chinese populations. Because these epidemics did not include the local rat population, they ended as soon as the climatic conditions ceased to favor spread of the infection from man to man.

Plague studies in China have confirmed the existence of foci in: a) inner Mongolia and southwest Manchuria, where *Citellus dauricus* is considered the reservoir, and b) north Manchuria, where the reservoir is believed to be *Marmota sibirica*. In south China, plague has persisted in commensal rodents *(R. norvegicus* and *R. rattus)* inhabiting the fields. In the north, *Meriones,* gerbils and *M. musculus* serve as facultative carriers—the last mentioned species also fulfilling the same role in the south. The last serious outbreak, in 1944, was centered in the Tungliao district and neighbouring areas of southwest Manchuria. Then a gradual decline set in and plague is now no longer reported in the south. However, it still persists in the north, several hundred strains having been isolated as late as 1951. Systematic observations according to the pattern adopted in the Soviet Union have been started.

In the Mongolian People's Republic, plague is enzootic in the Siberian marmot (tarabagan), which inhabits an area of some ten million hectares. This rodent is of great economic importance, being hunted for the sake of its fur, meat and fat. Plague outbreaks starting in persons hunting the animals or handling its fur, meat or fat are frequent and often pneumonic. This focus, which has remained fully active, is therefore potentially most dangerous and will prove difficult to control.

In the Mongolian People's Republic the fundamental plague carriers are marmots while in the southern zone independent roles are being played by gerbils and *Citellus* varieties. Commensal rats becoming secondarily infected from these field rodents act as temporary but active carriers of infection. Epizootics among *Microtus* and high mountain field mice *(Alticola worthingtoni semicanus)* have been observed.

As late as 1946 Burma reported 2,743 deaths from plague; in 1959 only ninety-eight cases were listed: of these thirty-six in four inland urban areas. In Saigon, in 1943, a plague epizootic among domestic mice, more heavily infected with *cheopis* fleas than were rats, was responsible for forty-two cases of bubonic plague (Hérivaux and Toumanoff, 1948).

The introduction of plague into Java in 1910 was ascribed to rice cargoes brought to the port of Surabaya. During the period 1920-27 there were 8,000 to 10,000 deaths annually: the rate was still very high in 1951: 4,292 cases, 1,993 deaths. Researches using techniques like those employed in Kurdistan and the northern provinces of India have revealed a permanent reservoir in a rodent now identified as *Rattus exulans,* which like *Tatera* is markedly resistant to plague and inhabits deep burrows in dry ground. The distribution of this rat coincides with the area of endemicity (Baltazard and Bahmanyar, 1960), domestic plague has turned wild, and feral plague has remained in Java as a residue of the original invasion.

For many years it was known that plague infection persisted in the interior of western Asia and was in part responsible for past plague invasions of Syria and Palestine. After study of two limited outbreaks of pneumonic plague in the south of Iranian Kurdistan in 1947, Baltazard and his colleagues (1960) added valuable information about this western Asiatic focus by finding the infection in three species of sand rats *(Meriones)* and a few other rodents. *M. tristrami* is not a subspecies of *M. shawi,* but an independent species existing in the area under investigation. *M. libycus erythrourus* included two speices, one of which was *M. libycus erythrourus* and the other *M. vinogradovi.* Of these species, *M. tristrami* and *M. vinogradovi* are extremely susceptible to plague. This makes it clear that in the plague focus of Kurdistan there are not only resistant wild rodents *(M. persicus* and *M. libycus),* but susceptible ones *(M. tristrami* and *M. vinogradovi).*

The persistence of plague in Kurdistan thus depends on the ecological interplay between susceptible and resistant rodent species living in close contact.

Further work in Turkey, Syria and Iraq has failed to reveal sylvatic plague. However, one of the human plague strains isolated near the Syrian border in Turkey had the same biochemical characters as the Iranian and south-west Russian strains (glycerol-positive and nitrite-negative).

At the meeting of the Expert Committee on Plague, Pastukhov (1960) and then Rall in his book on the epizootiology reviewed by Pollitzer (1960) presented information hitherto not available on the occurrence of wild rodent plague in the Soviet Union and also in Mongolia and China, summarized in Table 50.

TABLE 50

WILD RODENT FOCI IN THE SOVIET UNION ACCORDING TO RALL (1958b)

Location	Rodents Mainly Involved	Principal Fleas	Remarks
Pamir/Tien Shan area	*Marmota baibacina, M. caudata*	*Oropsylla silantiewi* (*Rhadinopsylla ventricosa, Citellophilus lebedewi*)	Recently plague also found in *Microtus gregalis* in the Tien Shan
Transbaikaue	*Marmota sibirica, Citellus dauricus, Ochotona daurica*	*Oropsylla silantiewi, Citellophilus tesquorum*	*Ochotona duarica* proved rather resistant to plague
Central Asiatic areas	*Rhombomys opimus* (with *Citellus fulvus* and *Meriones libycus erythrourus* as supplementary carriers)	*Xenopsylla* species	*Rhombomys opimus* proved resistant experimentally, but actually there was seasonal variation in the intensity of the epizootics
Volga-Ural area	In sandy stretches: *Meriones meridianus* and also *M. tamariscinus*	*Xenopsylla conformis, Nosopsyllus laeviceps* and some others	*M. wagneri* sometimes become involved and then are apt to spread plague to man
	In steppes: *Citellus pygmaeus,* Dipodidae	(*Citellophilus tesquorum, Neopsylla setosa*)	Also involved: *Citellus Citellus fulvus, C. major* and, in sandy enclaves, gerbils
Western Pre-Caspian area	*Citellus pygmaeus*	*Neopsylla setosa, Citellophilus tesquorum, Ctenophthalmus breviatus, Ctenophthalmus pollex*	Gerbils possibly play an important role in part of the area. Mice may become secondarily involved
Transcaucasian area	*Meriones libycus*	*Xenopsylla conformis, Nosopsyllus laeviceps*	Other gerbil species probably also involved in southern border region

(From Bull. World Health Organization.)

During 1957-58 plague was altogether absent from the Pre-Caspian area and Transbaikalia. However, the situation has remained serious in the Central Asiatic foci where over 4,000 plague strains were isolated, and to a lesser degree in Transcaucasus area where 600 strains were obtained.

Europe and Africa. Soon after the Second World War, Ajaccio on Corsica, Taranto in Italy, Malta and the Azores were the only places where plague appeared in Europe. North and northwest Africa recorded the infection in Egypt (712 cases in 1943 and 1944). Tunisia, Algeria, Morocco and French West Africa (639 cases in Dakar in 1944), central Africa—in particular Uganda, Kenya, Tanganyika and the Belgian Congo—plague foci of long standing, but the incidence of human infection is usually below 400 a year.

Striking reports from Africa on the discovery of wild rodent plague in Kenya have changed ideas on the epidemiology of plague in Central Africa, where it was formerly believed that *Rattus rattus* was the only primary reservoir. Heisch and co-workers (1953) concluded that *Arvicanthis* and the multimammate mouse *Rattus natalensis* were rather resistant to infection with *P. pestis* and formed, together with the moderately resistant swamp rats *(Otomys angoniensis),* the true plague reservoir in that focus. Infection in *Rattus rattus,* formerly considered the main culprit in Kenya, seemed secondary. During 1958, nineteen, 1959, fourteen, and 1960, two cases of human plague were observed in Kenya.

In the neighboring Belgian Congo which reported in 1959, twelve and in 1960, twenty-three cases of human plague with a high fatality rate, the multimammate mouse *(Rattus natalensis)* is considered the only commensal rodent in Blukwa; in Kivu this species coexists with *Rattus rattus* in the huts. In Kivu *X. brasiliensis* transmitted plague to man; in the Blukwa focus, both *X. cheopis* and *X. brasiliensis.* In studies in the outskirts of the infected villages plague was evidenced in wild rodents; the prevailing species were *Arvicanthis* and to a lesser extent *Otomys.* The epizootologic facts of rural and domestic plague existing side by side reviewed by Bonebakker (1960) leave little doubt that the two foci are a menace to the Central African hinterland. *R. rattus* has already invaded the interior along one of the large arterial roads and has obtained a firm footing in several centers of population. If it succeeds in maintaining itself and in multiplying, there is a real danger that when an infected rat is transported to one of these centers, it will create an epizootic among the domestic rats and a resulting explosion of human plague.

Important both historically and epidemiologically is the development of a permanent sylvatic plague area in South Africa. Plague gained a foothold in the Union in 1900 when the Boer War necessitated the importation of large amounts of forage from infected South American ports. The rats became infected and the disease broke out among people living in cities and towns; small human epidemics were the results. This "murine phase" terminated in 1912 (Davis, 1948). Direct transport of infected rats and fleas by rail or other means led to the establishment of three primary distributing centers of wild rodent plague in southwestern Transvaal and northwestern Orange Free State, in the Cape Midland and near Port Elizabeth from 1919 onwards. The continuous spread of plague among the wild rodents led to 556 human infections between 1919 and 1925, to 466 between 1925 and 1931 and to 687 between 1931 and 1937. Between 1937 and 1949, perennial or almost perennial outbreaks in hyperenzootic areas were responsible for 646 cases in man. The main reservoir of wild rodent plague in the Union of South Africa is formed by two species of gerbil associated with the fleas *Xenopsylla philoxera* and *X. pirei*. Human infections there again are not directly derived from the wild rodents nor their fleas; the semidomestic *Rattus (Mastomys) coucha natalensis* and *R. rattus* are the source, and *X. brasiliensis* acts as a vector between the primary gerbil reservoir and man. Nosogeographically the recent outbreaks in Basutoland, Bechuanaland and northern Rhodesia form a part of the enzootic area. The roots of the Rhodesian focus in wild rodents were in the south, traveling through the Kalahari Desert. There are no clear indications that there was old sylvatic plague; probably it was an example of feral plague, domestic plague turned wild.

This conclusion was reaffirmed by Davis (1953) in a valuable study on wild rodent plague in South Africa. The primary reservoir in the gerbils *(Tatera brantsi)* was the source of infection to the semidomestic *Rattus natalensis* (multimammate) mouse and the domestic *R. rattus* living in and around the farm buildings.

Since 1959 only ten cases of plague have been reported from South Africa.

On Madagascar the outbreaks in ports and along the coast are bubonic, but on the high plateaus the infections tend markedly to secondary lung involvement and on to pneumonic plague, 56.2 per cent of all cases seen there in 1946. The Plague Service of the Institut Pasteur de Madagascar for the period 1954-1955 reported fourteen, and for 1958-1959, twenty-five cases of bubonic, septicemic and pneumonic plague with eleven deaths; these figures compare favorably with the 291 cases recognized in 1951-1952. Between 29 and 30 per cent of the people on the island had been vaccinated with the living attenuated E. V. plague vaccine. A classical outbreak of penumonic plague in 1957 involving forty-one persons, spread from one district to another by a migrant case of bubonic plague complicated by secondary pneumonia, was terminated by chemoprophylaxis and the cure of six patients with streptomycin after an epidemic threatening the entire island (Brygoo and Gonon, 1958).

Plague in Morocco became manifest in 1909-1910; violent epidemics claimed 8,000 to 10,000 victims. Between 1940 and 1945 while Morocco was occupied by military missions the disease became quite serious, but by 1946 the state was free.

Blanc and Baltazard (1945) observed small epidemics of bubonic plague with a strong family character in Moroccan villages. This is quite different from the situations observed for example in India or Java, where in 70 per cent of cases, plague is restricted to a single case per family. The explanation is that in Morocco people cover themselves warmly in the cold season and seldom wash; the result is enormous numbers of fleas and lice. Although these human parasites are much less adequate vectors than the rat flea their density is so great (440 fleas and 12,740 lice per 100 persons), that plague may be transmitted from man to man by their own ectoparasites.

The permanent reservoir is a field rat or meriones that has its burrow near the human dwellings. Once man becomes infected, the disease spreads directly from man to man through human citroparantes. When a member of the family dies, his garments are divided among the relatives, some who may live in nearby villages. Thus the infected lice and fleas are carried in clothing to another village only to rekindle further cases of plague. As Swellengrebel (1953) points out there was no epizootic in 1946 in Marakech among the domestic rats, but there were several cases per family, and transmission to another family was followed by death elsewhere.

The contention by Blanc and Baltazard (1945) that human ecto-parasites, particularly the human flea, *Pulex irritans,* may be an effective vector in strict contrast to the views of the Plague Research Commission, has been seriously questioned. However in recent years, Bonebakker (1960) has brought forth further evidence that during the medieval epidemics in Europe, human ectoparasites may have had a part in the spread of the disease. According to an excellently documented article on plague in Venice in 1575-1577 by Rodennwaldt (1953) *P. irritans* evidently participated in the spread; the outbreaks ceased when wooden houses were supplanted by stone ones.

The Plague Experts of WHO were informed that in the Soviet Union *P. irritans* was a vector in areas where mice harbored *P. pestis* (Pastukhov, 1960).

North America. In the United States, plague was first recognized in San Francisco in 1900. Probably there is no more stirring account of the early efforts of sound public health and of the opposition to it by the press, citizens and courts than the correspondence dealing with this plague situation, published in the Annual Report of the Supervising Surgeon General of the Marine Hospital Service of the United States for the Fiscal Year 1900. Up to 1904, when San Francisco was declared plague-free, 121 persons had been infected and 113 of them died. Abundant epidemiological evidence associated rats with the outbreak. Then it broke out again between May 1907 and November 1908—159 cases, seventy-seven deaths. Infected rats, as many as 2 per cent of those trapped, were caught in badly infected districts of the city. Plague was found in rats in Seattle in 1912 and in New Orleans in 1914. In New Orleans, thirty persons became infected in 1914, twenty-five (11 deaths) in 1920. At the same time, Florida and Texas were reporting human plague (total of 41 cases). Effective suppressive measures apparently eliminated rat plague at that time, but in 1941 there were again infected rats in the San Francisco Bay area and in 1943 and 1944 in Tacoma, Washington. Whether these infections indicate recrudescence in old foci or re-introduction is not known. Murine plague now plays a negligible role in the United States. Between 1924 and 1951 there were no outbreaks of human plague of murine or urban origin. Just as in South Africa and some countries in South America, the "murine phase" at one time attracted attention.

TABLE 51

RAT-CAUSED EPIDEMICS OF PLAGUE IN U.S.A.

	Year	Cases	Deaths
San Francisco, California	1900–4	120	114
	1907–8	186	92
Seattle, Washington	1907	3	3
New Orleans, Louisiana	1914–15	31	10
	1919–21	25	11
Pensacola, Florida	1920	10	4
Galveston, Texas	1920	18	12
Beaumont, Texas	1920	14	6
Los Angeles, California	1924	41	34
Total		448	286

INFECTION CONTRACTED FROM WILD RODENTS

	Human Plague	Cases	Deaths	Infected Rodents Found
California	1908 to 1959	56	52	1908
Oregon	1934	1	1	1935
Utah	1936	1	0	1936
Nevada	1937	1	0	1936
Idaho	1940	1	1	1936
New Mexico	1949	12	5	1958 (1903)
Colorado (Texas)	1959	1	1	1941
Arizona	1950	1	0	1938
Total		74	60	

U.S.A. Total cases, 532; 346 (65%) deaths.

While investigating the origin of a case of fatal plague in 1903, Rupert Blue (1934) became impressed by the possibility that ground squirrels might be infected and five years later proof was obtained that mass mortalities among these rodents may be definitely caused by *P. pestis* (McCoy and Wherry, 1909). Occasional human infections have been traced to contact with squirrels or bites of their ectoparasites. A small outbreak of pneumonic plague (13 cases) in Oakland in 1919 was traced to a squirrel (Kellogg, 1920). A similar epidemic in Los Angeles in 1924, involving thirty-one mourners at a funeral, originated in rats that contracted their infection by association with squirrels. Until 1934, plague had been identified in only nine counties of California. With the discovery of an epizootic among ground squirrels in the foothills of the Sierra Nevada Mountains in the most northeasterly county of California and with a human case in the Great Basin in Oregon, intensive surveys were undertaken in the western states and led to the discovery of plague, acute or latent, among at least sixty-three species of wild rodents in

131 counties of fifteen states (Table 51). Plague infects wild rodents in wooded (giving it the designation "sylvatic plague"), desert and rural districts uninhabited or only sparsely settled by man. Aside from the three groups of rodents which constitute, according to Eskey and Haas (1940), the primary reservoir—ground squirrels in the Pacific coastal regions and the northern part of the Intermountain Plateau, wood rats in the southern deserts and prairie dogs in the plateau region of Arizona, New Mexico, Texas, the Dakotas and other states—the sagebrush voles and meadow mice are the indirect sources of the infection to man (Meyer, 1942; Mohr, 1951; Communicable Disease Center, 1949, Kartman *et al.*, 1958). Endemic rodent plague, now permanently established in this country, extends from the West Coast into North Dakota, Kansas and Texas, and from the Mexican to the Canadian border (Fig. 103) and on into Alberta (Humphreys *et al.*, 1951).

Plague may spread from this wild rodent reservoir to man by several routes. The sporadic cases in the West probably arose either from bites of infected rodents or through the broken skin of the hands during the skinning of infected squirrels or rabbits or from infected ectoparasites of rats or mice. A less direct way stems from the exchange of ectoparasites between wild and commensal rodents. Isolated instances of rat plague in urban (Los Angeles and Oakland) and rural areas of California exemplify this exchange. *P. pestis* was isolated from rats *(Rattus rattus rattus* and *R. norvegicus)* carrying ground squirrel fleas (Meyer and Holdenried, 1949). Since the wild rodents cannot be eliminated, the potential danger of this exchange is being met by efforts to keep rodents and fleas out of the human environment, particularly the rapid extension of urban areas.

In reality the danger of spread to man through direct contact with infected wild rodents or their fleas is slight, as the incidence summarized in Table 52 plainly shows. After nine years without any cases California reported in June 1956 a fatal case apparently contracted from ground squirrel fleas. In 1959, there were two successfully treated infections, one resulting from a flea bite in Yosemite Valley and the other probably through the handling of dead rodents. Two infections in 1960 in New Mexico resulted from skinning of infected cottontail rabbits (Kartman, 1960); the causes in two fatal and one nonfatal infections in the same state in 1961 could not be determined. In the midst of epizootics that litter pastures with cada-

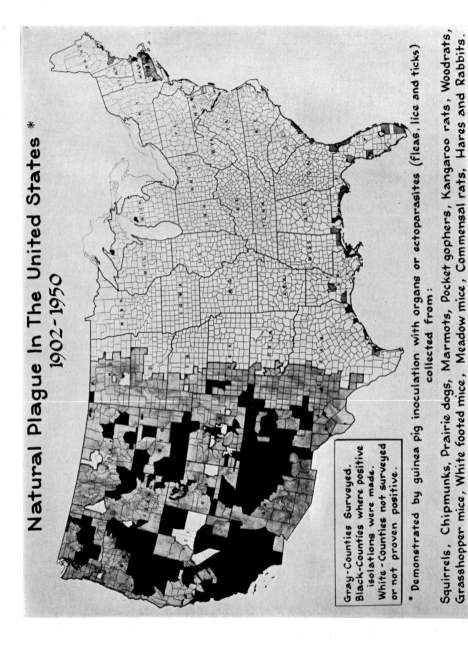

Fig. 103.

Natural Plague In The United States *
1902-1950

Gray-Counties Surveyed.
Black-Counties where positive
isolations were made.
White-Counties not surveyed
or not proven positive.

* Demonstrated by guinea pig inoculation with organs or ectoparasites (fleas, lice and ticks)
collected from:

Squirrels, Chipmunks, Prairie dogs, Marmots, Pocket gophers, Kangaroo rats, Woodrats,
Grasshopper mice, White footed mice, Meadow mice, Commensal rats, Hares and Rabbits.

vers of plague-infected wild rodents, particularly squirrels, when burrow openings are teeming with infected fleas, rarely if ever is a human being infected. The conditions in the United States are thus quite similar to those in South Africa and the Soviet Union.

TABLE 52

HUMAN CASES OF PLAGUE BY RODENT SOURCE IN CALIFORNIA 1900–1959

	Years	Total	Source		
			Rats	Wild Rodents	Unknown
Total	1900–1959	409–(419)	342	56	10
	1900	22	22		
	1901	32	32		
	1902	42	39		3
	1903	20	17	3	
	1904	10	10		
	1907	180	178	1	1
	1908	9	4	3	1
	1909	4		3	1
	1910	2		2	
	1911	5		3	2
	1913	2		2	
	1914	1		1	
	1915	1		1	
	1919	14		14	
	1920	1		1	
	1921	2		2	
	1922	2		2	
	1923	1			1
	1924	38	38		
	1925	2	2		
	1927	1		1	
	1928	3		3	
	1933	1		1	
	1934	1		1	
	1936	3		2	1
	1937	1		1	
	1941	2		2	
	1942	1		1	
	1943	1		1	
	1944*				
	1947	1		1	
	1956	1		1	
	1959	2		2	

Years in which no cases were reported are omitted.
*1 Laboratory infection—San Francisco.

Exhaustive studies on the occurrence and comparative importance of wild rodents and their fleas have been made in a plague-affected area around the San Francisco Bay by Miles and associates (1957), Murray (1957), Kartman and collaborators (1958). Of several field rodents, the vole *Microtus californicus* is thought to be the chief plague reservoir because of its high resistance to *P. pestis* and because of its parasitization by vector species and in fact by more than 90 per cent of all fleas of all species taken in the area. The fleas *Hystrichopsylla linsdalei* and *Malareus telchinium,* the two most prevalent species, both had relatively high natural plague-infection rates during epizootics. Most important is the confirmation that concerning enzootic-epizootic plague, "foci are quite limited; that the disease is actually transferred from wild rodents to rats; that an increase in plague incidence in fleas and in rodents is not necessarily accompanied by a decimation of the wild rodent population; in fact an apparent epizootic may occur simultaneously with a rise in the *Microtus* population; and that sylvatic plague may remain dormant and difficult, if not impossible, to demonstrate for periods of eighteen months or more, and then suddenly become resurgent" (Kartman *et al.,* 1958). One wonders how many thousand of such foci exist and perpetuate themselves throughout the Western States. Some are discovered when man or rats act as sentinels as they have in the human infections in recent years.

Mexico: Mexico was invaded by plague in 1902 and 1920. It has had a total of about 868 cases, 590 deaths, from plague in 1902-03 and 1920-23 in seventeen foci radiating from three seaports—Mazatlán, Veracruz and Tampico. Mexico is one of the few countries which has definitely succeeded in eradicating it. Owing undoubtedly to a spread of infections from adjacent parts of the U.S.A. plague was recently established in Mexico in the prairie dog. *Cynomys mexicanus* (Varela and Vázquez, 1954). Barrera (1957) recorded that this rodent had been found to harbor a few *Opisocrostis* fleas, but mainly *Pulex irritans dugesii* Baker. Thus the conditions for the persistence of plague enzootics in Mexico and the possibilities for an occasional spread of the infection to man markedly differ from those in the adjacent parts of the U.S.A. (Pollitzer, 1960)

South America. Plague is endemic in Brazil, Peru, Bolivia and Argentina. As a rule it is relatively benign, but pneumonic plague caused rapid aerosol infections among hospital nurses, attendants and doctors as late as 1939 (Murdock, 1940). The most comprehensive and authoritative report on the history of the plague in the Americas was written by Moll and O'Leary (1940-1942). Recent findings are presented by Pollitzer (1954). Venezuela has reported 218 cases of plague in the Miranda and thirty-seven in the Aragua State from 1910 to 1957. Commensal rats were no doubt responsible for the human infections. Natural plague was found also in two wild rodent species—*Heteromys anomalus* and *Sigmodon hirsutus.*

Brazil originally infected by the sea route continues to suffer from plague. Between 1899 and 1949, 9,248 cases were reported. In recent years, the WHO statistics list from sixteen to twenty-five cases annually in the Alagoas and Bahia States. There have been a few pneumonic epidemics but bubonic plague was preponderant. The mortality rate was generally low (Barreto and de Castro, 1946). A whole array of wild rodents are spontaneously infected there, but they are not primary reservoirs, they are secondarily or accidentally involved: the rat is the principal one.

In Argentina, with 6,428 human infections from 1899 to 1940, the role of commensal rats and of wild rodents is by no means clearly defined. During the past three years cases of plague have not been reported from Argentina. Plague transmission from commensal rats to wild rodents has been observed, but equally often the spread from wild rodents to commensal rats, the main sources of human infections, has been recognized. De la Barrera (1942) described opportunities for contact between the wild and the commensal rodents, particularly in the agricultural areas of North Argentina where both were attracted by the grain stores. Involvement of the commensal rats in the infection was far more frequently noted there than in the central provinces. According to Macchiavello, natural plague was found in the following wild rodent species: *Cavia pamparum, Galea musteloides* (2 subspecies), *Caviella australis, Graomys griseoflavus* (2 subspecies), *Hesperomys murillus cordovenis, Lepus europaeus, Sylvilagus brasiliensis gibsoni.*

Plague in southern *Bolivia* was bacteriologically confirmed in 1928 only, but little doubt outbreaks due primarily to its importation from North Argentina have occurred since 1921. A rat epizootic was responsible for an outbreak in the Tarija Department—it is believed that some of the subsequent epidemics were caused in the same manner. In the earlier plague manifestations, signs of rat epizootics seemed then to be absent; in later years a few wild rodents have succumbed to plague but there was no proof that the infection had become entrenched amongst them. In 1960, twelve cases were reported from Valle Grande province.

Peru: This country has the unhappy distinction of having had more plague than any other American country and no plague free year since its introduction in 1903. The total incidence reported from 1903 to 1952 is 22,254 cases, an annual average of 445; it reached 1,200 cases in 1926, 49 in 1948, 28 in 1959 and 128 in 1960. According to the classical study of Eskey, the most affected of any locality was the central part of Peru situated between 7° and 9° with an average mean temperature of 69° to 71° F. It suffered most from plague in rural and urban communities. The epidemics peaked during the summer months, but when the winter months were warm, the plague season began earlier. Human plague was mostly bubonic, but an outbreak of pneumonic plague has been reported. *R. norvegicus, R. rattus* and *R. rattus alexandrinus* were common and *X. cheopis* the most common flea and the only important vector. A plague outbreak in the mountainous region of Lambayeque was preceded by an epizootic among the guinea pigs in the home of the first patient which were infected with *P. irritans* as well as *X. cheopis*. Ramos Diaz (1938) thought that the former flea conveyed the infection to man and that transport in garments might lead to sporadic human infection without the intervention of rats. On the Peruvian Ecuadorian border, *Sciurus strammeus* squirrels and the flea *N. polygenis* were involved in the Andean region of Huancabamba; the *Cricetinae—Akodon dolores,* and *Oryzomys* species formed the primary reservoir of the infection, and a *Pleochaetis* species the principal vector.

Ecuador: The infection was established in Guayaquil in Ecuador as early as 1908, and it has spread from there to Chimborazo Loja Province, causing over 2,700 human infections between 1909 and 1940. Pneumonic epidemics are by no means infrequent there, 22.2 per cent of the 874 infections in Chimborazo were pneumonic.

Exclusively rural, the infection persists in the mountainous areas and is more rampant in December. Except in the pneumonic cases, the plague mortality in Ecuador is low. Two peculiar forms of the disease *angina pestosa* (tonsillar plague) and *viruela pestosa* (plague pox) were met there. Commensal rats are the most heavily infected, white guinea pigs play merely an auxiliary role. *X. cheopis,* possibly *Nosopsyllus londimensis* are the common vectors, and wild rodents did not cause plague (Macchiavello 1955).

Hawaii: Plague became manifest in Honolulu in November, 1899 and spread to adjacent districts and to Kauai, Maui and the Hawaiian Islands of the Archipelago. Between 1899 and 1949, the total cases reported was 416. In 1910, it was detected in the Hamakua District of Hawaii. A total of 112 human cases with 109 deaths and 1,161 infections in rodents and fleas have been recorded. None have occurred since 1949, nor have rodent and flea infections been detected since May 1957 in spite of intensive research (Wheeler and Gross, 1961).

EPIDEMIOLOGY AND ECOLOGY

Plague is primarily a disease of rodents, and man only accidentally and relatively rarely enters into the usual chain of transmission. The transfer of *P. pestis* from rodent to rodent, from rodent to man and possibly from man to man is accomplished by certain fleas. Epidemics in man are usually bubonic and flea-borne, but almost always include a few septicemic infections and secondary plague pneumonia, which may by aerogenic transfer give rise to the most fatal of all infectious diseases — pneumonic plague. Bubonic and pneumonic plague epidemics are caused by the same microorganisms, but the portal of entry and resulting symptoms differentiates them. Epidemiologically and clinically, pneumonic plague is a disease conspicuously different from bubonic plague. Age, sex or occupation play no role in incidence.

Epidemics of bubonic plague in man are preceded by or associated with epizootics in rats or other rodents. The great animal mortality so created favors the migration of fleas to man. This infection chain is heterogeneous: the animal host is usually a rodent and the insect vector is a flea.

The seasonal prevalence of the bubonic type depends largely on the influence of the weather on the breeding of rats and rat fleas. In temperate regions, outbreaks have occurred chiefly during the summer months. In hot, dry climates, on the other hand, it flourished during the winter, dying out in summer. Rats breed throughout the year in temperate climates, but breeding is retarded in extremes of heat or cold. With the influx of young susceptible rats, epidemics may flare up again. Similarly, breeding of rat fleas is retarded in the very cold or very hot months. Heat both interferes with deposition of eggs and prevents them from developing into larvae. A temperature of 85° F. causes the plague bacillus to disappear from the stomach of the infected flea rather rapidly. A temperature of 70° F. is optimum for propagation of an epidemic. Other factors in the epidemiology of plague in India have been described by Sharif (1951).

Brooks (1917) of the Indian Commission summarized his findings:

"1) Plague does not maintain itself in epidemic form when the temperature exceeds 80° F. and the saturation deficiency exceeds 0.30 inch.

"2) Plague epidemics are rapidly brought to an end when the saturation deficiency is high, even when the mean temperature throughout and after the termination of the epidemic has been considerably below 80° F.

"3) Plague epidemics may begin to be intensified when the mean temperature rises well above 80° F., provided the saturation deficiency is below 0.30 inch.

"4) In some districts in India and in certain tropical islands (e.g., Java and Mauritius) where climatic conditions favor the incidence and spread of plague throughout the year, outbreaks may be spaced indifferently at all seasons."

In North America, murine plague transmitted by the Oriental rat flea has in the past remained restricted to a narrow Pacific Coast area and the Gulf Coast area with smaller and spotty extensions in the southern river valleys. Where the *cheopis* flea populations reach high numbers and also affect a high percentage of domestic rats, murine plague may appear. In the northern, relatively cold cities, the annual mean of the flea population is too low to favor rat plague. The northern rat flea *(Nosopsylla fasciatus)* together with the fleas from wild field mice may have played a role in the murine epizootic of plague in Tacoma in 1942 (Mohr, 1951).

Meteorologic conditions also greatly influence the form plague will take in man. The severe epidemics of primary pneumonia have occurred during periods of constantly low temperature and high relative humidity. In Egypt, pure pneumonic plague is rare, while in Manchuria and Ural with the colder climate it is much more common. Secondary pneumonia complicating bubonic or septicemic plague is not as infectious as primary pneumonic plague, and unless crowding, social habits and the conditions for aerogenic transmission are favorable it rarely initiates large epidemics.

The means by which plague is carried over from one season to the next are not precisely known, but two tenable possibilities are that the bacillus lives through the winter in the digestive tract of the flea or that it leads a latent existence in the tissues of the rodent host.

Overcrowding, unsanitary conditions and social habits, in Los

Angeles intimate exposure at a funeral, favoring droplet transmission have contributed to epidemics. A tonsillar form occurs among groups that eat fleas and in the course of pneumonic plague epidemics when large size droplets produce a primary tonsillar process in cervical bubo followed by septicemia (Meyer and Larson, 1959). The bacilli may enter through the abraded skin of the feet, as in cow-dung floored houses in India.

A recent publication deals not with epidemiology *sensu strictu,* but with ecology (Pollitzer and Meyer, 1961). The ecology of an arthropod-borne disease is concerned with the localities of different size and extent where "natural plague" persists. These are rarely stationary phases; the dynamic flux in the living things involved and the effect of the environmental factors upon them accounts for the constant changes in the plague situations carefully investigated during the past ten years.

> Rodents with markedly different susceptibilities to plague are apt to coexist in the affected localities so that simultaneously there may be fuel for slowly progressing enzootics as well as for rapidly and widely spreading epizootics. The latter are apt to decimate the susceptible herds to such a degree that the infection becomes quiescent, or even absent, among them until the population density of the herds has been restored to a new level creating conditions suitable for a new epizootic wave. In addition to this long-term periodicity, the incidence of plague in wild rodents is also governed by seasonal influences, such as the appearance and dispersal of the young susceptible animals in spring and early summer, the comparative insusceptibility of the older animals which becomes manifest in late summer or autumn, and in the case of several of the species concerned also by aestivation or hibernation.
>
> Activities on the part of man, particularly agricultural operations, may exert a profound influence on plague in rodents. This may even be true in the case of natural plague foci, though, as justly pointed out by Meyer (1955), the ultimate disappearance of the infection, due to occupation of the localities in question by man, may be preceded by "an initial period of joint tenancy by people and wild and commensal rodents—a condition theoretically ideal for the propagation of plague." More frequently changes in the plague situation among commensal and peridomestic rodents may be brought about by the successive phases of agricultural work. Movements of the commensal species to the planted fields

are apt to reduce the population density of the animals in the settlements, but may at the same time bring these rodents into contact with infected peridomestic species. As a result the plague situation in the settlements may become exacerbated when, after the crops have been harvested, the commensal species and not rarely also peridomestic rodents invade compounds and houses.

Periodical changes in the plague situation will also be brought about by seasonal changes in the frequency of efficient vector fleas and/or the presence of climatic conditions promoting a high incidence of actually infective fleas. If many susceptible rodents are present under such circumstances, widespread epizootics are bound to occur and the resulting disproportion between a low number of rodents and a high number of fleas, which impels the latter to search for substitute hosts, may create a most dangerous situation for man.

Though no doubt the risk of contracting zootic plague is greatest under these circumstances, the chance or, one must often say, offchance of infection exists also under other conditions. An increased incidence of the disease may become manifest in certain occupational groups—for instance, as was observed in the past, among dock workers handling cargo from infected ports or among labourers using temporary shelters in rice fields. According to Pavlovski (1957), the infection may also be contracted by persons entering the natural plague foci or otherwise coming in contact with the reservoirs or vectors involved in their maintenance, for example, when skinning the carcasses of diseased animals or handling their furs.

Dealing with the problem of demic plague, Meyer (1961) drew attention to the occurrence of "purely" pneumonic epidemics, due to the arrival of patients with secondary or primary lung involvement in localities where the rodent populations were originally free from plague and where they remained entirely so even when the disease become rampant in man. The epidemic recently observed by Brygoo and Gonon (1958) in northeast Madagascar serves as a classic example of this type of the infection. It is consoling to note that all six patients with pneumonic plague met with after this outbreak had been notified, could be cured and that, more important still, the spread of the infection could be cut short by administration of sulfathiazole to the numerous contacts (Pollitzer, 1960).

Hosts

Plague in commensal or "domestic" rats differs epidemiologically from plague in wild rodents. This distinction is not always clear because chipmunks or other wild rodents may invade human habitation.

Plague in animals, especially rodents, can be detected by examination of the suspected reservoir hosts and/or their ectoparasites ("biotest"). Removing the ectoparasites, sacrificing and examining the rodent and excising samples of bubo, spleen, liver and lungs provide suitable specimens for study. Ectoparasites or pieces of the organs are ground separately in a mortar, with a little normal saline solution. The suspensions are then inoculated subcutaneously into guinea pigs, mice or other suitable animals. Plague-infected guinea pigs will succumb in about five days. Anatomical lesions are identified by microscopic examination, cultures, biochemical and serologic tests (Baltazard *et al.*, 1956; Brygoo, 1956).

Making a correct diagnosis of plague in animals found dead in enzootic areas has been facilitated by recent adaptation of the Ascoli test by Larson *et al.* (1951) and the complement-fixation test of extracts of tissues by Chen and his associates (1952). The complement-fixation test is more accurate than the precipitin test in this instance. For the rapid identification of *P. pestis* the fluorescent antibody method used by Winter and Moody (1959) and Hudson (1960) is highly specific even if contamination is heavy. Procedures recommended for improving the results of flea collection and examina-

TABLE 53

ROLES OF VARIOUS SPECIES OF RODENTS AND *Lagomorpha* IN THE MANIFESTATIONS OF PLAGUE

Category of Rodent Plague	Examples of Rodents (or Lagomorpha) Involved
Pestis nautica	*R. rattus*
P. urbana	*R. norvegicus*, etc.
P. urbanoruralis et *rodentium sylvestrium*	*R. rattus* and *Sigmodon peruanus*
P. murina ruralis	*R. r. alexandrinus*
P. murina campestris progressiva	Spreading, for example, from *R. rattus* to peridomestic *Cricetinae*
P. campestris regressiva	Reverting for example from *Cricetinae* to *R. r. frugivorus*
P. sylvestris	*Caviidae*, *Cricetinae*, *Leporidae*
P. sylvatica	*Sciuridae*, *Gerbillinae*, *Leporidae*

tion have been reported in Annex 6 to the report of the WHO Expert Committee on Plague (1959) and Pollitzer (1960, p. 350).

Plague can occasionally be demonstrated in animal tissues, from which no positive cultures could be obtained. Macchiavello (1955), in order to characterize the different roles of various species of rodents and *Lagomorpha* in the manifestation of plague, proposed the elaborate system of classification slightly modified by the reviewer in the *Tropical Diseases Bulletin* (1956, 53:584) (Table 53).

The classification is valuable because it calls attention to the fact that so-called wild rodent species or subspecies assuming peridomestic habits live near or with man, while on the other hand, commensal rats lead an independent existence well away from human settlements, for example, *R. hawaiiensis*. This species and *R. exulans* (or *R. concolor*) should therefore be placed in the wild rodent list.

Murine or Rat Plague

Plague has been observed in over 200 representatives of the order *Rodentia*. Rodents in pandemics are restricted to the family *Muridae*. Although over 1,300 species and varieties are known, only three *Murinae* are of universal importance in plague. The species of rat largely responsible for propagating it are the Norway or brown rat *(Rattus norvegicus)* and the English black rat *(R. rattus rattus)*, with its subspecies or varieties *(R. rattus alexandrinus, R. r. frugivorous)*. In Burma, *R. concolor,* in Java *R. r. diardii,* in the Hawaiian Islands *R. hawaiiensis* and in central and east Africa *R. coucha ugandae* and in South Africa the semidomestic *R. mastomys coucha natalensis* are hosts. Representatives of *Mus musculus, M. gentilis* and *M. azoricus* occasionally may become involved in the spread of plague.

The two responsible species and their varieties are found all over the world, often living together. The Norway rat is the largest, living in the ground under the floors and driving other rats to the upper stories. He may be found on shipboard. On the ground he is at home and flourishes exceedingly, outnumbering the other species by propagation. He is a migrant, often traveling many blocks in a night and several miles in a few days. The black rat and the roof rat find suitable quarters either on land between the walls or in the upper floors of buildings, in trees, fences and rock piles, or on ship-

TABLE 54

<small>WILD RODENT PLAGUE FOCI RESERVOIR HOSTS AND OTHER FAMILIES OR SUBFAMILIES FOUND NATURALLY INFECTED</small>

Plague Focus	Main Reservoir	Also Found Infected
Argentina	*Caviinae (Cavia*, etc.)	*Chinchillidae, Leporidae*
Central Africa (Belgian Congo, Kenya)	*Murinae (Arvicanthis, R. netalensis)*	*Otomyinae, Dendromyinae*
Iranian Kurdistan	*Gerbillinae (Meriones)*	*Dipodinae, Microtinae*
Java	*Murinae, Rattus (R. exulans)*	
India	*Gerbillinae (Tatera)*	*Murinae; Dipodinae, Microtinae*
Manchuria, Mongolia and Transbaikalia	*Sciuridae (Marmota)*, Ger- billinae (*Meriones*)	*Gerbillinae, Sciuridae, Ochotonidae*
Peru	*Cricetinae (Graomys), Cricetinae (Akodon)*	*Caviinae, Leporidae*
Peru/Ecuador border region	*Sciuridae (Sciureus)*	*Cricetinae*
South Africa	*Gerbillinae (Tatera)*	*Cricetinae, Dendromyinae, Leporidae, Murinae, Otomyinae, Pedetidae, Sciuridae*
U.S.A. Western States		
Arizona, New Mexico	*Sciuridae (Cynomys)*	*Leporidae, Cricetinae*
Coastal region and northern part of intermountain plateau	*Sciuridae (Citellus), Microtinae (Microtus), Cricetinae (Peromyscus)*	*Dipodomyinae, Geomyidae*
Southern Desert	*Cricetinae (Neotoma)*	*Leporidae, Sciuridae*
Washington	*Microtinae (Lagarus)*	*Cricetinae, Dipodomyinae, Sciuridae*
U.S.S.R. (Soviet Union)		
Pre-Caspian region in steppes	*Sciuridae (Citellus pygmaeus)*	*Dipodinae, Microtinae*
in sandy stretches	*Gerbillinae (Meriones* sp.)	
Central Asiatic focus in desert lowlands	*Gerbillinae (Rhombomys* and *Meriones)*	*Dipodinae*
high mountain area	*Sciuridae (Marmota* sp.)	
Transcaucasia	*Gerbillinae (Meriones)*	*Leporidae, Dipodinae*
Venezuela	*Heteromyinae (Heteromys), Cricetinae (Sigmodon)*	

board between walls, and in cargo and merchandise. The black rat *R. rattus rattus* is rare in Europe today, but is widespread and common in the tropics. *Rattus rattus alexandrinus* has participated in the spread of plague in Egypt and perhaps in the Pacific Islands. The ecology of the rats essential to plague in America is admirably detailed in the monograph *Rat-Borne Disease: Prevention and Control,* prepared by the Communicable Disease Center (1949).

In a note on the classification, origin and distribution of commensal rats, Schwarz (1960) maintains that both black and brown rats *(R. rattus* and *R. norvegicus)* were derived from wild forms of which *Rattus rattus* was typical. Both have world wide distribution; the *rattus* (black rat) series is generally more southern, the *nor-*

vegicus (brown rat) series more northern in distribution and found sporadically in the tropics and only along the coast in cities, never far inland. The *rattus* series includes indoor domestic commensals with grey bellies and the white-bellied outdoor peridomestic varieties. Both varieties are the common rats on ship. The Norway rat becomes shipborne occasionally which explains its occurrence in harbors all over the world. In Schwarz's opinion the grey-bellied domestic commensals are the most usual contacts for human plague. The white-bellied peridomestic commensals and the *norvegicus* maintain the contact between infected domestic commensals and human plague on the one hand and the wild reservoirs sylvatic (animal type) plague—on the other.

Natural Plague in Rats

Rats do not exhibit marked symptoms of plague until they near death. They are said to stagger and to be easy to capture; in cages they may seek a dark corner and try to hide.

The diagnosis is ordinarily based on macroscopic examination of the lesions, so characteristic as to leave small doubt in the mind of an experienced observer. In an epizootic, however, about half of the infected animals will have lesions so indefinite that it is necessary to resort to a microscopic examination or guinea pig inoculation. Diagnosis by animal inoculation is particularly useful because other plague-like bacteria also infect rats—organisms belonging to the *Salmonella* group, but in particular representatives of the *Pasteurella* group such as *P. pseudotuberculsois rodentium* and *P. multocida* var. *muricida* (Meyer and Batchelder, 1926). Cutaneous infection in guinea pigs is useful, but less sensitive than the subcutaneous. Gross lesions in infected guinea pigs resemble those in rats, but there are special features: a general subcutaneous edema is characteristic and the organs, especially the spleen, liver and lungs, are often studded with pseudotubercle-like nodules. The lungs may be congested, the areas range in diameter from 5 to 10 mm. A decrease in weight is a valuable sign that plague infection is in progress (Pollitzer, 1954, p. 192-200).

Typical lesions of acute plague in rats are five (Williams, 1920); not all will be present at one time, nor will any one appear alone. They are injection, bubo, granular liver, large, dark spleen and pleural effusion. Injection of the subcutaneous blood vessels, indicated by a dusky redness of the subcutaneous structures and muscles, will be apparent in about 75 per cent of the infected animals examined. Buboes in the rat are very suggestive of plague; they may be in the axilla, neck, groin or pelvis. If there is but one bubo, it may be in the neck, as it was in 75 per cent of such rats in India, or in the groin, as it was in 75 per cent of the rats in San Francisco. The proportion of rats with buboes varies markedly. In India 80 per cent of the infected rats examined had buboes; in San Francisco, 40 per cent; in New Orleans, 33 per cent. The liver is fatty and scattered sparsely with focal yellowish necrotic lesions (so-called granular liver) in 60 to 70 per cent of cases of acute plague. It is sometimes difficult to know whether the spleen is enlarged because the size of the normal rat spleen varies markedly, but different investigators consider that it is enlarged in 60 to 70 per cent of infected rats. Pleural effusion, often copious, occurs in more than 75 per cent, usually along with one or more other lesions.

A chronic form may be evidenced by very slight lesions—purulent or caseous foci taking the form of small abscesses of the liver, spleen or mesenteric glands. Plague bacilli may be very scanty in such lesions and can be detected only by guinea pig inoculation. Scars on some organs are sometimes the only evidence of chronic plague in rats that survive the disease. *P. pestis* has been isolated from rats without lesions in New Orleans and Galveston (Williams and Kemmerer, 1923).

Natural immunity is found in many old rats. The Haffkine Institute studied the susceptibility of Bombay rats and found that the number of susceptible rats declined between 1931 and 1936. The mortality rate among the rats after they were given a standard infective dose was only 20 per cent, while among rats from a nonendemic area in Madras it was 90 per cent. In San Francisco, 50 per cent of old rats and 15 per cent of young rats tested were resistant to virulent material inoculated. This immunity is natural, not acquired through previous attacks of the disease.

Plague in Wild Rodents Including Rabbits (Campestral and Sylvatic Plague)

A recent tabulation (Pollitzer and Meyer, 1961, using the standard nomenclature of Ellerman) lists 227 species or subspecies of rodents and lagomorpha, other than the cosmopolitan species of rats

(Rattus norvegicus and *R. rattus* subspp.) and of commensal mice proved naturally plague infected or strongly incriminated through positive findings in their ectoparasites. In an elaborate comparative study, Pollitzer (1954 and 1960) listed the families and subfamilies of rodentia and lagomorpha in which natural plague has been confirmed. Table 55, modified to include new data, shows: a) plague

TABLE 55

RODENTS AND LAGOMORPHA
HOSTS OF *P. pestis* IN U.S.A.

	Rodentia	
HETEROMYIDAE:	Kangaroo rat: *Dipodomys ordi*	Texas, Washington
	Pocket mouse: *Perognathus parvus*	Washington
MURIDAE:	8 species wood-rats: *Neotoma* species	California, Arizona, Nevada, New Mexico, Utah
Cricetinae	Pack-rat: *Neotoma micropus*	Texas
	Grasshopper mouse: *Onychomys leucogaster*	Western States
	5 species brush and deer mice: *Peromyscus*	Western States
	Harvest mouse: *Reithrodontomys megalotis*	California, Kansas, New Mexico
Microtinae:	4 species meadow mice: *Microtus californicus*	Western States
SCIURIDAE:	23 species squirrels: *Citellus* species	Regional distribution; also Canada
	7 species prairie-dogs: *Cynomys* species	Arizona, New Mexico
	4 species marmots: *Marmota* species	Wyoming, Colorado, Utah, New Mexico
	2 species chipmunk: *Tamias* species	California, Nevada
	Sierra Nevada chickaree: *Tamiasciurus douglasi albo-limbatus*	California
	Lagomorpha	
LEPORIDAE:	Black-tailed jack rabbit: *Lepus californicus*	California
	3 species cotton-tail rabbits: *Sylvilagus* species	California, New Mexico

foci where sylvatic plague is known to be, or to have been active; b) the principal species or main reservoir host which presides over the exchanges of the plague bacillus, and c) the families or subfamilies found infected and therefore subsidiary and, if living near man, able to act as intermediaries between the strict wild or commensal rodents.

The question of the relative importance of the different species and subspecies in harboring and perpetuating the infection has been debated at length. At one time the rodent species affected by wide-spread epizootics were generally considered the main reservoirs. But as early as 1910 McCoy and then Meyer in 1942 expressed the view that resistant rodents (rather than those apt to fall prey to the acute disease) functioned as the true reservoir or favored perpetuation of the infection. Valuable observations in Iranian Kurdistan (Baltazard *et al.*, 1960), in Kenya (Heisch *et al.*, 1953) and in California (Kartmann *et al.*, 1958) revealed variability among susceptible races in one and the same rodent species: susceptibility and resistance of a given species is uniform but subject to change. Factors governing the incidence and spread of wild rodent plague are discussed in the recent summary by Pollitzer and Meyer (1962). Habitat, range of movement, density of the wild rodent populations, seasonal influences and hibernation exert the effects in a manner expressed by Meyer (1942) in the following statement: "There is every reason to believe that the interplay between infection and immunity may be influenced by an infinite variety of ecological factors which accelerate or retard it. For example, even a coalescing epidemic spread of plague infection in a rodent population may fail to reach every colony. Thus, at the apparent termination of the epizootics, both susceptible and resistant rats or squirrels may survive and interbreed, furnishing sufficient hosts to maintain the infection in a smoldering nonreadily recognizable state!!"

Until 1934, the ground squirrel *Citellus beecheyi* (Fig. 104) was considered to be the sole reservoir of practical importance in California. Since then numerous species of *Citellus, Marmota* and prairie dogs (*Cynomys spp.*) (Fig. 105), hares (*Lepus spp.*) and rabbits (*Sylvilagus* spp.) have been hosts to spontaneous *P. pestis* infection.

These representatives of the *Sciuridae* and *Leporidae* preside over the exchange of the infective agent; small rodents (harvest mice *Microtus* sp., grasshopper mouse *Onychomys*, the Hawaii mouse *Reithrodontomys* sp., rice rats *Oryzomys-Hesperomys palustris*, cotton rats *Sigmodon hispidus* and *Neotoma floridana*) belonging to the *Murinae* act as complementary and auxiliary hosts. They support the epidemicity and aid in the dispersion of animal plague. Relatively little is known about this complex ecological interplay, the key to the solution of the plague problem in the United States. The inherent potentialities of the widespread sylvatic plague area cannot be defined until the natural histories of the rodents and their ecto-parasites in the exchange cycle of the plague bacillus is definitely understood. For details, the studies by Kartman and associates (1958) and Pollitzer (1960) should be consulted.

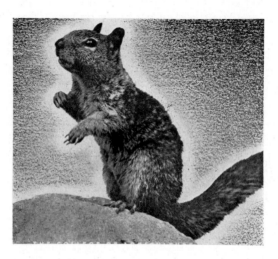

Fig. 104. Ground squirrel *(Citellus beecheyi)*, reservoir of plague in the United States.

Aside from the different wild rodent species and the receptivity to infection by members of the host herd the influence of hiberna-tion has been considered. Experiments, although suggestive, have, with one exception failed to imitate the supposed carry-over of any latent infection (Prince and Wayson, 1947). Among nonhibernat-ing wild rodents, other factors retard spread of the infection. Even in such species plague often shows a seasonal incidence. Periods in which epizootics are likely to occur alternate with periods in which the infection is enzootic and less fatal. This erratic behavior is par-ticularly well documented by the field studies of Kartman and as-sociates (1958 and 1960). In South Africa and to some extent in California, major epizootics have followed each other regularly every few years. Probably the vast sylvatic areas ensure persistence, because while the infection abates in one circumscribed zone, it may pass over to another area where the rodent population has not been impaired by recent epizootics.

In Russia in the northern steppes the summer epizootics among the sisels *(Citellus)* were regularly followed by high mortalities among mice in the southern sandy stretches. This circle favored continuity of the infection. Meyer and Eddie (1938) observed in San

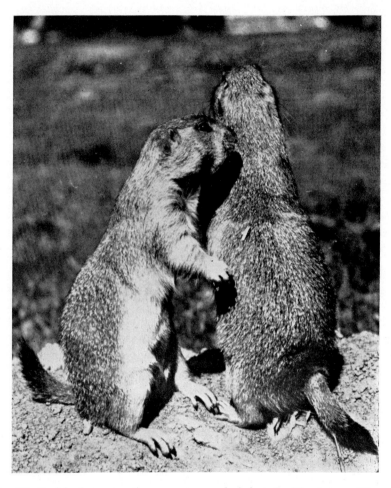

Fig. 105. Prairie dogs, sometimes spontaneously infected with plague. (Through the courtesy of the Fish and Wild Life Service, United States Department of the Interior.)

Mateo County, California, that two locations where infected ground squirrel fleas were found in 1936 were recognized as the same series of burrows proved to harbor diseased squirrels in the summer of 1916. Further suggestive evidence that sylvatic plague persists probably indefinitely in any area once invaded was supplied by Baltazard and his co-workers in the territories of the villages where human plague had been identified in 1871 and rodent plague was redetected in November 1948. It becomes more apparent that rodent fleas, far from being mere vectors, may be responsible for persistence and carry-over.

Pathologic changes in ground squirrels differ from those in rats. In the acute type a hemorrhagic caseous bubo is the prominent lesion; in the subacute or chronic type the bubo is purulent, and may be accompanied by caseous foci in the spleen and lungs. Pulmonary localizations are much more common in squirrels than in rats (Meyer 1942b), and latent infections are not infrequent. The lesions in other rodents are described by Pollitzer (1954).

Plague in Other Animals. Plague is rare among animals other than rodents. Rarely carnivores (badgers and cats), ruminants (camels and sheep) and birds (owls) have been incriminated. Brown monkeys *(Macacus radiatus)* have suffered outbreaks in India. Shrews, dogs and certainly cats may pass the plague bacillus directly to man. Ferrets *(Putorius furo)*, the suricate *(Suricata)* and the yellow mongoose *(Cynictis penicillata)* may also acquire plague.

Since the outbreak in Vetlianka in southeast Russia (1878) camels have been more or less definitely incriminated as hosts. Camels contract plague in the same way as other animals (Fedorov, 1960): through blood-sucking rodent ectoparasites, primarily fleas and in exceptional cases *O. tartakovskgi* ticks which have not long before sucked the blood of a plague-sick rodent. Vaccination with a single dose of 30,000 million living avirulent organisms induced an adequate immunity in adult camels. Experimentally calves and sheep are quite susceptible. Horses tolerate large doses of living *P. pestis*. But none of these animals is important in spreading the infection. Birds are quite generally resistant, but some share the burrows of wild rodents and may transport infected fleas.

Carnivora and birds of prey may spread plague; though they are resistant they may pick up and later disperse infected rodent fleas.

Insect Vectors. Members of the family *Pulicidae* and *Ceratophyllidae* are essential in the cycle of propagation. The flea was experimentally shown by Ogata (1897) and by Simond (1898) to be a possible agent for the dissemination of bubonic plague, either from animal to animal, animal to man, or man to man. The Commission for the Investigation of Plague in India (1905-10) in four classical experiments proved that rat plague in Bombay is fleaborne and cannot be transmitted continuously as an epizootic in the absence of rat fleas. The ecology of the wild rodent fleas has been well studied by Ioff (1941) in Russia, and by Eskey and Haas (1940), Wheeler and Douglas (1941), Burroughs (1947) and Kartman and associates (1958) in the United States. Comparatively few of the estimated 1,350 species of fleas can effectively transmit plague. Some of the usual fleas proved vectors are listed in Table 56.

TABLE 56

VECTORS OF PLAGUE

Flea (Known to Bite Man)	Distribution	Reservoir Hosts	Transmits Primarily to
Xenopsylla cheopis	Widely disseminated	*Rattus rattus*	Rats and man
Xenopsylla brasilensis	Uganda, Kenya, Nigeria	Rats	Rats and man
Xenopsylla hawaiiensis	Island of Hawaii	Field rats	Field rats
Xenopsylla astia	India, Ceylon, Burma, Mesopotamia, Mombasa	Rats	Rats
Xenopsylla nubicus	Tropical East and West Africa	Rats	Rats
Xenopsylla eridos	South Africa	Wild rodents	Wild rodents
Pulex irritans	Nearly cosmopolitan	Man, swine, rodents	Man, rodents
Nosopsyllus fasciatus	Temperate zone of Europe and America	*Rattus norvegicus*	Rats
Diamanus montanus	Western United States	Ground squirrels	Ground squirrels
Rhopalopsylla cavicola	South America	Cavies	Cavies or Cuis
Ceratophyllus tesquorum	Russian Steppes	*Citellus pygmaeus*	Ground squirrels
Oropsylla silantiewi	Manchuria	Rodents (tarbagans)	Rodents

Rat Flea Density. Early in the 20th Century observations in Australia and India suggested that the local flea census might give information about the plague potential. The average number of each flea found on the bodies of each species of rat is the figure—specific rat flea index—commonly reported. The *Xenopsylla cheopis* index is considered a significant figure in rat plague.

In fact, the *X. cheopis* infestation per rat in any given locality determines the extent of an outbreak. In parts of India where plague does not occur the predominating rat flea is not *Xenopsylla cheopis,* but other fleas (Cragg, 1921). In Colombo, which enjoys a relative absence of plague, the common rat flea is *Xenopsylla astia.* In the United States a survey by the Public Health Service showed that in New Orleans, where plague actually existed at the time, *X. cheopis* was the predominating flea; in New York and Boston this pest appeared for only a few months of the year.

The total number of fleas per rat varies with the climate, the season and other factors. In Belgaum, India, during July, August and September, the epidemic season, eighteen fleas per rat were found; in the colder, nonepidemic season, only four or five. In the United States in New Orleans in 1922 the average number of fleas in winter was about three; in the summer it mounted to nearly five. In New York City the average number of fleas on 4,756 rats for a two year period was 0.93, with the largest number from any single rat, thirty-eight. On the basis of epidemiologic comparisons, the species rat flea index is less valuable as an indicator of plague danger than the number of infected fleas that become blocked and therefore infective.

Many other observations have shown that climate and environment greatly influence the density of commensal rodent fleas.

In contrast to the commensal rodents infected by a few but, as a rule, widely distributed flea species, wild rodents in plague areas are usually parasitized by diverse flea species with almost invariably a local or at most a limited distribution.

Pollitzer (1960 and 1961) has compiled extensive tables and reviewed the prevalence of fleas actually or potentially involved in transmission in sylvatic plague areas. It has been tacitly assumed that each species of flea and each sex of each species is about equally efficient individually as a transmitter of the plague bacillus. But according to observations on the mechanism of plague transmission by fleas, transmitting power shows specific inequalities in the individual fleas.

Mechanism of Plague Transmission. Fleas feeding on an infected rat with bacteremia of 100,000,000 organisms per milliliter will at one feeding ingest about 5,000 organisms, and a high proportion will become infective. The organisms may multiply in the digestive tract of the flea and render it an infective vector. The flea is not merely a passive carrier. The transmitting mechanism is the so-called blockage phenomenon: a few days or even longer after the flea has fed on infected blood, clusters of plague bacilli become visible in its stomach. Later the proventriculus becomes plugged by gelatinous masses of bacilli, and its valvular action becomes inadequate. Because of this obstruction, the blood being sucked by the flea cannot find its way into the stomach. The esophagus containing virulent bacilli becomes distended. The elastic recoil of the walls of both pharynx and gullet when the flea stops sucking may drive highly infective blood back into the bite wound. This recoil sometimes extends through a partial blockage to the posterior end of the stomach. An infective flea may regurgitate between 11,000 and 24,000 organisms.

Many species of fleas merely become infected, blockage is never evident and they rarely if ever become pestiferous. Others remain infected throughout their entire lives and never become blocked. Others may carry plague bacilli in their intestinal tubes for a long time and become blocked later. In this last relationship between the flea and the plague bacillus may lie one explanation for the carry-over of plague from season to season in hibernating rodents.

Fleas that are feeble biological vectors in the way described may nevertheless be efficient mechanical vectors. Infection through bites of fleas with soiled probosci is frequent during epizootics in which mass transmission is the rule rather than the exception. There is experimental evidence that the combined action of a large number of fleas is as efficient as infection by a single blocked specimen.

Transmission by the blocked fleas as a biological vector is the primary means; it is followed by mechanical transmission; transfer to the mammalian host through flea feces into the skin or ingestion of infected fleas is very subordinate (Burroughs, 1947).

Vector Efficiency. The discoverers of the blockage phenomenon gained the impression that intestinal infection was more readily produced and that the obstruction of the proventriculus by the plague culture certainly occurred more readily in *X. cheopis* than in *N. fasciatus*.

This observation changed the position of the flea species factor, and many attempts have been made to determine more accurately the influences on specific vector efficiency. Wheeler and Douglas (1941) tried to combine a number of experimentally determined factors in a product called vector efficiency—the number of transmissions effected by a given number of any species of fleas. Among the factors are: 1) *the infection potential*—proportion of fleas of a given species harboring the plague bacillus after feeding on an infected rodent or the special apparatus of Kartman (1954); 2) *the blockage potential*—proportion of fleas with typical blockage; 3) *the vector potential*—the proportion of infected fleas to become infective; 4) *the transmission potential*—the mean number of transmissions effected by a like group of infected fleas; 5) the average *infection-in-fectivity intervals;* 6) *longevity of a) infected, and b) infective fleas* in similar climate; 7) the *relative proportions of the sexes of the species,* their comparative longevity when fully adult and the comparative vector efficiency of each sex. Other factors must be considered in determining the plague-vector potential—the blocking survival potential-ratio of the mean day of death of fleas after blocking over the mean day of blocking after the infectious meal (Kartman *et al.,* 1958). By including field data with the experimental index a very elaborate model for determination of the plague vector potential of fleas has been developed (Kartman 1957). Most comparative transmission experiments since the investigations by the Plague Research Commission established that *Xenopsylla cheopis* is paramount in the transmission of rat-caused plague. Less efficient vectors, such as *X. astia* and *X. brasiliensis,* in sufficiently large numbers may be subsidiary or even, to some extent, link independent participants. It is difficult to assess the place of wild-rodent fleas in the transmission of plague as systematically as was done in the case of commensal-rodent fleas. The species are numerous, and the individual vector capacities have not been uniformly well determined. Practically all the fleas species regardless of whether they could act as vectors individually, have conveyed the infection when attacking a susceptible rodent en masse (Kartman *et al.,* 1958). Recent comparative plague vector efficiency studies are well documented by Kartman, Prince and Quan (1956) and summarized by Pollitzer (1960).

With an ingenious apparatus for artificial feeding of fleas (Kartman, 1954; Cavanaugh *et al.,* 1956) blockage has been produced in *X. cheopis* and other fleas with avirulent plague strains. The organisms multiplied only in some instances, but transmission was successful. They did not change in virulence after one passage in the flea. When the bacteria count of the blood meal was increased to 920 million or more, 80 per cent of the fleas remained infected for more than five days and proventricular blocks developed.

P. pestis from blocked stomachs of fleas have been readily phagocytized by the human polymorphonuclear cells (Bacot and Martin, 1914). Why there was no such phagocytosis of the bacilli from the spleen of rats dying of plague has recently been explained by Cavanaugh and Randall (1959). Virulent strains of *P. pestis* resistant to phagocytosis by mouse polymorphonuclear leucocytes have Fraction

I antigen and additional fractions named V and W (Burrows and Bacon, 1956). Plague bacilli rapidly growing in the stomach of fleas have no detectable Fraction I or envelope slime and consequently are rapidly phagocytized by polymorphonuclear leucocytes and rapidly destroyed. But others are phagocytized by monocytes; they are not destroyed but multiply intracellularly, and by the time they are released by the monocytes they have developed resistance to both polymorphs and monocytes. Thus, the infectivity of any regurgitated plague bacilli appears to depend on the concentration of *P. pestis* rich in envelope slime and consequently resistant to phagocytosis by polymorphonuclear leucocytes but not to the action of the mononuclear cells.

Function of Fleas in the Perpetuation of Plague. The reported maximal life span of a regularly fed flea, *X. cheopis,* is 203 days, but this is shortened to twenty to thirty days when the vector is infective and has a blocked proventriculus. The starvation that results from blockage does not adequately explain the early deaths of infective fleas. In longevity experiments on wild-rodent fleas that have not ingested blood from plague-infected animals, unfed fleas lived longer than blocked fleas when held under favorable conditions. Nest fleas in general tolerate hunger better than fur fleas. Russian investigators infected fleas, buried them for varying periods and then removed and examined specimens at intervals. Although some fleas had no opportunity to feed during the winter, they were still infected when examined in the spring. The maximal length of life of the plague-infected fleas was 396 days. Wild rodent fleas, for example *Neopsylla setosa,* may readily carry the plague bacillus from one epizootic season to another. In a study in the Cumbum Valley, south India (George and Webster, 1934), *X. cheopis* could transmit infections after starvation for up to twenty-nine days at 79° F. Fleas infected in October can retain the infection and transmit it the following March (Prince and Wayson, 1947; Pirie, 1927; Meyer, 1942).

The necessity of rodent fleas to the perpetuation of the infection has been amply reaffirmed by many workers (Baltazard *et al.,* 1953; Davis, 1953; Macchiavello, 1957; Ioff, 1957 and Mikulin, 1957).

The external climate, temperature and saturation deficiency of the immediate surroundings of the flea determine their longevity. Certain climatic conditions favor an abundance of rat fleas and the spread of plague. The adult flea on the host is exposed to a fairly constant climate, but off the host it is subject to considerable variation. The microclimate of the subterranean burrow favors the spread of plague in the North beyond 35° latitude, ordinarily considered the limit for bubonic plague of rat origin. Within limits or until such high temperatures are reached that the flea dies regardless of the moisture content of the air, the saturation deficiency is the more influential of the two factors involved at low and medium temperatures, the life span of the flea being directly proportional to the saturation deficiency of the air. The highly efficient respiratory system of the flea is so constructed that during rest the trachea is nearly all closed, and the flea can retain moisture.

Flea Transport. Live infected fleas in all kinds of cargo can be transported when the time is not very long and climatic conditions are favorable. The Plague Research Commission assumed that the spread of the infection at a distance was effected by infected fleas carried either on the person or in the bedding of travelers who have lived in plague houses or had visited them. This mode is not major. Transport of infected fleas in goods, particularly grain, raw cotton, gunny bags, rags and hides, is far more threatening. How far the infection can be carried has been debated. It was claimed that proved infected fleas in baled jute bags from Calcutta were carried into Peru, but autochthonous plague was absent from Calcutta during the period of this alleged transport. In an assessment of the danger of importation of plague into the U.S.A., not a single flea was found (Norris *et al.,* 1953). In test transports of *X. cheopis* in the holds of vessels across the Pacific, the fleas failed to survive trips of a little more than three weeks. Pressure in baling apparently would sharply reduce the chances of survival of fleas trapped within the bale or jute products. The danger of long distance transport of plague-infected fleas in jute bale is rather remote or presumably even nonexistent.

Exchange of Fleas Between Commensal and Wild Rodents. The frequency and diverse character of the interchange of fleas between rodent species is being considered fundamental in all plague areas. Fleas may be exchanged from sylvatic to domestic environment interspecifically (Meyer and Holdenried, 1949; Kartman *et al.,* 1958). This may be fairly rare: rat plague has been found in the interior of the western states. On the other hand, at Roswell, New Mexico, in 1960 in all probability a plague epizootic in wood rats and white-footed mice had been transferred to rabbits *(Sylvilagus audoboni)* and created a focus of sylvatic plague. The means of this transfer has not been determined; in all probability it was through fleas. Two hunters who handled and skinned the cottontail rabbits contracted plague through direct transmission (Kartman *et al.,* 1960).

THE DISEASE IN MAN

Plague in man manifests itself in various forms, resulting in such designations as bubonic plague, septicemic plague, pneumonic plague, tonsillar ambulatory plague and pestis minor. The two chief types of clinical plague, the bubonic and the pneumonic, usually occur in separate epidemics, but occasionally they concur, as they have in Egypt and other parts of Africa.

Bubonic plague is by far the most common type, accounting for about 75 per cent of cases of plague. It takes its name from the fact that the lymph nodes draining the area through which the infection entered become enlarged (buboes). The incubation period varies from two to ten days, but usually averages four to six days. The onset is sudden. Its progression is accompanied by fever, depression and great prostration. The enlarged lymph nodes are extremely tender and painful. The buboes of the groin are most commonly affected because the legs are the usual site of flea bites; axillary and cervical glands follow in order.

Epidemiologists of human infections in sylvatic plague areas have made inquiries as to what extent wild-rodent fleas transmit plague to man. Meyer (1942) after studying the histories of fifty bubonic plague patients in the western states of the U.S.A. was convinced that seventeen patients with primary buboes in the groin had been infected through flea bites and that twelve with primary buboes in the axilla had contracted infection when handling sick or diseased rodents or through the bite of infected animals. If the infection is mild (pestis minor) the patient may be ambulatory. The chances of recovery, which may be tedious, protracted or rapid, are much improved after the seventh day. The case fatality rate varies from 50 to 90 per cent; it was as high as 93 per cent during the outbreak in San Francisco from 1900 to 1904. Despite the availability of effective drugs the death rate among the victims of plague contracted from wild rodents has been reduced only to 30 per cent.

In rare instances, meningeal complications lead to death late in the infection (Meyer *et al.*, 1937; Landsborough and Tunnell, 1947).

In septicemic plague there are no peripheral buboes. The patient is profoundly affected by plague toxins. Extreme prostration, with a temperature rarely above 100° F., may be accompanied by nose bleeds, diarrhea and other symptoms. It is always of short duration, eighteen hours to three days, and invariably fatal. The blood contains over 40 baccilli per 0.5 ml. of blood (Meyer, 1951).

In pneumonic plague the primary localization of the baccilli is in the lungs. The intense congestion of the air passages with hemorrhagic exudate in the alveoli and bronchi, but with little or no fibrin formation, is lobular, extending to involve entire lobes. Enormous numbers of *P. pestis* are always present. General malaise, severe headache, nausea, vomiting and temperature ranges from 102° to 105° F., difficult and hurried breathing, cough and expectoration characterize the disease. The sputum, at first watery and frothy, is tinged with blood, but rarely is it viscid or rusty as it is in lobar pneumonia. Pulmonary symptoms and cardiac distress increase, delirium supervenes, and death occurs on the fourth or fifth day, or earlier. The body exhibits cyanosis. From the accompanying cyanosis the disease takes the name Black Death. This is the most infectious form of plague, and it is highly fatal. Sporadic cases are likely to be missed and may give rise to outbreaks involving physicians, as the experiences in Oakland, California, in 1919 amply illustrate. In the course of any bubonic plague epidemic, secondary plague pneumonia may give rise to serious outbreaks during the colder seasons of the year.

During pneumonic outbreaks in China (Pollitzer and Li, 1943) and in Los Angeles (Meyer, 1961), patients were observed with what was designated "the non-pneumonic type of lung pest" or tonsillar plague. In experiments by Meyer and Larson (1959) healthy primates were exposed to cage mates with frank clinical plague pneumonia. Instead of the pneumonic or primary septicemic disease they had a primary tonsillar process in lymphatic tissues of the oropharynx with cervical buboes followed by bacteremia. The influence of infective particles or droplet size by the nose-breathing primate is suspected. Large particles (12 microns or above) impinged on the nasal mucosa, and the normal clearing mechanism brought the plague bacillus in contact with lymphatic tissues well suited for its multiplication. In other studies (Strong and Teague, 1912; Druett *et al.*, 1956) with single organism clouds only smaller particles produced typical primary pneumonia. Probably in man the entire respiratory tract can serve as a portal of entry for plague bacilli in the pestilential air.

Early diagnosis is essential not only to the patient, whose recovery may depend on the early administration of the sulfonamides or antibiotics, but also to his family, his physician and the community because of the seriousness of the disease. By puncturing the bubo in its earliest stages with an 18 gauge needle, a little gelatinous edema fluid may be readily aspirated for smears and cultures. In pneumonic plague the sputum usually contains the plague bacillus in great numbers (Baltazard *et al.*, 1956). Rapid identification of *P. pestis* is now assured by means of the fluorescent antibody technique (Winter and Moody, 1959).

Incision of buboes should be avoided until frank fluctuation occurs. Since plague is frequently not recognized during its course, it is imperative that postmortem examination be conducted in endemic areas and that specimens be collected from the liver, lungs and buboes in normal saline which preserves the virulence and vitality of *P. pestis* for ten days at 20° to 24° C. (Girard, 1952).

Intensive chemotherapy with antibiotics is the most effective treatment of plague. Experimental and field trials have assessed the value of chemotherapy of all forms of human plague (Meyer *et al.*, 1952). It is not surprising that modern workers use antibiotics rather than sulfonamides. No doubt, however, fully satisfactory results in the treatment of bubonic plague can be obtained with sulfa drugs. Excellent results in the treatment of pneumonic plague (McCrumb *et al.*, 1953; Brygoo and Gonon, 1958) with streptomycin and/or other antibiotics recognize the adequacy of this method of therapy, but in a few instances there was an inherent danger. The highly bactericidal streptomycin can produce severe, even fatal, Herxheimer reactions due to the liberation of the plague toxins. These reactions can be avoided if the dosages of the drug are carefully chosen or tetracyclines are used. This drug or sulfadiazine is used for the abortive treatment of contacts of pneumonic plague patients.

PREVENTION

The control of bubonic plague is accomplished: 1) by appropriate sanitary measures directed simultaneously against the vectors and the rodent reservoir; 2) by efforts to immunize the individual; and 3) by strict isolation of the sick and the handling of all infectious material with the greatest care (Pollitzer, 1954).

Rat ectoparasite control with the insecticide DDT (dichlorodiphenyltrichlorethane), introduced and tested during World War II, has achieved spectacular and consistent control of *X. cheopis* and other fleas that carry and transmit plague. Dusting rat runs with DDT has brought epidemics of plague under control. Today this is the method of choice to speed up a control program and to increase its effectiveness. Not only does it kill the ectoparasites on the rats, but some of the powder is carried by the rats back to their nests and harborages, and this is distributed over the breeding places of the fleas. Under certain circumstances the chemical kills even the rats. The methods of application of DDT dust are fully detailed in a publication of the Communicable Disease Center (1949). The use of DDT for patch dusting is recommended for plague control in India and has proven effective in South Africa, Kenya and the Soviet Union in the control of wild-rodent fleas. An insecticide bait box has been devised and found useful (Kartman, 1958). Ryckmann and associates (1954) report better results with dieldrin, aldrin and heptachlor than with 5 per cent DDT. Others found gamma isomer of benzene hexachloride in natives' huts and in burrows a long lasting insecticide (Heisch *et al.,* 1953).

The association of rats with the plague bacillus creates many problems rarely appreciated. In a very readable summary, Barnett and Bathard (1953) properly emphasizes the basic principles. All efforts to control rats must be planned ecologically, but since the data required for rational planning are still lacking it is very difficult indeed to strike a balance between a desirable and essential activity. The rat population must be watched closely, and the appearance of rodent plague, detected through autopsy of the rodents or inoculation of crushed fleas removed from them, must be met with adequate combative measures. In recent years, because of the general interest in rodent control, public health agencies and many citizens have undertaken rat-proofing and rat-eradication campaigns by properly trained personnel. Poisoning and fumigation are more effective than trapping for destroying large numbers of rodents. Red squill, phosphorus, barium carbonate, arsenic trioxide, zinc phosphide and thallium sulfate are some of the poisons commonly used. ANTU (alpha-naphthylthio-urea) and 1080 (sodium fluoro-acetate) proved more effective, but in recent years the lethal anticoagulant warfarin (alpha-phenyl-beta-acetylethyl, best known as 4-hydroxy coumarin), when used in cornmeal has shown great promise in consistently reducing rat populations consisting of *Rattus norvegicus, R. rattus* and *Mus musculus,* but not *R. hawaiiensis* (Hayes and Gaines, 1950; Gross *et al.,* 1951). Prebaiting has greatly enhanced the effectiveness of some poisons. Warfarin is a self-bating rodenticide and reasonable in cost. The poisons must be applied continually. Proper use of all rodenticides requires considerable skill and experience. Because some (1080, ANTU and others) are highly poisonous for mammals, including man, adequate safety precautions must be employed.

Before the introduction of DDT and warfarin, several fumigants (calcium cyanide, hydrocyanic acid gas, methyl bromide, sulfur dioxide, chloropicrin, carbon dioxide, carbon bisulfide) were used as supplementary measures to destroy rats and fleas in the nest and burrows. Only specially trained personnel should apply such materials. Cyanogas, the most useful, is a light powder that releases hydrocyanic acid on contact with moisture, and this acid is lethal to rats and to fleas. For stables, cellars and buildings, sulfur dioxide is serviceable, because it does not endanger human life as hydrogen cyanide does.

No rat control program is complete without supportive sanitation and until harborages are destroyed and buildings are rat-proofed. Rubbish, refuse and garbage—excellent harborages—must be eliminated. Wooden parts of houses should be reinforced with metal so that the rodents cannot gnaw through; concrete, stone or brick walls discourage rat harborage. Screening doors and openings around water, sewer and gas pipes helps prevent the entry of rats. In South America, small flame throwers using fuel oil are employed in cleaning burrows and adobe floors and walls.

Importation of rats from endemic areas should be guarded against by rat-proofing ships, applying measures to prevent the escape of rats from vessels and their entrance into ships from wharves. This is accomplished by rat guards on the hawsers. In the past all ships sailing from plague-infected ports were fumigated with cyanide gas before entering a port in the United States; today rat-proofing and the use of other rodenticides has made this procedure unnecessary.

Suppressing plague in rural districts is difficult. The areas is of unmanageable size and knowledge of the many ecologic factors that influence control operations is so inadequate that, except in a few small areas in California and, according to the Russians, in the Caucasian steppes, curtailment of the rodent population cannot yet liquidate plague among the squirrels. The anti-rodent measures adopted by the workers in the Soviet Union pay attention to the simultaneous extermination of the rodents and the ectoparasites by the combined use of "black cyanide" and "hexachlorocyclohexane" (Pastukhov, 1960). In the final evaluation of the results obtained in the Soviet Union Fenyuk (1960) admitted that the labor and money necessary for the campaigns had been so great as to render the methods used in the pre-Caspian area and Transbaikalia impracticable for the extensive natural foci of plague in the sparsely populated, high mountain, desert or semidesert districts of Asia, Africa and America.

During the early years of control work in California, the United States Public Health Service vaporized carbon bisulfide into the burrows of the squirrels. In recent years use of methyl bromide and in South Africa of DDT has proved valuable, particularly when it is accompanied by filling of burrows. Later, using grain as bait and poisoning it with thallium sulfate, strychnine or 1080 have proved effective. Experience has taught that a rise in the rodent population in canyons and draws to twenty to twenty-five ground squirrels per acre provides conditions particularly favorable for local epizootics. Control work must be continued indefinitely. The natural enemies of squirrels—the coyote, wolf, badger, skunk, hawk and mountain lion—even when little interfered with by man, have in recent years failed to influence the size of the rodent population appreciably, and consequently campestral plague has not infrequently assumed the function of checking their numbers.

In an outbreak, persons engaged in rat-control work should be immunized and should wear flea-proof clothing. Clothing impregnated with the repellent diethyltoluamide gives protection for one week.

Prophylactic vaccination or the injection of antigens made from killed virulent organisms has been advocated under certain circumstances. Various preparations have been used. The available statistics show that the ones available at this time do not prevent infection, but they do reduce the mortality rate. Workers in India, using the so-called Haffkine, heat-killed broth culture of a highly virulent strain, have repeatedly shown that the total number of cases and the death rates are lower in the injected than in the noninjected groups. For example, Beals (1920) reported that among 6,000 uninoculated in World War I there were 275 cases and 167 deaths, while among 4,378 given injections of Haffkine's antigen there were only thirty-nine cases and ten deaths. The next year among 6,000 uninoculated there were seventy-six cases and forty-seven deaths, while among the vaccinated there were seventeen cases with two deaths. On the other hand, these favorable results have not been duplicated by other workers, and the replies sent to the Office Internationale d'Hygiène Publique in 1931 and 1932 in answer to a questionnaire indicated that there was little confidence in the prophylactic value of the anti-plague antigens extracted from killed microorganisms. More recent studies only in part support this skepticism. For example, Patel and Rebello (1948) reported a mortality rate of 40.2 per cent in 410 inoculated against 59.2 per cent in 723 uninoculated persons in India. The socalled United States Army "vaccine" does stimulate antibodies in those injected with solutions containing 3,000 million formalin-killed plague bacilli. By coating the killed virulent bacilli with aluminum hydroxide the immunogenicity of this vaccine has been improved. It is sound practice to repeat the injections when the population remains under exposure (Meyer, 1960).

As early as 1907 the value of living avirulent plague cultures had been demonstrated (Strong, 1908), but it was not until 1934 in Java that this method of protection was evaluated carefully (Otten, 1941). By 1941, 10,000,000 vaccinations had been given there. In carefully controlled series, in which family after family was injected alternately with 1,000,000,000 live organisms, the mortality in the vaccinated was 1.0 per 1,000 against 4.76 per 1,000 in the nonvaccinated. The steady decrease of plague in Java has been attributed to the use of vaccines consisting of living avirulent organisms. Equally favorable results have been reported from Madagascar (Girard and Robic, 1936; Girard, 1948) where over 2,000,000 vaccinations have been performed and from South Africa (Grasset, 1946). Conclusive statistical results are not available yet from these areas, but the workers claim many advantages: single injections allowing mass inoculations in much shorter time, comparatively little undesirable local reaction in natives, and economical production because the vaccines can be lyophilized and hence handled readily. Vaccination with live avirulent organisms, like other vaccines, has never controlled an outbreak, but it definitely does reduce the number of deaths. The Expert Committee on Plague of the World Health Organization concluded that vaccination is too slow and unreliable for immediate prophylaxis.

Pneumonic plague has not been apparently influenced by vaccination nor inoculation of antigens.

Antiplague serum produced in horses with living virulent or avirulent plague strains was recommended by Yersin (1894) and since by others; such sera have been low in protective antibodies. In experiments sera of rabbits properly immunized have been more promising. There is little proof that antiplague sera has noteworthy prophylactic properties.

Human infections constitute important sources of other human infections. Strict isolation of the patients in insect-proof rooms is essential. The patient's clothing must be disinfected and disinfested of fleas in a steam sterilizer. All those who come in contact with patients must wear gloves and gowns. If the infection is pneumonic or suspected of being pneumonic, physicians, nurses and any others in contact with the patient must be protected by complete overalls, gloves, hoods equipped with goggles and face masks of eight layers of gauze covered by a deflection mask. The chance of infection through droplets or droplet nuclei is quite high and occupational infection not infrequent. Persons accidentally exposed to unsuspected plague pneumonia must be quarantined for seven days, and chemoprophylaxis with sulfadiazine or tetracycline should be instituted. The air of the room in which patients with pneumonic plague are housed, preferably under an oxygen tent, should be kept dry; the use of ultraviolet light screens and possibly other auxiliary protective measures against aerogenic infection deserve consideration. In contrast to the tedious, if not difficult, procedures involved in the prevention and control of rodent-caused and flea-borne plague, control of the pneumonic form is comparatively simple, provided that chemoprophylaxis is started as soon as the disease is diagnosed.

ITEMS OF NOTE

1) Plague is primarily a disease of rodents.

2) Bubonic plague is usually a disease of tropical or semitropical climates.

3) Pneumonic plague in epidemic form is a disease of cold and temperate climates.

4) The control of fleas and rats is sufficient to control epidemics of bubonic plague in man.

5) Pneumonic plague lends itself to no practical control methods, although chemoprophylaxis offers a practically infallible means of protecting contacts against manifest attacks of the disease.

6) In the United States, squirrels, chipmunks, prairie dogs, marmots, meadow mice, pocket mice, white-footed mice, grasshopper mice, deer mice, harvest mice, wood and pack rats, kangaroo rats, and jack and cottontail rabbits, are naturally infected in fifteen Western states extending from the Pacific Coast to Texas, and from Arizona across the Canadian border into British Columbia and Alberta, also Mexico.

7) No practical means are available for controlling the endemic reservoir of plague in rural areas, so rodent-free belts around human habitations offer the best preventive measure.

8) Treatment with sulfadiazine, tetracyclines, streptomycin, chloramphenicol, in carefully chosen doses is effective against human plague.

REFERENCES

ADVISORY COMMITTEE: *J. Hyg.,* 7:324-358, 1907a.

ADVISORY COMMITTEE: *J. Hyg.,* 7:694-723, 1907b.

BACOT, A. W. and MARTIN, C. J.: *J. Hyg., Plague Suppl. III, 13*:423-439, 1914.

BALTAZARD, M. and BAHMANYAR, M.: *Bull. World Health Organ., 23*:169-215, 217-246, 1960.

BALTAZARD, M. and SEYDIAN, B.: *Bull. World Health Organ., 23*:157-167, 1960.

BALTAZARD, M., BAHMANYAR, M., MOSTACHFI, P., EFTEKHARI, M. and MOFIDI, C.: *Bull. World Health Organ., 23*:141-155, 1960.

BALTAZARD, M., DAVIS, D. H. A., DEVIGNAT, R., GIRARD, G., GOHAR, M. A., KARTMAN, L., MEYER, K. F., PARKER, M. T., POLLITZER, R., PRINCE, F. M., QUAN, S. F., and WAGLE, P.: *Bull. World Health Organ., 14*:457-509, 1956.

BARRERA, A.: *Acta zool. mex., 1*, 4 pp., 1956. (Abstract: *Rev. Applied Entomol., 45:*153, 1957.)

DE LA BARRERA, J. M.: *Proc. Am. Sc. Cong. (1940), 6:*291-292, 1942.

BARRETO, J. DE B. and DE CASTRO, A.: *Mem. Inst. Oswaldo Cruz, 44:*505-527, 1946.

BEALS, L. H.: *J.A.M.A., 75:*955-956, 1920.

BLANC, G. and BALTAZARD, M.: *Compt. rend. Acad. sc., 213:*813-816, 1941.

BLUE, R.: *California & West. Med., 40:*363-365, 1934.

BONEBAKKER, A.: *Trop. & Geogr. Med., 12:*47-53, 1960.

BROOKS, R. S.: *J. Hyg., Plague Suppl. V*, 881-889, 1917.

BRYGOO, E. R.: *Bull. Soc. path. exot., 49:*409-414, 1956.

BRYGOO, E. R. and GONON, M.: *Bull. Soc. path. exot., 51:*47-58, 1958.

BURROUGHS, A. L.: *J. Hyg., 45:*371-396, 1947.

BURROWS, T. W. and BACON, G. A.: *Brit. J. Exper. Path., 37:*286-299; 381-393, 1956.

CAVANAUGH, D. C. and RANDALL, R.: *J. Immunol., 83:*348-363, 1959.

CAVANAUGH, D. C., WHEELER, C. M., SUYEMOTO, W., SHIMADA, T. and YAMAKAWA, Y.: *J. Infect. Dis., 98:*103-106, 1956.

CHEN, T. H., QUAN, S. F. and MEYER, K. F.: *J. Immunol., 68:*147-158, 1952.

CLEMOW, F. G.: *Brit. M. J., 1:*1141-1146, 1900.

COMMUNICABLE DISEASE CENTER: *Rat-borne Disease. Prevention and Control*, 292 pp., 1949.

CRAGG, F. W.: *Indian J. M. Research, 9:*374-389, 1921.

CROCKER, T. T., CHEN, T. H. and MEYER, K. F.: *J. Bact., 72:*851-857, 1956.

DAVIS, D. E.: *Quart. Rev. Biol., 28:*373-401, 1953.

DAVIS, D. H. S.: *Ann. Trop. Med. & Parasitol., 42:*207-217, 1948.

DAVIS, D. H. S.: *J. Hyg., 51:*427-449, 1953.

DEVIGNAT, R.: *Bull. World Health Organ., 4:*247-263, 1951.

DRUETT, H. A., ROBINSON, J. M., HENDERSON, D. W., PACKMAN, L. and PEACOCK, S.: *J. Hyg., 54:*37-48, 1956.

ESKEY, C. R. and HAAS, V. H.: *Pub. Health Bull.*, No. 254, 83 pp., 1940.

FEDOROV, V. N.: *Bull. World Health Organ., 23:*275-281, 1960.

FENYUK, B. K.: *Bull. World Health Organ., 23:*263-273, 1960.

GEORGE, P. V. and WEBSTER, W. J.: *Indian J. M. Research, 22:*77-104, 1934.

GIRARD, G.: *Proc. Internat. Cong. Trop. Med. & Malaria, 1:*257-263, 1948.

GIRARD, G.: *Bull. World Health Organ., 5:*109-116, 1952.

GIRARD, G. and ROBIC, J.: *Bull. Office internat. d'hyg. pub., 28:*1078-1087, 1936.

GRASSET, E.: *Tr. Roy. Soc. Trop. Med. & Hyg., 40:*275-294, 1946.

GROSS, B., BAKER, R. H., and BONNET, D. D.: *Pub. Health Rep., 66:*1727-1733, 1951.

HAESER, H.: *Lehrbuch der Geschichte der Medicin und der epidemischen Krankheiten. Dritte Bearbeitung. Dritter Band. Geschichte der epidemische Krankheiten.* Jena: Verlag von Gustav Fischer, pp. 24, 37, 97, 1882.

HAYES, W. J. and GAINES, T. B.: *Pub. Health Rep., 65:*1537-1555, 1950.

HEISCH, R. B., GRAINGER, W. E. and D'SOUZA, J. S. A.: *Tr. Roy. Soc. Trop. Med. & Hyg., 47:*503-521, 1953.

HÉRIVAUX, A. and TOUMANOFF, C.: *Bull. Soc. path. exot., 41:*318-325, 1948.

HIRST, L. F.: *The Conquest of Plague.* Oxford: Clarendon Press, 478 pp., 1953.

HUDSON, B. W.: *Bull. World Health Organ., 24:*291-292, 1961.

HUMPHREYS, F. A., CAMPBELL, A. G. and SMITH, E. S.: *Canad. J. Pub. Health, 42:*68, 1951. (Abstract)

IOFF, I. J.: *Problems in the Ecology of Fleas in Their Relation to Their Epidemi-*

ological Importance. Pyatigorsk: Ordjhonikidze Regional Publishing House, 1941. (In Russian)

IOFF, I. J.: *Zh. mikrobiol., epidemiol. i immunobiol. (Moskva) 28:*91-99, 1957.

KARTMAN, L.: *Exper. Parasitol., 3:*525-537, 1954.

KARTMAN, L.: *Exper. Parasitol., 6:*599-609, 1957.

KARTMAN, L.: *Zoonoses Research, 1:*1-27, 1960.

KARTMAN, L., MILES, V. I. and PRINCE, F. M.: *Am. J. Trop. Med. & Hyg., 7:*112-124, 1958.

KARTMAN, L., PRINCE, F. M. and QUAN, S. F.: *Bull. World Health Organ., 14:*681-704, 1956.

KARTMAN, L., PRINCE, F. M. and QUAN, S. F.: *Am. J. Trop. Med. & Hyg., 7:*317-322, 1958.

KARTMAN, L., PRINCE, F. M., QUAN, S. F. and STARK, H. E.: *Ann. New York Acad. Sc., 70:*688-711, 1958.

KAUL, P. M.: *Epidemiol. & Vital Statistics Rep., 2:*143-165, 1949.

KELLOGG, W. H.: *Am. J. Pub. Health, 10:*599-605, 1920

LANDSBOROUGH, D., and TUNNELL, N.: *Brit. M. J., 1:*4-7, 1947.

LARSON, C. L., PHILIP, C. B., WICHT, W. C. and HUGHES, L. E.: *J. Immunol., 67:*289-298, 1951.

LINK, V. B.: *Am. J. Trop. Med., 31:*452-457, 1951a.

LINK, V. B.: *Pub. Health Rep., 66:*1466-1472, 1951b.

LISTON, W. A.: *Brit. M. J., 1:*950-954, 1924.

LLOYD, B. J.: *J.A.M.A., 85:*729-733, 1925.

MACCHIAVELLO, A.: *Bol. Ofic. san. panam., 39:*339-349, 1955.

MACCHIAVELLO, A.: *Bol. Ofic. san. panam., 43:*225-250, 1957.

MACCHIAVELLO, A.: *Bol. Ofic. san. panam., 44:*484-512, 1958.

McCOY, G. W. and WHERRY, W. B.: *J. Infect. Dis., 6:*670-675, 1909.

McCRUMB, F. R., MERCIER, S., ROBIC, J., BOUILLAT, M., SMADEL, J. W., WOODWARD, T. E., WOODWARD and GOODNER, K.: *Am. J. Med., 14:*284-293, 1953.

MEYER, K. F.: *Medicine, 21:*143-174, 1942a.

MEYER, K. F.: *Am. J. Trop. Med., 22:*9-36, 1942b.

MEYER, K. F.: *Ann. New York Acad. Sc., 48:*429-467, 1947.

MEYER, K. F.: Plague. In: *Modern Practice in Infectious Fevers.* Edited by H. S. Banks. New York: Paul B. Hoeber, Inc., vol. 1, pp. 478-496, 1951.

MEYER, K. F.: Pasteurella. In: *Bacterial and Mycotic Infections of man.* Edited by R. Dubos. Ed. 3, Philadelphia: J. B. Lippincott Co., pp. 400-436, 1958.

MEYER, K. F.: *California Vector Views, 2:*41; 43, 1955.

MEYER, K. F.: *Pub. Health Rep., 72:*705-719, 1957.

MEYER, K. F.: *Schweiz. med. Wchnschr., 90:*1392-1398, 1960.

MEYER, K. F.: *Bact. Rev., 25:*249-261, 1961.

MEYER, K. F. and BATCHELDER, A.: *Proc. Soc. Exper. Biol. & Med., 23:*730-734, 1926.

MEYER, K. F. and EDDIE, B.: *Proc. Soc. Exper. Biol. & Med., 38:*333-334, 1938.

MEYER, K. F. and HOLDENRIED R.: *Puerto Rico J. Pub. Health, 24:*201-209, 1949.

MEYER, K. F. and LARSON, A.: *Proc. Symp. Diamond Jubilee Haffkine Inst.,* pp. 1-12, 1959.

MEYER, K. F., QUAN, S. F., McCRUMB, F. R. and LARSON, A.: *Ann. New York Acad. Sc., 55:*1228-1274, 1952.

MIKULIN, M.: *Zh. mikrobiol., epidemiol. i immunobiol. (Moskva), 28* (10):142-144, 1957.

MILES, V. I., KINNEY, A. R. and STARK, H. E.: *Am. J. Trop. Med. & Hyg.*, 6:752-760, 1957.

MOHR, C. O.: *Am. J. Trop. Med.*, 31:355-372, 1951.

MOLL, A. A. and O'LEARY, S. B.: *Bol. Ofic. san. panam.*, 19:451-461; 576-584; 759-771; 878-887; 1081, 1940; 20:139-149; 254-262; 365-374; 697-714; 1149-1155, 1941; 21:245-252; 780-785; 874-883; 980-1000, 1942.

MURDOCK, J. R.: *Pub. Health Rep.*, 55:2172-2178, 1940.

MURRAY, K. F.: *Am. J. Trop. Med. & Hyg.*, 6:1068-1086, 1957.

NORRIS, E. W., SCHNEIDER, L. B., HANCHETT, L. J., KOHLER, C. E. and BUREN, W. F.: *Pub. Health Rep.*, 68:802-804, 1953.

OGATA, M.: *Centralbl. f. Bakt.*, 21:769-777, 1897.

OTTEN, L.: *Mededeel. dienst. volksgezondh. in Nederl.-Indië*, 30:61-110, 1941.

PASTUKHOV, B. N.: *Bull. World Health Organ.*, 23:401-404, 1960.

PATEL, T. B. and REBELLO, J. L.: *Indian M. Gaz.*, 83:151-155, 1948.

PAVLOVSKI, E. N.: *Zh. mikrobiol., epidemiol. i immunobiol. (Moskva)*, 28 (11):11-18, 1957.

PIRIE, J. H. H.: *Pub. South African Inst. M. Research*, 3:109-118, 1927.

PODACH, E. F.: *Schweiz. med. Wchnschr.*, 82:40-42, 1952.

POLLITZER, R.: *Plague*. WHO Monograph Series, No. 22, 698 pp., 1954.

POLLITZER, R.: *Bull. World Health Organ.*, 23:313-400, 1960.

POLLITZER, R. and LI, C. C.: *Chinese M. J.*, 61:212-216, 1943.

POLLITZER, R. and MEYER, K. F.: The ecology of plague. In. *Studies in Disease Ecology.* Volume II in the series Studies in Medical Geography. Edited by J. M. May. New York: Hafner Publishing Company, Inc., pp. 433-501; 582-590, 1961.

PRINCE, F. M. and WAYSON, N. E.: *Pub. Health Rep.*, 62:463-467; 1167-1168, 1947.

QUAN, S. F. and KARTMAN, L.: *Tr. Roy. Soc. Trop. Med. & Hyg.*, 50:104-105, 1956.

QUAN, S. F., VON FINTEL, H. and McMANUS, A. G.: *Am. J. Trop. Med. & Hyg.*, 7:411-415, 1958.

QUAN, S. F., KARTMAN, L. and McMANUS, A. G.: *Science*, 120:1101-1102, 1954.

QUAN, S. F., MILES, V. I. and KARTMAN, L.: *Am. J. Trop. Med. & Hyg.*, 9:85-90, 1960.

QUAN, S. F., KARTMAN, L., PRINCE, F. M. and MILES, V. I.: *Am. J. Trop. Med. & Hyg.*, 9:91-95, 1960.

RALL, I. M.: *Zh. mikrobiol., epidemiol. i immunobiol. (Moskva)*, 29 (2):74-78, 1958.

RALL, I. M. and FEDOROV, V. N.: *J. Microbiol., Epidemiol. and Immunobiol.*, 31:228-235, 1960.

RAMOS DÍAZ, A.: *Bol. Ofic. san. panam.*, 17:776-789, 1938.

RODENWALDT, E.: *Pest in Venedig, 1575-1577. Ein Beitrag zu der Frage der Infektionskette bei den Pestepidemien Westeuropas.* Sitzungs Berichte der Heidelberger Akademie de Wissenschaften, 1952. II. Zwei Abhandlungen. Heidelberg: Springer Verlag, p. 151, 1953.

RYCKMAN, R. E., AMES, C. T., LINDT, C. C. and LEE, R. D.: *J. Econ. Entomol.*, 47:604-607, 1954. (Abstract: *Rev. Applied Entomol.*, 43:116, 1955).

SCHWARZ, E.: *Bull. World Health Organ.*, 23:411-416, 1960.

SHARIF, M.: *Bull. World Health Organ.*, 4:75-109, 1951.

SIMOND, P.-L. *Ann. Inst. Pasteur*, 12:625-687, 1898.

SIMPSON, W. J.: *A Treatise on Plague Dealing with Historical, Epidemiological, Clinical, Therapeutic and Preventive Aspects of the Disease.* Cambridge: University Press, 490 pp., 1905.

STEWART, J.: *Nestorian Missionary Enterprise.* Edinburgh: Clarke, 1928.

STICKER, G.: *Abhandlungen aus der Seuchengeschichte und Seuchenlehre I. Band: Die Pest. 1. Teil: Die Geschichte der Pest.* Giessen: A. Töpelmann, 478 pp. 1908.

STICKER, G.: *Abhandlungen aus der Seuchengeschichte und Seuchenlehre. I. Band: Die Pest. 2. Teil: Die Pest als Seuche und als Plage.* Giessen: A. Töpelmann, 542 pp., 1910.

STRONG, R. P.: *J. M. Research, 18:*325-346, 1908.

STRONG, R. P. and TEAGUE, O.: *Philippine J. Sc., 7:*173-180, 1912.

SWELLENGREBEL, N. H.: *J. Hyg., 48:*135-145, 1950.

SWELLENGREBEL, N. H.: *Docum. Med. Geog. Trop., 5:*151-156, 1953.

VARELA, G. and VÁZQUEZ, A.: *Rev. Inst. salub. y enferm. trop., 14:*219-223, 1954.

WHEELER, C. M. and DOUGLAS, J. R.: *Proc. Soc. Exper. Biol. & Med., 47:*65-66, 1941.

WHEELER, C. W. and GROSS, B.: Paper read at the Pacific Science Congress, Honolulu, 1961.

WILLIAMS, C. L.: *Am. J. Pub. Health, 10:*851-864, 1920.

WILLIAMS, C. L. and KEMMERER, T. W.: *Pub. Health Rep., 38:*1873-1881, 1923.

WINTER, C. C. and MOODY, M. D.: *J. Infect. Dis., 104:*274-294, 1959.

WORLD HEALTH ORGANIZATION: Expert Committee on Plague. Third Report. *World Health Organ. Tech. Rep. Ser.,* No. 165, 42 pp., 1959.

YERSIN: *Ann. Inst. Pasteur, 8:*662-667, 1894.

Chapter 22

TULAREMIA

H. J. Shaughnessy, Ph.D.

Tularemia is primarily a disease of wild mammals and birds, spread by arthropods. Man becomes secondarily infected but ordinarily does not enter into the chain of causation. The causative agent is *Pasteurella tularensis,* an organism closely related to *P. pestis,* the plague bacillus.

HISTORY

What may be the first description of tularemia is found in a paper by Horne[1] describing studies of lemmings carried out in 1896 and 1903. He produced a disease resembling tularemia, clinically, bacteriologically, and pathologically in mice, rabbits and guinea pigs by inoculating them with tissues of dead lemmings collected in Norway.

Since 1910, the disease now called tularemia has been recognized under various names according to the circumstances in which it was encountered. Thus McCoy designated it as a "plague-like disease of rodents"; in Utah it was known as "deer-fly fever" and in Washington, D. C., as "rabbit fever"; in Idaho, Lamb referred to it as "the glandular type of tick fever," and in Japan it has been reported as "Ohara's disease."

In 1911,[2] McCoy working in Tulare County, California, described a "plague-like disease of rodents" in California ground squirrels. The next year he and Chapin isolated the causative agent of the disease and named it *Bacterium tularense.*[3] Both Chapin and a laboratory assistant had gone through an obscure attack of fever in the course of their work and it was found afterwards that their blood serum agglutinated this organism.

In 1914, Vail described an eye infection from which Wherry and Lamb[4] isolated the tularemia organism, this being the first human case of tularemia on record to be diagnosed bacteriologically. In 1915, Sattler[5] and in 1917 Lamb[6] described similar cases of conjunctivitis. The natural reservoir of infection in wild rabbits, and its important relation to human disease, were also first disclosed by Wherry and Lamb.[7,8]

In 1920, Francis isolated the tularemia organism from seventeen jack rabbits and seven human cases of "deer-fly fever." This disease had been known in Utah since the publication of a paper by Pearse[8] in 1911, and was so named because it was popularly supposed that infection was due to the bite of the blood-sucking fly, *Chrysops discalis*, commonly found on horses. Francis[10] proved that the deer-fly actually did transmit the tularemia organism. He named the disease tularemia because of the presence of the causative organism in the blood.

Francis[11] also demonstrated that "rabbit fever," a disease prevalent among sellers of wild rabbits in Washington, D. C., was tularemia contracted by contact with the carcasses of these animals. The role of ticks as vectors was demonstrated by Parker and Spencer and others.

THE ETIOLOGIC AGENT

Pasteurella tularensis is a pleomorphic, nonmotile, Gram negative and nonsporulating microorganism whose morphologic units are represented by globules, globi, bacilliary forms, and minimal reproductive units, any or all of which may at times be filamentously interconnected. The size of units ranges from 90 millimicrons to almost 3 microns for globular units, and from 0.5 micron to 4 microns or more for bacillary forms.

Growth does not take place on ordinary culture media; the standard solid medium is glucose cystine blood agar. Abundant growth may be obtained in a variety of liquid media, peptone cysteine broths, hydrolyzate media, and purely synthetic media made with the fourteen amino acids for which the organism has an obligate requirement.

The organism is easily killed by heat in ten minutes at 56° C. to 58° C. Cooking therefore renders infected tissue harmless. Chemical disinfectants destroy the organism easily—tricresol 1.0 per cent in two minutes and formalin 0.1 per cent in twenty-four hours. Glycerin, pure and undiluted, is suitable for preserving spleens for laboratory inoculations, the organisms remaining alive many days at room temperature when the spleen of an affected rabbit or guinea pig is thus treated.

When glycerinated spleens are stored at a temperature of —14° C. or lower, the viability and virulence of *P. tularensis* is prolonged indefinitely. Four strains of the organism stored in this way were still of maximum virulence, two after a period of thirteen years and two after ten years. When the organs of infected animals were frozen at —14° C. without glycerin, the organism remained virulent for forty-two months in the spinal cord, thirty-six months in the brain, eighteen months in the spleen, twelve months in the muscle and six months in the bone marrow. Pure cultures are preserved by lyophilization but with less success than with other bacteria.

GENERAL EPIDEMIOLOGY

Tularemia probably can be transmitted by more different routes than any other infectious disease. There are also probably more natural reservoirs of tularemia than in most other diseases. In addition to animal reservoirs infection is maintained in several species of ticks by transovarian passage to succeeding generations. With all these sources and modes of infection it is remarkable that only 30,851 cases of tularemia have been reported in the U.S.A. through 1960. It is also interesting that there has been a steady decline in the number of reported cases in the U.S.A. from 1401 in 1947 to 390 in 1960.

People of all ages and races are susceptible so that the infection rate is determined by the degree of contact with infected animals or their carcasses, infected arthropods, contaminated water or food and dust. Occupational exposure is important. Incidence rates are higher in agricultural and forestry workers, especially in Russia, and among laboratory investigators working with cultures or infected animals. In North America infection occurs often among rabbit hunters or those handling rabbit carcasses; thus housewives are often involved. Vacationers in areas where transmission by ticks is important may also have relatively high incidence rates.

The epidemiology of tularemia in the United States differs by regions. In most areas contact with infected rabbit carcasses is the principal source of infection. In some areas, such as Arkansas, more than half of the cases are attributed to ticks. Transmission by deerflies in the Rocky Mountain area is so well known that it requires only passing mention. Although streams and drainage ditches in that area are contaminated by *P. tularensis,* human cases from contact with them or drinking water from them have rarely occurred. Jellison *et al.*[12] described an outbreak involving four people in Montana who drank water contaminated with *P. tularensis.*

In Europe rodents (mice and rats) are the principal reservoirs of infection, although hares are infected to some extent. Human infection occurs by contact with infected animals or their hides and carcasses but outbreaks from contaminated water or food have been prominent.

Before streptomycin therapy was employed the fatality rate for tularemia in North America was 5 to 7 per cent whereas in Europe the fatality rate has been very low, probably under 1 per cent. It appears that this difference may be accounted for by the different reservoirs of infection in Europe and America. *P. tularensis* strains isolated from rabbits, ticks or sheep are of maximum virulence but those from rodents or water, in both the USSR and the United States, are of much lower virulence.

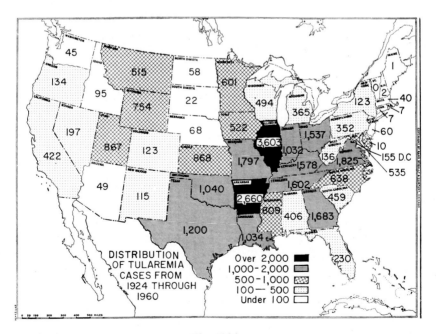

Fig. 106A.

GEOGRAPHIC DISTRIBUTION

Tularemia has been reported from practically all parts of the United States. The Central and South Atlantic areas have more cases than others whereas few cases have been reported from the New England and Middle Atlantic States. Vermont and Hawaii are the only states from which no cases of tularemia have been reported. Alaska has had one questionable case.

Tularemia has been reported from many other countries, including Austria, Belgium, Canada, Czechoslovakia, France, Germany, Italy, Japan, Mexico, Norway, Poland, Russia, Sweden, and Turkey. Laboratory infections have occurred in England but natural occurrence of the disease has not been reported from the British Isles.

SEASONAL PREVALENCE

The seasonal prevalence of tularemia is determined by the source of infection and the area concerned. Laboratory infections may occur at any time. Human cases are more prevalent in summer time in the western states where ticks and deer flies are the cause of infection (*Dermacentor andersoni,* March to August; *Chrysops discalis,* June to September). Human cases, due to infection from dissecting jack rabbits, are likewise most prevalent during April to October because these are the months of greatest destruction of these pests. East of the Mississippi River cottontail rabbits are responsible for most human cases and since they are generally protected by law except during a few winter months, the seasonal prevalence is apt to be November to January, when the hunting season is on.

VECTORS

The following arachnids and insects have been shown to be capable of transmitting tularemia:

Wood tick	*Dermacentor andersoni*
Dog tick	*Dermacentor variabilis*
Pacific Coast tick	*Dermacentor occidentalis*
Lone star tick	*Amblyomma americanum*
Argasid ticks	*Ornithodorus turicata, O. parkeri, O. moubata, O. hermsi*
Rabbit tick	*Haemaphysalis leporis-palustris*
Rabbit louse	*Haemodipsus ventricosus*

Rabbit flea	*Cediopsylla inaequalis*
Squirrel flea	*Diamanus montanus*
Rat flea	*Xenopsylla cheopis*
Mouse flea	*Malaraeus telchinum*
Mouse louse	*Polyplax serratus*
Deer fly	*Chrysops discalis*
Stable fly	*Stomoxys calcitrans*
Mosquitoes	*Aedes cinereus, A. excrucians*
Bed bug, feces, not by bite	*Cimex lectularius*

The human body louse, *Pediculus humanus,* has also been experimentally infected and might be capable of transmitting infection from man to man.

ANIMALS SUSCEPTIBLE

Tularemia has been found in the United States in the following wild animals in their natural state: beaver, chipmunk, coyote, deer, fox, ground hog, snowshoe hare, deer mouse, field mouse, meadow

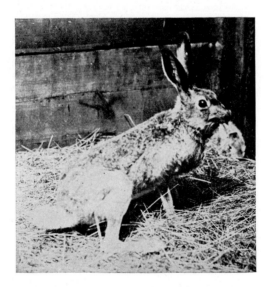

Fig. 106B. Jack rabbit, common host and transmitter of tularemia west of the Mississippi River.

mouse, mink, muskrat, opossum, prairie dog, cottontail rabbit, jack rabbit, raccoon, wild rat, shrew, skunk, bull snake, ground squirrel, tree squirrel, and weasel.

Tularemic infection occurs in several of the domestic animals including the cat, dog, hog, horse, sheep and cow. Domestic rabbits are highly susceptible but rarely, if ever, become infected, probably because they do not ordinarily come in contact with infected wild animals. Sheep are apparently the only domestic animals in which epizoötics occur but dogs may be an important reservoir in some areas.

Wild birds, such as the Columbian grouse, ruffed grouse, sharp-tailed grouse, Franklin gull, chicken hawk, sage hen, pheasant, horned owl, and quail are naturally infected, but the tularemia organism seems to be of lower virulence.[11] The domestic hen, pigeon, and turkey are apparently immune.

THE DISEASE IN ANIMALS

Transmission of tularemia from animal to animal is probably carried on by means of blood sucking insects, especially fleas, lice, and ticks. The rabbit tick is one of the chief agents in perpetuating the disease in nature. It is estimated that in an average year about one per cent of wild rabbits are infected with tularemia. Rabbit lice are active the year around; wood ticks are a menace during the spring and summer in not only carrying the infection from rabbit to rabbit directly but also in transmitting it to its offspring through the egg. The deer fly, while usually found around horses, may bite rabbits, mechanically transmitting the infection from animal to animal through its infected mouth parts. The mouse louse is probably the cause of the spread of the disease in mice.

While the gross lesions vary somewhat in different animals they resemble very closely bubonic plague in the guinea pig. Guinea pigs readily contract the disease if a minute amount of the culture is placed upon the shaved skin, death occurring in five to seven days. The site of the inoculation is necrotic; the contiguous lymph glands are hemorrhagic or caseous while a secondary chain of lymph glands may be caseous; the liver is covered with small yellowish-gray necrotic foci, the spleen is enlarged and thickly studded with miliary necrotic granules, so thick that large areas of the spleen are at times necrotic (Figure 107).

A chronic form of the disease has been reported in guinea pigs inoculated with attenuated cultures. There is a marked enlargement of lymph nodes and other organs which, with necrotic foci, suggests tuberculosis. Animals killed early in the disease, the first or second day after illness, exhibit no gross pathologic lesions although the infection is present in the liver as well as in all other tissues of the body.

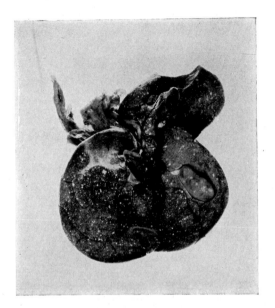

Fig. 107. Rabbit's liver in tularemia.

Greene[13] has shown that natural passage of *P. tularensis* in birds tends to lower the virulence of the organism. Guinea pigs inoculated with strains isolated from naturally infected grouse lived for fifteen days, while guinea pigs inoculated with rabbit strains lived for only six days. The grouse strains passed through guinea pigs increased in virulence to equal that of the rabbit strains.

SOURCES AND MODES OF HUMAN INFECTION

There are twenty methods, according to Francis,[14] by which man may be infected with tularemia. Among the more important of these are: handling infected carcasses of infected rabbits and rodents; bites of infected arthropods; ingestion of contaminated water or partially cooked infected meat; inhalation of aerosols or dust containing *P. tularensis*.

Rabbits. Snowshoe hare, *Lepus bairdii;* cottontail rabbit, *Sylvilagus floridanus;* jack rabbit, *Lepus sp*. Rabbits are the most prolific source of infection, being responsible for over 90 per cent of human cases in the United States, with only 0.3 per cent of the cases occurring beyond the range of *Sylvilagus sp*.[15] Persons who dress rabbits with bare hands are most likely to contract the disease, such as market men, hunters and housewives. The organism may enter through a wound or cut or abrasion or directly through the unbroken skin. No human case has been traced to domestic rabbits.

Ticks. Dog tick, *Dermacentor variabilis;* Wood tick, *Dermacentor andersoni* and lone star tick, *Amblyomma americanum*. The wood tick has caused many cases in Montana and surrounding states, while the dog tick is responsible for much of the disease in the southern and eastern states. An outbreak of fifty cases among soldiers in Tennessee was attributed to the lone star tick.[16]

Flies. Deer fly, *Chrysops discalis*. The deer fly is the principal source of infection in Utah. It bites on exposed parts of the body. An outbreak of thirty cases was reported among 170 members of a camp of the Civilian Conservation Corps who worked stripped to the waist because of the heat.[17]

Other Insect Bites. The work of Olin in Sweden,[18] and of Karpov and others in Russia,[19] leaves no doubt that both endemic cases and human epidemics have occurred owing to mosquito-born infection. *Aedes cinereus* and *A. excrucians* were found naturally infected. The Russians further incriminate *A. caspius, Anopheles maculipennis, Culex apicalis,* and both midges *(Chironimidae)* and buffalo-gnats or black flies *(Simuliidae)*.[20]

Animal Bites. Tularemia has followed bites from the following animals: cat, kitten, wild boar, coyote, dog, hog, lamb, muskrat, opossum, raccoon, white rat, skunk, Montana ground squirrel, tree squirrel, snapping turtle, and weasel. It is assumed that the mouth parts of the animal had been contaminated by feeding on infected material.

Laboratory Infections. Laboratory workers have been infected in many instances, more than 100 in this country alone. In many cases the route of infection was conjectural, but the frequent occurrence of dysphagia and mediastinal node enlargement indicated inhalation as an important one. Primary lesions are always rare in this group, most patients presenting the typhoidal clinical type of disease.

Ingestion. Many cases in the United States have followed the ingestion of partially cooked rabbit meat. Among twenty cases in five families there were twelve deaths.[21] In Russia, in 1935, there was an epidemic of forty-three cases among peasants who drank water from a brook thought to have been contaminated by water rats.[22] Streams in the United States have been found contaminated with *P. tularensis*.[23]

Inhalation. Many thousands of cases occurred during the last war in South Russia owing to inhalation of dust from grains containing infected rodent carcasses.[24]

Rats. Water rat, *Arvicola amphibius*. Water rats caused more than a thousand cases in Russia in 1928 among persons who skinned the animals for their pelts. The water rat is the chief reservoir host in Russia, and a common chain of infection is water rat to field mouse to house mouse to man. Wild rats in Los Angeles and field mice in other parts of California have been found naturally infected and human cases may have been traced to them.

Squirrels. Tree squirrels have caused a number of cases among persons who dressed the animals. California ground squirrels and the ground squirrels in Utah and Montana are infected, but have caused few human cases.

Sheep. Outbreaks have been reported in sheep in Canada[25] and in Montana and Idaho.[26] Infection apparently occurs in early spring when sheep pass through sagebrush where wood ticks are abundant. Since only about half the tick-infested sheep become ill, it appears that these animals are rather resistant to tularemia. Only one authenticated human case has been reported from contact with sheep; in this instance a sheepherder was apparently infected while skinning carcasses.

Dogs. Calhoun, *et al.*[27] have demonstrated that in Arkansas dogs may be a primary reservoir of *P. tularensis* and a principal disseminator of the lone star tick. However, only a few cases of human infection have been attributed to direct contact with dogs.

Opossum. Several cases are reported among persons who had killed and skinned opossums.

Birds. A few human cases of tularemia have followed contact with pheasants and sage hens[28] as well as with the Columbian grouse, chicken hawk, horned owl and quail. Tularemia infection has been demonstrated in sharp-tailed grouse and ruffed grouse in Minnesota and those birds are potential sources of danger.

Miscellaneous Animals. Human cases also have followed contact with the following animals: beaver, catfish, coyote, deer, red fox, ground hog, mink, muskrat, pig, raccoon, skunk, bull snake and mountain ground squirrel. In many instances the victim of the disease had skinned or dressed the animal. Several human cases followed the scratch of the cat, the infection apparently being on the claws from contact with an infected animal.

Eye Infections. A considerable number of eye infections have been reported, the organism being transferred to the eye by the hands while the person was dressing rabbits or after crushing flies or ticks. Several cases resulted from infected material squirting into the eye from the animal being dressed.

THE DISEASE IN MAN

The incubation period of tularemia is about three days, varying from one to nine days. The onset is sudden often occurring while the patient is at work. There is headache, chilliness, vomiting, fever, and aches and pains in various parts of the body. The sore at the site of the initial lesion develops, while the associated lymph nodes become enlarged and tender. The duration of the disease is about three to four weeks with sweating, loss of weight and much debility. Convalescence is slow, covering a period of two or three months. Cases without complications usually recover with no bad after effects and usually with a solid immunity against a second attack. Several second attacks with production of systemic disease and recovery of the organism have occurred among heavily exposed laboratory workers. Foshay[29] reported a case that was apparently recovered but which developed a local lesion several months later from which tularemia organisms could be cultivated. He drew attention to the danger of tularemic infection in those with preexisting vascular disease. Tularemic pneumonia is being reported more and more often and is a serious complication.[30] The tularemia organism is present in the sputum, not only of persons with pneumonic lesions, but also of those suffering from other types of the disease.[31] This situation, involving an organism with known ability to penetrate unbroken skin and mucosa, would ordinarily arouse concern about the likelihood of cross infections in wards and secondary infections among bedside attendants and family. However, the actual forty year experience is that no such secondary cases have yet occurred, even despite the customary hospital practice of not enforcing isolation of tularemic cases.

Several clinical types of tularemia have been reported.

1) Ulceroglandular, the primary lesion being a papule, later an ulcer of the skin and accompanied by enlargement of the regional lymph nodes.

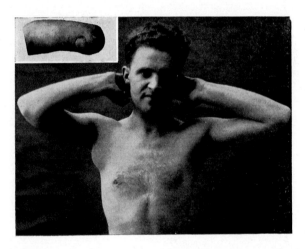

Fig. 108. Ulcer of right finger with axillary abscess in case of tularemia.

2) Oculoglandular, the primary lesion being a conjunctivitis and accompanied by enlargement of the regional lymph nodes. Fulminant cases, running a rapid course, with death, have been noted in the oculoglandular type.

3) Glandular, without primary lesion, but with enlargement of the regional lymph nodes.

4) Typhoidal, without primary lesion and without glandular enlargements.

5) Pneumonic, usually without primary lesion and without glandular enlargements.

6) Meningitic, a rather rare occurrence in this country[32] but not infrequent in Asia under certain conditions of insect transmission.[33]

7) Oropharyngeal, described as occurring often in Russia where drinking infected water is common, is less rare in U.S.A. than thought.[34]

Diagnosis of tularemia may be confirmed by several laboratory procedures. The most rapid is the fluorescent antibody test which

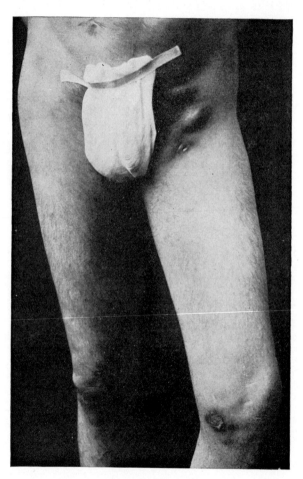

Fig. 109. Tularemia due to tick bite.

can be applied to organisms in sputum or local lesions. *P. tularensis* may be cultivated from lesions during the first two weeks of the disease in appropriate culture media or may be isolated from exudates or sputum by animal inoculation. Because the handling of live cultures of virulent *P. tularensis* is so hazardous to laboratory personnel, serologic tests are usually employed. Agglutination or flocculation tests usually become positive during the third week of the disease. The agglutination test remains positive for many years and may, therefore, be a source of error in diagnosis. Tularemia may also stimulate anamnestic reactions with brucella agglutinins which may lead to erroneous conclusions in regard to diagnosis.

TREATMENT

Streptomycin is quite effective in daily doses of 0.5 to 1.0 gram, and has completely replaced Foshay's antiserum. The tetracyclines and chloramphenicol are also effective in doses of 2.0 to 3.0 gm. per day given orally. The use of these drugs probably has caused the fatality rate to decline markedly; since 1950 it has been under 2 per cent in the U.S.A.

PREVENTION

Man can protect himself by avoiding contact with infected animals. It is probable that many cases of tularemia could be prevented ·if the opening of the rabbit hunting season would be delayed until after the onset of freezing weather in areas where this is feasible.[35]

In areas where ticks are important vectors of tularemia there is added reason for avoiding infestation with these arthropods and in removing them from the body as soon as possible.

Because of the possibility of water-borne infection with tularemia, it is advisable not to drink raw surface water especially in areas where tularemia is quite prevalent in wildlife.

Laboratory workers should wear rubber gloves and take all possible precautions known to medical science. Hunters, market men and cooks should wear rubber gloves while skinning and dressing rabbits. The hands should be thoroughly washed with soap and water after handling rabbits, even though only the fur is touched. Scratches and abrasions on the hands should be treated with a disinfectant.

Thorough cooking destroys infection, thus rendering a rabbit safe for eating purposes, even though it may have harbored the disease.

Isolation and quarantine of human cases are not necessary since the transmission of tularemia from person to person is extremely rare and then usually by easily preventable accidents.

An ordinance prohibiting the sale of wild rabbits has been used in some cities to reduce the morbidity and mortality of the disease during the rabbit hunting season.

IMMUNITY

Immunization is recommended for those exposed by occupation such as microbiologists and those in the wild rabbit industry and persons who hunt wild rabbits or spend a good deal of time in areas where the infection is spread by deerflies or ticks. Vaccination with killed cultures of *P. tularensis* achieved some success but apparently could not be relied upon to protect laboratory scientists exposed to aerosols of the highly virulent *P. tularensis* strains such as those isolated from the cottontail rabbit. It appears, however, that solid immunity against even this type of infection can be accomplished by inoculation with the recently developed live-culture vaccine.[36,37] Mass immunization of human beings with aerosolized attenuated *P. tularensis* has been employed in Russia.[38] Recently reported experiments[39] indicate that monkeys and guinea pigs develop greater immunity from aerogenic immunization than from dermae inoculations.

Those who have recovered from a naturally occurring infection are solidly immune and may engage in occupations leading to exposure with little danger of re-infection although an occasional second attack of the disease has been reported.

ITEMS OF NOTE

1) Tularemia is primarily a disease of rodents and rabbits, although many other animals are infected and act as hosts.

2) The disease is quite prevalent in North and Central America, Europe, and Asia. It is not known to be present in South America, Africa, or Australasia.

3) About 90 per cent of human cases in the U.S.A. are acquired from rabbits, chiefly the cottontail.

4) Ticks are an increasing source of infection in the U.S.A.

5) In Europe and Asia human infections are acquired usually from rodents or from water contaminated by them.

6) Strains of *P. tularensis* from rabbits, ticks or sheep are much more virulent than those isolated from rodents, birds or water.

7) Prevention of tularemia depends on avoidance of infection and, in highly exposed groups, vaccination with attenuated vaccine.

REFERENCES

1. HORNE, H.: *Zbl. Bakt. I. Orig., 66:*169-178, 1912.
2. McCOY, G. W.: U.S. Pub. Health Service. *Pub. Health Bull., 43:*1911.
3. McCOY, G. W. and CHAPIN, C. W.: U. S. Pub. Health Service. *Pub. Health Bull., 53:*1912.
4. WHERRY, W. B. and LAMB, B. H.: *J. Infect. Dis., 15:*331-340, 1914.
5. SATTLER, ROBERT. *Arch. Ophth., 44:*265-269, 1915.
6. LAMB, F. W.: *Ophth. Rec., 26:*221-226, 1917.
7. WHERRY, W. B.: *Pub. Health Rep., 29:*3387, 1914.
8. WHERRY, W. B., and LAMB, B. H.: *J.A.M.A., 63:*2041, 1914.
9. PEARSE, R. A.: *Northwest Med., 3:*81-84, 1911.
10. FRANCIS, E.: Tularemia Francis 1921. *Hyg. Lab. Bull., 130,* 1922.
11. FRANCIS, E.: *Pub. Health Rep. 38:*1391-1396, 1919.
12. JELLISON, W. L., EPLER, D. C., KUHNS, E. and KOHLS, G. M.: *Pub. Health Rep., 65:* 594-597, 1950.
13. GREENE, R. J.: *Am. J. Hyg., 38:*282-292, 1943.
14. FRANCIS, E.: *Pub. Health Rep., 52:*103-113, 1951.
15. JELLISON, W. L. and PARKER, R. R.: *Am. J. Trop. Med., 25:*349-362, 1945.
16. WARRING, W. B. and RUFFIN, J. S., JR.: *New England J. Med., 234:*137-140, 1946.
17. HILLMAN, C. C. and MORGAN, M. T.: *J.A.M.A., 108:*538-540, 1937.
18. OLIN, G.: *Bull. Off. Internat. Hyg. Pub., 30:*2804-2807, 1938.
19. KARPOV, S. P., POPOV, V. M., SLINKINA, A. G., CHERNYSHEV, F. I. and RIAZANTSOV, M. I.: *J. Microbiol. Epidemiol. Immunobiol., 7/8:*24-28, 1943.
20. GLASS, G. B. J.: *Am. J. M., Sc., 216:*411-424, 1948.
21. AMOSS, H. R. and SPRUNT, D. H.: *J.A.M.A., 106:*1078-1080, 1936.
22. KARPOV, S. P. and ANTONOV, N. I.: *J. Bact., 32:*243-258, 1936.
23. JELLISON, W. L., KOHLS, G. L., BUTLER, W. J. and WEAVER, J. A.: *Am. J. Hyg., 36:* 168-182, 1942.
24. MAISKY, I. N.: *J. Microbiol. Epidemiol. Immunobiol., 7/8:*32-38, 1945.
25. GWATKIN, R.: *Canad. J. Comp. Med., 6:*163, 1942.
26. JELLISON, W. L. and KOHLS, G. M.: *Pub. Health Monograph, 28:*1-17, 1955.
27. CALHOUN, E. L., MOHR, C. O. and ALFORD, H. I.: *Am. J. Hyg., 63:*127-135, 1956.
28. KURSBAN, N. J. and FOSHAY, L.: *J.A.M.A., 131:*1493-1494, 1946.
29. FOSHAY, L. and MAYER, O. B.: *J.A.M.A., 106:*2141-2143, 1936.
30. STUART, B. M. and PULLEN, R. L.: *Am. J. M. Sc., 210:*223-236, 1945.
31. LARSON, C. L.: *Pub. Health Rep., 60:*1049-1053, 1945.
32. STUART, B. M. and PULLEN, R. L.: *Arch. Int. Med., 76:*163-166, 1945.
33. GLASS, G. B. J.: *M. Clin. North America,* May:769-778, 1948.
34. HUGHES, W. T. and ETTELDORF, J. N.: *J. Pediat. 51:*363-372, 1957.
35. YEATTER, R. E. and THOMPSON, D. H.: *Bull. Ill. Nat. Hist. Survey, 25:*351-382, 1952.
36. HITCHNER, S. B. and REISING, G.: *Proc. Am. Vet. M. A.,* 89th Annual Meeting, 258, 1952.
37. GORHAM, J. R., LEADER, R. W. and GUITERREZ, J. C.: *Science, 119:*125, 1954.

38. ALEKSANDROV, N. I., GEFEN, N. Y., GARIN, N. S., GAPOCHKO, K. G., DAAL-BERG, I. I. and SERGEYER, V. M.: *Voyenno-Meditsinskiy Zhurnal, 12:*134-142, 1958.
39. EIGELSBACH, H. T., TULIS, J. J., OVERHOLT, E. L. and GRIFFITH, W. R.: *Proc. Soc. Exper. Biol. & Med., 108:*732-734, 1961.

Chapter 23

PSEUDOTUBERCULOSIS

WILLIAM H. FELDMAN, D.V.M., D.SC.
and ALFRED G. KARLSON, D.V.M., PH.D.

PSEUDOTUBERCULOSIS is a disease of guinea pigs, wild rodents and wild birds caused by *Pasteurella pseudotuberculosis.* This microorganism is capable of producing natural infections with varying degrees of severity in a long list of fowls and mammals including man.*

It is generally believed that infection in guinea pigs with *Pasteurella pseudotuberculosis* was first observed by Malassez and Vignal[33] who, in 1883, described lesions in guinea pigs inoculated with a cutaneous lesion from the forearm of a child who had died of tuberculous meningitis. The lesions in the guinea pig resembled those of tuberculosis although tubercle bacilli were not demonstrable by staining. These workers thought that the disease in the guinea pigs was due to a transitional form of tubercle bacilli.[34] Presumably Malassez and Vignal were not aware of the fact that guinea pigs are sometimes naturally infected with a purulent granulomatous disease. It seems likely that these workers did observe pseudotuberculosis in guinea pigs but did not recognize the true nature of the etiologic agent.

Subsequent to the reports of Malassez and Vignal, Eberth[17,18] recorded his observations on a naturally acquired tuberculosislike disease in guinea pigs[17] and in rabbits[18] which he designated as "pseudotuberculosis." The microorganism was observed subsequently and described by others, and in 1894 Preisz named the disease "pseudo-

---

*The term "pseudotuberculosis" sometimes is used in veterinary pathology to designate several infections occurring in different species. Caseous lymphadenitis in sheep caused by *Corynebacterium pseudotuberculosis* is commonly called "pseudotuberculosis." In mice, infection with *Corynebacterium kutscheri* is called "pseudotuberculosis." For a brief discussion of so-called pseudotuberculosis of different species the account by Topley and Wilson[61] may be consulted.

tuberculosis rodentium" to emphasize its predominant occurrence in rodents such as guinea pigs and rabbits. Preisz also noted that this infection had been seen in animals other than rodents and that it was widespread in nature.

The microorganism has been designated by a variety of names such as *Bacillus pseudotuberculosis, Streptobacillus pseudotuberculosis rodentium, Corynebacterium rodentium, Corynebacterium pseudotuberculosis,* and *Shigella pseudotuberculosis rodentium.* It was placed in the genus *Pasteurella* by Topley and Wilson.[60] McDiarmid has written that pseudotuberculosis is of greater importance in birds than in mammals and, therefore, the term "rodentium" is justifiably dropped from the name of the microorganism. It has been recommended by Loghem that a separate genus, *Yersinia,* be established for the microorganisms of plague and of pseudotuberculosis because these two bacteria have many features unlike pasteurellae in general.

BACTERIOLOGIC FEATURES

Morphologically and biologically the microorganism is capable of many variations depending on the duration of artificial cultivation, the age of the culture, the type of medium used and the temperature of incubation. Many of the variables are not necessarily significant but should be recognized when one attempts to identify newly isolated cultures. As a standard of reference the following description is paraphrased in part from Bergey's Manual.[8]* *Pasteurella pseudotuberculosis* is a small pleomorphic, gram-negative rod of varying sizes (Fig. 110). Single cells may be ellipsoid, coccoid, or rod-shaped with rounded ends occurring singly or in short chains; occasionally long curved filamentous forms are seen. Bipolar staining is variable in occurrence.

Studies by Preston and Maitland on motility of *Pasteurella pseudotuberculosis* may be summarized as follows: The microorganism is motile and has one to six flagella when grown at 22° C.; it is nonmotile and nonflagellated when grown at 37° C. This change from a motile to a nonmotile form takes place at approximately 30° C. Nonmotile strains grown at 37° C. may develop flagella and

---

*For a description of the growth characteristics of newly isolated strains from a variety of different species the following references may be consulted: Bishop, Blaxland, Eieland, Topping, Watts and Lillie, Moss and Battle, Thal, and Knapp.[27]

become motile when grown at 22° C. A review of the literature on motility of *Pasteurella pseudotuberculosis* plus electron micrographs of flagellated cells is provided by Knapp.[27]

Growth usually occurs readily at 37° C. on ordinary medium but the optimal temperature for rapid growth is 30° C. Some observers report that occasionally isolations of *Pasteurella pseudotuberculosis*

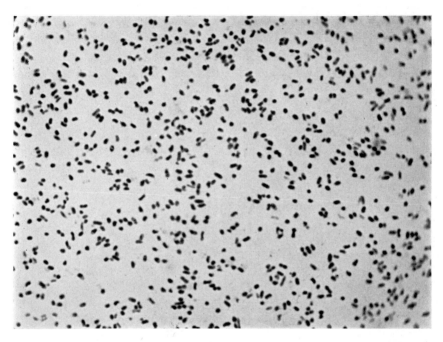

Fig. 110. *Pasteurella pseudotuberculosis* from human source. Bacterial cells stained with dilute carbol-fuchsin and showing pleomorphic, coccoid and bipolar forms. Twenty-four hour subculture grown on blood serum agar slant at room temperature (x1,800). (Culture obtained through courtesy of Dr. K. F. Meyer, University of California.)

from lesions may succeed only by incubation at room temperatures; it is therefore recommended that incubation temperatures of 22° C. and 37° C. be used.[27] On agar the growth is seen in twenty-four to forty-eight hours as confluent, raised, grayish, translucent, glistening colonies with irregularly lobate edges. Hemolysis does not occur on blood agar. In broth, moderate turbidity is seen after twenty-four hours; later it clears to form a viscous sediment and a ring pellicle. Litmus milk becomes alkaline; indole is formed; nitrates are reduced; acetyl-methyl-carbinol is not formed, and results of the methyl red test are positive.

Pasteurella pseudotuberculosis splits urea, whereas *Pasteurella pestis* does not; this is an important differential characteristic.[1,59] On desoxycholate citrate agar the microorganism of pseudotuberculosis grows abundantly to form large opaque yellowish colonies; in contrast, *Pasteurella pestis* grows scantily on this medium in the form of pin-point reddish colonies.[1] The occurrence of pseudotuberculosis as well as plague in rodents and the similarities between the lesions necessitate accurate bacteriologic diagnoses. Some differential characteristics of the pasteurellae that may be found in animals are given in Table 57.

TABLE 57

Some Distinguishing Features of Three Members of the Genus Pasteurella*

	Pasteurella Pseudotuberculosis	*Pasteurella Pestis*	*Pasteurella Multocida*
Growth on agar plates	Rapid, luxuriant and spreading	Slight, confluent, limited to line of inoculation	Fine, transparent
Motility	Nonmotile at 37° C. Motile at 18° to 22° C.	Nonmotile	Nonmotile
Litmus milk	Definitely alkaline	No change or slightly acid	No change
Urease	+	−	±
Indole	−	−	+
Acid fermentation			
Maltose	+	±	−
Rhamnose	+	−†	−
Sorbitol	−	−	+
Sucrose	−‡	−	+
Melibiose	+	−	−
Virulence for wild rat	+	+	−
Virulence for albino rat	−	+	−

*Data compiled from various sources.[1,8,27,50,53,57]
†According to Pollitzer,[42] *Pasteurella pestis* almost invariably fails to acidify rhamnose, but in some instances delayed acidification may occur.
‡A few strains produce acid from sucrose.

RESISTANCE TO PHYSICAL AND CHEMICAL AGENTS

The resistance of *Pasteurella pseudotuberculosis* to desiccation is slight,[53] but lyophilized cultures have remained alive for at least two years.[27] In tissue the microorganisms have been found after storage for eighteen days at 40° C.[40] Studies by Knapp[27] on the resistance of *Pasteurella pseudotuberculosis* may be summarized as follows: Viable bacilli were found in organs after three months' storage at 2° C., for ten to twenty days at 22° C., and for three to five days when stored at 37° C. For suspensions in milk, an exposure to 60° C. for 70 minutes killed only two of ten strains. In 0.85 per cent solutions of sodium chloride, exposures of 50° to 60° C. for 180 minutes did not regularly kill all strains; exposures of 70° to 80° C. for five minutes were required for sterilization of bacterial suspensions. The microorganisms were killed in 0.5 minute by 5 per cent phenol, 5 per cent formalin, 0.1 per cent mercuric chloride and by 75 per cent alcohol.

Harisijades used the tube-dilution method to examine seven strains of *Pasteurella pseudotuberculosis* and found them to be inhibited by the following antibacterial agents in concentrations of micrograms per milliliter of medium as follows: terramycin, 3.1 to 6.3; aureomycin, 12.5; streptomycin, 1.6 to 3.1; chloromycetin, 1.6 to 3.1; and by 12.5 to 50 units of penicillin. Additional studies on the in vitro effect of various antibacterial drugs have been summarized by Knapp.[27]

ANTIGENIC FEATURES AND IMMUNITY

Thal[57] examined 186 cultures of *Pasteurella pseudotuberculosis* and found that they could be classified into five types, designated I, II, III, IV and V based on the presence of group specific somatic or 0 antigens. Types I, II, III and V have a common flagellar or H antigen and all have a common R antigen. Strains of types II and IV have antigens in common with *Salmonella* of group B and D respectively.[28,58] Of particular importance is the occurrence of antigens in common with *Pasteurella pestis* which has been studied by many workers.[3,11,14,58]

Burrows and Bacon found that antigens essential for high virulence of *Pasteurella pestis* were possessed by many strains of *Pasteurella pseudotuberculosis*. These investigators were of the opinion that this finding supported the hypothesis that *Pasteurella pestis* sporadically is derived from *Pasteurella pseudotuberculosis* in nature, which may account for the alternation of epidemics of plague.

Thal[57] found that an exotoxin was formed in vitro by some strains of *Pasteurella pseudotuberculosis* of type III. A toxoid prepared from the toxin stimulated the production in animals of an antitoxin. Thal found that under experimental conditions two kinds of immunity to pseudotuberculosis could be induced: 1) Avirulent live cultures produced a solid anti-infectious immunity against virulent strains but did not protect against the toxin. 2) The development of antitoxin afforded protection against the toxin but not against infection with nontoxic strains.

Active immunization of experimental animals has been demonstrated by many workers, but the results of vaccination with live or heat-killed cultures is not predictable; failures may occur if antigenically impotent strains are used. Of particular interest is the fact that in experimental animals *Pasteurella pseudotuberculosis* may produce immunity against infection with *Pasteurella pestis;* the reverse has not been achieved, however. The important aspects of immunity in infections due to *Pasteurella pseudotuberculosis*, particularly cross-immunity with *Pasteurella pestis,* have been reviewed by Pollitzer[42] and by Knapp.[27]

PATHOGENICITY FOR ANIMALS

Few bacteria are capable of infecting a greater number of animal species than is *Pasteurella pseudotuberculosis*. The following reports are cited to illustrate the geographic distribution and the many kinds of animals from which the microorganism has been isolated. In Sweden, Karlsson recorded that during the years 1938 through 1945 pseudotuberculosis had been diagnosed in swine, fox, mink, rabbits, nutria, guinea pigs, mice, and in four different species of birds. More recently Borg and Thal reported that in Sweden the disease had been seen in deer, otter, an owl, pheasants, and partridge; pseudotuberculosis was demonstrable in 154 (6.2 per cent) of 2500 wild hares examined in Sweden from 1948 to 1960. In Switzerland pseudotuberculosis accounts for 58 per cent of the septicemic disseases of hares and has also been seen in deer.[7] In France the microorganism was isolated from 300 of 683 (44 per cent) hares examined from 1931 to 1939.[64]

Girard and Chevalier studied a collection of *Pasteurella pseudotuberculosis* obtained in France from 1929 to 1958 which included cultures from cats, swine, monkeys, hares, guinea pigs, turkeys, a swan, a canary, and a duckling. A veritable epizootic of infection was seen in a group of monkeys in a menagerie in France.[63]

In Scotland the microorganism was demonstrated by bacteriologic studies in cases of orchitis in rams[24] and it has been isolated from a goat in India.[47] In Australia,[46] *Pasteurella pseudotuberculosis* was found to be the cause of a serious outbreak of infection in sheep characterized by hepatic abscesses. The microorganism also was isolated from dead magpies found in the vicinity of the sick and dead sheep.

An outbreak of infection in doves with a high mortality was described in England, and the microorganism was demonstrable in other birds in the immediate area.[12] In England also, the infection was seen in bats.[36] *Pasteurella pseudotuberculosis* has been isolated from a variety of wild rodents in Russia and has been studied extensively there in relationship to plague.[43] A report from Germany[56] records the finding of pseudotuberculosis in cats, turkeys, rabbits, and in an anteater. In the Netherlands, where the disease exists in hares and in guinea pigs, it was also demonstrated in a lion in a zoologic garden.[16] In North America few reports have been made of finding *Pasteurella pseudotuberculosis* in animals. It has been reported in guinea pigs,[4] a black bird,[2] turkeys,[35,49] and chinchillas.[30]

The summary is by no means complete; it merely emphasizes that infection with *Pasteurella pseudotuberculosis* is widespread and involves many kinds of wild and domestic animals and fowl. Additional reports are referred to by Knapp,[27] Stephan, Stafseth, Borg and Thal and Pallaske and Krahnert.

Considering the large number of species of animals susceptible to natural infection with *Pasteurella pseudotuberculosis,* it seems strange that this disease is not reported more frequently. It is of course possible that the infection does exist but that, as yet, it has not been widely recognized. A survey of many cases reveals: 1) that the disease rarely has been recognized in animals in North America, 2) that the reports have pertained predominantly to instances of its occurrence in western Europe, 3) that the disease usually has appeared sporadically except in guinea pigs, hares, and turkeys in which it may be epizootic, and 4) that the disease is of a low order of contagiousness except in a few instances.

Nothing is known about the means of transmission of this disease. McDiarmid suggested that green crops may be contaminated by infected animals and thus may be a source of infection. It is assumed by most writers on the subject that transmission occurs via the oral route by means of food and water contaminated by feces of infected animals.

Pathologically, pseudotuberculosis, as it occurs naturally in animals, is essentially a necrotizing purulent granulomatous disease. It is characterized by the formation of a few to innumerable nodular foci of variable sizes. The lesions occur most frequently as grayish white or as white discrete nodules in the liver and spleen (Fig. 111). The lungs are affected less frequently than the other organs. The lesions contain purulent or caseous material. Diarrhea may occur, and

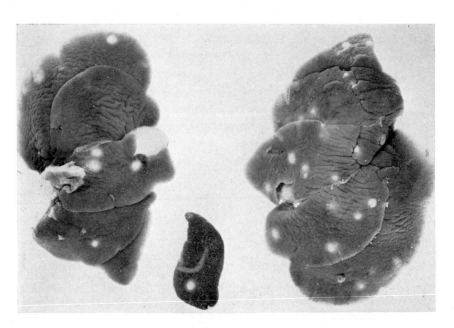

Fig. 111. Naturally acquired pseudotuberculosis in guinea pigs. The well-delineated multiple whitish nodules in the livers and the nodules in the spleens are characteristic of the disease following natural infection. (Photograph furnished through the courtesy of Dr. W. L. Boyd, Division of Veterinary Medicine, University of Minnesota.)

the lymphoid deposits of the intestine and mesentery are likely to be swollen and confluent and to contain purulent or caseous abscesses. The infection is usually septicemic, especially during the early or active phase of the pathogenesis, and *Pasteurella pseudotuberculosis* can be cultivated from the blood as well as from the morbid tissues.

Experimental transmission of the infection is readily achieved in susceptible animals such as guinea pigs or white mice. In guinea pigs the character of the resultant infection depends on the route of inoculation and the dose of the inoculum[4] (Fig. 112).

Briefly, the microscopic appearance of the lesion is that of a necrobiotic process of the parenchyma with a subsequent influx of neutrophils which, in turn, necrose and undergo fragmentation.

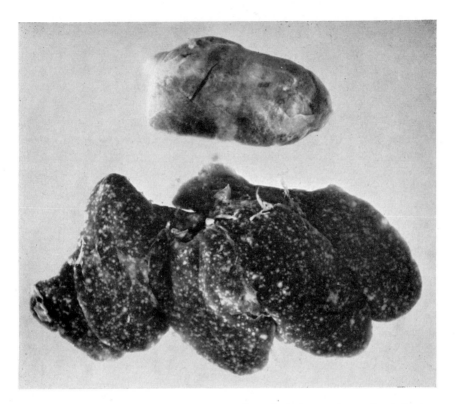

Fig. 112. Experimentally induced pseudotuberculosis in a guinea pig. Infection induced by subcutaneous inoculation of suspension of *Pasteurella pseudotuberculosis*. Note the enlarged spleen with fibrinous exudate. The lesions in the liver are miliary and are more numerous than those shown in Figure 111. (Photograph obtained through the courtesy of Dr. W. L. Boyd, Division of Veterinary Medicine, University of Minnesota.)

Bacteria are frequently numerous in the midst of the cellular detritus. Epithelioid cells appear rarely except in lesions of considerable duration. Bacterial emboli may form in the smaller vascular channels. As the pathogenesis becomes quiescent, peripheral fibrocytic proliferation indicative of healing characteristic of a chronic infectious granulomatous process is apparent. Giant cells are not observed.*

PATHOGENICITY FOR HUMAN BEINGS

In 1951, Meyer reported that there were only seventeen cases of *Pasteurella pseudotuberculosis* infection in man on record and that, of these seventeen, only four had been encountered in the United States. Knapp and Masshoff could find only fourteen cases that had been bacteriologically proved prior to their report in 1954. In 1955, Feldman stated that pseudotuberculosis is one of the rarest diseases of human beings; he gave a synoptic review of fourteen cases from the literature from 1910 to 1949 which may be summarized as follows: Twelve of the fourteen patients were men; the youngest patient was fourteen years of age and the oldest sixty years, seven of the fourteen patients having been from thirty to forty-nine years of age. The duration of illness ranged from four days to nine weeks. However, all but two patients died. With two exceptions, death occurred within three weeks of onset of disease.

Among the symptoms noted in various cases were headaches, chills, vomiting, diarrhea, leukocytosis, fever, icterus, and enlarged liver and spleen with abdominal tenderness or pain, especially in the right upper quadrant.

The important necrospy findings which characterized these fourteen cases collected from 1910 to 1949 concerned changes in the liver, the spleen, and the mesenteric lymph nodes. Less frequently, ascites and ulcerative enteritis were noted. The liver and spleen usually were swollen, and one or both of these organs contained few to innumerable circumscribed nodular lesions variable in size and grayish white or yellow (Fig. 113). The nodules were necrotic and usually contained purulent or caseous material from which *Pasteurella pseudotuberculosis* was isolated (Fig. 114). Lymph nodes, when affected, had circumscribed diffuse areas of necrotic material in which the microorganism was present.

Aside from the rare and usually fatal form of pseudotuberculosis in adults, there has been recognized in the last decade a commoner

---

*Additional information on the pathologic changes of experimental and naturally occurring pseudotuberculosis in animals may be found in the following references: Topping, Watts and Lillie, Moss and Battle, Pallaske and Krahnert and Communal.

and more benign infection which occurs primarily in children and which Mair and associates have aptly described as "acute mesenteric adenitis mimicking appendicitis." Interest in this form of pseudotuberculosis was stimulated by the report in 1954 of Knapp and Masshoff who recorded the isolation of *Pasteurella pseudotuberculosis* from enlarged mesenteric lymph nodes of children operated on for appendicitis but whose appendices were found to be normal.

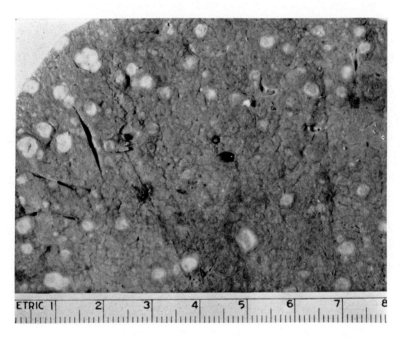

Fig. 113. Pseudotuberculosis in liver of woman seventy-three years of age. Cut surface of organ showing the distribution and gross appearance of numerous discrete lesions of variable sizes. (Photograph supplied by Dr. David G. Mason, Pathologist, Providence Hospital, Seattle, Washington.)

In addition, agglutinins specific for the microorganism were demonstrable in the blood. Knapp and Masshoff described the principal lesion as an "abscess-forming reticulocytic lymphadenitis."

A few cases of this kind of pseudotuberculosis had been reported previously, and since the publication of the paper by Knapp and Masshoff in 1954 there have been reports from various European countries. The diagnosis of pseudotuberculosis has been made by culture of the microorganism or by demonstration of specific agglu-

tinins. In 1958, Knapp[26] wrote that the new disease complex had
been seen in 117 patients in one institution in Germany. A detailed
description and review of the literature were provided by Knapp[27]
in 1959. In 1960, Mollaret[38,39] and Destombes and Mollaret reviewed
the world literature pertaining to acute mesenteric adenitis caused
by *Pasteurella pseudotuberculosis* and presented data from thirty

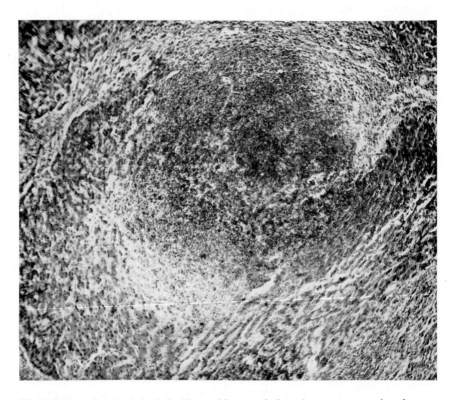

Fig. 114. Pseudotuberculosis in liver of human being. Severe progressive destructive process with a minimum of peripheral reaction. Same case as Figure 113
(x27). (Illustration prepared from material supplied by Dr. K. F. Meyer, University of California.)

cases encountered in France. The first cases reported in the English
language were those of Mair and associates in 1960.

Briefly, the characteristic features of mesenteric adenitis due to
Pasteurella pseudotuberculosis are as follows: The infection is seen
oftenest in young males. Of thirty cases reported by Mollaret,[38]
twenty-five patients were males. The range in age was three to seven-

teen years except for two patients who were three months and thirty years old respectively. The presenting symptoms are those of acute appendicitis; leukocytosis and elevation of temperature are common. Operation discloses a normal appendix but there are enlargement and congestion of a single node or of groups of mesenteric lymph nodes, usually at the ileocecal valve or on the medial aspect of the ascending colon. The histopathologic picture, while not specific, is characteristic (Fig. 115). A single abscess or multiple small abscesses with central necrosis are found as well as a peripheral zone of proliferating reticulum cells with no evidence of fibrosis.[15,27,32] Specific agglutinins are demonstrable at titers up to 1 to 12,800 which may persist for several months after removal of the affected mesenteric lymph nodes.[26,32] No specific treatment is known.

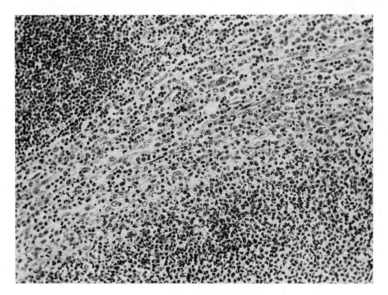

Fig. 115. Histopathology.

DIAGNOSIS

It has been emphasized that infections due to *Pasteurella pseudotuberculosis* can be established with certainty only by bacteriologic procedures.[57] The clinical signs are not characteristic, and their proper interpretation may constitute a diagnostic dilemma. In one instance in which[40] the diagnosis was not established while the patient was living, the following disease entities were considered: typhoid fever, tularemia, malaria, spinal epidural abscess, perinephric abscess, hepatic amebiasis, abdominal Hodgkin's disease, lymphosarcoma, relapsing fever, rat-bite fever and other spirochetal infections. Reimann and Rose also have drawn attention to several features that pseudotuberculosis has in common with tularemia. The commoner form of the infection in man, acute mesenteric lymphadenitis, must be differentiated from appendicitis and from other acute or subacute abdominal conditions.[32,38] In a resumé of fifteen bacteriologically proved cases of this nature, a preoperative diagnosis of appendicitis had been made in twelve; for the others, tuberculous mesenteric lymphadenitis, salmonellosis, splenomegaly, neoplasm, and pericecal abscess had been considered.[27]

If a culture is obtained either directly from the patient or from guinea pigs inoculated with material from the patient which can be identified as belonging to the genus *Pasteurella,* the differentiating features listed in Table 57 may be useful in distinguishing *Pasteurella pseudotuberculosis* from *Pasteurella pestis* and *Pasteurella multocida.* From a bacteriologic point of view, *Pasteurella pestis* and *Pasteurella pseudotuberculosis* are similar in many respects. This is especially true as regards fermentation reaction with certain sugars. Furthermore, occasionally, atypical strains have been observed that have not conformed in all details to the characteristics that serve to establish identification. Consequently, the value of tests dependent on changes in the reaction of culture mediums cannot be accepted unequivocally as differential criteria in distinguishing the bacillus of plague from *Pasteurella pseudotuberculosis.*

Since it is recognized that strains of *Pasteurella pestis* and of *Pasteurella pseudotuberculosis* capable of certain atypical biochemical reactions may occur, it would seem desirable to subject new or freshly isolated strains suspected of being *Pasteurella pseudotuberculosis* to several tests of dissimilar character before a conclusion is reached.

An important diagnostic aid for pseudotuberculosis with acute abdominal symptoms is the agglutination test. The value of the test is based on the finding that agglutinins specific for *Pasteurella pseudotuberculosis* do not occur in normal persons nor in children with appendicitis.[26,27,52] Agglutination tests must be done with each of the five types of microorganisms. When reactions occur with antigens of types II and IV, the serums must be absorbed with salmonellae of groups B and D, respectively, because of the cross reactions that exist. Most cultures isolated from human beings having pseudotuberculosis have been type I.

During the acute stages of the illness and before removal of the affected lymph nodes, agglutination titers up to 1 to 12,800 have been recorded.[26,27,32,51] The titer may wane and disappear in one to four months, which, with the characteristic clinical signs and the histopathologic picture, is of great diagnostic value. The persistence of a high titer after surgical extirpation of the enlarged nodes may mean that a focus of infection persists. The agglutination test is particularly important in those cases in which attempts to isolate *Pasteurella pseudotuberculosis* have failed.

Gunnison, Larson and Lazarus proposed a rapid method for distinguishing *Pasteurella pestis* from *Pasteurella pseudotuberculosis* by means of bacteriophage specific for *Pasteurella pestis*. When the tests were done at 20° C. a distinction could be made between bacilli causing plague and those causing pseudotuberculosis. The results were less definitive when the tests were carried out at 37° C. Detailed descriptions for bacteriophage identification tests for bacilli causing plague are given by Baltazard and associates who, in 1956, wrote that some experts are inclined to ascribe greater value to differentiation by bacteriophage than by the biochemical tests. The Russian workers have not found the differentiation of plague and pseudotuberculosis microorganisms by bacteriophage to be wholly reliable.[43] The test requires a proper dilution of culture and a definite temperature. Some strains of *Pasteurella pseudotuberculosis* are lysed by bacteriophages for bacilli causing plague, especially if the concentration of microorganisms is too great. Knapp[27] has written that not enough experience has been obtained to judge the reliability of the test.

TREATMENT

Since practically all patients with a diagnosis of pseudotuberculosis of the septic form have died, it is obvious that therapeutic measures have been inadequate. The fact that two patients recovered[9,54] after treatment with sulfonamide and streptomycin, respectively, indicates the use of a similar approach. It should be recognized, however, that a well-established septic pseudotuberculosis represents more than bacteremia. The multiplicity of the lesions which may exist in the liver, spleen, and abdominal lymph nodes presents a formidable therapeutic problem even for a bactericidal agent of high potency.

In most cases of relatively benign mesenteric adenitis due to *Pasteurella pseudotuberculosis,* surgical treatment has been used because of the mistaken preoperative diagnosis of appendicitis. Removal of the affected lymph nodes usually is followed by an uneventful recovery. The value of antibacterial agents is difficult to assess. Mair and associates recommended that when the administration of antibiotics is considered necessary, the broad spectrum antibiotics are the drugs of choice.

ITEMS OF NOTE

1) Pseudotuberculosis due to *Pasteurella pseudotuberculosis* is a relatively rare disease. Many species of mammals and birds are susceptible to infection by this organism; yet the disease seldom has been recognized in man in America.

2) Pseudotuberculosis occurs occasionally in guinea pigs and may be sporadic or epizootic in character. The naturally occurring infection in guinea pigs must be recognized when these animals are used as an aid to diagnosis. In guinea pigs the disease must be differentiated from tuberculosis and brucellosis.

3) The septic form of human infections with *Pasteurella pseudotuberculosis* is exceedingly uncommon and appears to be limited to men. Most of the proved cases have occurred in Europe. Clinically, the disease has presented a difficult diagnostic problem, the true character of the illness finally being established by bacteriologic procedures. The organism has a predilection for the liver, spleen, and the lymph nodes of the mesentery. In practically all of the reported cases the patients have died.

4) The relatively benign form of infection usually attacks children, particularly boys. The presenting symptoms are those of an acute abdominal illness and a preoperative diagnosis of appendicitis is often made. Operation discloses a normal appendix but enlarged mesenteric lymph nodes. Microscopically, the lesions consist of small abscesses with proliferating reticulum cells surrounding a central zone of necrosis. The diagnosis is based on isolation of *Pasteurella pseudotuberculosis* or, more commonly, on the demonstration of specific agglutinins.

REFERENCES

1. BALTAZARD, M., DAVIS, D. H. S., DEVIGNAT, R., GIRARD, G., GOHAR, M. A., KORTMAN, L., MEYER, K. F., PARKER, M. T., POLLITZER, R., PRINCE, F. M., QUAN, S. F., and WAGLE, P.: Recommended laboratory methods for the diagnosis of plague. *Bull. World Health Org., 14:*457, 1956.

2. BEAUDETTE, F. R.: A case of pseudotuberculosis in a blackbird. *J.A.V.M.A., 97:*151, 1940.

3. BHAGAVAN, N. V., CHEN, T. H., and MEYER, K. F.: Further studies of antigenic structure of *Pasteurella pestis* in gels. *Proc. Soc. Exper. Biol. & Med., 91:*353, 1956.

4. BISHOP, LUCILLE M.: Study of an outbreak of pseudotuberculosis in guinea pigs (cavies) due to *B. peudotuberculosis rodentium. Cornell Vet., 22:*1, 1932.

5. BLAXLAND, J. D.: Pasteurella pseudotuberculosis infection in turkeys. *Vet. Rec. 59:* 317, 1947.

6. BORG, K. and THAL, E.: Pseudotuberkulosen Pasteurella (pseudotuberculosis) som zoonos. *Svenska läk.-tidning. 58:*1923, 1961.

7. BOUVIER, G., BURGISSER, H., and SCHNEIDER, P. A.: Les maladies des ruminants sauvages de la Suisse. Service Veterinair Cantonal et Institut Galli-Valerio Lousanne, 1958, 132 pp.

8. BREED, R. S., MURRAY, E. G. D., and SMITH, N. R.: *Bergey's Manual of Determinative Bacteriology,* Ed. 7. Baltimore, Williams & Wilkins, 1957, p. 399.

9. BURIANEK, J., MALKOVA, J., and TION, F.: Sepsis due to Pasteurella pseudotuberculosis. *Časop. lék. česk. 88:*775, 1949.

10. BURROWS, T. W., and BACON, G. A.: V and W antigens in strains of *Pasteurella pseudotuberculosis. Brit. J. Exper. Path., 41:*38, 1960.

11. CHEN, T. H., and MEYER, K. F.: Studies on immunization against plague. X. Specific precipitation of *Pasteurella pestis* antigens and antibodies in gels. *J. Immunol., 74:*501, 1955.

12. CLAPHAM, P. A.: Pseudotuberculosis among stock-doves in Hampshire. *Nature, 172:*353, 1953.

13. COMMUNAL, RENÉ: La pseudo-tuberculose du chat. Paris, Imprimérie R. Foulon, 1945, 125 pp.

14. DAVIES, D. A. L.: The smooth and rough somatic antigens of *Pasteurella pseudotuberculosis. J. Gen. Microbiol., 18:*118, 1958.

15. DESTOMBES, P., and MOLLARET, H. H.: L'adénite mésentérique aiguë à "Pasteurella pseudo-tuberculosis" (bacille de Malassez et Vignal). III. Étude anatomopathologique. *Presse méd., 68:*1485, 1960.

16. VAN DORSSEN, C. A.: Oriënteerende proeven over therapie en vaccinatie bij pseudotuberculosis van knaagdieren. *Tijdschr. voor Diergeneesk., 77:*235, 1952.

17. EBERTH, C. J.: Zwei Mykosen des Meerschweinchens. *Virchows Arch. path. Anat., 100:*15, 1885.

18. EBERTH, C. J.: Der Bacillus der Pseudotuberculose des Kaninchens. *Virchows Arch. path. Anat., 103:*488, 1886.

19. EIELAND, ERLINGS Infeksjon hos rev med Pasteurella (Bacterium)-pseudotuberculosis rodentium. *Norsk. vet. Tidsskr., 59:*1, 1947.

20. FELDMAN, W. H.: Pseudotuberculosis. In HULL, T. G.: *Diseases Transmitted From Animals to Man,* Ed. 4. Springfield, Thomas, 1955, pp. 358-377.

21. GIRARD, G., and CHEVALIER, A.: Classification sérologique de 56 souches de *Pasteurella pseudotuberculosis* dont 52 isolées en France. *Ann. Inst. Pasteur, 88:*227, 1955.

22. GUNNISON, J. B., LARSON, A., and LAZARUS, A. S.: Rapid differentiation between *Pasteurella pestis* and *Pasteurella pseudotuberculosis* by action of bacteriophage. *J. Infect. Dis., 88:*254, 1951.

23. HARISIJADES, S. S.: I. The action in vitro of some antibiotics on Pasteurella pseudo-tuberculosis. *Acta med. Jugoslavica, 7:*34, 1953.

24. JAMIESON, S., and SOLTYS, M. A.: Infectious epididymoorchitis of rams associated with Pasteurella pseudotuberculosis. *Vet. Rec., 59:*351, 1947.

25. KARLSSON, K. F.: Pseudotuberkulos hos hönsfåglar. *Skandinav. vet. tidskr., 35:*673, 1945.

26. KNAPP, WERNER: Mesenteric adenitis due to *Pasteurella pseudotuberculosis* in young people. *New England J. Med., 259:*776, 1958.

27. KNAPP, WERNER: Pasteurella pseudotuberculosis unter besonderer Berücksichtigung ihrer humanmedizinischen Bedeutung. *Ergebn. Hyg., Bakt., Immunitätsforsch, exper. Therap., 32:*196, 1959.

28. KNAPP, W.: Über weitere antigene Beziehungen zwischen Pasteurella pseudotuberculosis und der Salmonella-Gruppe. *Zeitschr. f. Hyg., 146:*315, 1960.

29. KNAPP, W., and MASSHOFF, W.: Zur Ätiologie der abszedierenden retikulozytären Lymphadenitis: Einer praktisch wicktigen, vielfach unter dem Bilde einer aktuen Appendizitis velaufenden Erkrankung. *Deutsche. med Wchnschr., 79:*1266, 1954.

30. LEADER, R. W., and BAKER, GRACIA, A.: A report of two cases of *Pasteurella pseudotuberculosis* infection in the chinchilla. *Cornell Vet., 44:*262, 1954.

31. VAN LOGHEM, J. J.: La classification du Bacille pesteux (*Yersinia* gen. nov.). *Ann. Inst. Pasteur, 72:*975, 1946.

32. MAIR, N. S., MAIR, HÉLÈNE J., STIRK, E. M., and CORSON, J. G.: Three cases of acute mesenteric lymphadenitis due to *Pasteurella pseudotuberculosis*. *J. Clin. Path., 13:*432, 1960.

33. MALASSEZ, L., and VIGNAL, W.: Tuberculose zoogloéique (forme ou espèce du tuberculose sans bacilles). *Arch. de physiol. norm. et path., s.3, 2:*369, 1883.

34. MALASSEZ, L., and VIGNAL, W.: Sur le micro-organisme de la tuberculose zoogloéique. *Arch. physiol. norm. et path., s.3, 4:*81, 1884.

35. MATHEY, W. J., JR., and SIDDLE, PHYLLIS, J.: Isolation of *Pasteurella pseudotuberculosis* from a California turkey. *J.A.V.M.A., 125:*482, 1954.

36. McDIARMID, A.: Diseases of free-living wild animals. FAO Working Document, Animal Health Branch Monograph No. 1, Rome, 1960, 91 pp.

37. MEYER, K. F.: Perspective concerning infections in animals transmissible to man. *Northwest Med., 50:*333, 1951.

38. MOLLARET, HENRI: L'adénite mésentérique aiguë à "Pasteurella pseudo-tuberculosis." (Bacille de Malassez et Vignal): A propos de 30 observations. I. Étude clinique sérologique et bactériologique. *Presse méd., 68:*1375, 1960.

39. MOLLARET, H. H.: L'adénite mésentérique aiguë à "Pasteurella pseudo-tuberculosis" (Bacille de Malassez et Vignal): À propos de 30 observations. II. Étude épidémiologique. *Presse méd., 68:*1447, 1960.

40. MOSS, EMMA S., and BATTLE, J. D., JR., Human infection with Pasteurella pseudotuberculosis rodentium of Pfeiffer. *Am. J. Clin. Path., 11:*677, 1941.

41. PALLASKE, G., and KRAHNERT, R.: Die durch Bakterien und pflanzliche Parasiten hervorgerufenen Infektionskrankheiten. I. Bakterien. 15: Pseudotuberkulose, sog. Nagertuberkulose. In COHRS, PAUL, JAFFÉ, R. and MEESSEN, H.: *Pathologie der Laboratoriumstiere*. Berlin, Springer-Verlag, 1958, vol. 2, pp. 22-28.

42. POLLITZER, R.: Plague. World Health Monograph Series, Geneva, No. 22, 1954, 698 pp.

43. POLLITZER, R. M.: Review of Russian papers on plague. Bethesda, Maryland. Na-

tional Institutes of Health, Russian Scientific Translation Service Program, 1958, 65 pp.

44. PREISZ, HUGO: Recherches comparatives sur les pseudotuberculoses bacillaires: Et une nouvelle espèce de pseudotuberculose. *Ann. Inst. Pasteur, 8:*231, 1894.

45. PRESTON, N. W., and MAITLAND, H. B.: The influence of temperature on the motility of *Pasteurella pseudotuberculosis*. *J. Gen. Microbiol., 7:*117, 1952.

46. PULLAR, E. M.: Pseudo-tuberculosis of sheep due to P. pseudotuberculosis rodentium (so-called pyemic hepatitis). *Australian Vet. J., 8:*181, 1932.

47. RAJAGOPALAN, V. R., and SANKARANARAYANAN, N. S.: A case of pseudotuberculosis (*Pasteurella pseudotuberculosis* infection) in the goat. *Indian Vet. Sci., 14:*34, 1944.

48. REIMANN, H. A., and ROSE, W. J.: The similarity of pseudotuberculosis and tularemia. *Arch. Path., 11:*584, 1931.

49. ROSENWALD, A. S., and DICKINSON, E. M.: A report on Pasteurella pseudotuberculosis infection in turkeys. *Am. J. Vet. Res., 5:*246, 1944.

50. SCHIPPER, G. J.: Unusual pathogenicity of Pasteurella multocida from the throats of common wild rats. *Bull. Johns Hopkins Hosp., 81:*333, 1947.

51. SCHMIDT, JOACHIM: Über Pasteurella pseudotuberculosis-Infektionen des Menschen. *Arch. f. Hyg., 143:*262, 1959.

52. SCHMIDT, JOACHIM: Untersuchungen über Durchseuchung der Bevölkerung mit Pasteurella pseudotuberculosis. *Zentralbl. Bakt., 180:*530, 1960.

53. SCHÜTZE, H.: B. pseudotuberculosis Rodentium Preisz. In Medical Research Council: *A System of Bacteriology in Relation to Medicine*. London, His Majesty's Stationery Office, 4:474, 1929.

54. SNYDER, G. A. C., and VOGEL, NAOMI J.: Human infection by Pasteurella pseudotuberculosis: Report of case with recovery. *Northwest Med., 42:*14, 1943.

55. STAFSETH, H. J.: Brucellosis, Anthrax, Pseudotuberculosis, Tetanus, Vibrio Infection and Avian Vibrionic Hepatitis. In BIESTER, H. E., and SCHWARTE, L. H.: *Diseases of Poultry*. Ed. 4, Ames, Iowa, Iowa State College Press, 1959, pp. 338-342.

56. STEPHAN, J.: Über die Ausbreitung des Bacillus pseudotuberculosis rodentium Pfeiffer, und seine Differenzierung. *Tierärztl. Rdsch., 47:*52, 1941.

57. THAL, ERNST: *Untersuchungen über Pasteurella pseudotuberculosis unter besonderer. Berücksichtigung ihres immunologischen Verhaltens*. Lund, Berlingska Boktryckeriet, 1954, 69 pp.

58. THAL, E.: Relations immunologiques entre *Pasteurella pestis* et *Pasteurella pseudotuberculosis*. *Ann. Inst. Pasteur, 91:*68, 1956.

59. THAL, E., and CHEN, T. H.: Two simple tests for the differentiation of plague and pseudotuberculosis bacilli. *J. Bact., 69:*103, 1955.

60. TOPLEY, W. W. C., and WILSON, G. S.: *The Principles of Bacteriology and Immunity*. New York, Wood, vol. 1, 1929, p. 482.

61. TOPLEY, W. W. C., and WILSON, G. S.: *Principles of Bacteriology and Immunity*, Ed. 4, vol. 2. (Revised by G. S. WILSON and A. A. MILES.) Baltimore, Williams & Wilkins, 1955, p. 1858.

62. TOPPING, N. H., WATTS, C. E., and LILLIE, R. D.: A case of human infection with B. pseudotuberculosis rodentium. *U. S. Pub. Health Rep., 53:*(pt. 2):1340, 1938.

63. URBAIN, A., and NAUVEL, J.: Epidémie de pseudotuberculose constatée sur des singes patas *"Erythrocelus patas"* (Schreber). *Bull. Acad. nat. de méd., 133:*299, 1949.

64. VAUTRIN, ANDRÉ: Contribution à l'étude de la pseudotuberculose du lièvre. (Thesis, Faculté de Médecine de Paris.) Paris, Imprimérie R. Foulon, 1949, 74 pp.

Chapter 24

LEPTOSPIROSIS

KARL R. REINHARD, D.V.M., PH.D.

LEPTOSPIROSIS is an etiological designation applied to a variety of syndromes caused by infection with parasitic members of the genus *Leptospira* of the order *Spirochaetales*. The clinical manifestations in man and animals are protean, varying from unapparent infection, to fever with malaise and meningismus, to severe renal and ictero-hemolytic disease. Pathological changes vary from inconspicuous lesions to severe parenchymatous degeneration, cellular infiltration and physiological derangement in the major solid viscera. More than forty types of *Leptospira* and a large, undetermined number of animal species are involved in this disease complex. The distribution of leptospirae and occurrence of leptospirosis, in its varied forms are world-wide, from subarctic to tropical areas.

The leptospiroses are zoonotic diseases; they extend to man from natural animal reservoirs, which are governed, in turn, by profound bionomic factors. A large number of domestic and wild animals are involved as hosts and reservoirs in the natural history of this disease complex. Synonyms are multitudinous; for example, Weil's Disease, mud fever, trench fever, swineherd's disease, rice-field fever, cane-cutters' fever, pea-pickers' fever, swamp fever, spirochaetal jaundice, Japanese autumnal fever, Japanese seven-day fever, Canicola fever, and flood fever.

The first clinical description of human leptospiral disease is ascribed to Weil,[1] who, in 1886, presented four cases in detail, which were characterized by hepatomegaly, splenomegaly, hemorrhagic tendencies and renal failure. Microbiological findings were not part of this description. In 1907, Stimson[2] first demonstrated spirochaetes, undoubtedly leptospirae, in histopathological specimens from a fatal case of "yellow fever." Leptospirae were not recovered in pure culture from human cases until 1915. At that time Inada and Ido,[3]

Huebnar and Reiter,[4] and Uhlenmuth and Fromme,[5] all accomplished the cultivation of leptospirae from cases of Weils Disease. In the years since these initial microbiological recoveries, factual information on the *Leptospira* and the leptospiroses have accumulated rather slowly. The leptospiroses remain one of the less-well understood zoonotic disease groups, despite their ubiquitous occurrence and the world-wide distribution of the agents and reservoirs.

CHARACTERISTICS OF LEPTOSPIRA

The organisms of this genus are well described morphologically by the name; lepto:thin; spira:spiral. They are cylindrical organisms about 0.1 micron or less in thickness, and four to twelve, or sometimes 30 to 40 microns in overall length. The organisms are con-

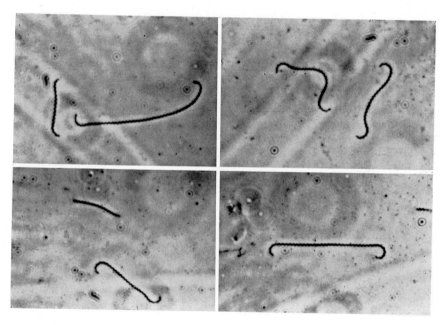

Fig. 116. Leptospira organisms.

voluted, forming regular, tight spirals about 0.5 microns in amplitude (see Figure 116). Electron microscopic pictures show the organism to have a filament or axistyle, around which the protoplast is wound.[6] They are hooked at one or both ends and are moderately flexible. Locomotion is achieved in fluid medium by a whirling motion around the longitudinal axis and by a serpentine or corkscrew motion in semisolid medium. They are intensely active, even in large aggregates, but movements have no apparent directional trophism. A few species are free living saprophytes in natural waters, but most of the known types are obligate parasites and persist for relatively short periods of time outside of the animal host.

No valid morphological or biochemical means have been found for taxonomic differentiation of species of the parasitic *Leptospira*. They are distinguished as serotypes, by virtue of antigenic differences. They stain with difficulty, and cannot be seen in the live state by brightfield microscopy. Darkfield or phase contrast microscopy must be used and, of the two, the darkfield technique is the easier and more generally used. In tissue, leptospirae are generally demonstrable by silver impregnation methods.[7] The difficulty in visualization by the ordinary bacteriological, tinctorial, and microscopical approach accounts for the frequent failures to diagnose leptospiral infections and this is aggravated further by highly fastidious cultural requirements which render the usual bacteriological media unsuitable for leptospiral culture. They grow well, but slowly, at pH ranges of 6.2 to 7.4, at temperature ranges of 25 to 38° C. in media that contain serum or similar biological materials in addition to customary nitrogen, carbohydrate and mineral salt components.[8] Once cultures are grown, they will remain viable for many weeks or months as long as the medium is kept from desiccation. Fluid and semisolid media are generally used for leptospiral cultivation, but a plate method for colony growth and counting has been devised.[9] Means of quick-freezing leptospiral cultures for long-term preservation have also been developed.[10-11]

Comparatively little work has been done to determine the exact nutritional requirements and intermediary metabolism of the *Leptospira*. Two studies of the amino-acid requirements of *L. canicola*[12,13] showed that glycine, lysine, tryptophane, arginine, aspartic acid, methionine, serine, and phenylalanine were utilized. One of these studies also demonstrated a rise in the amino acid content of media during leptospiral growth, indicating the presence of proteases and peptidases. Green and associates[14] developed a semisynthetic medium composed of dialyzed rabbit serum, mineral salts, amino acids, vitamins, and purine and pyrimidine bases, which supported growth of *L. canicola* through many serial transfers. Helprin and Hiatt[15] found that fatty acids stimulated respiration in L. icterohemorragiae, but that a serum fraction which serves as a "detoxifier" was required to support the reaction. Fulton and Spooner[16] demonstrated the production of minute quantities of fatty acids in leptospiral cultures. They also demonstrated a cytochrome oxidation system in the organisms. Nucleic acid, polysaccharide and lipid fractions of leptospira have been discerned by Schneider.[17] A hemolytic toxin has been found in some serotypes in several independent investigations.[18,19,20,21] The hemolysin was found to be thermolabile, non-dialyzable, and was more active at 37-38° C. Blood from ruminants was highly sensitive to leptospiral hemolysin although human and rabbit erythrocytes were also susceptible to some extent. Hemolysin prepared in culture showed *in vivo* activity in animals in the experiments of Kemenes.[22] The foregoing assorted nutritional, biochemical and physiological information on *Leptospira* represents only a fragment of that which is needed as a basis for understanding the pathogenetic activities and natural history of these organisms.

PATHOGENESIS AND SYMPTOMATOLOGY

The site of entry of leptospirae into the host is presumed to be through mucosal surfaces (conjunctival, nasal, oral and vaginal), and abraded or lacerated skin. These views are supported by experimental and epidemiological evidence. The initial locus of leptospiral proliferation, once entry has been made, has not been determined. There is abundant evidence from both experimental and clinical studies that the disease becomes septicemic early in the prodromal stage and that the proliferating leptospirae are thus disseminated throughout the body. The role of the lymphatic system in the distribution of the invasive leptospirae has not been determined, although pathological evidence has indicated lymphatic involvement. Within the first few days, the leptospirae are established in the various organs such as the spleen, liver, and kidney, and pathological changes are initiated. At the end of the prodromal stage, at the time serum antibodies become evident, the leptospirae are in the parenchyma of the liver and spleen, and are found between the tubules as well as in the tubule lumens in the kidneys, where they may persist and propagate for many weeks, and be shed in the urine.

The symptoms of leptospirosis are referable to pathologic involvement of the central nervous system, the erythropoietic system, the liver and the kidneys, and, at times, the eyes. The degree of involvement of the various systems varies from case to case. To some extent the serotype and strain of infecting Leptospira determines the pathological and clinical features of the disease. For instance, infections by *L. icterohaemorrhagiae* tend to cause icteric and renal symptoms in man, while *L. pomona* tends to produce aseptic meningitis. The host type may condition the symptomologic response; for example, *L. pomona* in cattle frequently produces hemolytic anemia, while in man the aseptic meningitis picture predominates. Other physiological conditions may condition response; to illustrate, epidemiological and experimental evidence has shown that abortions may tend to occur in animals which become infected in late pregnancy.[23,24] These are generalizations. For detailed discussions of the symptomatology, reviews such as those by Broom,[25] Ashe,[26] Van Thiel,[27] Gsell,[28] and the Symposium On The Leptospiroses (Walter Reed Army Medical Center),[29] should be consulted. For the purposes of this paper the pathogenesis will be discussed under five headings: 1) Hemolytic Anemia, 2) Hepatitis, 3) Nephritis, 4) Meningitis, and 5) Abortion.

Hemolytic anemia is the easier of the categories to discuss rationally because of the previously mentioned experimental evidence that certain strains produce a hemolysin or hemotoxin and that hemolysis can be produced *in vivo* by intravenous injection of culturally-prepared hemotoxin. The current thought on the mechanism of this reaction is that primary intravascular hemolysis produces secondary response in the hemapoietic system in the effort to replace the destroyed erythrocytes. The products of hemolysis lead to splenic congestion, may cause splenic, hepatic and renal hemosiderosis and produce general icterus. Should the hemolytic anemia become profound, systemic hypoxia leads to other metabolic derangements and possibly death.

The degree of pathologic involvement of the liver is quite variable in leptospirosis, and may have little correlation with the degree of functional change found in the diseased subject.[30] Centrolobular necrosis, dissociation of liver cords, and a general serous hepatitis may be found, but the cause is not apparent and the clinical hepatologic signs may greatly exceed, in degree, the relative amount of histopathologic liver damage. Erythrocyte destruction, due to hemolytic anemia may add to hepatic embarrassment due to the load of degradation products. Renal failure with uremia may also provoke hepatic dysfunction. All these factors contribute to liver damage, and even when icterus is not a feature of the disease, some hepatic pathology is present. A leptospiral cytotoxin other than hemolysin has been suggested, but never demonstrated conclusively.

Nephritis is one of the more constant and probably the most important pathologic involvement in leptospirosis, for it is through the urinary system that the disease is disseminated and perpetuated. The characteristic lesion is focal interstitial nephritis, with round cell infiltration and tubular necrosis. Leptospirae are found in the lesions, both in the parenchyma and in the tubule lumens. Glomerular ischemia, possibly due to intra-renal vascular shunt, complicates the pathophysiological picture.[25] Renal infection may persist for many months in convalescent animals and the leptospirae may be shed in urine, maintaining the cycle of disease. In the mild, unapparent cases, only a few foci of nephritis may form, but in more aggravated cases, when a major proportion of the renal tissue is affected, renal function may be so impaired that uremia, with its many systemic repercussions, may set in. Massive nephritis with uremia is thought to be a major cause of death in malignant leptospirosis. In dogs, and possibly some rodents, a chronic, progressive, cirrhotic nephritis may set in and cause debility or death eventually. The mechanism by which leptospirae stimulate nephritis is entirely unknown.

A very mild encephalitis has been found post mortem in some human patients.[26] However, the most common central nervous system involvement is serous meningitis, which is pathologically, relatively mild, but which can cause temporary debility. Temporary reduction in reflexes and regional paresis may occur. Nuchal rigidity is characteristic. Since almost all cases recover, histopathological evidence is scant. Cerebrospinal fluid shows the changes characteristic of non-suppurative meningitis.

Ocular complications warrant special discussion. These have been found more frequently in man and the horse than in the other animal species involved. Epidemiological, clinical and experimental evidence have shown that recurrent iridocyclitis of horses can be caused by leptospiral infection. Iridocyclitis (uveitis) has occurred as a complication in a large number of human cases of leptospirosis and some cases developed secondary glaucoma and cataract. An excellent discussion of ocular complications is given by King.[31]

Abortion has been observed in human, porcine, bovine and ovine cases of leptospirosis, and has been demonstrated experimentally in cattle,[23] sheep,[32] pigs,[33] and guinea pigs.[24] The more mature fetuses are more liable to be infected and aborted. The leptospirae are capable of penetrating the placental barrier and even capable of stimulating antibody response in fetuses that live for a number of days after infection.[23] Abortion, then, can be considered to be due to active intrauterine infection of the fetus and not secondary to maternal debility caused by leptospiral infection.

Susceptibility of various hosts to leptospiral infection and the degree of disease produced are not directly related. Rats, the smaller field rodents, and mature pigs seem to be quite susceptible to leptospiral infection, develop nephritis and may shed large numbers of leptospira in the urine, yet may give few or no overt signs of disease. Cats are resistant to infection. Ruminants, horses, dogs, and man are apparently highly susceptible to infection, a proportion develop severe and sometimes fatal disease, but, except for dogs, the convalescent renal shedding of leptospira is usually not massive. Recent epidemiological evidence indicates that earlier reports of a high mortality rate of leptospirosis in man and animals were in error, because only the more severe cases received clinical, serological, and microbiological attention, while the large proportion of mild or unapparent leptospiral infections were not perceived. A list of the range of symptomatology encountered in leptospiral infections is given in Table 58. The exhibition of all the listed signs in any one individual would be extremely rare. Most cases are relatively mild, and exhibit only a few clinical signs. A large proportion of leptospirosis in animals may be missed because the signs are mild and escape detection. Mild leptospirosis in people may mimic influenza or some of the more common bacterial or viral diseases, and thus be misdiagnosed.

THERAPY

Before the advent of the antibiotics, no specific chemotherapeutic agents were available for the treatment of leptospirosis. Arsenic and bismuth compounds were tried, to no avail, and in severely ill persons these drugs proved to be dangerous. Treatment with equine-origin antiserum or serum from recovered human cases was tried—

also with equivocal results. The studies by Larson[35] demonstrated that antiserum was effective only if administered in the prodromal period in experimental animals. Few natural cases are detected and diagnosed early enough to make specific antiserum therapy useful.

TABLE 58

SPECTRUM OF SYMPTOMATOLOGY OF LEPTOSPIROSIS INFECTIONS IN MAN AND ANIMALS

General Physical Signs

Fever	Chills
Depression	Rash
Weakness	
Weight loss	Retarded growth

Enteric Signs

Anorexia	Nausea
Emesis	Abdominal pain
Diarrhea or enteric stasis	

Hemorrhagic Signs

Increased capillary fragility
Submucosal, subserosal hemorrhage
Hemorrhage into body cavities and
  tissues
Hemoptysis, hematochesia
Hematemesis   Epistaxis

Hemolytic Signs

Pale mucosa and sclera
Hemoglobinemia
Hemoglobinuria
Increased erythrocyte fragility
Icterus
Urobilinuria

Nephritic Signs

Polydipsia	Polyuria
Albuminuria	Uremia
Oliguria (in severe cases)	
Elevated blood non-protein nitrogen	

Pulmonary Signs

Hyperpnea (in fever or advanced anemia)
Cough
Pulmonary congestion

Neurological Signs

Headache	Vertigo
Incoordination	Paresis
Hyperirritability	Coma
Hyperesthesia	Paresthesia
Opisthotonus (in severe cases)	
Delerium	Myalgia

Ophthalmic Signs

Episcleral injection
Conjunctivitis
Iritis
Uveitis

Reproductive Disorders

Fetal death	Abortion
Neonatal death	Placentitis
Delayed conception	

Disorders of Lactation

Oligogalactia
Agalactia
Dysgalactia

Clinical Pathology

Serum protein changes
Increased erythrocyte sedimentation rate
Leucocytosis (granulocytosis)
Leucopenia in cattle

Cardiovascular Signs

Tachycardia
Peripheral circulatory disturbances
Cardiac failure (in advanced cases)

Secondary Infections

Stomatitis   Pharyngitis   Herpes
Pneumonia   Enteritis

The sulfonamide compounds also proved to be therapeutic failures in treatment of leptospirosis.

Soon after penicillin became available, Larson and Griffitts[36] evaluated its therapeutic usefulness in extensive controlled studies in experimental animals. They found that antibiotic treatment was highly effective only when administered in the prodromal stage. After gross symptoms appeared, treatment with penicillin had little effect on the course of the disease. Chloramphenicol, streptomycin, chlortetracycline, tetracycline, and erythromycin also have been tested in experimental animals by a number of workers with essentially the same results: to be effective, the antibiotics must be administered early in the disease, before the end of the septicemic phase. Once the leptospira are well established in the tissues, the course of the disease seems to be predestined.

Various case reports, dealing with human and animal cases, have left the impression that antibiotic therapy is effective; however, the studies were not conducted under controlled conditions. Spontaneous remissions of the disease were not ruled out. Controlled therapeutic trials in natural human cases in Malaya[37] and Puerto Rico[38] showed that penicillin, streptomycin, chlortetracycline, tetracycline, bacitracin and chloramphenicol, were equally incapable of changing the clinical course of patients who were first treated when symptomatic. This experience serves to indicate that most symptomatic cases may not be amenable to antibiotic therapy. However, antibiotic administration, in maximum dosage, is a reasonable approach to therapy in any suspected case of leptospirosis, in the hopes that the disease is still septicemic and that the leptospiral spread can be checked. The matter of therapeutic ineffectiveness of antibiotics in the fully developed disease leads to consideration of the histologic location of the leptospirae and pathologic progress of the disease. With regard to the former question, we do know that histological response to the presence of leptospirae is non-suppurative, consisting mostly of dense infiltrations of round-cells. Neutrophilic responses are late, apparently to deal with cellular debris. The leptospirae are frequently seen in the intercellular spaces, and have been seen within cells. One might speculate whether these peculiarities of tissue reaction may impair antibody or antibiotic activity. A more logical hypothesis is that the pathological damage is well developed by the end of the septicemic stage and is beyond amelioration by antimicrobial therapy. Treatment other than antibiotic should be adjusted to the organic systems involved, and to the severity of the symptoms. Evidently anemia and renal failure with uremia are the most lethal factors in the disease. These should be monitored by appropriate clinical pathological tests and treated by the most effective means currently available.

In an interesting experiment reported by Ringen and Okazaki,[39] calves fed chlortetracycline at a level of 0.5 mg. per pound body weight, for a week previous to and two weeks after inoculation with virulent leptospira, remained free of symptoms of leptospirosis, although seven out of the nine subjects developed antibodies and may have been infected. In a therapeutic and prophylactic trial reported by Stoenner and associates,[40] a large laboratory mouse colony was freed from endemic leptospirosis by administration of chlortetracycline in the feed, for a period of ten days, coupled with introduction of specific hygienic precautions in the husbandry of the colony. Ringen and associates,[41] reported some decrease in the renal shedding of leptospira in cases of bovine leptospiroses, both natural and experimental, after administration of dihydrostreptomycin. These reports suggest that antibiotics may be valuable in prevention of disease, and in the reduction of the spread of leptospira from domestic carrier animals in the course of epizootic or epidemic leptospirosis.

IMMUNOLOGY-SEROLOGY

A strong persistent antibody response is characteristic of leptospiral disease in man and animals. Circulating antibodies are detectable as early as four days after infection and persist for many years. Six methods of serum antibody measurement have been used: these are: 1) the Microscopic Lysis-Agglutination Test, employing live leptospirae as antigen, 2) the Microscopic Agglutination Test, with chemically killed antigen; 3) the Macroscopic Agglutination Test, using a dense suspension of killed leptospirae, which is prepared and read in capillary tubes, or on glass plates; 4) the Erythrocyte-Sensitizing Test, in which sheep red cells are sensitized by exposure to leptospiral extracts and then hemolyzed by the action of leptospiral antibodies and complement; 5) the Complement Fixation Test, employing whole or fractionated leptospirae as antigens; and 6) Animal Protection Tests, which determine the effectiveness of graded antiserum doses in prevention of disease in experimental animals which receive a standard infective or lethal dose of leptospirae. None of these tests have been standardized nationally or internationally, and all have their peculiar technical encumbrances, limitations in interpretation, or sources of error.

The Lysis-Agglutination Test is the generally accepted reference test in leptospiral serology. It is conducted by mixing specific dilutions of antiserum with a standardized suspension of live leptospira. Reactions are read microscopically after several hours or overnight incubation. It has been used longer and more widely than any other test. It is, quantitatively, the most sensitive test available and will detect much lower levels of antibody than the other tests mentioned. Its disadvantage lies in the reading, which requires that samples of each dilution of the antiserum-antigen system be examined under the microscope. Two phenomena can be observed. One is the disintegration of leptospirae observed in that part of the test run with the less-diluted serums. The other is agglutination which occurs throughout the reactive dilutions of the test series. Agglutination differs qualitatively in different grades of serum dilution. For example, in an antiserum which reacts with leptospira throughout tenfold serum dilutions, from 1:10 to 1:100,000, lysis may occur only in the 1:10 and 1:100 dilutions. Agglutination will occur throughout the reactive range, but in the less diluted antiserum—perhaps 1:10 to 1:1,000—clumps may be loosely woven and flocculent. The agglutinated leptospirae in the more diluted antiserum will tend to form granular, spherical and compact aggregates. Figure 117 presents, comparatively, these types of agglutination. This qualitative difference in agglutination clumping has not been explained. It might involve different antigen and antibody components or be caused by quantitative relationships between antigen and antibody. Lysis proceeds slowly, and apparently is not dependent upon complement— but this point has not been closely investigated. The end product of lysis is an irregular mass of granular material which is quite different from the compact balls of fully-formed leptospira seen in the more diluted sera and end points. The titers which have been reported for agglutination test end-points are astounding; as high as 1×10^{-5} or 1×10^{-6}. It is possible that these excessively high titers are caused by the incomplete flushing of pipettes in preparation of serial serum dilutions for routine tests. Whether or not these extremely high reported titers are completely valid, it is still obvious that the agglutination-lysis test with live antigen is extremely sensitive. It is the test most likely to detect residual serum antibodies, years after the active disease. It is also highly specific for the infective serotype and for this reason the agglutination-lysis test, using a single serotype of *Leptospira* as antigen, cannot be used as a screening test for antibodies against other serotypes. However, because of its specificity, the test is useful in determining serotype-etiology and also in distinguishing and classifying cultures of leptospiral isolates.

The second type of test—microscopic agglutination—employs antigens composed of leptospiral cultures which have been killed and preserved, usually by addition of formalin. This test is prepared and read in the same way as the one first described, but lysis does not occur, and the reaction is read only as agglutination. The sensitivity

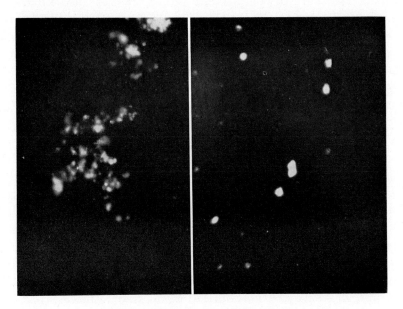

Fig. 117. Types of Agglutination.

of the microscopic agglutination test with formalinized antigen is not as great as that found with live antigen. The killed antigen also tends to clump spontaneously, which may lead to false positive tests, especially when inexperienced workers use the technique.

Macroscopic agglutination tests have been devised which employ concentrated, buffered suspensions of leptospirae in hypertonic saline solutions. Test systems employing such antigens can be set up and read in capillary tubes or on glass plates. Visualization of the reactions may be enhanced by staining of the antigen.[42,43,44] The most sensitive and carefully standardized macroscopic agglutination antigen was developed by Hoag, Gochenour and Yager.[45] Because of the greater concentration of antigen, the macroscopic agglutination tests suffer in sensitivity, and because of decreased sensitivity they are less likely to detect low, residual titers. However, they are useful for large-scale screening for current or recent cases of leptospirosis. They are also serotype-specific.

In recent years an erythrocyte-sensitizing test has been developed, arising from the discovery that leptospiral extracts could be absorbed on sheep blood red cells and render the latter susceptible to hemolysis in the presence of complement and leptospiral antibodies.[46,47,48] This is a useful screening test because of the convenient hemolysis indicator system and because the sensitizing antigen is genus specific, even to the extent that extracts from saprophytic leptospirae can be used to sensitize erythrocytes. The sensitivity is less than that of the macroscopic agglutination test. It is useful as a serological test for relatively recent infection by the genus *Leptospira,* but it will not distinguish leptospiral serotypes.

Complement fixation tests have been devised using whole,[49] disintegrated[50] and chemically fractionated leptospira.[51,52] The tests employing the first two types of preparation are genus-specific, while the chemical fractionation work has yielded both pentosan preparations which act as serotype-specific antigens and alcohol-soluble fractions which are genus-specific antigens. The former fraction is an incomplete antigen in that antibodies developed in response to pentosans do not agglutinate whole leptospirae. Complement fixation tests are rather insensitive, and complement-fixing antibodies are quite transitory, sometimes falling to undetectable levels in a few weeks or months after infection. The tests are useful, however, and can serve as indication of recent leptospiral infections.

Protection tests are not used diagnostically, but are valuable to determine immunologic cross reactions between serotypes, and to test the effectiveness of therapeutic antisera.

There is a great need to develop standard, simple, generally-acceptable techniques and reagents for diagnosis of leptospirosis and for the definition of serotypes. At present few laboratories can compare results because of individual variations of techniques and reagents. Borg-Petersen and Fagroeus did much to standardize a live-antigen test by their careful work to show the effect of antigen density and quality on the level of the end-titer.[53] More comprehensive and detailed information on the immunochemical composition of leptospirae is needed to elucidate taxonomic relations, demonstrate the chemical basis of biological variation and to improve diagnostic procedures.

TABLE 59

MAJOR LEPTOSPIRAL SEROGROUPS, SEROTYPES AND TYPE STRAINS

Sero-group		Serotype	Type Strain
I	1.	*L. icterohaemorrhagiae* AB	Wijnberg
	2.	*L. icterohaemorrhagiae* A	Kantorowicz
	3.	*L. naami*	Naam
	4.	———	Mankarso
II	5.	*L. javanica*	Rat Batavia 46
	6.	———	Poi
III	7.	*L. sarmini*	Sarmin
IV	8.	*L. schuffneri*	Vleerm 90-C
V	9.	*L. canicola*	Hond Utrecht
VI	10.	*L. benjamini*	Benjamin
VII	11.	*L. ballum*	Mus 127/S. 102
VIII	12.	*L. pyrogenes*	Salinam
	13.	*L. australis* B	Zanoni
IX	14.	*L. cynopteri*	Vleerm 3868
X	15.	*L. sentoti*	Sentot
XI	16.	*L. autumnalis* AB	Akiyama A
	17.	*L. autumnalis* A	Rachmat
	18.	———	Bankinang I
XII	19.	*L. djasimani*	Djasiman
XIII	20.	*L. australis* A	Ballico
	21.	———	Munchen C90
XIV	22.	*L. pomona*	Pomona
XV	23.	*L. grippotyphosa*	Moscow V
	24.	———	Duyster
	25.	———	Bernkopf
XVI	26.	*L. hebdomadis*	Hebdomadis
	27.	*L. medanensis*	Hond HC
	28.	*L. wollfi*	3705
	29.	———	Harjoprajitno
	30.	*L. sejroe*	M 84
	31.	*L. saxkoebing*	Mus 24
XVII	32.	*L. bataviae*	Van Tienen
	33.	———	Paidjan
XVIII	34.	*L. semaranga*	Veldrat
XIX	35.	*L. adaman* A	CH–11
XX	36.	*L. hyos* (mitis)	Mitis Johnson

Other serotypes and strains recently described, but not yet officially placed, are not cited here.
Adapted from Wolff, refs. (8) and (29).

Antibodies also have been demonstrated in the urine and milk of infected individuals by means of the agglutination, hemolysis or lysis test.[54,55,56,57] Tests employing urine and milk have distinct clinical pathological value in the acute and early convalescent stage.

The antigenic relationships among members of the *Leptospira* have served as a means of taxonomic division in the absence of criteria for speciation. More than forty serotypes have been established upon the basis of antigenic differences[8,30] and a number of variant, unclassified strains are still to be analyzed.[25] Most of the established types are listed in Table 59. Experiments in deliberate production of serologic mutation[58,59,60] indicate that evolutionary development of new types may occur normally in the natural history of the *Leptospira*. Therefore the need for development of simpler serologic diagnostic tests is quite evident, particularly tests which are adaptable to the operational needs of the small public health or hospital diagnostic laboratory.

It is evident from the foregoing discussion that a laboratorian must select the serological techniques to be used with view of the objectives of the project. If confirmation of current or recent leptospiral infections is desired, the genus-specific complement fixation or erythrocyte sensitization tests may be adequate. If definition of the etiologic serotypes is desired, the agglutination tests must be used. Of these the macroscopic tests, using concentrated antigen, are less sensitive than the microscopic tests, but are useful for detection of current or relatively recent infection, but for epidemiological studies requiring the longest possible retrospect and exact definition of serotypes, the microscopic tests are the most applicable, particularly the lysis-agglutination test employing live antigen. The latter test is also used for sero-taxonomic determinations by agglutinin absorption and cross-agglutination. In recent years fluorescent antibody procedures have been developed for the detection of leptospirae and leptospiral antigens in tissue and body fluids,[61,62] but have not been applied widely.

ECOLOGY AND EPIZOOLOGY

The bionomics of the leptospirae and the leptospiroses have always been a function of the ecology of scientific workers interested in the disease. Twenty years ago leptospirosis was thought to be endemic in certain parts of Europe, particularly in the Netherlands and some middle European countries and in Indonesia and in Japan. Weil's disease and canicola fever were considered to be ubiquitous because of the world-wide distribution of rats and dogs. In the last twenty years, however, ecological information has accumulated rap-

TABLE 60

ANIMAL HOST SPECTRUM OF MORE COMMON LEPTOSPIRAL SEROTYPES
SMALL RODENTS EXCLUDED

HOST ANIMALS	Leptospiral Serotypes											
	L. ictero-haemorrhagiae	L. canicola	L. pomona	L. bataviae	L. mitis (hyos)	L. sejroe (saxkoebing)	L. autumnalis A	L. grippo-typhosa	L. australis	L. ballum	L. hebdomadis	Others
Domestic Animals												
Dog — Canis familiaris	X	X*	X	X		X	X		X	X	X	L. mediensis
Cat — Felis domestica	X	X	X*	X		X	X		X	X	X	L. javanicae
Cattle — Bos sp.	X	X	X	X		X		X		X		
Swine — Sus domestica	X	X	X*		X*			X				
Horses — Equus caballus								X				
Donkeys — Equus sp.								X				
Sheep — Ovis sp.								X				
Goats — Capra sp.								X				
Wild Animals												
Deer — Dama virginiana	X	X	X		X	X		X		X		
Jackal — Canis aureus		X							X			
Grey Fox — Urocyon cinereoargenteus	X	X	X					X		X		
Red Fox — Vulpes fulva	X		X					X		X		
Wildcat — Lynx rufus				X								
Raccoon — Procyon lotor	X	X		X			X		X		X	
Mongoose — Herpestes griseus	X				X							
Skunk — Mephitis mephitis			X				X	X	X	X	X	
Opossum — Didelphis virginiana			X					X		X		
Bandicoot — Bandicoota bengalensis						X			X			L. poi
Hedgehogs — Erinaceus europas europas							X	X		X		L. esposito
Erinaceus europas transcaucasicus		X										
Erinaceus roumanicus							X	X				
Hamichinus auritus		X							X	X		
Muskrat — Ondatra zibethicus	X											
Nutria — Myocaster coypus												L. bonariensis
Bats — Various species												*L. cynopteri, L. schuffneri

*Based on cultural and serological evidence of reports from Europe, Israel, Indonesia, Malaya, United States and South America.
X indicates cultural or serological evidence of infection has been obtained.

idly; so much so that the standard monographs are obsolescent, and a comprehensive, detailed concept of distribution and prevalence of leptospirosis must be assembled piecemeal from many sources. Approximately a third of the recognized serotypes of *Leptospira* are now known to be world-wide in distribution. Much broader host-spectrums have been found with all the common serotypes, and the "primary hosts" for a number of serotypes have become more difficult to define. To illustrate this point, Table 60 presents the present host spectrum, excluding rodents, of a number of leptospiral serotypes. The "primary host," according to former concepts is marked by an asterisk, except for those serotypes which were supposed to have had rodents as primary hosts. With the accelerated leptospirological research, definition of even broader host spectrums can be expected. Table 61 lists types of rodents that are known to serve as reservoir hosts of various leptospiral types. This is an imposing array, but can be considered only part of the eventual rodent reservoir that will be delineated as studies of leptospirosis extend into new areas.

TABLE 61

Leptospiral Species Recovered from Various Species of Rodents

Rodent Species	Letospiral Serotype
Microtus arvalis	grippotyphosa
Microtus guentheri	grippotyphosa
Microtus hirtus	sejroe or saxkoebing, ballum
Microtus montebelloi	autumnalis, hebdomadis
Evotomys glareolus	grippotyphosa
Peromyscus maniculatus	hyos
Mus musculus	sejroe, ballum, bataviae, icterohaemorrhagiae
Micromys minutis sorcinus	bataviae
Avicanthis abessinicus	ndambi
Apodemus agrarius	pomona
Apodemus flavicollis	saxkoebing
Apodemus speciosus spec.	autumnalis
Apodemus sylvaticus	ballum, sejroe, saxkoebing
Rattus brevicaudus	semaranga, pyrogenes, javanica, autumnalis
Rattus concolor	javanica
Rattus mulleri	grippotyphosa
Rattus rajah	schuffneri
Rattus rattus	icterohaemorrhagiae, pyrogenes
Rattus r. alexandrinus	icterohaemorrhagiae
Rattus r. culmorum	australis A, australis B
Rattus r. decumanus	icterohaemorrhagiae
Rattus r. diardii	autumnalis, bataviae, icterohaemorrhagiae
Rattus r. norvegicus	icterohaemorrhagiae, bataviae
Rattus sabanus	species undetermined
Rattus whiteheadie	mankarso

Data gathered from reports from Europe, United States, Israel, Asia and Australia.

The growing complexity of the taxonomy of *Leptospira* is illustrated by the fact that more than forty serotypes are now recognized currently. These fall into twenty serogroups. A number of strains have not been classified,[8,25,63] and are recognized to be different from the established serotypes.

The natural history of leptospirosis is governed by a host of factors, geologic, climatologic and biologic, which affect the establishment and maintenance of animal reservoirs, as well as the viability of pathogenic leptospirae outside of the animal host. Foci of enzootic and epizootic leptospirosis have always been associated with moist or watery conditions—for leptospirae do not survice under dry conditions or in highly acid or alkaline environment. In the absence of favorable physical environmental conditions, maintenance of enzootic or epizootic leptospirosis requires close association of large numbers of host animals.

Available publication space does not permit detailed and expansive discussion of the factors in the natural history of leptospirosis. For this the reader is referred to general reviews on the subject,[27,28,29] and a concise discussion will be presented here. Geographic factors, both general and local include such items as topography and watersheds, which govern the extent and nature of bodies of water, the type and concentration of flora and fauna, and microclimatic conditions. The soil type, its physical and chemical characteristics, is an important consideration. Climatologic and meteorlogic conditions are of extreme importance, both general and local. These include factors such as average and seasonal rainfall, sun exposure, average mean temperature, seasonal temperature extremes, daily temperature variation, and natural disasters such as floods, storms and droughts. Botanical environmental factors are poorly defined, although lush vegetation frequently serves to support large concentrations of animals, and prevents desiccation of the soil and evaporation of pools of water. Zoological factors include the diversity, density and kind of animals, the natural population cycles, migrations (both seasonal and daily), range overlap, longevity, predation, social habits, and possibly exoparasitism.

The preceding delineation of factors might be made more meaningful by practical illustration. In the mountain and high plains region of the American west, epizootic leptospirosis has not been a problem among cattle that are sparsely distributed on the arid or semiarid range, but it does become a problem when these animals are assembled in large groups in wintering quarters, feed lots, or perhaps around watering holes. In a number of studies, epizootic leptospirosis in field mice—from which human infections were derived—was favored by the coincidence of several factors, such as moist soil conditions and lush vegetation caused by unusually heavy rainfall or floods, dense concentration of field mice due to a peak in population cycle, and mild ambient temperatures, both average and in daily variations. Population density and longevity have an effect on rate of infection and animal reservoir size: Many surveys have shown that the prevalence of *L. canicola* infection in dogs and *L. icterohaemorrhagiae* infection in rats increases with age and local concentration of the animal population. Food habits are important— leptospirosis of rodent origin seems to be an "occupational" disease among some domestic and natural predators of rodents such as rat terriers, cats and mongooses. Animal "social" habits are sometimes of critical importance—there is no doubt that the habits of dogs associated with micturition and sexual aggressiveness lead to spread of leptospirosis by direct contact with urine. The observation of concurrent existence of bovines and *Apodemus agrarius* in two islands of Denmark, and the existence of *L. pomona* infection in both hosts illustrates the importance of natural range overlap.[64] In Israel, the occurrence of *L. canicola* infection in domestic animals has been linked to nocturnal invasion of agricultural compounds by jackals.[65] The effect of warm climate is illustrated by the general hyperendemicity of leptospirosis in tropical countries, as compared with its seasonal and sporadic occurrence in more northerly climes.

A few studies have been conducted on the persistence of leptospira in natural environments. Kirschner and Maguire[66] demonstrated that pathogenic leptospirae were viable as long as three weeks in wet, urine-contaminated soil with a pH of 6.6. In abattoir sewage affluent they survived only a few hours, but when this sewage was diluted with rainwater and filtered, it served as a good growth medium. In self-digested sewage, the survival was one month. Sea water was highly leptospirocidal. Okazaki and Ringen[67] demonstrated that *L. pomona* survived in natural waters between the pH levels of 6.0 and 8.4 and between 7° and 36° C. Survival at lower temperatures was favored by pH levels in the acid range. They also demonstrated that leptospirae survived only thirty minutes in air-dried soil, but as long as 183 days in super-saturated soil. Survival in natural waters was about seven days. Gillespie and associates[68] indicated that, on an experimental basis. *Leptospira pomona* survival times in natural pools and running waters could be as long as fifteen days. There is ample evidence, therefore, that suitable ambient conditions will allow pathogenic leptospirae to survive in natural environment, outside of the host animal, for a few weeks or months.

EPIDEMIOLOGY

Infection of man is an integral part of the natural history of the leptospiroses. The human animal is susceptible to most of the known serotypes of *Leptospira,* and in many instances has yielded the first cultural recovery or serological indication of the existence of individual leptospiral serotypes. Under civilized conditions of living, man probably does not return infective leptospirae to the environment as a result of infection, but under primitive and aboriginal conditions, he may serve as a source of contamination of his environment with urine-borne leptospirae.

The epidemiology of leptospirosis, like the epizoological phase, is governed by environmental and ecological factors. Infection occurs when the host and infectious leptospirae are brought together under conditions that favor initiation of infection. Civil life adds some artifactual conditions, by virtue of occupational, social and recreational activities, but these then become part of the bionomic system. Some occupational groups with high liability for leptospiral infection are butchers, fish workers, miners, sewer workers, dockhands, cooks—all persons who are liable to work in rat-contaminated environments. These persons are likely to contract Weil's Disease caused by *L. icterohaemorrhagiae,* which is carried by *R. norvegicus, R. rattus* and the other large rats harbored by civilization. Abattoir workers, animal husbandmen, and agricultural workers of many kinds, such as ricefield planters, canefield and peafield harvesters, are subject to exposure to the sylvatic forms of leptospirosis which have reservoirs in small field rodents, horses, cattle, swine, sheep and goats. Military operations in endemic leptospirosis areas have led to many cases of sylvatic origin. In the Netherlands, Weil's Disease has often occurred when people were accidentally immersed in rat-contaminated canals or ponds. Epidemics of leptospirosis have occurred among people who bathed or swam in ponds or slow-moving streams which had been contaminated with leptospirae by diseased or dead domestic or wild animals.[69,70,71] The intimate relationship of man and dog has led to many cases of human canicola fever, for urban dog populations show high morbidity rates. In a number of surveys, antibodies to *L. canicola* have been found in 20 per cent to 40 per cent of urban dogs. At times, immediate contact with the infected animals or contaminated premises may not be necessary to cause infection. Gsell[74] cites an instance where pea-harvest workers contracted *L. grippotyphosa* infection by handling pea haulm brought from fields that were heavily infested with leptospirotic voles. Local practices and technology may alter the rate and prevalence of leptospirosis. In Switzerland, Gsell made a study of the distribution of swineherds disease by cantons, and found that morbidity rates were much greater in those areas where farms kept large herds of pigs. Comparing the swine-raising industry in Switzerland and the United States, one would expect a high prevalence of swineherds disease in the latter because of the magnitude of the swine-raising industry and the very large herds. But it is surprising to find a relatively low incidence of swineherds disease in the U.S.A. This may be due to the fact that much of the husbandry is mechanized, that range-feeding is generally practiced, and that contact between swine and the herdsmen is not intimate. The same may apply to the beef-cattle industry. The epidemics of swine- and cattle-borne leptospiroses in the United States are largely due to bathing in bodies of water contaminated by diseased animals.

Leptospirosis is a "doctors' disease." It is found mostly by those who seek it. It can mimic influenza, enteric viral infections, infectious gastroenteritis, adenovirus infections and various etiologically undefined syndromes. On the American scene, clinicians generally are not aware of the protean nature of this disease, and the widespread reservoirs for human infection shown by veterinary research. For this reason the true incidence of leptospirosis is not known. It would be well to have at least a genus-specific leptospirosis serological test available in every medical laboratory as part of the battery used for the definition of fevers of undetermined etiology.

RECOVERY OF LEPTOSPIRAE FROM FIELD SOURCES

The existing monographs[8,28,29] present ample basic information on diagnostic methods, and the literature cited under the microbiological and serological sections of this paper contain information on newer developments in cultural procedures and serological measurements. However some general comments may be in order.

The cultural approach to diagnosis and epidemiology should be broadly based, for greater assurance of success. Nutritional requirements of the genus are poorly understood, therefore cultural search and control should employ two or three kinds of media, including a semisolid type. Young hamsters and weanling guinea pigs are the more useful of the common laboratory animals. Attempts at isolation of leptospirae employing animals should be thorough, including daily checks for weight loss and twice daily checks on body temperature. In the absence of fever and lesions, two or three blind passages should be made at seven- to ten-day intervals. Embryonated chicken eggs (at 7 to 8 days of incubation) are useful for cultivation,[75] but the sure establishment of culture lines may require several blind passages after five- to seven-day incubation, post inoculation, before the organism becomes adjusted to the medium. Embryonic fluids must be examined closely in the early passages, since prolific growth usually does not occur until a number of serial passages have been accomplished. The cultural handling qualities of leptospirae, in animals and embryos is much like that of viruses. The highly parasitic forms may have to adjust to artificial media and hosts, they cannot be expected to grow profusely. After adjustment to the new medium, animal or artificial, leptospirae usually become stabilized in their new growth pattern and increase in pathogenic potential for the new host. Figure 118 demonstrates the pathogenic activity of *L. pomona* stabilized in serial guinea pig passage. The lesions shown were manifest at five to seven days after intraperitonial injection of emulsified viscera samples taken within ten days of inoculation, or blood taken during the febrile period of the previous animal passage.

PREVENTIVE MEDICINE

From the foregoing discussions it should be evident that prevention of leptospirosis is not a simple problem, but a multifaceted one that involves interacting complexes of environmental factors, available hosts and resident infective leptospirae. Were all these complexes completely understood, formulation of preventive medical procedures would be more certain. However, as we have seen, the

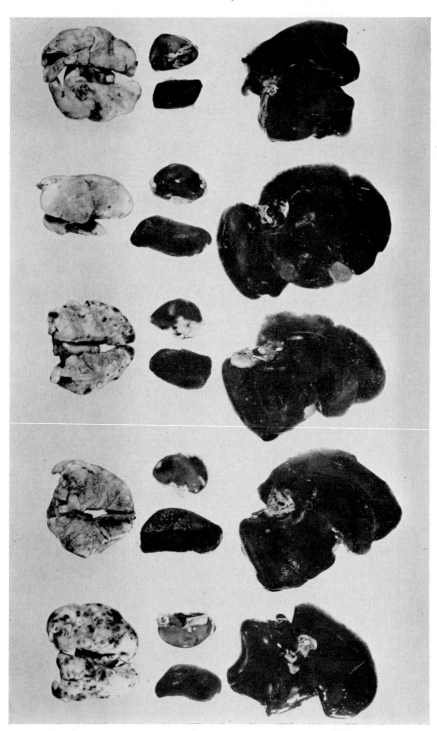

Fig. 118. Pathogenic activity of *L. pomona* stabilized in serial guinea pig passage.

bionomics of the leptospiroses are far from full delineation. New hosts and new serotypes are being discovered. Recent work with ticks[76,77] gives indications that they also may serve as reservoirs and vectors. If this is true naturally, another large bionomic factor will require concerted study.

With the leptospiroses of domestic rat and dog origin some sanitary steps can lead to reduction of prevalence. The most obvious of these is a stringent, continuing community-wide rat eradication program. The elimination of rats will eliminate a reservoir. The second procedure for reduction of "domestic" leptospirosis, hygienic control of the dog population, is much more difficult because of the exaggerated sentimental value of this animal in the esteem of part of the public. There is no doubt that elimination of stray dogs and strict adherence to a policy of tethering or confining all owned dogs would lead to a drastic reduction of both canine and human canicola fever. An effective vaccine to prevent leptospirosis in dogs would also serve to curb human infections.

The occurrence of leptispirosis in agricultural animals and consequent reduction of leptospirosis in slaughterhouse, farm workers, and swimmers, etc., would be more difficult to attain. Agricultural animals can contract infection from natural sources. However, much agricultural animal leptospirosis could be eliminated by more hygionic approaches to animal husbandry, based on epizoological principles. A proved, effective vaccine is also desirable for agricultural animals. The most difficult phase of control of leptospirosis in agricultural areas is that dealing with wild animals and natural environment. Animal population, such as wild carnivores and rodents, cannot be destroyed ruthlessly without upsetting natural balances, leading to conditions worse than the original problem. At the present rudimentary state of our knowledge of natural population dynamics and epizoology, little can be recommended beyond local farm and camp hygiene to prevent contamination of water, food and implements, coupled with procedures to limit, to a reasonable extent, the overlap of domestic and wild animal habitation. Good public health education in endemic leptospirosis areas could lead to reduction in the incidence of exposures of men and domestic animals to reservoirs of leptospirae.

Vaccination against leptospirosis in domestic animals and in human high-risk occupational groups is highly desirable for the prevention of endemic and epidemic episodes of this disease. A re-sume of progress in the development of vaccines for people has been given by Borg-Petersen.[78] An antigen has been developed and tested experimentally in human volunteers and experimental animals, which seems to be effective. Its epidemiological effectiveness, how-ever, has not been established because of necessarily small sample groups. Vaccine reactions are rigorous enough with this product to prevent wide-scale use.

Much work has been done on the development of vaccine for do-mestic animals, particularly swine and cattle. Commercial bacterins have been on the market for ten years or longer. However, the true effectiveness of the vaccines—mostly against *L. pomona*—has not been assessed. The earlier field trials employed vaccine in herds in the midst of enzootic or epizootic leptospirosis, and credited the vaccine for abatement of disease—without consideration of the probability that the outbreaks had abated naturally. In some experimental stud-ies animals were challenged within a few weeks of injection of an-tigen—at a time when immunologic response was naturally at its peak. Thus no evaluation of long term effectiveness was obtained.

Recent studies by Kenzy and associates,[79] using rigid criteria for evaluation of infection, and challenges at varying and remote periods from vaccination, have yielded encouraging progress towards devel-opment of an effective vaccine. Among the many interesting facts shown by this group is the fact that vaccinated animals can become infected by the same type of leptospira used in the vaccine, show little or no physical affects, yet develop leptospiruria. Their more re-cent studies point towards the potential of the use of live, pathogene-tically attenuated leptospiral strains as vaccines. This had been dem-onstrated earlier in experimental pathogenesis studies by other authors.[80]

Once effective vaccines for single leptospiral strains have been developed, then the problem of multiple-type vaccines must be solved. The immunity developed from inoculation or infection with one leptospiral serotype will not protect against infection by an anti-genically heterologous strain.[81] A basic approach to this issue lies in immunochemical studies such as that started by Hoag,[82] with the end view of deriving broad spectrum or genus-specific antigens.

CONCLUSION

The studies of recent years have shown that leptospirosis is a zoonotic disease problem of large proportions and world-wide distribution, involving microbiological, ecological and environmental factors of rather profound nature. The agricultural and public health implications are serious and require that a commensurate part of veterinary, medical and biomedical scientific endeavors be devoted to solution of the many problems of the field. If research on leptospirosis continues to grow at the rate of the past fifteen years, we shall have solved many of the practical issues by the end of the next fifteen.

BIBLIOGRAPHY

1. WEIL, H. A.: *Deutsches Arch. f. Klin. Med., 39:*209, 1886.
2. STIMSON, A. M.: *Public Health Reports, 22:*541, 1907.
3. INADA, R., IDO, Y., HOKI, R., KANEKO, R., and ITO, H.: *J. Exper. Med. & Hyg., 23:*377, 1916.
4. HÜBNER, E. A., and REITER, H.: *Deutsch. Med. Wochschr., 41:*1275, 1915.
5. UHLENMUTH, P., and FROMME, W.: *Med. Klinik, 44:*1202, 1915.
6. SIMPSON, C. L., and WHITE, L. H.: *J. Infect. Dis. 109:*243, 1961.
7. PARA, M.: *Archives of Pathol., 42:*649, 1946.
8. WOLFF, J. W.: *The Laboratory Diagnosis of Leptospirosis.* Springfield, Thomas, 1954.
9. LARSON, A. D., TREICK, R. W., EDWARDS, C. L., COX, C. D.: *J. Bact., 77:*361, 1959.
10. SHIGEKAWA, J. M., and STOCKTON, J. J.: *Am. J. Vet. Res., 16:*619, 1955.
11. ANNEAR, D. D.: *Australian J. Exper. Biol., 36:*1, 1958.
12. GERHARDT, M., BALL, M. G.: *J. Bact., 77:*17, 1959.
13. MARSHALL, P. B.: *J. Infect. Dis., 84:*150, 1949.
14. GREENE, M. R., CAMIEN, M. N., and DUNN, M. S.: *Proc. Soc. Exper. Biol. & Med., 75:*208, 1950.
15. HELPRIN, J. J., HIATT, C. W.: *J. Infect. Dis., 100:*136, 1957.
16. FULTON, J. D., and SPOONER, D. F.: *Exper. Parasitol., 5:*154, 1956.
17. SCHNEIDER, M. D.: *Proc. Soc. Exper. Biol. Med., 85:*32, 1954.
18. ALEXANDER, A. D., SMITH, O. H., HIATT, C. W., and GLEISER, C. A.: *Proc. Soc. Exper. Biol. & Med., 91:*205, 1956.
19. BAUER, D. C.: *Proc. Soc. Exper. Biol. & Med., 98:*505, 1958.
20. REINHARD, K. R.: *Bovine Leptospirosis.* Thesis, Cornell University, 1950.
21. RUSSELL, C. M.: *J. Immunol., 77:*405, 1956.
22. KEMENES, F.: *Acta Veterinaria, 8:*143, 1958.
23. FENNESTAD, D. L., BORG-PETERSEN, C.: *J. Infect. Dis., 102:*227, 1958.
24. REINHARD, K. R.: *Symposium on Reproduction and Infertility.* Michigan State University Centennial, 1955, p. 19.
25. BROOM, J. C.: *Trans. Roy. Soc. Trop. Med. & Hyg., 47:*273, 1953.
26. ASHE, W. F., PRATT-THOMAS, H. R., KUMPE, C. W.: *Medicine, 20:*145, 1941.
27. VAN THIEL, P. H.: *The Leptospiroses.* Leiden, Univ. Press, 1948.
28. GSELL, O.: *Leptospirosen.* Bern, Hans Huber, 1952.

29. *Symposium on the Leptospiroses. Med. Publ. #1.* AMSGS, Walter Reed Army Med. Center, 1952.

30. KOPPISCH, E., BOND, W. M.: *Symposium on the Leptospiroses (Ref. #29)* 1952, P. 83.

31. KING, J. H.: *Symposium on the Leptospiroses (Ref. #29)* 1952, P. 72.

32. SMITH, E. R., REYNOLDS, I. M., and SAKAI, T.: *The Cornell Veterinarian, 50:*34, 1960.

33. RYLEY, W. J. and SIMMONS, G. C.: *Queensland J. Agric. Sci., 11:*61, 1954. Also *Australian Vet. J., 30:*203, 1954.

34. FENNESTAD, K. L.: *Proc. XIII Nord. Congr. Path. & Bakt.,* Turku, June, 1961. Also *Nature, 180:*1210, 1957.

35. LARSON, C. L.: *Pub. Health Reports, 58:*10, 1943.

36. LARSON, C. L., and GRIFFITS, J. J.: *Pub. Health Reports, 60:*317, 1945.

37. FAIRBURN, A. C., and SEMPLE, S. J. G.: *The Lancet, 270/6906:*13, 1956.

38. HALL, H. E., HIGHTOWER, J. A., DIAZ-RIVERA, R., BYRNE, R. J., SMADEL, J. E., WODWARD, T. E.: *Ann. Int. Med., 35:*981, 1951.

39. RINGEN, L. M., OKAZAKI, M. S.: *J.A.V.M.A., 133:*214, 1958.

40. STOENNER, H. G., GRIMES, E. F., THRAILKILL, F. B., and DAVIS, E.: *Am. J. Trop. Med. & Hyg., 7:*423, 1958.

41. RINGEN, L. M., BRACKEN, F. K., KENZY, S. G., GILLESPIE, R. W. H.: *J.A.V.M.A., 126:*272, 1955.

42. STOENNER, H. G.: *Am. J. Hyg., 57:*316, 1953.

43. STOENNER, H. G.: *Am. J. Vet. Res. 15:*434, 1954.

44. GALTON, M. M., POWERS, D. K., HALL, A. D., CORNELL, R. G.: *Am. J. Vet. Res., 19:*505, 1958.

45. HOAG, W. G., GOCHENOUR, W. S., JR., YAGER, R. H.: *Proc. Soc. Exper. Biol. & Med., 83:*490, 1953.

46. CHANG, R. S., McCOMB, D. E.: *Am. J. Trop. Med. & Hyg., 3:*481, 1954.

47. COX, C. D.: *Proc. Soc. Exper. Biol. & Med., 90:*610, 1955.

48. RINGEN, L. M.: *U. S. Livestock San. Assoc., 63rd Ann. Proc.* 1959, P. 120.

49. YORK, C. J.: *Am. J. Vet. Res., 4:*117, 1952.

50. RANDALL, R., WETMORE, P. W., WARNER, A. R.: *J. Lab. & Clin. Med., 34:*1411, 1949.

51. SCHNEIDER, M. D.: *Proc. Soc. Exper. Biol. & Med., 82:*655, 1953.

52. ROTHSTEIN, N., WOLMAN, F.: *J. Infect., Dis., 105:*280, 1959.

53. BORG-PETERSEN, C., FAGROEUS, A.: *Act. Path. & Microbiol. Skand., 26:*555, 1949.

54. VAN DER HOEDEN, J.: *Bull. Res. Council, Israel, 6E,* 1956.

55. VAN DER HOEDEN, J.: *Cornell Veterinarian, 45:*190, 1955.

56. STUART, R. D.: *Canad. J. Microbiol., 2:*288, 1956.

57. RINGEN, L. M.: *J. Immunol., 84:*582, 1960.

58. BESSEMANS, A., DEROM, R.: *Rev. Belge Path. Med. Exptl., 18:*391, 1948.

59. SCHLOSSBERGER, H.: *Z. Hyg. Infekt. Kr., 131:*152, 1950.

60. PIKE, R. M., SCHULZE, M. L.: *J. Immunol., 81:*172, 1958.

61. SHELDON, W. H.: *Proc. Soc. Exper. Biol. & Med., 84:*165, 1953.

62. WHITE, F. H., STOLIKER, O. H. E., GALTON, M. M.: *Am. J. Vet. Res., 89:*650, 1961.

63. ALEXANDER, A. D., WETMORE, P. W., EVANS, L. B., JEFFRIES, H., and GLEISER, C. A.: *Am. J. Trop. Med. & Hyg., 4:*492, 1955.

64. FENNESTAD, K. L.: *Nordisk. Veterinaermedicin, 8:*325, 1956.

65. VAN DER HOEDEN, J.: *J. Am. Vet. M. A., 126:*207, 1955.

66. KIRSCHNER, L., and MAGUIRE, T.: *New Zealand M. J., LVI:*385, 1957.

67. OKAZAKI, W., and RINGEN, L. M.: *Am. J. Vet. Res., 18:*219, 1957.

68. GILLESPIE, R. W. H., KENZY, S. A., RINGEN, L. M., and BRACKEN, F. K.: *Am. J. Vet. Res., 18:*76, 1957.

69. SCHAEFFER, M.: *J. Clin. Invest., 30:*670, 1951.
70. COCKBURN, T. A., VAVRA, J. D., SPENCER, S. S., DUNN, J. R., PETERSON, L. J., REIN-HARD, K. R.: *Am. J. Hyg., 60:*1, 1954.
71. WILLIAMS, H. R., MURPHY, W. J., McCROAN, J. E., STARR, L. E., WARD, M. K.: *Am. J. Hyg., 64:*46, 1956.
72. ZAHARIJA, I.: *Report, Yugoslavian Center for Leptospirosis* Zagreb, 1952.
73. BRUNNER, T. K.: *North Am. Vet., 30:*517, 1949.
74. GSELL, O.: *Symposium on the Leptospiroses (Ref. 29),* P. 34.
75. BAKER, J. A., LITTLE, R. B.: *J. Exper. Med., 88:*295, 1948.
76. VAN DAR HOEDEN, J.: *Bull. Research Council of Israel, 6E:#*3, 1957.
77. BURGDORFER, WILLY, *Exper. Parasitol., 8:*502, 1959.
78. BORG-PETERSEN, C.: *Symposium on the Leptospiroses,* 1952, P. 193.
79. KENZY, S. G., GILLESPIE, R. W. H., LEE, J. H.: *J.A.V.M.A., 139:*452, 1951.
80. REINHARD, K. R., HADLOW, W. J.: *Proc. 91st. Ann. Meeting. Amer. Vet. Med. Assoc.* Published by *Am. Vet. M. A.,* Aug., 1954.
81. Author's data, unpublished.
82. HOAG, W. G., BELL, W. B.: *Am. J. Vet. Res., 16:*381, 1955.

Chapter 25

RAT-BITE FEVER

(Sodoku and Haverhill Fever)

WILLIAM L. JELLISON, PH.D.

THIS CHAPTER is prepared in two sections on the premises: 1) that rat-bite fever in man is a clinical syndrome following the bite of rats, mice, and other rodents, and rarely from bites of carnivores or other sources of infection; 2) that two independent etiological agents are involved, one known as *Spirillum minus* and the other as *Streptobacillus moniliformis;* and 3) that although the two infections have some differential characteristics a definite etiological diagnosis can only be established by laboratory means.

An anomalous situation exists in regard to *Streptobacillus moniliformis* infections. In a single epidemic at Haverhill, Massachusetts, in which the etiological agent was repeatedly demonstrated, eighty-six human cases were attributed to contaminated milk. In a very similar milk-borne epidemic at Chester, Pennsylvania, about 600 cases were involved but the etiological agent was not isolated. These two epidemics involved about four times as many people as all the rat-bite fever cases of both types reported in the United States up to the present time. In spite of this preponderance of milk-borne cases the history of rat-bite is usually the clue to diagnosis of sporadic human cases of infection with either organism. Furthermore, there had been no good name proposed for *Streptobacillus* infections until the Haverhill epidemic. Thus we are obliged to use the name Haverhill fever. This name connotes a newly recognized epidemic disease, spread through milk, with cows presumably the reservoir of infection, whereas, the common manifestation is a sporadic case, contracted from rat bite with rats the well-known reservoir of infection.

SODOKU

Rat-bite fever due to Spirillum minus

The term "sodoku" is from the Japanese (*So*, a rat, *doku*, poison) and is being resorted to more commonly by American workers to avoid controversy and confusion over the correct application of the term rat-bite fever.

Sodoku is primarily an infection of rats, mice, and other rodents. Secondarily, man is infected following the bite of a rodent. When infection has been attributed to the bite of a weasel, ferret, cat, or other carnivore, it has been assumed that these animals were recently contaminated by predatism on rodents and acted as mechanical carriers. Experimental infection in cats has been demonstrated and transient natural infection in small carnivores is a possibility. Intentional infection of man, "Sodoku inoculata," for treatment of general paresis, a procedure no longer practiced, has further demonstrated the pathogenicity of the organism. The mode of human infection may sometimes be obscure, such as infection in an abrasion from inanimate objects.

History

Sodoku is said to have been known in the fourth century B.C. in India. Its principal reservoirs, *Rattus* spp. and *Mus* spp., are indigenous rodents in Asia and Africa and as they are definitely introduced species in the New World, they probably introduced the infection to this continent. Infection has been found to a limited extent in our native rodents where they are in contact with *Mus* or *Rattus* populations.

Miyake brought this disease to the attention of the Western World, where very few cases had been reported, in 1900. Hata; Surveyor; and Dalal, who successfully treated cases with salvarsan, tried this drug because the periodic fever, local lesion, and peculiar eruption suggested that the disease was one caused by an infective agent allied to the spirochetes.

A spirochete-like organism was seen in the initial lesion of one rat-bite fever patient and in the lymph node of another out of four cases observed by Futaki, Takaki, Taniguchi, and Osumi in 1915. They briefly described and pictured the organism and established the infection in monkeys, guinea pigs, and white rats. On the basis of microscopic findings, similarity of the disease to other spirochete infections and response of the patients to spirochetocidal drugs they claimed this to be the etiological agent of rat-bite fever. They further described the organism, demonstrated it directly in two more patients and one wild rat and named it *Spirochaeta morsus muris* in 1917. They cited the work of Carter who in 1887 had seen a similar organism in the blood of a rat *"Mus decumanus"* (= *Rattus norvegicus*) in India and had named it *Spirillum minor*. Carter's organism had not been associated with any human disease. They also cited the work of Schottmüller who had isolated *Streptothrix muris ratti* from a rat-bite fever patient. Their claims to culture without successful transfer probably represented only survival.

The Japanese discovery found ready confirmation. With the recognition of the wide distribution of the disease and its prevalence in rats, the name *Spirillum minus*, adapted from *Spirillum minor* of Carter 1887, has been accepted.

Prevalence and Distribution

Sodoku is probably of world-wide distribution coincidental with its natural reservoirs, *Rattus* spp. and *Mus* spp., which have been spread by human commerce. Cases attributed to *S. minus* infection have been recognized in Japan, India, Malaya, England, and the United States. It is not apparent that different distributional patterns exist for sodoku and Haverhill fever, but this may be possible.

Brown and Nunemaker list 125 cases, including eighty-one cases compiled by Bayne-Jones, of rat-bite fever of both types in the United States from 1916, when *S. minus* was found to be a human pathogen, through 1940, the date of their study. They repeat claims, with reservations, that *S. minus* was demonstrated by direct examination in five cases. In seventeen instances the organism was seen after animal passage but only one worker checked his animals before inoculation. Eleven of the seventeen cases were definitely and one supposedly attributed to rat bite. The others were from mouse bite, contact with dogs, cat bite, cat scratch, and trauma without known animal contact.

Three cases of rat-bite fever in Washington, D.C. were studied by Larson, who searched for both etiological agents. He demonstrated *S. minus* in one by animal inoculation and attributed the others to *Streptobacillus* infection on the basis of culture in one case and serological evidence in the other. He concluded that either organism may cause the disease in that area.

Several writers have stated that cases are scarce or nonexistent in the Rocky Mountain area. However, Jellison *et al.* reported a case from Bozeman, Montana, in which infection was attributed to the bite of a house mouse, *Mus musculus,* a host not previously charged with human infection although known to be naturally infected. House mice were abundant on the premises and the first 16 house mice examined were all infected with *S. minus. S. minus* was also found in one of the many specimens of *Microtus* from the premises. Another case occurred at Silver Star, Montana, and was reported by Seidenstricker in August 1949. The patient, a young girl, was bitten by a field rodent which probably was not *Mus musculus.* Numerous field rodents and house mice were trapped on the premises but *S. minus* was found only in one *Mus musculus* from the barn. Rats, *Rattus* spp., are entirely absent from these sections of Montana.

S. minus was demonstrated in the blood of two rat-bite fever patients in Atlanta, Georgia, by Beeson with animal passage. Experimental animals were carefully checked before inoculation. They were examined repeatedly but were not found positive until the 17th day after injection.

The Etiological Agent

The causative agent of sodoku is *Spirillum minus.* It is a rather short thick cell, 0.5 micron wide and 3.0 microns long, having two or three windings which are thick, regular, and spiral. They are actively motile by means of bipolar tufts of flagella. They stain readily with Giemsa's and related stains and with silver impregnation techniques. The organisms have been found abundantly in the wound at site of bites, in the lymph nodes, salivary glands, peritoneal fluid, and circulating blood of man and animals. There are numerous failures, however, in attempts to demonstrate their presence in patients. Inoculation of white mice or guinea pigs with blood or exudate from the initial lesion is recommended for diagnosis. Experimental animals must be carefully checked before inoculation because of frequent natural infections in them. After about two weeks the organisms may be demonstrated in the blood by dark-field or in stained films. Successful culture of *S. minus* on artificial media has been claimed several times but so far the results have not been consistently reproducible by others. Although differences in pathogenicity are recognized and many names have been proposed for similar organisms in rodents, it is generally considered that all refer to the ones species, *S. minus*.

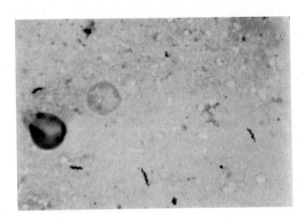

Fig. 119. *Spirillum minus* from heart muscle of a mouse. (*Rocky Mountain Laboratory, United States Public Health Service, Hamilton, Montana.*)

Eight other valid species in the genus *Spirillum* as recognized by Bergey's Manual are free-living bacteria-like organisms and have nothing to do with rodents or rat-bite fever. In fact, many would remove *S. minus* from the genus *Spirillum* except that it does not fit in well elsewhere, although it shows some relationship with the true spirochetes.

Susceptible Animals

Mice, white rats, guinea pigs, and rabbits have been found readily susceptible to infection. Mice and young guinea pigs are the animals of choice for isolation of strains or diagnosis of human cases. Organisms appear in the blood in three to seventeen days after inoculation, persist for a few weeks, and gradually diminish in number. After the bacteremia is passed the organisms can be found abundantly in impression smears of heart muscle. Mice do not usually show any symptoms of infection but some strains produce fatal infections in mice according to Robertson.

Rats are likewise susceptible. McDermott describes concentrations of the organism in gummatoid lesions of the lungs and lymph nodes comparable to the tertiary-stage lesions of syphilis in man.

Guinea pigs are very susceptible and are killed by some strains of *S. minus*. Conjunctivitis, keratitis, and alopecia are conspicuous signs of infection in guinea pigs, and characteristic syphilis-like lesions follow inoculation in the genitals of guinea pigs and rabbits. Robertson mentioned interstitial mycocarditis in guinea pigs but did not associate it with concentrations of the organism.

A number of other animals, including cats, ferets, and monkeys, have been experimentally infected. Birds were found refractive to infection.

The Disease in Animals

Natural infection in rats and mice with *S. minus* does not seem to inconvenience them. The organism is present in the blood stream for an unknown period in natural infections and for several weeks or longer in experimental infection in rats and mice. No special concentration of the organisms has been shown in the oral tissues of rats, and it is assumed that infection takes place from organisms in the saliva or blood of the reservoir. Oral contamination may come from naso-pharyngeal concentrations of the organisms. Peritoneal fluid of infected animals is usually a richer source of organisms than blood.

Hughes (see Jellison *et al.*), of the Rocky Mountain Laboratory, discovered that organisms were abundant in the Giemsa-stained impression smears of heart muscle from naturally infected wild mice when they could not be found in the blood, spleen, or liver. This observation has been verified many times and promises a technique suitable for survey work. Experimental white mice show eight to twenty organisms per microscopic field in heart impression smears after the bacteremia has passed and up to one year after infection. There has been no opportunity to determine whether this tissue predeliction exists in man or can be associated with any human symptoms or pathology.

Robertson; Francis; and Knowles *et al.* have found spontaneous infection in laboratory mice, and Das Gupta has found it in guinea pigs. Such natural infections have no doubt been responsible for erroneous diagnosis of some human cases when the experimental animals were not checked before inoculation.

Several surveys of rat populations for *S. minus* infection are cited by Brown and Nunemaker presumably based on examination of stained blood smears or dark-field preparations (see Table 62).

TABLE 62

INFECTION OF RATS WITH *S. minus* IN VARIOUS SURVEYS
(CITED BY BROWN AND NUNEMAKER)

Japan............................	5.9 per cent infection
	8.3 per cent infection
	11.2 per cent infection
	13.8 per cent infection
Bombay, India....................	4.3 per cent infection
Calcutta, India..................	3.0 per cent infection (stained films)
	21.7 per cent infection (dark-field preparations)
London...........................	about 25 per cent infection
Rochester, New York..............	0 per cent infection
Atlanta, Georgia.................	0 per cent infection

The Disease in Man

Rat-bite fever in man is characterized by complete healing of the primary lesion until about the time of onset of systemic symptoms, one to three weeks later, when there is an inflammation of the tissues surrounding the wound, involvement of regional lymph nodes, localized pain and often ulcer formation. Organisms are demonstrable in the serous exudate of the wound at this stage. There is a sudden onset of fever accompanied by muscular pain and malaise. A rash, usually maculo-papular, may appear with the initial fever but more often appears in the febrile relapses. After two to five days of fever there is a remission of symptoms to be followed by one or many relapses of diminishing severity at intervals of seven to ten days, unless treatment is effective. Robertson emphasizes that the cardinal symptoms are "recurring inflammation at the site of bite and in regional lymph system, the remittent nature of the fever and the characteristic rash." Arthritis is not a prominent symptom in soduku case reports except in intentional inoculations for paresis therapy. Robertson states it occurred in 25 per cent of a series of cases.

Early records of rat-bite fever in Japan given by Miyake indicated a mortality of about 10.5 per cent, and Robertson estimates specific treatment has reduced this to about 2.0 per cent. In the United States the mortality has been estimated at 10 per cent.

However, Bayne-Jones after a critical review of 81 reported cases of both types reduced this to 6 per cent. Brown and Nunemaker state for the United States "death has never been reported in a case of rat-bite fever from which *S. minus* has been isolated."

Serological tests for the diagnosis of *S. minus* infection include one in which immune serum immobilizes a living preparation of the organism. It is not dependable according to Francis and apparently not routinely run by any laboratory in the United States. The Wassermann test has been reported positive in many cases and negative in others. This discrepancy may be due to confusion of the etiological agents. An active lytic principle has been observed in immune sera and this would suggest the possibility of a mouse protection test. *S. minus* infection in rabbits gives rise to a positive Weil-Felix reaction with *Proteus* OXK strains according to Savoor and Lewthwaite.

Treatment

Based on the premise that sodoku resembled the spirochete diseases, treatment with salvarsan and other arsenical compounds was tried and found effective by Hata; Surveyor; and Dalal even before the etiological agent was discovered. Savoor stated that neoarsphenamine has been the drug of choice for many years but that penicillin was also effective in the treatment of one case. Streptomycin was found effective in a single case reported by Jellison *et al.*

Prevention and Control

The prevention of sodoku is entirely dependent on the control of rats and protection of babies and small children from rats. Rat-bite wounds should be treated promptly with disinfectants and antispectic dressings. A protective dose of penicillin would seem indicated. If infection develops and *S. minus* is identified, either arsenical drugs or penicillin is effective. Penicillin has the advantage of being therapeutic for either sodoku or Haverhill fever. Considering the low mortality of the disease and the few cases of either sodoku or Haverhill fever in which the etiology has been established beyond any doubt, the writer suggests that the first consideration be specific diagnosis of the etiology even if it means the patient must go untreated for several days.

HAVERHILL FEVER

(Erythema Arthriticum Epidemicum)

Rat-bite fever due to Streptobacillus moniliformis

Haverhill fever (erythema arthriticum epidemicum) takes its name from the city in Massachusetts where a milk-borne epidemic occurred in 1926. The bite of a rat is a common mode of infection, although about as many cases were involved in this one epidemic as have been attributed to rat bite in the United States in thirty-five years. An even larger milk-borne epidemic, involving about 600 cases occurred at Chester, Pennsylvania, in 1925 and has been generally accepted as Haverhill fever though the etiological agent was not identified from any of the cases.

History

Haverhill fever was described as a clinical entity in 1926 by Place, Sutton, and Willner and later by Place and Sutton after a study of the Massachusetts epidemic. Infection was traced to milk and milk products from one dairy. Parker and Hudson recovered from eleven of the patients an infectious agent which they named *Haverhillia multiformis* but they did not recognize the relationship or identity of the organism to *Streptobacillus moniliformis,* which had been isolated from a previous case of "acute erythema multiforme," or to any of the organisms named and isolated from rodents or rat-bite fever cases. Certainly there was little in the epidemiology of Haverhill fever to suggest rat-bite fever. In 1934, Scharles and Seastone reported a case of "Haverhill fever following rat bite" and due to *H. multiformis.* It was soon established that *Haverhill multiformis* and *Streptobacillus moniliformis* were identical.

It appears that this agent was identified with cases of rat-bite fever before the Spirillum organism, *"Spirochaeta morsus muris,"* was described by Futaki *et al* in 1917. Schottmüller is credited with the isolation of an organism which he named *"Streptothrix muris ratti"* from a rat-bite fever patient in 1914. In the next few years there were several other isolations of *Streptothrix*-like organisms from rat-bite fever patients and from rodents, and a variety of names were proposed for the organisms cultured. Evidence favoring *Streptobacillus* as the cause of rat-bite fever grew while considerable doubt developed as to the role of *S. minus.* This concept persists as indicated by Dolman *et al.* who state in 1951 "The conclusion is reached that *S. moniliformis* is the true causal agent in this disease, and that *S. minus* plays only a minor or negligible role, or may not even be transmissible to man."

Streptobacillus moniliformis, the name temporarily accepted for the organism, was proposed by Levaditi, Nicolau, and Poincloux in 1925 for an organism isolated from a case of "acute erythema multiforme" unassociated with rat bite. However, Lemierre *et al.,* in 1937, first reported the organism from the blood of a patient with rat-bite fever. *S. moniliformis* is then the first name applied to the organism associated with a syndrome later described as Haverhill fever. With the present recognition of Haverhill fever as only one epidemiological form of disease caused by this agent a good claim can be made for recognition of one of the earlier names for the organism. In fact, some other name or combination of names appears necessary as Bergey's Manual (Breed *et al.*) states "The genus name *Streptobacillus* is invalid." The organism is not definitely placed in another genus.

Geographic Distribution

Haverhill fever is probably widespread although world-wide reports are much fewer than for sodoku. Cases resembling the disease and from which organisms similar to *Streptobacillus* have been isolated are reported from Russia, Germany, France, England, Scotland, and Norway, as well as from various parts of the United States. Dolman *et al.* have recorded the first two cases of *"Streptobacillus* infection" in Canada (Vancouver, B.C.), and state that eight previous cases of rat-bite fever in Canada were attributed to *Spirillum minus* infection. Milk epidemics have been limited to Pennsylvania and Massachusetts. Sporadic cases have been listed by Brown and Nunemaker from Massachusetts, Connecticut, Tennessee, Illinois, Maryland, Pennsylvania and New York. The only case confirmed by culture from any of the Western States was in a baby from Stockton, California as reported by Frank and Bower.

The Etiological Agent

Streptobacillus moniliformis is a gram-negative, nonmotile rod 2 to 5 microns in length and 0.1 to 0.4 micron in width. It is extremely pleomorphic and under favorable conditions may grow in long filaments. It grows best in media enriched with blood, serum, or ascitic fluid. Cultural characteristics have been well studied by Brown and Nunemaker who emphasize the need of special though simple culture techniques. Larson used a veal infusion broth enriched with 20 per cent rabbit serum.

In liquid media, growth appears in the bottom of the tube. Typical "fluff balls" appear along the inoculation channel in semisolid media.

Organisms do not always grow well on original isolation but later transfers give conspicuous growth. Frequent transfer, even every twenty-four hours, is recommended. Cultures may be kept viable at low temperatures, $-25°$ C., for months at a time. Cultures may be isolated directly from the patient's blood during the first three weeks of illness. Such primary isolations are more conclusive than those resulting from animal passage because of the high incidence of natural infection in laboratory animals. White mice are preferable to rats for experimental animals as they are more free of spontaneous infection.

A culturable organism forming microscopic colonies has been referred to as a variant, symbiont, pleuropneumonia-like organism, L_1 form or component of *S. moniliformis,* respectively.

The following names used in the literature probably all refer to this organism according to Brown and Nunemaker:

> *Streptothrix muris ratti* Schottmüller, 1914
> *Streptothrix teraxeri cepapi* Schottmüller, 1914
> *Streptothrix longus* Litterer, 1917
> *Streptothrix brevis* Litterer, 1917
> *Streptothrix putorii* Dick and Tunnicliff, 1918
> *Bacillus actinoides* Smith, 1918
> *Actinomyces actinoides* (Smith) Bergey *et al.,* 1923
> *Streptobacillus moniliformis* Levaditi, Nicolau and Poincloux, 1925
> *Haverhillia multiformis* Parker and Hudson, 1926
> *Actinobaccillus actinoides* (Smith) Topley and Wilson, 1929
> *Bacillus actinoides* variety *muris* Nelson, 1930
> *Actinomyces muris* (Nelson) Topley and Wilson, 1936
> *Actinobaccillus actinoides* (Smith) Bergey *et al.,* 1939

Actinobacillus muris Nelson, 1940

Murimyces streptobacilli-moniliformis Sabin, 1941 (for L_1 component)

Astericoccus muris (Nelson) Heilman, 1951

Musculomyces streptobaccilli-moniliformis (Sabin) (for L_1 component) is used in the 1948 edition of *Bergey's Manual*.

Milk Epidemics

The epidemic studied by Place, Sutton, and Willner occurred in Haverhill, Masachusetts, in January 1926. There were eighty-six cases in thirty-nine families, all living in a small area. The ages of the patients varied from two years to fifty-four years. All were users of raw milk from a small dairy. When the milk was pasteurized the epidemic stopped. The source of contamination for the milk was not definitely known but it was assumed that rats were involved. One cow showed serum antibodies for the organism isolated and this animal had a small healed lesion on one teat suggestive of a rat bite. In this epidemic, Parker and Hudson isolated the etiological agent from eleven of seventeen patients studied. Serum antibodies were demonstrated in some of the patients. In a more complete report on Haverhill fever, Place and Sutton also refer to a previous epidemic with about 600 cases of undetermined etiology that occurred at Chester, Pennsylvania, in May and June 1925. Ninety-two per cent of the patients used raw milk from a single source. The similarity of onset, symptoms, course of disease, and epidemiology were comparable to the Haverhill episode.

No other milk-borne epidemic of Haverhill fever has been reported. It should be noted that Evans reported a streptothrix present in cows' udders but not associated with any recognized disease condition. It may be questioned whether the name Haverhill fever should be retained for sporadic cases of a disease following rat bite when the clinical symptoms, mode of infection, and etiological agent were quite well known long before Haverhill fever was described. There appears to be no other appropriate name. It may seem presumptuous to include a discussion of these epidemics under rat-bite fever; however, as they were attributed to infection with *Streptobacillus moniliformis*, one of the recognized agents of rat-bite fever, there appears to be no alternative.

The Infection in Rats

Rats, *Rattus* spp., appear to be the principal reservoir of *S. moniliformis* although a squirrel and a weasel were included in the sources of human infection listed by Brown and Nunemaker. Organisms presumably of this species had been recovered from calves dying of pneumonia and from laboratory mice showing spontaneous infectious rheumatism.

Rats are not greatly inconvenienced by chronic infection but severe inner ear involvement causes partial loss of balance and discomfort in some individuals. Infectious material from rats is often contaminated with other organisms but can be freed of contaminants by passage through mice. Some strains produce fatal infections in mice while others produce low-grade infections with arthritis as the chief manifestation (Brown and Nunemaker).

Other experimental animals have been little used. Rabbits are refractive to infection but are useful for production of immune serum.

Strangeways found that 50 per cent of the wild rats carried *S. moniliformis* in their naso-pharynx. The middle ear and lungs of either wild or laboratory rats are also consistent sources of infection.

An epizootic in laboratory white mice with a fairly high morbidity and mortality rate was reported by Freundt at the State Serum Institute in Copenhagen. Infection was attributed to apparently healthy albino rats kept in the same animal room. This epizootic prompted a study of the modes of transmission and the author concluded the portal of entry of infection was the throat and mouth.

The Disease in Man

In two instances, one confirmed by laboratory tests and one diagnosed by clinical symptoms and epidemiology, Haverhill fever was characterized by epidemic outbreaks. The conspicuous symptoms were abrupt onset, with chills, fever, malaise, vomiting and headache; an early eruption, rubellaform or morbilliform, occurring on the extremities and tending to become hemorrhagic; a multiple arthritis of varying intensity but often severe and crippling; a fever curve of abrupt rise, with remission in from two to five days, and after a few days of relative freedom from symptoms a recurrence with which the arthritic manifestations appeared.

The disease due to rat bite does not differ in its clinical features from milk-borne infection. Abrupt onset, nausea, and vomiting are as prominent symptoms in such cases as in the epidemic where infection was presumably from ingestion. In rat-bite cases the initial wound is said to heal promptly without a delayed reaction of pain, inflammation or ulcer formation, differing in this respect from sodoku.

The incubation period usually is from two to ten days but sometimes is longer.

The death rate is low. In the tabulation of 125 cases of rat-bite fever (both types) by Brown and Nunemaker (1942), only two cases attributed to *"Streptothrix"* (= *Streptobacillus*) were fatal. No fatalities are mentioned in the two Haverhill fever epidemics involving eighty-six and "about 600" cases, respectively.

In reporting a case of acute bacterial endocarditis caused by *S. moniliformis* from the bite of laboratory white rat, Hamburger and Knowles (1953) cite reports of seven other cases, six of which were fatal. The only case which recovered received large doses of penicillin. Their patient recovered following penicillin and streptomycin therapy.

Prevention and Control

Prevention of Haverhill fever as of sodoku depends on the control of rats. Milk-borne epidemics are probably due indirectly to rat contamination. Compulsory pasteurization of milk is an added precaution for this and for so many other serious diseases that there is no justification for the general distribution of raw milk.

Penicillin is recommended for therapy.

ITEMS OF NOTE

1) Sodoku is caused by *Spirillum minus*.

2) *Spirillum minus* causes no symptoms of disease in natural infections in its animal reservoirs, rats and mice.

3) Human cases of sodoku in the United States confirmed beyond reasonable doubt number less than thirty.

4) Sodoku in man results from the bite of an infected rat, mouse, or other animal.

5) The prevention of sodoku consists in the elimination of rats and mice.

6) Sodoku is probably much more common than published reports indicate.

7) Haverhill fever is caused by *Streptobacillus moniliformis*.

8) The rat is the chief reservoir of Haverhill fever.

9) Sporadic cases of Haverhill fever result from rat bites.

10) Epidemics of Haverhill fever arise from use of unpasteurized milk apparently directly or indirectly contaminated by rats.

11) Prevention of Haverhill fever is dependent on rat control, pasteurization of milk, and protection of food supplies from rodent contamination.

REFERENCES

ALTEMEIER, W. A., SNYDER, H. and HOWE, G.: *J.A.M.A.*, *127*:270-273, 1945.

BAYNE-JONES, S.: *Inter. Clinics.*, *3*:235-253, 1931.

BEESON, P. B.: *J.A.M.A.*, *123*:332-334, 1943.

BREED, R. S., MURRAY, E. G. D. and HITCHENS, A. P.: *Bergey's Manual of Determinative Bacteriology*. 6th Edition, Baltimore, Williams & Wilkins, 1948.

BROWN, T. M. and NUNEMAKER, J. C.: *Bull. Johns Hopkins Hosp.*, *70*:201-328, 1942.

CARTER, H. V.: *Sc. Mem. by Med. Officer of the Army of India.* 1887, part 3, p. 45.

DALAL, A. K.: *Practitioner, 92*:449, 1914.

DAS GUPTA, B. M.: *Indian Med. Gaz., 73*:140-141, 1938.

DOLMAN, C. E., KERR, D. E., CHANG, H. and SHEARER, A. R.: *Canad. J. Pub. Health, 42*:228-241, 1951.

EVANS, A. E.: *J. Infect. Dis., 23*:373-376, 1918.

FRANCIS, E.: *Pub. Health Rep., 51*:976-977, 1936.

FRANK, W. P. and BOWER, A. G.: *California Med., 74*:42, 1951.

FREUNDT, E. A.: *Acta Path. & Microbiol. Scand., 38*:231-245, 1956.

FUTAKI, K., TAKAKI, I., TANIGUCHI, T. and OSUMI, S.: *J. Exper. Med., 23*:249-250, 1916.

FUTAKI, K., TAKAKI, I., TANIGUCHI, T. and OSUMI, S.: *J. Exper. Med., 25*:33-44, 1917.

HAMBURGER, M. and KNOWLES, H. C.: *A. M. A. Arch. Int. Med., 92*:216-220, 1953.

HATA, S.: *Münch. Med. Woch. 59*:854, 1912.

JELLISON, W. L., ENEBOE, P. L., PARKER, R. R. and HUGHES, L. E.: *Pub. Health Rep., 52*:1661-1665, 1949.

KNOWLES, R., DAS GUPTA, B. M. and SEN, S.: *Indian Med. Gaz., 71*:210-212, 1936.

LARSON, C. L.: *Pub. Health Rep., 56*:1961-1969, 1941.

LEMIERRE, A., REILLY, J., LAPORTE, A. and MORIN, M.: *Bull. Acad. Med. Paris, 117*:705-713, 1937.

LEVADITI, C., NICOLAU, S. and POINCLOUX, P.: *Compt. rend. Acad. Sc., 180*:1188-1190, 1925.

MCDERMOTT, E. N.: *Quart. J. Med., 21*:433-458, 1928.

MIYAKE, H.: *Mitt. Grenzgeb. D. Med. U. Chir., 5*:231-262, 1900.

PARKER, F., JR. and HUDSON, N. P.: *Am. J. Path., 2*:357-379, 1926.

PLACE, E. H. and SUTTON, L. E.: *Arch. Int. Med., 54*:659-684, 1934.

PLACE, E. H., SUTTON, L. E. and WILLNER, O.: *Boston Med. & Surg. J., 194*:285-287, 1926.

ROBERTSON, A.: *Ann. Trop. Med. & Parasit., 24:*367-410, 1930.

SAVOOR, S. R.: *Studies from the Institute for Med. Res., Federation of Malaya. 25:*303-304, 1951.

SAVOOR, S. R. and LEWTHWAITE, R.: *Brit. J. Exper. Path., 22:*274-292, 1930.

SCHARLES, F. H. and SEASTONE, C. F., JR.: *New England J. Med., 211:*711-714, 1934.

SCHOTTMÜLLER, H.: *Dermdt. Wohnschr. (Supp.), 58:*77-103, 1914.

SEIDENSTRICKER, J. C.: Correspondence and unpublished data at Rocky Mountain Laboratory, 1949.

STRANGEWAYS, W. I.: *J. Path. & Bact., 37:*45-51, 1933.

SURVEYOR, N. F.: *Lancet, 185:*1764, 1913.

Chapter 26

THE ENDEMIC RELAPSING FEVERS

GORDON E. DAVIS, S.M., Sc.D.

THE RELAPSING fevers are acute infectious diseases caused by spirochetes of the genus *Borrelia* which are transmitted through the agency of the body louse, *Pediculus humanus corporis* (epidemic form) and by several species of ticks of the genus *Ornithodoros* (endemic form).

HISTORY

Although the clinical features of the disease are recorded in the writings of Hippocrates (b. 460 B.C.), not much further information was obtained until the middle of the eighteenth century when Rutty, in 1741, observed the same type of disease associated with typhus in Dublin. The term "relapsing fever" was first given during an epidemic in Edinburgh in 1843, at which time it was differentiated from epidemic typhus. During an epidemic in Berlin in 1868, Obermeier first observed relapsing fever spirochetes in patients' blood. However, due to the influence of his chief, Virchow, and further because of his failure to reproduce the disease in the available laboratory animals, which included dogs, rabbits, and guinea pigs, he did not publish these findings until he had confirmed them during a second epidemic in 1873.

The term *Protomycetum recurrentis* was given to the organism by Lebert in 1874, and *Spirochaete obermeieri* by Cohn the following year. Since the demonstration of tick-transmission numerous specific names have been given, some of which may be retained for the sake of convenience, and others for more special reasons. Mackie, in 1907, on an epidemiological basis, concluded that the louse was the vector in India. Experimental evidence for this conclusion was afforded by Sergent and Foley in 1910, and by Nicolle and his colleagues in 1912, by the infection of monkeys with the triturates of lice removed from relapsing fever patients.

Among the earliest references to the tick-borne type is that of R. Drury in 1702, in Madagascar. David Livingstone (1857) recorded it in the Congo, and Cook (1904) reported the disease in Uganda. Tick-borne transmission *(O. moubata)* was independently proved by Ross and Milne in Uganda in 1904 and by Dutton and Todd in the Congo (1905). The latter two authors also reported transovarial transmission.

In 1913, Dschunkowsky demonstrated the presence of the disease in Iran, and during the middle twenties its exstence in the U.S.S.R. and in the region east of the Caspian Sea was fully established. De Buen reported it in Spain in 1926. In a letter to the editor of the Lancet, Adler, Theodor, and Schieber (1936) reported the tick-borne type in Palestine, for the first time. The most recently reported areas in Asia are Kashmir and Jammu in India (Rao and Kalra, 1949). During World War II several new foci of infection were reported, one of which was in Cyprus. This seems of special interest, as the term "Cyprus fever" appeared in the literature as early as 1878.

In the Western Hemisphere the first reports came from Colombia, Venezuela, and Panama in the early part of the present century, later from Guatemala and Mexico, and very recently from Ecuador. The disease, as reported from Peru, Uruguay and Cuba is not authenticated as tick-borne. However, two species of *Ornithodoros (O. aragaoi* and *O. davisi)* have been described from Peru. One indigenous case has been reported from Argentina.

In the United States, the disease which is now known to be tick-borne but was thought to be louse-borne, was reported from Colorado by Meader in 1915 and by Waring in 1918. It was then recognized in other states in rapid succession and is now known to be present in twelve of the western states and in British Columbia. Increased interest in the disease in the United States began in 1930, when Weller and Graham first called attention to the tick, *O. turicata,* as a vector in Texas.

SEASONAL PREVALENCE

The louse-borne form which occurs in parts of Europe, Asia, Africa, and Latin America has its greatest prevalence in winter and spring.

The seasonal prevalence of the tick-borne form varies considerably in different parts of the world. In warmer countries the disease occurs throughout the year. Such prevalence is also true when the vectors are house-inhabiting such as *O. moubata, O. rudis, O. talaje,* etc. In Kashmir and Jammu, where *O. crossi* is the vector, ticks are reported as active in the huts throughout the winter. In California, cases occur mostly in June, July, and August. In Texas, cases have been reported every month in the year, with the largest number occurring in October and equal numbers in January and August.

AGE AND SEX

Neither age nor sex is exempt. In the louse-borne form both sexes are about equally attacked, while in the tick-borne form there is an apparent preponderance in males.

El-Ramly, in Egypt, tabulated 2682 cases of epidemic relapsing fever as to age and sex. There were 1422 males and 1260 females. The ages ranged from intrauterine to sixty years, with the highest incidence in the fifteen to twenty-five year groups. Of 107 cases tabulated by Herms and Wheeler (1936) in California, where *O. hermsi* is the chief vector, sixty-seven were males and forty females. The ages ranged from two to sixty-eight years. Morrison and Parsons (1941) have reported the disease in a six-day-old infant in Nevada. This infection may have occurred *in utero* or during passage through the birth canal.

DISTRIBUTION AND TICK VECTORS

Endemic relapsing fever is present in all continents with the exception of Australia.

In the Western Hemisphere it is present in Argentina, Venezuela, Colombia, Ecuador, Panama, Guatamala, and Mexico. At least twelve of the western United States (Arizona, California, Colorado, Idaho, Kansas, Nevada, New Mexico, Oregon, Oklahoma, Texas, Utah, Washington) and British Columbia, Canada, have reported cases of relapsing fever. The distribution of potential tick vectors is much wider than is indicated by these areas, as spirochetes have been recovered from ticks collected in areas from which cases of relapsing fever have not been reported.

In the Western Hemisphere there are three important vectors: *O.*

hermsi, O. turicata, and *O. rudis.* Only one case has been attributed to *O. parkeri,* which is normally a burrow tick. (Table 63)

O. talaje, found in houses, is considered a fourth vector. It is the only species of the genus known in Guatemala where the disease is present. It is also found in dwellings in Mexico and Panama and spirochetes have been recovered from this species in Mexico as well

TABLE 63

DISTRIBUTION OF *Borrelia* SPECIES AND TICK VECTORS IN THE WESTERN HEMISPHERE

Borrelia *Species*	*Normal* *Tick Vectors*	*Reported Geographic* *Distribution*	*Remarks*
B. hermsii	O. hermsi	U. S. A.: Calif., Colo., Idaho, Nev., Ore., Wash., and in British Columbia, Canada	Vector in named areas
B. turicatae	O. turicata	U. S. A.: Ariz., Calif., Colo., Fla., Kansas, New Mexico, Okla., Utah, Texas. Mexico: Aquascalientes and Jalisco	Vector in Kansas, New Mexico, Okla., Texas, and in Mexico
B. parkeri	O. parkeri	Calif., Colo., Idaho, Mont., Nev., Ore., Wash., Wyoming, Utah	Vector in Calif. Spirochetes recovered: Calif., Idaho, Mont., Nev., Ore., Wyo., Utah
B. mazzottii	O. talaje	U. S. A.: Calif., Ariz., Nev., Kans., Texas, Fla., and southward to Argentina	U. S. A. spirochetes recovered from Ariz., Kans., and Texas. Also Mexico
B. venezuelensis	O. rudis	Panama, Colombia, Ecuador, Venezuela and Paraguay	Vector in first four Republics
B. brasiliensis	O. brasiliensis	Brazil	State of Rio Grande do Sul

as from several areas in the United States where it has a wide distribution. However, here, the chief hosts are the pack rats. *Neotoma* spp. and the kangaroo rats, *Dipodomys* spp. It appears that in Panama the normal host of the larvae is the commensal rat, *Rattus* sp., as is also true of the very closely allied species, *O. puertoricensis* in Puerto Rico, from which spirochetes have not been recovered. Another closely related species, *O. dugesi,* in Mexico, from which spirochetes have been recovered, was reported as being found on "ratas silvestris." It should be remembered that the "*O. talaje*" reported in houses in New York, Wisconsin, and Minnesota by Matheson (1931), Herrick (1935), and Riley (1935), has been described as a new species, *O. kelleyi,* Cooley and Kohls (1941). The normal hosts of this tick are bats, *Myotis* spp., and *Pipistrellus* spp.

In the Eastern Hemisphere there are four important vectors: *O. moubata, O. tholozani, O. erraticus* (large form), and *O. crossi.* Most ixodologists consider *O. papillipes* and *O. crossi* as synonyms of *O. tholozani,* but there are still differences of opinion. The distribution of the disease is coincident with the distribution of these species as indicated in Table 64.

TABLE 64

DISTRIBUTION OF *Borrelia* SPECIES AND TICK VECTORS IN THE EASTERN HEMISPHERE

Borrelia Species	*Normal Tick Vectors*	*Reported Geographic Distribution*	*Remarks*
?	*O. crossi*	India: Kashmir and Jammu	Only known vector
B. duttonii	*O. moubata*	In Africa from Lake Chad eastward to the coast and southward to Cape Colony. Also in Madagascar	Vector throughout this area
B. hispanica	*O. erraticus*	Spain and Portugal	
B. marocana	*O. erraticus*	Morocco	
B. persica	*O. tholozani*	Cyrenaica, the Egyptian Western Desert, Cyprus, the Eastern Mediterranean, Iran, Iraq, and the southern USSR eastward to the western border of China	Vector in named areas, probably also in Afghanistan

Question mark indicates that it is the writer's belief that these spirochetes have not been named. Should *O. crossi* finally be conceded as a synonym of *O. tholozani,* then the organism would be *B. persica. B. novyi* has been omitted, as nothing is known of this spirochete in relation to the louse or any species of tick. The frequent reference to *B. novyi* as "the American strain" is entirely unwarranted. Neither *O. savignyi* nor *O. lahorensis* has been incriminated in nature.

There is still little agreement as to the validity of *B. usbekistanica* and *B. sogdianum,* both of which have been applied to spirochetes normally transmitted by *O. tholozani.* The organisms thus named differ chiefly in virulence for the guinea pig.

The recently recognized "small" form of *O. erraticus* is of considerable interest, as several specific names have been given to the spirochetes recovered from this form and its hosts in different geographical locations. These are listed in Table 65. Little is known concerning their relation to the disease in man. These two forms of *O. erraticus* require very different conditions for rearing in the laboratory.

TABLE 65

Borrelia Species	Normal Tick Vector	Reported Geographical Distribution
B. caucasica	O. verrucosus	The Caucasus
B. crocidurae	O. erraticus	Senegal
B. dipodilli	O. erraticus	Kenya
B. dugesii	O. dugesi	Mexico
B. merionesi	O. erraticus	Morocco
B. microti	O. erraticus	Iran
B. latyschewi	O. tartakovskyi	U. S. S. R. Fergana, Usbekistan
B. normandi	O. normandi	Tunisia

THE ETIOLOGIC AGENTS

The causative agent was described by Obermeier in 1873. The relapsing fever spirochetes have been claimed by both protozoologists and bacteriologists, while some would place them in an intermediate group. They have also been placed in several genera, including *Spirilla, Protomycetum, Treponema, Spironema, Spirochaeta, Borrelia,* etc. The classification of spirochetes is still in a fluid state. Not even the two families within the Order as given in Bergey's Manual of Determinative Bacteriology are in general acceptance. For the present purpose, the agents will be considered as bacterial in the genus *Borrelia,* as it does not seem fitting to place the blood spirochetes in the genus *Spirochaeta* which was created for a free-living species. It is generally stated that morphologically the several "species" are indistinguishable. However, when several "species" are studied closely in the same mammal unmistakable differences become apparent.

The organisms stain easily with aniline dyes, but some modification of the Romanowsky method, such as Giemsa's stain, is frequently used. In stained preparations the length is from 8 to 16 microns. Larger forms are the result of incomplete division. The spirals vary in number and are coarse, shallow, or irregular. The presence or absence of flagella has long been a question. The election microscope and several staining methods have demonstrated structures which may be flagella. If these structures can be shown to be constant in number and arrangement they may well aid in classification. There has been a feeling on the part of some workers over a considerable period of time that the life-cycle of the spirochetes is not a simple one.

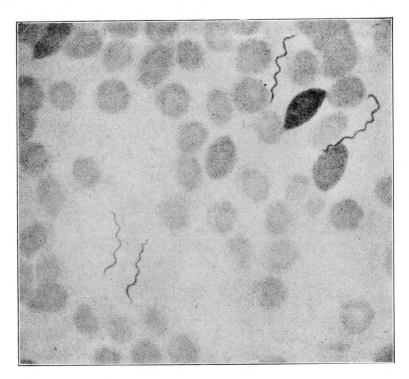

Fig. 120. *Borrelia turicatae,* Texas strain, in blood of white mouse. (A. M. M. 50437.)

Many recipes for media for cultivation have appeared in the literature, but none of them seem to be uniformly successful. A natural method for maintenance within specific tick vectors is possible, and often the spirochetes survive throughout the life of the tick. The longevity of some tick vectors is phenomenal. One female *O. turicata* in the writer's collection survived for nine and one-half years without feeding, and a further three years after one blood meal. One *O. parkeri* has transmitted spirochetes over a period of twelve years.

A list of named spirochetes with their natural tick vectors is presented in Tables 63, 64 and 65. There is little agreement concerning specific epithets. However, within the United States there is a 100 per cent specificity between the tick vector and the spirochete naturally transmitted by it. As an example, *O. hermsi* from any area will transmit spirochetes from this species of tick from any other area, but none of the other tick vectors will transmit the spirochetes. It was for this reason that *O. hermsi* spirochetes were given the name *B. hermsii*, *O. parkeri* spirochetes the term *B. parkeri*, and for the same reason Brumpt named the spirochetes of *O. turicata*, *B. turicatae*. There has been a notable exception. In a limited number of experiments *O. hermsi* from Utah failed to transmit *O. hermsi* spirochetes from other areas.

MODES OF TRANSMISSION

It is rather generally agreed that the epidemic type of relapsing fever is transmitted through the agency of the crushed body louse *Pediculus humanus corporis*, and not through feeding. The head louse, *Pediculus humanus humanus*, may also be implicated. As transovarial transmission in the louse is not generally accepted, it must be assumed that man is the only reservoir.

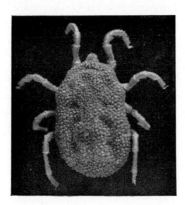

Fig. 121. Argasid tick. *Ornithodoros turicata*. (*U. S. Dept. Agriculture, Bureau of Entomology* and *Plant Quarantine*.)

In the endemic type, transmission is by ticks. According to a recent classification (Cooley and Kohls, 1944) the family Argasidae contains four genera: *Octbius, Antricola, Argas,* and *Ornithodoros*. There are two species within each of the first two genera, about a dozen species in the genus *Argas*, and approximately fifty-five species in the genus *Ornithodoros*.

Little or nothing is known concerning the biology of many species of the genus. At least fourteen species are proved vectors of relapsing fever spirochetes.

The spirochetoses of some larger mammals are transmitted by ixodid ticks and names have been given to the spirochetes such as *Spirochaeta ovis, S. equi,* etc. The spirochetes of ducks, geese, and fowls are transmitted by ticks of the genus *Argas.* However, for the most part we are interested in ticks of the genus *Ornithodoros.* The species of *Ornithodoros* may be divided into two groups: species known to be vectors to man, and species from which spirochetes have been recovered but which seldom come in contact with man. These are indicated in the accompanying tables.

Several methods of infection have been reported: by feeding, through the secretion of the salivary glands; by means of the coxal fluid which is passed copiously by some species while feeding; and by the excreta from the malpighian tubules.

Although spirochetes have been demonstrated microscopically in the malpighian tubules, "excreta" on the host have been observed rarely and only in *O. moubata.* In *O. hermsi* the coxal fluid crystallizes very rapidly and is normally seen only as a white deposit. There are other species which seldom or never pass coxal fluid while on the host. It must therefore be concluded that such species also transmit by bite. There are other species, such as *O. moubata* and *O. talaje,* which almost invariably pass the fluid while nearing repletion, and as spirochetes have been demonstrated in the fluid either by dark-field examination or by animal inoculation, it appears that transmission is, in part, through this medium.

The much discussed problem of the importance of, or necessity for, animal "reservoirs" can be evaluated only by the study of each species of tick. In some species (*O. turicata,* Davis, 1943) trans-ovarial transmission has been shown up to 100 per cent, while in other species this type of transmission has never been demonstrated. On the other hand, when a series of ticks is allowed to feed on an infected host, there is a wide range in the number of ticks of different species which will subsequently transmit spirochetes. Through the combination of transovarial transmission and feeding on infected hosts, survival of the organisms is assured.

Nicolle postulated the maintenance of infection by ticks and the spread of it by lice. Experimental studies by several workers over a period of years on the survival of tick-borne spirochetes in lice tend to confirm this opinion. The results of these studies materially alter some older concepts as to the origin of epidemics.

THE DISEASE IN ANIMALS

Ticks of the genus *Ornithodoros* have a wide range of hosts, including numerous species of mammals, as well as birds and reptiles. Spirochetes have been recovered from many hosts, including armadillos, opossums, weasels, chipmunks, tree squirrels, hamsters, several species of gerbilles, mice, bats, horses, cattle, an insectivore, and from several species of monkeys and chimpanzees. However, with the exception of the marmoset, *Leontocebus geoffroyi* (Pucheron), and the armadillo in Panama (Clark, Dunn, and Benavides, 1931), (Dunn, L. H., and Clark, H. C., 1933), very little is known concerning the disease in these animals. In the young marmoset, the disease almost invariably proves fatal.

In the laboratory the animals most frequently used are white mice, white rats, guinea pigs, and hamsters. Various species of monkeys have afforded important data, but it is obvious that they cannot be used when large numbers of animals are required.

The course of the disease in these laboratory animals varies widely in the different species, as well as with the strains of spirochetes and methods of infection. In the white mouse there is an incubation period of from about three to eight days. Frequently the only evidence of infection is the appearance of spirochetes in the peripheral blood. However, infection with some strains may prove fatal. Spirochetemia may be continuous for many days, or the course of infection may be the relapsing type with a rapid multiplication of spirochetes. This is followed by their sudden and complete disappearance, and their reappearance a few days later. In the United States, the guinea pig has been ignored for the most part. However, when susceptible to the species of spirochetes, the course of the disease in guinea pigs more nearly approximates the disease in man than with any other laboratory animal (with the possible exception of the monkey) in that there are repeated febrile relapses, at which times spirochetes reappear in the peripheral blood (Davis, 1939). The guinea pig is not susceptible to certain strains, but is the animal of choice for *O. tholozani* and *O. crossi* spirochetes. On the Gold Coast, Russell (1936), working with louse-borne spirochetes and the pouched bush rat, *Cricetomys gambianus,* reported that the disease in this animal closely resembles the disease in man.

At present, new-born mice, rats, rabbits, and guinea pigs are being used, as they are more susceptible to some strains than are the adult animals.

THE DISEASE IN MAN

The disease in man is characterized primarily by alternate febrile and afebrile periods. The onset is usually sudden with an initial feeling of being cold. There rapidly follows a high fever with frontal headache and an acute chill with profuse sweating, at which time the temperature falls by crises. There may be intense pains in the back, limbs, and joints. A petechial rash is sometimes seen. The patient then returns to near normal for a week or more, when a relapse occurs. From one to fourteen relapses have been reported.

The incubation period has been definitely established in a number of cases. Some selected cases representing different vectors are as follows: Adler, Theodor, and Scheiber (1936) reported thirteen cases in Israel in which the period varied from five to nine days following the bites of *O. tholozani* in a cave. In the attempted treatment of neurosyphilis and nonsyphilitic psychoses by feeding infective *O. turicata* on 147 patients (Lawrence and Terrell, 1942), the incubation period varied from four to nine days, with an average of 6.5 days. In a laboratory infection, symptoms occurred on the eighth day following the attachment of an *O. turicata* larva (Davis, 1948). Following the contamination of a field worker's hands with the blood of an infected rodent (*O. hermsi* spirochetes), the incubation period was six days (Legge, 1933).

In the tick-borne forms there are frequently neurologic symptoms, even to the impairment of vision and hearing, and a prolonged and painful generalized peripheral neuritis.

Russell (1932), in a study of the spleen in fifteen cases of louse-borne relapsing fever on the Gold Coast, concluded that "the miliary lesions, which consist of a zone of congestion and cell infiltration round the malpighian bodies, are characteristic of human relapsing fever" and that these lesions "appear to be the most important guide to the pathologist in the differential diagnosis of fatal relapsing fever, short of actually finding spirochetes."

TREATMENT

The arsenicals have long been considered as specific in the treatment of the relapsing fevers, but the standard textbook statements are being seriously challenged. It was early noted in North Africa that certain cases did not respond to the arsenicals. In the United States, Francis (1938) found that neoarsphenamine failed to show therapeutic value in the treatment of three patients infected with a Texas *Ornithodoros turicata* strain, and considered that the opinion concerning this drug as a "specific" must be radically modified. These strains have since been considered peculiar in that they were "arsenic-fast." However, when case reports of the adherents of arsenical therapy are evaluated, it is easily seen that in many cases there were as many relapses as there would have been without therapy. In a post-war review (Davis, 1948), which included both louse-borne and tick-borne types, reported from many areas, the concensus was not in favor of the arsenicals. In one recent report on 400 cases among native troops in East Africa, Quinn and Perkins (1946) reported that "N.A.B. therapy in doses up to 0.6 gm. appeared to have little effect on the course of the disease." The tick vector in this area is *O. moubata.*

During a louse-borne epidemic in Cairo Egypt, in 1946 Ingraham and Lapenta in carefully controlled experiments on fifty-two patients found that 25,000 units of penicillin administered every three hours until 1,000,000 units had been given, resulted in no relapses; while the relapses occurred in 87 per cent of the untreated patients. A considerable number of cases of the tick-borne disease from widely separated areas have been reported as treated successfully with antibiotics, especially aureomycin, terramycin and streptomycin.

PREVENTION

There is only one general rule, which is the avoidance of ticks. However, it should be remembered that methods of prevention are quite different from the ones given for disease agents transmitted by ixodid ticks. While the ixodid ticks require several days for engorgement in all stages, and may readily be found by careful examination shortly after attachment, ticks of the genus *Ornithodoros* [with the exception of the larval stage of a few species (including *O. talaje*)], engorge and voluntarily detach within a few minutes up to an hour, and that in the larval stage some species may transmit spirochetes in as short a time as thirty seconds after attachment. It may be added that there is no "feeling" while the tick is feeding. The first evidence that a tick has fed is the appearance of a small area of erythema, followed by a papule, and subsequently by necrosis. There may be intense itching some hours after the bite of ticks of some species.

In *O. moubata* territory, avoidance of ticks might mean a change in the mode of living, or in a frequent burning of the "home" as this species is a "tick of the hut." The bamboo-type of bed so frequently used in northern South America, and in Panama, affords excellent harborage for *O. rudis* and *O. talaje*. As caves are a source of infection (*O. turicata* in Texas, *O. tholozani* in Cyprus and Palestine, etc.), one might suggest the suppression of the explorer instinct! One very practicable suggestion is the rodent-proofing of summer homes in *O. hermsi* areas, and the destruction of logs, stumps, etc., which obviously are nesting places for rodents in nearby areas.

Some of the newer "insecticides" may be shown to be effective, but there is little definite information at the present time.

ITEMS OF NOTE

1) The endemic relapsing fevers are present in all continents, with the exception of Australia.

2) The etiologic agents are spirochetes of the genus *Borrelia,* which are transmitted by ticks of the genus *Ornithodoros.*

3) The spirochetal reservoirs are the hosts on which the ticks feed, or the ticks themselves.

4) The generally accepted concepts of treatment by the arsenicals are being seriously challenged. The antibiotics have not been sufficiently tested, but some of them appear to be efficient.

5) The demonstration of the survival of tick-borne spirochetes within the louse over a sufficient period of time to initiate an epidemic in a louse-infested population may explain the origin of epidemics.

REFERENCES

ADLER, S., THEODOR, O. and SCHIEBER, H.: *Lancet,* 448, (Feb. 22), 1936.
ADLER, S., THEODOR, O. and SCHIEBER, H.: *Ann. Trop. Med. & Parasit, 31*:25, 1937.
CLARK, H. C., DUNN, L. H. and BENAVIDES, J.: *Am. J. Trop. Med., 11*:243, 1931.
COHN, F.: *Beitrage z. Biol., 1*:196, 1875.
COOK, A. R.: *J. Trop. Med.,* 7:24, 1904.

Cooley, R. A. and Kohls, G. M.: *Pub. Health Rep., 56*:910, (April 25) 1941.

Cooley, R. A. and Kohls, G. M.: *The American Midland Naturalist.* Notre Dame, Ind., University Press, Monograph No. 1 (1944).

Davis, G. E.: *Pub. Health Rep., 54*:1721, (Sept. 22) 1939.

Davis, G. E.: *Pub. Health Rep., 58*:839, 1943.

Davis, G. E.: *Ann. Rev. Microbiology, 2*:305, 1948.

de Buen, S.: *Ann. Parasitol., 4*:185, 1926.

Drury, R.: In: Neel, R., Payet, M. and Gonnet, C.: *Bull. Soc. Path. Exot., 42*:384, 1949.

Dschunkowsky, E.: *Deutsch. med. Wchnschr., 39*:419, 1913.

Dunn, L. H. and Clark, H. C.: *Am. J. Trop. Med., 13*:201, 1933.

Dutton, J. E. and Todd, J. L.: Memoir 17, Liverpool School of Trop. Med., Liverpool. 1905.

El-Ramly, A. H.: *J. Egypt. Pub. Health A., 21*:125, 1946.

Francis, E.: *Pub. Health Rep., 53*:2220, 1938.

Herms, W. B. and Wheeler, C. M.: *California State Dept. Pub. Health,* 1936, Special Bull. No. 61.

Ingraham, H. S. and Lapenta, R. G.: *Naval Med. Bull., 46*:1719, 1946.

Lawrence, D. H. and Terrell, J. L.: *A.A.A.S.* Bull. No. 18, Washington, D. C. 1942, p. 109.

Lebert, H.: Ziemssen's Handbuch, *Spec. Path. u. Therap., 2*:243, 1874.

Legge, R. T.: *California & Western Med., 38*:370, 1933.

Livingstone, David: *Missionary Travels and Researches.* London, John Murray, 1857, p. 382 and p. 628.

Mackie, F. P.: *Ann. Trop. Med. & Parasitol., 1*:157, 1907.

Meader, C. N.: *Colorado Med., 12*:365, 1915.

Morrison, S. K. and Parsons, L. P.: *J.A.M.A., 116*:220, 1941.

Nicolle, C., Blaizot, L. and Conseil, E.: *Compt. rend. Acad., Paris, 155*:481, 1912.

Obermeier, O.: *Berlin. klin. Wchnschr., 10*:349, 364, 1873.

Quinn, C. E. and Perkins, E. S.: *J. Trop. Med. & Hyg., 49*:30, 1946.

Rao, K. N. A. and Kalra, S. L.: *Indian J. Med. Res., 37*:385, 1949.

Ross, P. H. and Milne, A. D.: *Brit. M. J.*, p. 1453, (Nov. 26) 1904.

Russell, H.: *Tr. Roy. Soc. Trop. Med. & Hyg., 26*:259, 1932.

Russell, H.: *Tr. Roy. Soc. Trop. Med. & Hyg., 30*:179, 1936.

Sergent, E. and Foley, F. H.: *Ann. Inst. Pasteur., 24*:337, 1910.

Waring, J. J.: *Am. J. Med. Sc.,* New Series, *155*:819, 1918.

Weller, B. and Graham, G. M.: *J.A.M.A., 95*:1834, 1930.

Chapter 27

MURINE TYPHUS FEVER

R. E. DYER, M.D.

RICKETTSIAL DISEASES

TYPHUS FEVER belongs to the group of diseases caused by Rickettsiae. Rickettsiae may be classified as falling between the filterable viruses on one side and the true bacteria on the other. They are minute organisms appearing as coccoid or bacillary forms within the cells of animal tissues. They are non-motile, measure about half a micron in diameter, and are readily stained with Giemsa, Castaneda, or Macchiavello stains. Unlike the viruses, they are not filtrable.

Rickettsiae have never been cultivated in media free from living cells, but grow rapidly in tissue cultures. The rickettsial diseases are usually regarded as being animal diseases which are transmitted from animal to animal, including man, by various arthropods. As a matter of fact, the evidence is equally as good that Rickettsiae are arthropod parasites, and that animals are only incidentally infected while acting as a source of food for infected arthropods. Whatever may be the original host of the parasite, it is known that, in these diseases, the infections are present in certain animals in nature, and that certain species of arthropods may be infected by feeding upon such infected animals. Four of the identified rickettsial diseases which occur in man, typhus, Rocky Mountain spotted fever, tsutsugamushi, and rickettsial pox, have been shown to be separate entities, although closely related. There are several other diseases which belong to the Rickettsial group, the relationship of which to the other members of the group as yet has not been definitely determined, as trench fever, boutonneuse fever, Kenya typhus, certain South African tick fevers, Russian tick typhus, and North Queensland tick typhus. The various tick fevers may be considered as falling into a sub group of the rickettsial diseases with Rocky Mountain spotted fever. Yet another disease, Q fever, is usually classified as a rickettsial disease. However, in the epidemiology of this disease, the characteristics of the causative organism and the clinical picture, Q fever stands a little apart from the true rickettsial diseases. With the exception of Q fever, the epidemiology of each rickettsial disease is determined by the life history and feeding habits of its arthropod vector (see Table 66).

TABLE 66

RICKETTSIAL DISEASES TRANSMITTED FROM ANIMALS TO MAN

Disease	Etiologic Agent	Common Vector	Animal Reservoir
Epidemic typhus	R. prowazeki	Body louse Pediculus humanus corporis	Man
Murine typhus fever	Rickettsia mooseri	Rat flea Xenopsylla cheopis	Rat
Rocky Mountain Spotted fever	R. rickettsi	Wood tick Dermacentor andersoni Eastern dog tick Dermacentor variabilis	Rodents and other animals
Brazilian and Columbian spotted fevers	R. rickettsi	Cayenne tick Amblyomma cajennense	Dog
Boutonneuse fever and Kenya typhus	R. conori	Brown dog tick Rhipicephalus sanguineus	Dog
South African tickbite fever	R. pijperi	Haemaphysalis leachi	Dog
Tsutsugamushi Disease	R. tsutsugamushi (R. orientalis)	Kedani mite Trombicula akamushi	Field rats and mice
Rickettsial pox	R. akari	Mite Allodermanyssus sanguineus	Mice
Q fever	Coxiella burneti	Ticks Haemaphysalis humerosa Ixodes holocyclus Boophilus annulatus Dermacentor andersoni Amblyomma americana	Bandicoot, rats, cattle, sheep, goats

TYPHUS FEVERS

There are two epidemiological types of typhus which are determined by the identity of the arthropod vector: Epidemic typhus transmitted from man to man by lice, and murine typhus transmitted by fleas from rodent hosts to man. In man, the clinical symptoms of the two diseases are similar, the epidemic or louse-borne form being more severe.

EPIDEMIC TYPHUS—HISTORY AND GEOGRAPHIC PREVALENCE

It is possible that typhus may have occurred in human beings in the early civilizations, but it is not until the middle ages that a written description of a pestilence is definite enough to warrant the assumption that typhus was present. In 1083, an epidemic occurred in Italy, which probably was typhus. A few years later, in 1106, another epidemic apparently of the same disease, occurred in Bohemia. In both of these epidemics, the outbreaks followed famine. This tendency for epidemics of typhus to accompany human misery, as during war, civil revolution, and times of famine, has been the chief epidemiologic characteristic of this form of the disease. The popular names that have been given to the disease attest this fact—gaol fever, famine fever, ship fever. In the many military campaigns, typhus has killed more soldiers than has the enemy—the seige of Granada, the Thirty Years' War, and the Napoleonic campaigns, especially the Russian expedition, for example. In civilian populations, Ireland, Southeastern Europe, and Russia were chief endemic centers of the disease in the past century. In Ireland, it was particularly associated with the failure of the potato crops. More recently, typhus became epidemic in Siberia during World War I, when it caused over 100,000 deaths in six months. It took an estimated toll of upwards of 3,000,000 lives in Russia in the years following the revolution. During World War II, typhus fever caused epidemics in North Africa and Naples. Many cases occurred in and around prison camps in Germany during this last war.

In civil populations, typhus in its epidemic form occurs most often in the poorer sections of cities where cold and poverty result in a crowded and dirty population. Under such conditions, lice abound and readily move from one person to another. With the introduction of typhus into such a population, the disease spreads rapidly from person to person, frequently attacking those in attendance on the sick. The morbidity and mortality rates among doctors and nurses were very high, before the development of typhus vaccine.

Epidemic typhus has been introduced into America from time to time in the past four centuries in connection with immigration. It was present in Mexico shortly after the Spanish conquest, probably being introduced with the Spanish troops. In North America, outbreaks occurred in practically all of the northern Atlantic ports during the 19th century. All of these outbreaks were more or less self-limited, the disease never gaining a permanent lodging in North America as an endemic disease.

A form of typhus now known as Brill-Zinsser disease has been present in New York and Boston for many years. In 1898 Brill described mild typhus-like infections occurring in New York City. These cases differed from louse-borne typhus in epidemiological characteristics, particularly by the lack of communicability and dissociation from poverty, dirt, and lice. In 1912, Anderson and Goldberger found that strains of typhus, isolated in Mexico, were identical with a strain isolated from a case of Brill's disease in New York City. In 1934, Zinsser isolated strains of typhus from cases of Brill's disease. These strains corresponded in every respect with European typhus. Since these cases occurred among immigrants from Europe, Zinsser advanced the hypothesis that cases of Brill's disease were recrudescenses of typhus fever acquired earlier in life during residence in epidemic foci in Europe and that lice might be infected if fed on patients with Brill's disease.

In 1951, Murray and Snyder isolated rickettsiae from seven patients with Brill's disease and found they were identical with epidemic typhus strains. It was also shown that these newly isolated strains would infect lice. In 1952, Loeffler and Mooser suggested that the name of Brill's disease be changed to Brill-Zinsser disease.

In further support of Zinsser's hypothesis, Price in 1955, using tissue culture medium, succeeded in isolating strains of epidemic typhus from two patients who had come to this country from Russia more than twenty years before the isolations were made. The rickettsiae were recovered from lymph nodes taken during abdominal operations. The patients showed no symptoms suggesting typhus infection at the time of the operations and gave no clinical history suggesting typhus for at least six years before the operations. As Price points out, the final problem in the solution of Brill-Zinsser disease is the "mechanism that causes the recrudescence of the illness."

SEASONAL PREVALENCE

The peak of prevalence of epidemic typhus is in the winter and spring. This form of the disease is very severe, the case fatality rates varying from 25 to 60 per cent of those attacked (Fig. 122).

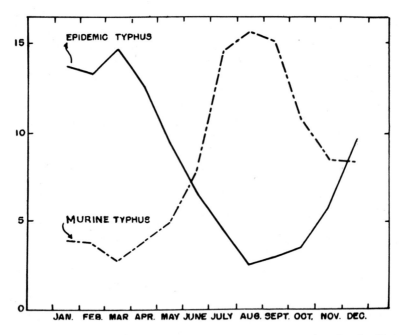

Fig. 122. Seasonal distribution of 5,334 cases of murine typhus in the United States, compared with 180,000 cases of epidemic typhus in Europe, during the same period.

THE VECTOR OF EPIDEMIC TYPHUS

For many years, it was suspected that the body louse was the transmitting agent of epidemic typhus, but it remained a suspicion until 1909 when Nicolle succeeded in transmitting the infection to monkeys by means of body lice. Head lice have also been shown capable of transmitting the infection experimentally, but the epidemiologic evidence indicates that the body louse is the principal vector in nature. Human body lice feed naturally only upon man, and under conditions that bring about the crowding of human beings in close quarters, as cold and poverty, lice multiply rapidly (Fig. 123).

The typhus rickettsiae multiply in the body of the louse in the cells lining the intestine, becoming infectious in four or five days. The infection in the louse reaches its height in about 10 days, finally killing its host. The rickettsiae are present in the feces of infected lice, and may be transmitted through this medium. It has not been definitely shown that the infection can be transmitted by the bite alone. The rickettsiae are not transmitted through the egg to succeeding generations of lice.

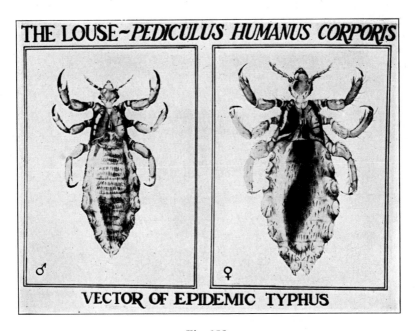

THE LOUSE~*PEDICULUS HUMANUS CORPORIS*

VECTOR OF EPIDEMIC TYPHUS

Fig. 123.

MURINE TYPHUS: HISTORY AND GEOGRAPHIC DISTRIBUTION

Just as the epidemiology of epidemic typhus is bound up with the life cycle and feeding habits of human lice, so is the epidemiology of murine typhus determined by the life cycle and feeding habits of the rat flea.

After the description of mild typhus by Brill, similar cases were described in several of the southern cities from time to time until 1923 when Maxcy undertook a study of this disease in the Southeastern States. He found that the infection was fairly common in those states, particularly the ports and towns bordering the coast from Baltimore south along the Atlantic and Gulf Coasts, and in the Rio Grande Valley. In his study, he noted an absence of lice, a lack of communicability from person to person, and no tendency to attack the poorer sections of cities. In addition, he pointed out that the disease was more prevalent in the late summer and fall, and was more apt to occur among those who were engaged in the handling of foodstuffs: grocery men, warehouse men, and the like. This latter observation was extended and confirmed by Rumreich who found that a high percentage of the cases investigated by him occurred in men who had lived or worked in rat infested quarters.

In the years 1930 to 1945, there was an apparent spread of the disease to many of the towns and cities of the interior of the South Atlantic and Gulf States, and an extension into certain rural sections of the same states. The accompanying map (Fig. 124) will give an idea of the distribution of the disease in this country in 1945, approximately 5,000 cases being reported in that year. Subsequent to the introduction of the DDT control program in 1945 there has been a sharp decline in the number of reported cases to less than 500 in 1951 and to fifty-one in 1959. Following the investigations in this country, the disease has been encountered at various places throughout the world.

RESERVOIR IN NATURE

Many animals, chiefly rodents, have been found susceptible to typhus, and the infection has been recovered from species of rats, and field mice trapped in nature. Many rodent species have been experimentally infected with the disease; it is probable that the disease may be present in nature in other species of rodents. The animals susceptible to typhus fever are shown in Table 67.

THE VECTOR OF MURINE TYPHUS

Experimentally, it has been shown possible to infect the human louse, the rat louse and several species of fleas with murine typhus. The evidence at present indicates that the rat flea and the rat louse are the vectors from rodent to rodent, and that the flea transmits the infection to man. Of the species of rat fleas experimentally capable of transmitting the infection, the species *Xenopsylla cheopis* is prob-

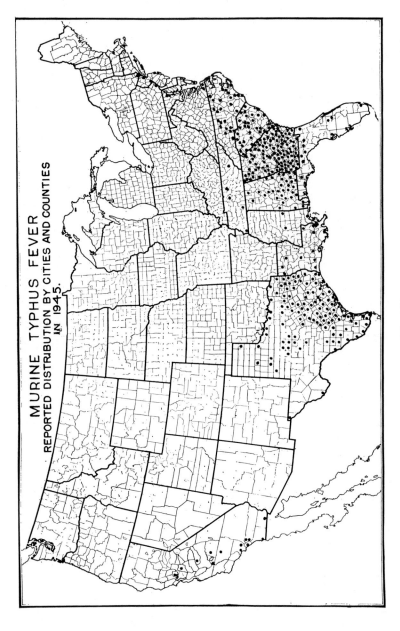

MURINE TYPHUS FEVER
REPORTED DISTRIBUTION BY CITIES AND COUNTIES
IN 1945.

Fig. 124.

ably the most common vector to man, since the curve of prevalence of this flea fits closely the curve of incidence of the disease in man.

Dyer recovered murine typhus from rat fleas taken from rats caught in areas in Baltimore where human cases of murine typhus were present. Mooser recovered similar strains from the brains of rats trapped in Mexico during an epidemic of typhus. Dyer found that when rat fleas are infected by feeding on murine-typhus infected

TABLE 67

ANIMALS SUSCEPTIBLE TO TYPHUS FEVER

Laboratory and domestic animals:
  Cat, dog, guinea pig, rabbit (laboratory), white rat, white mouse

Animals not native in the United States:
  Chimpanzee
  Monkey—two species (*Macacus sinicus, Macacus rhesus*)
  Hedgehog,* gerbil,* garden mouse,* wood mouse*
  Spermophile (*Citellus citellus*)
  Squirrel (*Xerus-atlantoxerus-getulus*)
  Dwarf mouse (*Mus minutus*)
  Meadow mouse (*Microtus terrestris*)

Animals introduced into the United States:
  Grey rat, house mouse

Animals native in the United States:
  Flying squirrel (*Glaucomys volans saturatus*)
  Opossum (*Didelphis virginiana*)
  Woodchuck (*Marmota monax monax*)
  Cotton rat (*Sigmodon hispidus hispidus*)
  Rice Rat (*Orzyomys palustris palustris*)
  Wood rat (*Neotoma floridana rubra*)
  Cotton mouse (*Peromyscus gossypinus gossypinus*)
  Golden mouse (*Peromyscus nuttalli aureolus*)
  Meadow mouse (*Microtus pennsylvanicus pennsylvanicus*)
  Old-field mouse (*Peromyscus polionotus polionotus*)
  White-footed mouse (*Peromyscus leucopus noveboracensis*)

*Subspecies not identified.

rats, the infection multiplies in the flea, reaching its height in two or three weeks. The feces of infected fleas are infectious, and the infection may gain entrance through flea bites or through abrasions caused by scratching. A more common mode of transmission may be the inhalation of dried flea feces or by contamination of mucous membranes by such infected material. All attempts to transmit the infection by the bite alone have been negative. Unlike the louse, the flea does not succumb to the infection. The virus is not transmitted through the egg to succeeding generations of fleas (Figs. 125 and 126).

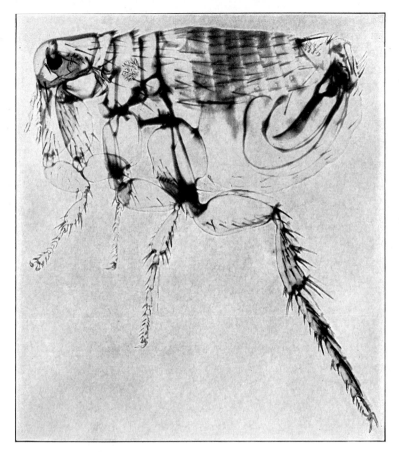

Fig. 125. Rat flea, *Xenopsylla cheopis* (male).

TYPHUS IN LABORATORY ANIMALS

Of the animals known to be susceptible to typhus fever, the guinea pig is the most satisfactory for experimental use. Although excepting the severity of the attack there are no recognizable differences in the clinical reaction of man to murine typhus or epidemic typhus, there are certain differences in the reaction of guinea pigs to these two types. In the murine type, a fever develops a few days after intra-peritoneal inoculation of infectious material. The duration of this incubation period from the time of inoculation to onset of fever varies somewhat with the material used for inoculation. If infectious guinea pig blood is used, the incubation period is usually five to

nine days in duration, occasionally longer. The fever is apt to be irregular in type, seldom going higher than 40° C. to 40.2° C., and
commonly lasts from one to five days. Occasionally, guinea pigs show
fever a few days longer without other evidence of the presence of
secondary infections. Uncomplicated typhus does not kill the guinea

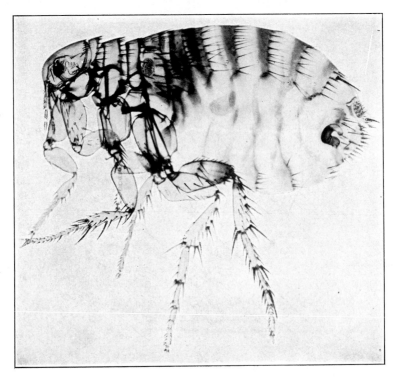

Fig. 126. Rat flea, *Xenopsylla cheopis* (female).

pig. Following intraperitoneal inoculation of murine typhus into
the male guinea pig, and usually coincident with the fever, there is
a swelling of the genitalia and a reddening of the scrotum. From
oedema of the underlying tissues the scrotum is tightly stretched,
and the testicles can not be pushed through the rings into the abdominal cavity, a reduction readily accomplished in the normal animal. This involvement of the genitalia usually disappears with the
fever. Autopsy of animals at the height of the infection will show a
congestion of the blood vessels of both layers of the tunica covering
the testicles, often with hemorrhages, and a filmy exudate on the

surface. Rickettsiae are readily demonstrable in the cells of this exudate.

In guinea pigs infected with epidemic typhus, the incubation period is about the same as that noted for the murine type. The fever is more uniform since days on which the animal shows no fever are not as common. The fever usually lasts from five to nine days. As in murine typhus, the animals do not appear sick and do not die unless other infections are also present. Transient reddening and swelling of the scrotum occasionally is seen in guinea pigs infected with an epidemic type strain, but usually this reaction is lacking.

Rabbits and monkeys, when infected with typhus rickettsiae of either form (epidemic or murine) develop the Weil-Felix reaction, usually with a titre of 1:40 to 1:320. Guinea pigs do not show this reaction.

White rats develop a fever following inoculation with the murine strains, but fail to do so in response to epidemic strains. Rats occasionally develop the Weil-Felix reaction in low titres. Animals develop complement-fixing antibodies following infection with either form of typhus.

In white mice, the rickettsiae of the murine disease can be passed from mouse to mouse indefinitely, but epidemic rickettsiae often die out after a few passages in the same species. Complete cross immunity exists between the two types of typhus in laboratory animals.

THE DISEASE IN MAN

In man, typhus fever runs a febrile course of about fourteen days. The most definite diagnostic sign is the rash which appears about the fifth day. The rash consists of rose-red macules, 2 to 3 mm. in diameter, which become definitely petechial and darker as the disease progresses. The rash first appears over the lower chest or upper abdomen, spreading from this location to the upper arms, shoulders, back, and thighs. In severe cases, the forearms, lower legs, and palms and soles may be involved. The rash seldom appears on the face.

In the murine form of the disease, serious complications are rare, the fatality rate being below 5 per cent, with most of the deaths occurring in those over fifty years of age. Complications, particularly pneumonia, are more common in the epidemic disease, and the case fatality may reach 60 per cent in severe epidemics.

In treatment, aureomycin, chloramphenicol, and terramycin are of value.

DIAGNOSTIC AIDS

The Weil-Felix reaction is constantly positive in both forms of typhus in man. This reaction is the agglutination of certain *B. proteus* X strains by the serum of the infected individual. The strain of this organism commonly used is known as X_{19}, and is not concerned with the etiology of the disease. The agglutinins appear in the second week and reach their height about the time of defervescence, often reaching a titre of 1:1280 or more. Titres of 1:320 or less should not be regarded as diagnostic unless the clinical picture is compatible with typhus and other diseases can be excluded. Unfortunately for the diagnosis of typhus, this reaction is also present in other of the rickettsial diseases. In the section of the United States where Rocky Mountain spotted fever and typhus both exist, the Weil-Felix, consequently, gives no aid in the differential diagnosis.

The complement-fixation and agglutination tests using rickettsiae grown in the yolk sac of the developing chick embryo have proved of great value in the diagnosis of rickettsial diseases and in addition, differentiate between the various rickettsial infections.

PREVENTION

The prevention of epidemic typhus is based on vaccination and the eradication of the body louse by personal cleanliness—bathing and change of clothing. In a measure this makes the prevention of typhus in civil populations a social problem—education and the alleviation of squalor. In the control of epidemics of typhus, the patients should be freed of all vermin and segregated in surroundings where they may be kept free from vermin. Rooms from which typhus patients have been removed should be disinfected to insure the destruction of all lice.

The use of the chemical DDT has proved to be the method of choice for delousing. This compound is prepared in a dusting powder which by use of hand or power duster can be thoroughly disseminated in the clothing without disrobing.

In the prevention of murine typhus, the same measures should be applied which have been found of value in the control of bubonic plague—the destruction of rats and rat harbors. The rat flea, *Xeno-*

psylla cheopis, when hungry, feeds readily upon man. These fleas spend part of their time away from their normal hosts along rat runs and in the rat nests, from which locations they may infest man when occasion offers. The value of DDT in the destruction of fleas in murine typhus foci has been demonstrated in recent years.

Vaccines have been prepared against typhus, both in Europe and this country. The vaccine with which the American armed forces were inoculated during World War II is prepared from rickettsiae grown in the yolk sac of the developing chick embryo. This vaccine has been used on a large scale, and the accumulated evidence shows that it will definitely modify the severity of a subsequent attack of typhus. As far as is known at present, no death from typhus has occurred in a previously vaccinated individual. The reactions following the use of this vaccine are usually mild. Persons known to be allergic to chicken or eggs should be skin-tested before vaccination to determine sensitivity.

ITEMS OF NOTE

1) Typhus fever is one of the Rickettsial diseases.
2) There are two epidemiologic types of typhus, epidemic or louse-borne, and murine, or flea-borne.
3) The epidemiologic features of epidemic typhus are:
   (a) Great prevalence in winter and spring;
   (b) Communicability from man to man;
   (c) Tendency to attack distressed populations;
   (d) Association with lice.
4) The epidemiologic features of murine typhus are:
   (a) Greater prevalence in late summer and fall;
   (b) Lack of communicability from man to man;
   (c) Association with rats and rat harbors.
5) A known reservoir of murine typhus exists in species of rodents.
6) The rash in both forms of typhus begins on the body, and spreads to the extremities, avoiding the face.
7) The Weil-Felix reaction is present in practically all cases.
8) The complement-fixation and agglutination reactions develops in infected animals including man.
9) Prevention and control of epidemic typhus are based on vaccination and delousing.

10) Prevention and control of murine typhus are based on the elimination of rat harbors and the destruction of rats and fleas.

REFERENCES

BRILL, N. E.: *New York State J. Med., 67*:48 and 77, 1898.

BRIGHAM, G. D.: *Pub. Health Rep., 52*:659, 1937.

COX, H. R.: *Pub. Health Rep., 53*:2241, 1938.

DYER, R. E., *et al.: Pub. Health Rep., 46*:334, 1869, 2481, 1931; *Ibid., 47*:131, 1932.

GOLDBERGER, JOSEPH and ANDERSON, J. F.: *Pub. Health Rep., 27*:29, 1912.

JELLISON, W. L.: *Ann. Rev. Entomology, 4*:389, 1959.

LOEFFLER, W. and MOOSER, H.: *Schweiz. Med. Wchnschr., 82*:493, 1952.

MAXCY, K. F.: *Pub. Health Rep., 41*:2967, 1926.

MOOSER, H., *et al.: J.A.M.A., 97*:231, 1931.

MURRAY, E. S. and SNYDER, J. C.: *Am. J. Hyg. 53*:22, 1951.

NICOLLE, C., COMPTE, C. and CONSEIL, E.: *Copt. rend. Acad. sc., 149*:486, 1909.

PRATT, H. D.: *Ann. N. Y. Acad. Sc., 70*:516, 1958.

PRICE, W. H.: *J. Bact., 69*:106, 1955.

RUMREICH, A., *et al.: Pub. Health Rep., 46*:1192, 1931.

SADUSK, J. F., JR.: *J.A.M.A., 133*:1192, 1947.

SMADEL, J. E.: *Am. J. Med., 7*:671, 1949.

SMADEL, J. E.: *Ann. Int. Med., 51*:421, 1959.

WEIGL, R.: *Arch. Inst. Pasteur, 22*:315, 1933.

WHEELER, C. M.: *Am. J. Pub. Health, 36*:119, 1946.

ZINSSER, H., *et. al.: J. Exper. Med., 53*:325, 493, 1931; *Ibid., 57*:381, 391, 1933.

ZINSSER, H.: *Am. J. Hyg., 20*:513, 1934.

Chapter 28

ROCKY MOUNTAIN SPOTTED FEVER

R. E. DYER, M.D.

ROCKY MOUNTAIN spotted fever is one of the two rickettsial diseases endemic in the United States. (See Typhus Fever, Chapter 27). The rickettsiae described in connection with this disease have been named *Rickettsia rickettsii* or *Dermacentroxenus rickettsii*. The disease is transmitted to man by ticks of two or more species.

HISTORY

Rocky Mountain spotted fever is known to have been present in certain sections of the northern Rocky Mountain regions at the time that country was first settled by white men. It is probable that the disease occurred among the Indians prior to white settlement, but no accurate data of the earlier period are available. The disease was well recognized among the settlers in the eighties and nineties of the last century, but was first noted in the medical literature by Maxey in 1899.

Until 1930, spotted fever was thought to be limited to the northwestern states, as, with the exception of a single case which occurred in Indiana in 1925, no cases had been recognized east of a north and south line drawn through the center of the Dakotas. In 1930, the disease was recognized by Rumreich, and clinically and epidemiologically differentiated from murine typhus in Maryland and Virginia. At the same time, Badger, by laboratory studies, definitely established the identity of the eastern cases with the northwestern cases of spotted fever. Later study of the records of earlier cases in the eastern states has led to the conclusion that spotted fever existed in the east for at least fifteen years before recogniion. A disease described in Sao Paulo, Brazil, under the name, exanthematic typhus of Sao Paulo, was identified as Rocky Mountain spotted fever, by cross immunity and protection tests. The disease has also been identified in Colombia and Mexico. Other closely related diseases are: Boutonneuse fever of the Mediterranean basin, Kenya typhus of East Africa, Russian tick typhus, South African tick typhus, and North Queensland tick typhus.

GEOGRAPHIC DISTRIBUTION

Following the establishment of the fact that spotted fever was not limited to the northwestern states, there has been a recognition of cases in forty-six states. It is seldom reported inland in New England, New York or in the West-North Central states. The greatest number of cases during the years 1951-1955 were reported from the South Atlantic states, particularly Virginia, Maryland, and North Carolina (Fig. 127). Cases have been recognized in two of the provinces of Canada, Alberta and British Columbia, and in Panama, Mexico and Brazil. The number of cases reported in the United States was 596 in 1947, 295 in 1955, and 199 in 1959.

SEASONAL PREVALENCE

As in the other rickettsial diseases, the epidemiology of Rocky Mountain spotted fever in man is dependant upon the life history and feeding habits of the vector, in this instance, a tick. The disease occurs most frequently among those whose occupations expose them to the bites of ticks, such as sheepherders, agricultural workers, surveyors, foresters, and the like. A number of cases occur each year among campers, vacationists, picknickers, and others whose occupations or pleasures take them into rural areas. Occasional cases occur in urban dwellers from contact with ticks in vacant lots or with ticks brought home by pets. In several instances, persons have acquired the infection by crushing ticks with their fingers while removing them from dogs. The great majority of cases of spotted fever occur in the late spring and early summer with an occasional case developing in late summer and fall. There is some variation in this seasonal prevalence in the different sections of the country. In the northwest, the disease is practically limited to the months of March to July, inclusive, with April, May, and June, the months of greatest incidence. In the states along the Atlantic seaboard, cases occur during the same months noted for the northwest with an extension to include the first part of August. The season of greatest incidence in the east falls a

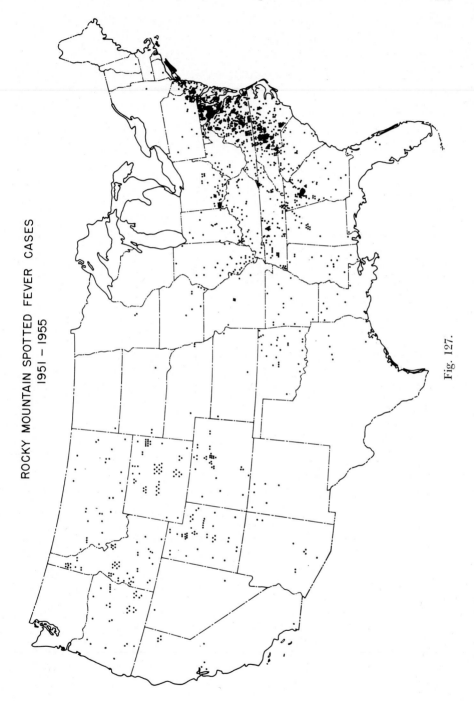

ROCKY MOUNTAIN SPOTTED FEVER CASES
1951 – 1955

Fig. 127.

little later than in the west, the months of May, June and July being the height of the spotted fever season.

Age and sex have no influence on susceptibility to the disease. There is a greater incidence among males than females and among children of both sexes than among adult females, a fact which is explained by the greater risk of exposure to ticks by reason of the occupations of adult males, and the more frequent excursion of children into tick infested areas in the course of their play (Fig. 128).

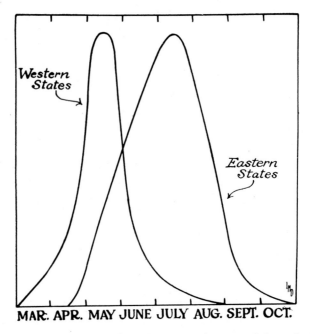

Fig. 128. Seasonal distribution of Rocky Mountain spotted fever in the United States.

In general, it may be stated that all cases occur following conditions under which exposure to ticks was probable, and that definite history of tick contact (bites or crushing of ticks) precedes the onset of the disease in man in the great majority of cases.

THE VECTOR

The role of ticks in the transmission of Rocky Mountain spotted fever was largely worked out by Ricketts in 1906, prior evidence being supplied by the work of McCalla, Wilson, and Chowning, and supplemental data added by the work of Fricks, Spencer, Parker, and others. King experimentally transmitted the disease by ticks about the same time that Ricketts successfully carried out the same experiments. Ticks of several species have been found capable of being infected, and of transmitting the infection experimentally while infected ticks of three species have been found in nature.

Tick species found infected in nature in the United States are:

> Western Wood Tick *(Dermacentor andersoni)*
> Eastern Dog Tick *(Dermacentor variabilis)*
> Rabbit Tick *(Haemaphysalis leporis-palustris)*

In addition to the three species listed above, the following species have been shown to be capable of transmitting the infection experimentally:

> Pacific Coast Tick *(Dermacentor occidentalis)*
> Brown Dog Tick *(Rhipicephalus sanguineus)*
> Lone-star Tick *(Amblyomma americanum)*
> Cayenne Tick *(Amblyomma cajennense)*
> Rabbit Dermacentor *(Dermacentor parumapertus)*

Of the above ticks, *D. andersoni* and *D. variabilis* are of the greatest importance in transmitting the disease to man in North America. Accumulated evidence indicates that the rabbit tick, *Haemaphysalis leporis-palustris,* although not feeding on man, plays a greater part than any other tick in the dissemination of this disease in nature, being the only tick which occurs in all parts of this continent where spotted fever has been recognized in man.

In each of the species listed above, the experimental data show that stage to stage transmission of spotted fever rickettsiae takes place. In other words, the infection may be acquired by the tick in one stage of its life cycle and retained through subsequent moults to succeeding stages and from infected adult females through the egg to the larvae (Fig. 129).

The two ticks held accountable for most of the human cases of spotted fever in this country, *D. andersoni* and *D. variabilis* are "three host" ticks, spending the periods between feedings away from the hosts. The larval or nymphal stages are found on the smaller animals, especially rodents, while the adults are found more frequently on the larger animals, wild and domestic. The adult tick conveys the infection to man since the two immature stages are seldom found on man.

The known distribution of *D. andersoni* include the states of Washington, Oregon, Idaho, Montana, Wyoming, Nevada, Utah, Colorado, northern sections of California, New Mexico, and Arizona, and the extreme western part of South Dakota, while *D. variabilis* has been reported from the remaining states of the Union. California, Colorado, Oregon, South Dakota, and Montana have reported both species.

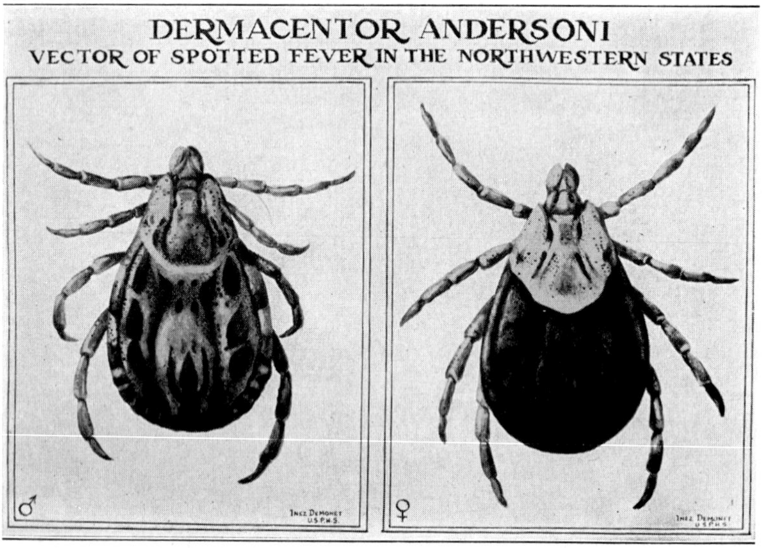

Fig. 129.

The life cycle and feeding habits of the two Dermacentors are as follows: the adult tick normally attaches to one animal and feeds to engorgement, taking seven to ten days. The female increases enormously in size during feeding and after becoming detached, she drops to the ground, lays her eggs, two to six thousand in number, and dies without feeding again. From the eggs hatch six-legged larvae. These larvae find a host, presumably in most instances a small rodent, and feed to engorgement during a period of four to six days. The larvae then detach, drop to the ground, and after a small period of sluggish activity become quiescent and moult to eight-legged nymphs. These nymphs in their turn find a host and feed to engorgement, taking six to eight days in the process. They then moult to the eight-legged adult, male and female.

In nature, these ticks pass the winter in one of the flat or unfed stages and probably consume two years in completing the cycles from adult to adult. Unfed adult ticks are said to be able to survive up to four years.

The percentage of infected ticks found in nature varies from year to year in known infected localities. In certain small sections of the northwest, the percentage of ticks examined and found infected has reached 2 per cent in certain years while no infected ticks have been found in the same areas in other years. Out of about one thousand ticks taken from small areas in the east where spotted fever was occurring in human beings, the rickettsiae were recovered only once.

SUSCEPTIBLE ANIMALS

Studies made by Wilson and Chowning in 1902 led to the conclusion that a reservoir of Rocky Mountain spotted fever existed in nature in rodents. It is known that infected animals exist in nature, and play an important part in the perpetuation of the disease since protective antibodies have been demonstrated in the blood of certain wild rodents and *Rickettsiae ricketsii* have been recovered from meadow mice and cottontail rabbits trapped in Virginia. Laboratory studies have shown that many species of animals are susceptible to this disease, and while infected, are capable of transmitting the infection to their tick parasites. The list of animals found susceptible embraces several species of rodents, squirrels, rats, mice, and woodchucks, and of the larger animals, the dog and the sheep. It should be noted that the dog is possibly the chief reservoir of boutonneuse fever which is closely related to spotted fever.

THE DISEASE IN LABORATORY ANIMALS

Rhesus monkeys, rabbits, white rats and guinea pigs are susceptible to Rocky Mountain spotted fever, and of these the guinea pig is the most satisfactory for experimental or diagnostic investigations.

To establish the infection in guinea pigs from a human case, 2 to 4 cc. of blood taken from the patient at the height of the disease should be injected intraperitoneally. In examining ticks for the presence of the infection, they may be ground up in a mortar suspended in a little saline and this suspension injected into the guinea pigs intraperitoneally. Experience has shown that attempts to disinfect the outside of the ticks prior to grinding them up are unnecessary as secondary infections of the animals seldom follow the injection of tick suspensions without preliminary disinfection.

The incubation period in guinea pigs following intraperitoneal injection of blood varies somewhat with the virulence of the strain. The highly virulent strains produce the disease in guinea pigs two to three days after inoculation. These animals show listlessness, progressive loss of weight and high fever, usually 105° F. or a little above. About 90 per cent of the animals die around the end of the first week. If the animal survives, defervescence occurs after a variable period of five to fifteen days. In a majority of male guinea pigs infected with a virulent strain, a scrotal reaction develops about the third day of fever. This reaction begins as a macular rash on the skin of the scrotum. Edema of the underlying tissues and swelling of the testicles are absent on gross inspection, the reaction being largely confined to the skin. The rash becomes petechial and coalescence of the spots occurs. As the reaction progresses, necrosis of the affected skin areas follows which is in turn followed by sloughing. As the guinea pig recovers, healing takes place by scar formation. Necrosis of the tips of the ears frequently occurs. At autopsy of guinea pigs at the height of the infection, the most noticeable finding is an enlarged and darkened spleen. This organ is enlarged in all diameters and may be from two to five times its normal size.

In less virulent strains in guinea pigs, the percentage of deaths may fall as low as 5 per cent, and the scrotal reaction be absent. The strains from Sao Paulo, Brazil, have shown scrotal reactions identical with those caused by virulent strains isolated in the United States.

Monkeys and rabbits develop the Weil-Felix reactions when infected with spotted fever. Monkeys often develop a rash similar in character to the rash seen in human cases. The rash in monkeys is found on the face, over the lower back and the outside of the thighs. Necrosis of the ears sometimes occurs in monkeys. Virulent spotted fever is highly fatal in monkeys.

Rabbits develop a fever and quite frequently show a scrotal reaction similar to that seen in guinea pigs.

THE DISEASE IN MAN

The diagnosis of spotted fever in the human being is usually made on clinical grounds and the complement-fixation test.

In man the disease has an incubation period of two to twelve days, most often being a week or a little less. The actual onset may be preceded by a few days of ill-defined prodromata-loss of appetite, listlessness and headache. The onset is usually sudden with a chill or chilly sensations, and rapidly rising fever. Prostration is usually marked. In the more severe cases, nosebleed may occur early. Soreness of the muscles and joints is commonly present. The temperature rises rapidly and reaches its highest point usually in the second week. The termination is by rapid lysis after a febrile period of about three weeks.

The most distinguishing characteristic of the disease is the rash. This appears between the second and fifth days, usually on the third or fourth. The eruption is macular, rose red in color at first, and becomes fainter, almost disappearing during the morning remission of fever early in the disease. The macules become more distinct each day, becoming definitely petechial early in the second week in all but the mildest cases. In the severe cases, the spots become deep red or purplish and confluent. Necroses may develop. The rash usually persists throughout the febrile period and into convalescence, becoming brownish in color. A branny desquamation often occurs over the areas where the rash was thickest. The site of first location of the rash and its spread and final distribution are important in the diagnosis of the disease. The rash first appears usually on the wrists and ankles. It spreads rapidly in the first twenty-four to forty-eight hours to the back, then arms, legs, chest, and last to the abdomen, where it is least marked. The palms and soles are frequently involved, and occasionally the face and scalp are included.

The case fatality rate varies with the age of the patient, being much higher in the older age groups. Average for all ages is about 20 per cent in untreated cases. Chloramphenicol and the tetracyclines are of value in treatment.

PREVENTION AND CONTROL

Methods for prevention of spotted fever have been directed at the eradication of ticks. To date these attempts have not been very successful. The difficulty of the problem may be recognized when the variety of hosts on which this parasite may feed is considered. In Montana, the poisoning of rodents has been tried in the hope of limiting the food supply available for the immature stages of the ticks. The adult ticks have been attacked by the dipping of domestic stock. The clearing away of brush and the burning over of tick infested areas are doubtless of assistance in reducing the number of ticks both by removing common sources of food for the ticks, and by actual destruction of the ticks themselves.

Two types of vaccines have been prepared for spotted fever. The original method utilized rickettsiae harvested from infected ticks. A vaccine similar to the typhus yolk-sac vaccine is now in use. In the production of immunity there is no choice between the two vaccines. The yolk-sac vaccine should be avoided if sensitization to chicken or egg is present in the individual to be examined. Sensitization to ticks occurs, but is relatively uncommon.

Vaccine may be administered to those whose occupations expose them particularly to tick bites in known infected areas. Two or three inoculations of the vaccine give a degree of protection usually sufficient to last through one tick season, but the immunity apparently is not permanent. Occasional cases of spotted fever have developed in vaccinated persons, but the vaccine apparently lessens the severity of the disease and seems to insure recovery. For its full protective value the vaccine should be taken at least ten days before exposure to tick bite. The vaccine is of no value in the treatment of the disease.

Probably the most effective method of prevention is the exercise of personal care. Known infected areas should be avoided insofar as possible during the tick season. Those who must visit such areas should frequently examine their clothing and body for ticks. The tick usually does not become attached to its host at once, but often times crawls around for several hours. It has been shown also that the chance of receiving infection from the bite of an infected tick is directly proportional to the length of time the tick has fed on the exposed individual.

ITEMS OF NOTE

1) Rock Mountain spotted fever is one of the Rickettsia diseases.

2) It has been recognized in most states of the United States, and in Brazil, Colombia, Mexico, and Canada.

3) The disease is transmitted to man by ticks.

4) Several species of ticks are capable of transmitting the infection. The two most important species in the United States are *D. andersoni* in the northwest, and *D. variabilis* in the east.

5) Animals furnish food supply for ticks, and infected animals exist in nature.

6) The disease is not transmitted from person to person.

7) The disease is rural in nature, and is practically limited to the spring and early summer, although "out of season" cases do occur.

8) Ticks once infected remain so for life, and pass the infection to succeeding generations.

9) The prevention of the disease is largely one of personal care in avoiding ticks, plus the use of vaccine in known infected areas where it is not feasible to avoid ticks.

REFERENCES

BADGER, L. F., *et al.: Pub. Health Rep., 46:*463, 1931.

COX, H. R.: *Viral and Rickettsial Infections of Man,* Rivers and Horsfall, 3rd Edition. Lippincott, 1959, p. 828.

DYER, R. E.: *Pub. Health Rep., 48:*521, 1933.

FRICKS, L. D.: *Pub. Health Rep., 31:*516, 1916.

GOULD, D. J. and MIESSE, M. L.: *Proc. Soc. Exper. Biol. & Med., 85:*558, 1954.

KING, W. W.: *Pub. Health Rep., 21:*863, 1906.

LaBIER, C. L.: *J. Indiana M. A., 18:*418, 1925.

MAXEY, E. E.: *Med. Sentinel, 7:*433, 1899.

McCALLA, L. P.: *Med. Sentinel, 16:*87, 1908.

PARKER, R. B. and DAVIS, G. E.: *Pub. Health Rep., 48:*501, 1933.

PHILIP, C. B.: *Pub. Health Rep., 74:*595, 1959.

RICKETTS, H. T. and WILDER, R. M.: *Contribution to Medical Science.* Chicago, Univ. of Chicago Press, 1911.

RUMREICH, A., *et al.: Pub. Health Rep., 48:*501, 1931.

SHIRAI, A., *et al.: Proc. Soc. Exper. Biol. & Med., 107:*211, 1961.

SMADEL, J. E.: *Ann. Int. Med., 51:*421, 1959.

WILSON, L. B. and CHOWNING, W. M.: *J.A.M.A., 39:*131, 1902.

Chapter 29

TSUTSUGAMUSHI DISEASE

(Mite Typhus)

R. E. DYER, M.D.

TSUTSUGAMUSHI DISEASE is an infection of rodents caused by *Rickettsia tsutsugamushi*. Man is infected by the bite of the rat mite.

HISTORY

Tsutsugamushi disease has been known, according to Williams since the sixth century. In an extensive review of the literature, Blake, Maxcy, Sadusk, Kohls, and Bell state that it was encountered by the natives of South China in the sixteenth century.

Hashimoto described the disease in Japan in 1810, calling it "tsusuga." Palm, in 1878, added further evidence, calling it "shimamushi." Clinical and epidemiological evidence was added by Tanaka in 1899 and later by workers of the Kitasato Institute for Infectious Diseases. Kitashima and Miyajima, in 1918, demonstrated that field mice in Japan were rodent hosts. The etiologic agent was suspected by Hayoshi, in 1920, and named *Rickettsia tsutsugamushi*. Various other workers described the organisms under other names. Nagayo and his associates in 1930 identified it under the name of *Rickettsia orientalis*.

Little attention was paid to the disease in occidental countries up to the Second World War when American troops invaded the islands of the Southwest Pacific.

Among the various designations by which the disease has been known are tsutsugamushibyo, shimamushi, Japanese river fever, flood fever, kedani fever, mite fever, scrub typhus (K form), rural typhus, tropical typhus, pseudo typhus and Mossan fever. By priority, tsutsugamushi disease is the accepted term, although the name scrub typhus is often used.

GEOGRAPHIC DISTRIBUTION

Tsutsugamushi disease has been found over a wide-spread area in the Asiatic-Pacific region. Originally, it was thought to be confined to Japan, but later experience showed that it existed also in China, Korea, Nansei Islands, Formosa, Pescadores Islands, Philippine Islands, Indo-China, Cambodia, Malay Peninsula, Ceylon, Maldive Islands, Sumatra, Java, Borneo, New Guinea, North Queensland (Australia), Bako Islands, Burma, and India.

There are probably other areas also where the disease exists. There is also the possibility, because the vector is a mite, that areas now known to be free of the disease will later become infected. The disease is tropical in nature, however, and according to Cook does not occur at temperatures less than 65° F.

SEASONAL PREVALENCE

No seasonal variation in the incidence of tsutsugamushi disease occurs in the tropics. In cooler climates, such as Japan and Formosa, a seasonal variation has been noted with cases occurring mostly during the months of July and August.

ETIOLOGIC AGENT

The etiologic agent of tsutsugamushi disease is *R. tsutsugamushi* (*R. orientalis, R. nipponica, R. akamushi*). Blake and his co-workers confirmed the rickettsial nature of the organism in New Guinea. Early in the course of the illness it can be recovered from the patient's blood stream. Injection of white mice produces a fatal infection, and intra- and extra-cellular bodies frequently occurring in pairs may be demonstrated in Giemsa-stained smears.

Cultures in bacteriological media (broth or agar slants) remain sterile, but the organism may be grown on yolk-sac tissue of fertile hens' eggs in a manner similar to the other rickettsia of the typhus group.

Strains of *R. tsutsugamushi* isolated from different geographic areas vary in virulence, but are identical in cross immunity tests.

Mite Vectors

Tsutsugamushi disease is transmitted by the bite of the larval form of a mite of the genus *Trombicula*. In the development of the

mite from the egg to the adult, only the larval forms are parasitic on
vertebrate hosts. The metamorphosis from larva to nymph requires
a meal of blood from the host. The nymph and adult forms are not
parasitic on man or animals, but live on the ground, feeding on
plants. The adults lay their eggs on the ground, where the new larvae
hatch out (Fig. 130).

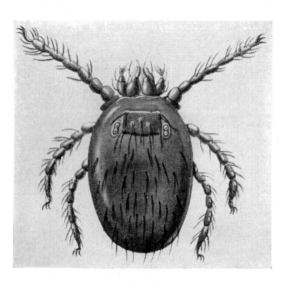

Fig. 130. Kedani mite, *Trombicula akamushi*. (Courtesy, Sharp and Dohme.)

The larval forms which attack man are reddish in color, but of almost microscopic size, about 0.2 to 0.3 mm. in length. They are six-
legged, resembling tiny spiders. They attach themselves to the skin
by means of their hooked mouth parts. One meal of blood is all that
is necessary for the metamorphosis from larva to nymph, and apparently the larva does not feed a second time. If the larva of a preceding
generation, however, has fed upon an infected rodent, the new larva
will probably be capable of causing infection in the new host, for the
rickettsiae are transmitted through the egg from generation to
generation.

Williams lists the following mites responsible for the transmission
of tsutsugamushi disease:

Trombicula akamushi in Japan, China, Formosa, Malaya, Pescadores Islands and Sumatra.

Trombicula deliensis in Australia, India, Malaya, New Guinea and Sumatra.

Trombicula minor in Australia and New Guinea.

Trombicula acuscutellaris in India.

Numerous species of mites infest rodents in the Orient, and islands of the Southwest Pacific, and additional investigation has shown that others than those listed above are capable of transmitting tsutsugamushi disease. Some mites are merely nuisances, causing a severe dermatitis, called "scrub itch." In North America, *Trombicula irritans* causes "harvest itch."

Ticks such as the genus *Amblyomma* in Sumatra, have been suspected in the transmission of this disease, but definite evidence is lacking.

RODENT HOSTS

A variety of rodent hosts of tsutsugamushi disease are found in nature. Rickettsial organisms have been found in the following rats:

Melomys littoralis, Rattus assimilis, Rattus conatus, Rattus novegicus (white strain), *Rattus norvegicus* (black and white strain), *Rattus rattus, Rattus losea, Rattus concolar growni,* and *Mus rattus rufescens.* The vole, *Microtus montebelli,* and the bandicoot, *Isoodon torosus,* also carry the organisms. Numerous other rodents are infested with mites, and experience may show that they are reservoirs of rickettsial infection.

The laboratory animals which are subject to infection include white mice, white rats, guinea pigs and rabbits.

Birds have been reported as possible hosts of the disease, since they are infested with mites, but this has not been confirmed. Wild birds are capable, however, of distributing infected mites over wide areas, and to distant countries in migration.

Mites feed upon dogs, cats, wild pigs, swamp hens, bush fowls, parrots, buffaloes, monkeys, lizards, and probably many other animals. Gunther lists seventeen such hosts. Few of them probably compare with rodents as reservoirs of tsutsugamushi disease.

THE DISEASE IN MAN

The mites which cause tsutsugamushi disease attack regions about the waistline, scrotum, groin, and armpits where they find the moisture favorable. The most common site of the primary lesion, according to Ahlm and Lipshutz is found in the scrotal area, though the inguinal and ankle areas are frequently involved. Cook found 92 per cent on the trunk, arm, or thigh. The bite is painless and usually overlooked.

The primary lesion, or eschar, where the mite causes the infection, has a pinched out appearance about three to ten mm. in diameter, covered with a black crust and surrounded by a small erythematous border. After an incubation period of seven to fourteen days, the patient suffers from headache, backache, weakness, chilliness, fever, and insomnia. The fever rises to about 104° F. or 105° F. About the fourth or fifth day after symptoms appear, there is a macular or maulopapular rash on the trunk. Mild cases begin to improve in twelve to fourteen days. Severe cases may develop atypical pneumonia or encephalitis.

Diagnosis is confirmed by the appearance of the eschar, when it can be found, by the recovery from the blood stream of *R. tsutsugamushi* during the febrile period, and by a positive Weil-Felix test with Proteus OXK after the twelfth or fourteenth day of illness. A negative Weil-Felix reaction does not rule out the disease, however.

The complement-fixation reaction using antigens prepared from infected yolk sacs of developing chick embryos is a definite diagnostic aid.

Various other diseases occur in regions where tsutsugamushi disease is found, such as malaria, dengue, and infectious hepatitis, which often make a differential diagnosis difficult.

The mortality rate varies from 2 to 10 per cent, depending on various factors such as age, the condition of the patient, etc. Above the age of forty years, the mortality rate is much higher. Tsutsugamushi disease is not transmitted from person to person.

PREVENTION

There is no vaccine of proven value against tsutsugamushi. Persons going into mite-infested areas where the disease exists incur some risk of infection. This risk may be minimized by precautions learned by the military forces during World War II.

Camp sites should be cleared of grass and debris, the ground burned over, and then sprayed with oil. Cots or hammocks should be used for sleeping purposes, rather than the ground. Clothes should be sprayed or rubbed with an anti-mite fluid, such as di-methyl phthalate or dibutyl phthalate. McCulloch found that dibutyl phthalate was very efficient. At a dosage rate of one fluid ounce per set of clothes, it gave protection for twenty-two days, the clothes being washed eight times in cold water during that period. The hands should be smeared with an anti-mite fluid at frequent intervals when in tick-infested areas, and care should be taken to protect the ankles. At the earliest time possible after exposure, a bath should be taken with thorough soaping and scrubbing of the skin.

DDT is not effective against mites.

ITEMS OF NOTE

1) Tsutsugamushi disease is one of the Rickettsia group of diseases. The causative agent is *R. tsutsugamushi.*

2) The disease exists over a large area of Southeast Asia from Korea to India and in the islands of the Southwest Pacific from Japan to northern Australia.

3) The vector is the rat-mite, *Trombicula akamushi,* or related species.

4) Only the larval forms of the mite are parasitic and transmit the disease.

5) Mites once infected, pass the rickettsia on to the next generation through the egg.

6) The reservoir of infection is found in wild rats and mice.

7) Mortality in persons suffering from the disease varies from 2 to 10 per cent, depending on such factors as age, condition of the patient, etc.

8) Prevention consists in protection against mite bites. There is no protective vaccine.

REFERENCES

AHLM, C. E. and LIPSHULTZ, J.: *J.A.M.A., 124:*1095, 1944.

BERRY, M. G., JOHNSON, A. S., JR. and WASHAUER, S. E.: *War Med., 7:*71, 1945.

BLAKE, F. G., MAXCY, K. F., SADUSK, J. F., KOHLS, G. M. and BELL, E. J.: *Am. J. Hyg., 41:*243, 372, 1945.

COOK, C. E.: *M. J. Australia, 2:*539, 1944.

KOHLS, G. M., ARMBRUST, C. A., IRONS, E. N. and PHILLIP, C. B.: *Am. J. Hyg., 41:*374-399, 1945.

LIPMAN, B. L., CASEY, A. V., BYRON, R. A. and EVANS, E. C.: *War Med., 6:*304, 1944.

McCULLOCH, R. N.: *M. J. Australia, 1:*717, 1946.

SMADEL, J. E., BAILEY, C. A. and DIERCKS, F. H.: *Am. J. Hyg., 51:*229, 1950.

WILLIAMS, R. W.: *Am. J. Trop. Med., 24:*355, 1944.

Chapter 30

Q FEVER

R. E. Dyer, M.D.

Q fever is at present classified with the rickettsial diseases, although its usual mode of transmission to man is not characteristic of the other infections in this group. In addition, the causative organism is more resistant to physical and chemical agents than are the true rickettsiae.

HISTORY

The occurrence of an obscure fever among meat workers and slaughterhouse employees in Brisbane, Australia, in 1935, was studied by Burnet and others of the Queensland Department of Health. The disease was designated as "Q" fever (the letter "Q" standing for "Query"), and the causative agent was named *Rickettsia burneti.*

In 1938, Davis and Cox in the United States reported the isolation of rickettsia-like organisms from wood ticks collected near Nine Mile Creek, Montana, and Dyer reported the first case of human infection in this country. The disease was designated as American Q fever, and the organism was first named *Rickettsia diaporica.*

The organisms encountered in Australia and in the United States were shown to be immunologically identical by Dyer and Bengston.

GEOGRAPHIC DISTRIBUTION

Q fever was first reported in Australia by Derrick in 1937. The next report of a naturally acquired infection was made by Hesdorffer and Duffalo in Montana in 1941. Since that time, the disease has been found in many areas throughout the world. Greece, where it was first called Balkan Grippe, Bulgaria, Roumania, Italy, Panama, Switzerland, Great Britain, Turkey, Portugal, Algeria, Israel, South Africa, Mexico, Germany, France, Spain, and Yugoslavia. In the United States, Q fever has been recognized in Montana, Texas, Illinois, Arizona, California, Pennsylvania, Massachusetts, New York, and Washington, D.C. The disease has been identified in cattle in thirty-five states.

In addition to cases occurring in the general population, many infections have occurred among those working in laboratories where the causative agent of Q fever has been under investigation. The first laboratory infection was reported in connection with the original Australian outbreak. Since that time, many laboratory infections have occurred in practically every laboratory throughout the world where studies of Q fever have been undertaken.

ETIOLOGIC AGENT

The causative agent of Q fever was first classified as a rickettsia, and was named *Rickettsia burneti,* the disease itself being regarded as belonging to the rickettsial group of diseases. However, on account of certain differences in the mode of transmission and clinical aspects, the causative organism has been renamed *Coxiella burneti,* and the disease itself is regarded as being closely related to, but somewhat distinct from the true rickettsial diseases. The differences between *Coxiella burneti,* and the true rickettsiae rest in the filterability of *C. burneti,* and its greater resistance to physical and chemical agents.

VECTORS

The tick of chief importance in Australia in the spread of Q fever is *Haemaphysalis humerosa,* but there are several other possible vectors (Table 68). *H. humerosa* probably is an important source of infection among bandicoots, but it does not bite man. A possible method of human infection is inhalation or wound contamination with the dried feces of the tick. The coxiellae are confined to the lining of the epithelium and the lumen of the gut, and the feces are highly infective. Hereditary transmission of the coxiellae has not been demonstrated in *H. humerosa.*

In the United States, *Coxiella burneti* has been found in nature in nymphal and adult forms of the lone star tick, *Amblyomma americanum* in Texas, and the wood tick, *Dermacentor andersoni,* in Montana and Wyoming. Experimental transmission has been accomplished with the argasid ticks, *Ornithodoros moubata* and *O. hermsi.* The former remained infective for 670 days and transmitted the coxiellae through the egg; the latter conserved the coxiellae in the tissues for 979 days, but failed to pass the infective agent through the egg in the few experiments tried.

TABLE 68

TICKS OF POSSIBLE SIGNIFICANCE IN THE TRANSMISSION OF Q FEVER IN AUSTRALIA

Tick	Principal Host	Other Reported Hosts	Relation to Q Fever
Haemaphysalis humerosa	Bandicoot	*Rattus rattus, Rattus culmorum youngi*	Proved vector among bandicoots
Haemaphysalis bispinosa	Cattle	Opossum, cattle, horse, sheep, horse, dog, man	Potential vector
Boophillus annulatus microplus	Cattle	Sheep	Can be infected
Ixodes holocyclus	Bandicoot	Most bush and domestic animals, and man	Probable vector
Rhipicephalus sanguineus	Dog	Sheep, cattle, horse, cat, man	Potential vector can be infected
Ornithodorus gurneyi	Kangaroo	Man	Unlikely vector

ANIMAL RESERVOIRS

The chief reservoir of Q fever in Australia is the bandicoot, a small marsupial. Agglutination tests showed 34 per cent were infected in nature. Derrick found other bush animals (two marsupials and seven rodents) susceptible to infection, and he considers them factors in spreading the disease. Experimental infection in all of them was mild, and often inapparent.

The animal reservoirs serving as the chief sources of infection for man are cattle, sheep, and goats. Man contracts the infection by inhalation of coxiellae being carried in air laden with dust containing offal of the infected animals. As a result many cases have occurred among cattlemen, slaughterhouse workers, wool-sorters, and among residents adjacent to cattle and sheep stockyards. Raw milk is also a source of infection.

THE DISEASE IN ANIMALS

Isolation of the agent from the blood of the patient in guinea pigs is usually successful. After the strain is established in guinea pigs, a spleen emulsion from the infected animals may be use to inoculate the yolk sac of developing chick embryos using defibrinated blood and serum from the patient. Mice may also be used for the initial isolation. In the guinea pig, the incubation period varies from five to fourteen days. After the expiration of the incubation period, these animals develop temperatures ranging from 40° C. to 41° C. This temperature usually lasts from one day to one week. The death rate varies with the strain. The most characteristic gross finding on the autopsy of the guinea pig is an enlarged spleen, sometimes being three to five times above the normal size. The identification of Q fever in the animal is made by serological tests, or by the development of immunity against a challenge dose of a proven strain of C. burneti. The complement-fixation test is the test of choice using either the technique described by Bengston, or a modification of the Kolmer technique.

THE DISEASE IN MAN

There have been many cases of Q fever recognized since the disease was first described. There is no definite seasonal incidence. The majority of the cases have occurred among those exposed to domestic livestock, cattle, sheep and goats, or their products, such as: slaughterhouse employees, dairy workers, and those living in the neighborhood of dairies or consuming raw milk from infected cows. Coxiellae have been recovered from the air around infected herds.

The actual mode of transmission from animals to man has not been learned. Since the organisms withstand drying, and remain viable for long periods at ordinary temperatures, the inhalation of dust particles contaminated with material from infected animals, or the contamination of the abraded skin or of the mucous membranes would seem to be important.

There is little evidence of transmission from person to person. The mortality rate is very low.

The disease manifests itself by an acute onset, with chills, prostration, and fever. Headache is pronounced in most cases. The fever is continuous, lasting from a few days to two or three weeks.

The headache is most often frontal, and is often accompanied by pain in the neck and photophobia. Burning of the eyes, lacrimation, and conjunctival infection have been noted in some cases. Stiffness of the neck, aching of the lower extremities, soreness of the joints, and sense of the fullness behind the sternum are not uncommon. Cough is present in practically all cases having pneumonitis.

As stated earlier, the absence of a rash is one of the characteristics which has placed this disease a little apart from the true rickettsial diseases.

On physical examination of the chest, abnormal physical findings are often negative for the first few days, with the later development of slight rales and mild dullness, usually over the lower part of the chest. Chest pains when present are usually minimal in character. A majority of the cases develop lesions which are sometimes found only upon roentgen ray examination. On x-ray examination the findings resemble very closely those seen in cases of primary atypical pneumonia, pneumonic consolidation shown by x-ray being one of the findings in many of the cases. A soft, infiltrative lesion is visible on the film. This lesion is not of the uniform density seen in lobar pneumonia. The areas of consolidation are patchy in character with a ground glass appearance, and usually only a portion of a lobe is involved.

PREVENTION

The prevention of Q fever is difficult, because complete knowledge concerning the mode of transmission of the disease is lacking. Vaccines have been prepared which are experimentally effective. Their value for the protection of exposed populations has not as yet been thoroughly tested.

ITEMS OF NOTE

1) Q fever is caused by the *Coxiella burneti (Rickettsia burneti, R. diaporica).*

2) It may be transmitted by ticks or through tick feces.

3) It has been encountered widely throughout the world.

4) Bandicoots, cattle, sheep, goats, and rodents are the chief reservoirs of infection. Coxiellae usually infect man by the inhalation of dust-carrying organisms from infected areas.

5) Infection often results in an atypical pneumonia.

6) The death rate is very low.

7) Prevention is difficult due to inadequate knowledge of the mode of transmission.

REFERENCES

BELL, J. A., BECK, M. D., and HUEBNER, R. J.: *J.A.M.A., 142:*868, 1950.
BENGSTON, I. A.: *Pub. Health Rep., 56:*272, 1941.
BURNET, F. M. and FREEMAN, M.: *M. J. Australia,* 2:299, 1937.

Cox, H. R.: *Am. J. Trop. Med., 20:*463, 1940.

Davis, G. E. and Cox, H. R.: *Pub. Health Rep., 53:*2259, 1938.

Delay, P. D., *et al.: J. Immunol., 65:*211, 1950.

Derrick, E. H.: *M. J. Australia, 2:*281, 1937.

Derrick, E. H.: *J. Hyg., 43:*357, 1944.

Derrick, E. H., *et al.: Australian J. Exper. Biol. & Med. Sc., 18:*409, 1940.

Dyer, R. E.: *Pub. Health Rep., 53:*2277, 1938.

Dyer, R. E.: *Pub. Health Rep., 54:*1229, 1939.

Hornibrook, J. W.: *Pub. Health Rep., 55:*1936, 1940.

Irons, J. V., *et al.: Pub. Health Rep., 61:*784, 1946.

Jellison, W. L., *et al.: Pub. Health Rep., 65:*395, 1950.

Lennette, E. H., and Welsh, H. H.: *Am. J. Hyg., 54:*44, 1951.

Luoto, L.: *Pub. Health Rep., 75:*135, 1960.

Luoto, L.: *Am. J. Pub. Health, 49:*334, 1959.

Philip, C. B.: *Am. J. Hyg., 37:*301, 1943.

Shepard, C. C.: *Am. J. Hyg., 46:*185, 1947.

Stoenner, H. G., *et al.: Am. J. Hyg., 69:*202, 1959.

Chapter 31

RICKETTSIALPOX

R. E. Dyer, M.D.

Rickettsialpox is a rickettsial disease which was first discovered in New York City. It is characterized by an initial lesion similar to that seen in tsutsugamushi and boutonneuse fever, and by the later appearance of a varicelliform rash.

HISTORY

In the summer of 1946, cases of this hitherto unrecognized disease occurred in housing developments in New York City. Some of the original cases were diagnosed as chicken pox on account of the character of the rash; consequently this new disease was named Rickettsialpox. In addition to New York City, this disease has been found along the Atlantic seaboard from Boston to Philadelphia and also in Cleveland, Ohio. Approximately 200 cases are diagnosed annually throughout these areas. The transmitting arthropod, *A. sanguineus*, has been identified in the above locations and also in the District of Columbia, Indianapolis, and Arizona. A closely related infection has been described in Russia and is known as Vesicular Rickettsiosis.

SEASONAL PREVALENCE

The cases reported in the New York City outbreak occurred in the late summer and early fall. No other data are available to assist in determining the seasonal prevalence.

ETIOLOGIC AGENT

The etiologic agent of rickettsialpox has been recovered from mites and human patients. This agent has been named *Rickettsia akari*.

VECTORS OF THE DISEASE

The mite, *Allodermanyssus sanguineus,* has been shown to be a vector. This mite feeds on rodents particularly house mice. In addition to house mice, laboratory mice, and guinea pigs have been shown to be susceptible to infection. It is probable that other species of rodents are also susceptible.

THE DISEASE IN ANIMALS

Four or five days following intraperitoneal inoculation of *R. akari* into guinea pigs these animals develop an irregular low-grade fever lasting from one to four days. The onset of fever is accompanied by an inflammatory reaction of the tunica vaginalis which lasts about two weeks. The scrotum becomes swollen and red, without necrosis as in Rocky Mountain spotted fever.

Gross pathology in the guinea pig sacrificed at the height of the infection shows a thickened and inflamed tunica vaginalis with adherence of the testes. The spleen usually shows moderate enlargement. In some instances, indurated subcutaneous nodules are found at the site of inoculation.

THE DISEASE IN MAN

In man, the disease shows some similarity to boutonneuse fever in that a primary lesion occurs at the site of the infecting mite bite. This lesion in appearance resembles the tache noir of boutonneuse fever. The lesion begins as a small red papule about a week before onset of other symptoms, reaching its maximum size about the second or third day of fever at that time being about 10 mm. in diameter. The papule develops a vesicle at the top, which eventually breaks with the subsequent formation of a dark colored scab. The lesion may be present as long as three weeks from the time of first appearance. Nearby lymph nodes may become enlarged and tender.

The onset of illness is marked by fever, headache, and chills or chilly sensations. The fever is irregular in character, seldom exceeding 103.5° F., and lasts about one week.

Two or three days after the onset of fever, a varicelliform rash appears, first on the trunk and face, later extending to the extremities. Lesions may be present in the mouth, tongue and soft palate, but apparently do not appear on the palms and soles. The lesions first appear as papules developing vesicles at the summit within forty-eight hours. There is little erythema around the lesions. The vesicles dry up in about a week.

PREVENTION AND CONTROL

The outbreaks of rickettsialpox which have been identified have occurred in dwellings heavily infested with mice. There has been a definite association with premises where garbage collection or destruction has been careless, particularly where neglected incinerators were present in the basements. Rodent proofing of dwellings and proper disposal of garbage are the essential factors in the control of this infection.

ITEMS OF NOTE

1) Rickettsialpox is a relatively mild infection which is characterized by a varicelliform rash.

2) The causative agent is *Rickettsia akari*.

3) The vector is a mite, *Allodermanyssus sanguineus*.

4) The common host in nature as far as is known at present is the house mouse.

5) Prevention and control rest on proper disposal of wastes and protection of food supplies against access of mice.

REFERENCES

GREENBERG, M., PELLITTERI, O., KLEIN, I. S. and HEUBNER, R. J.: *J.A.M.A., 133*:1947.

HUEBNER, R. J., JELLISON, W. L., and ARMSTRONG, C.: *Pub. Health Rep., 62*:777, 1947.

HUEBNER, R. J., JELLISON, W. L. and POMERANTZ, C.: *Pub. Health Rep., 61*:1677, 1946.

HUEBNER, R. J., STAMPS, P. and ARMSTRONG, C.: *Pub. Health Rep., 61*:1605, 1946.

SMADEL, J. E.: *Ann. Int. Med., 51*:421, 1959.

SUSSMAN, L. N.: *New York Med., 2*:27, 1946.

ZHDANOV, V. M., *et al.*: *Zh. Mikrobiol. Epidemiol. Immunobiol., 6*: 1954.

Chapter 32

LYMPHOCYTIC CHORIOMENINGITIS

Charles Armstrong, M.D.

Lymphocytic choriomeningitis (LCM.) is a rarely fatal acute infectious disease of man occasioned by a specific virus described in 1934. The disease which in man produces varied clinical manifestations has been found occurring spontaneously in man, white mice, house mice, monkeys, dogs, guinea pigs, roaches, cotton rats, foxes, chinchillas and possibly in ticks and mosquitoes.

HISTORY

The virus of lymphocytic choriomeningitis was first isolated by Armstrong and Lillie (1934) during study of the brain from a patient who had died presumably of encephalitis (St. Louis type). The virus was later isolated from the spinal fluid of a laboratory worker by Scott and Rivers (1936) and has subsequently been found in widely separated countries and it is probably present in all densely populated areas where mice exist.

THE ETIOLOGIC AGENT

While strains of LCM. virus from different sources may vary in their virulence for man and experimental animals and in their affinity for various organs, they have all been found to be immunologically similar. The supposedly exceptional strain isolated by MacCallum, Findlay and Scott (1939) which they designated pseudo-choriomeningitis was found to be, in fact, ectromelia virus. (MacCallum, Scott, Dalldorf and Gifford 1957).

Choriomeningitis virus passes through Seitz, Berkefeld and Chamberland filters. The size of the virus is usually given as 40 to 60 millimicrons. It is readily preserved in 50 per cent buffered glycerine at a temperature of 3° C. or in infected mouse brains suspended in water and rapidly frozen and stored at the temperature of dry ice. Saline is deleterious to the virus.

EXPERIMENTAL ANIMALS

In addition to the above named susceptible animals, rabbits, hamsters, ground squirrels, moles, horses and deer have been experimentally inoculated and while they show little or no recognizable symptoms the virus has been found in their blood or organs for varying numbers of days thereafter.

Cattle, calves, canaries, hedge hogs, cats and chickens are apparently insusceptible. It is interesting that Bengtson and Wooley (1936) succeeded in carrying the infection through a number of embryo passages. Some of the infected embryos hatched but the chicks seemed slow and drowsy for a time but soon became normal.

Choriomeningitis in Mice

Normal adult mice may be infected by intracerebral, intraperitoneal, subcutaneous or intragastric routes, or by natural exposure. Such infected mice may die or may recover with the development of complement fixing or virus neutralizing antibodies with or without showing signs of illness. The offspring of such mice are infectable. However, when female mice become infected during pregnancy, the embryos become infected, probably by way of the blood stream, or if newborn mice are inoculated during the first seven or eight days after birth they are rendered tolerant to the viruses (Traub 1936, 1938, 1939, 1941). That is, the virus will be found in their blood streams and organs for as long as they live. Such tolerant mice appear normal in every respect but they develop no circulating antibodies, nor have attempts employing adjuvants and other means been successful in inducing them to do so. Such mice are resistant to experimental LCM. infection, the resistance being due to other than circulating antibodies.

The offspring of such tolerant mice give birth to tolerant offspring and they in turn do the same and so on indefinitely; male mice tolerant to the virus may also convey infection to normal females (Traub 1936, 1938, 1939). The blood and organs of such tolerant mice contain the virus in high concentration as do their urine, feces and nasal secretions. It is therefore apparent that this latent form of infection has great significance in perpetrating the virus. Armstrong, Wallace and Ross (1940) trapped several choriomeningitis infected, apparently normal, mice from a home where a human case had developed. Twenty years later, a normal appearing mouse was trapped from the same home and LCM. virus was recovered from its blood. That the presence of latent infection with LCM. virus may tend to favor the development of lymphomatosis in mice is suggested by the work of Traub (1941), who observed two groups of mice for one year, one group of normal mice and one of mice with latent LCM. infection. At the end of the year there were 123 of the normal group of mice surviving, 5 per cent of which had developed lymphomatosis and of the group of mice with latent infection 104 survived of which 21 per cent had developed tumors.

OUTBREAKS IN MAN

There are few instances of multiple infection in a family and little or no evidence of infection from person to person. Dalldorf, Jungeblut and Umphlet (1946) described the occurrence of three cases in a multiple family building and a fourth case in a near neighbor. Verlinde, van der Werff and Briet (1948) described an epidemic which occurred in a convalescent home during the winter of 1946/47. From the spinal fluid, blood and throat of some of the cases they isolated a strain of virus which at first induced choriomeningitis only in guinea pigs but after a few passages in this species it did affect mice. Another peculiarity of this virus was that it affected only females; women patients, nurses and servant girls. There was no indication that mice were the source of infection. These characteristics suggest that this was an exceptional strain of LCM. virus, conveyed in an exceptional manner or that some other virus was complicating the picture.

ROUTE OF INOCULATION IN MAN AND PREVENTION

There is some experimental evidence indicating that monkey lice, mosquitoes, bedbugs and Rocky Mountain wood ticks may convey infection under special conditions of temperature, feeding, etc. However, the occurrence of cases throughout the year in the temperate zones suggests that arthropods are not an important means of spread.

The close association frequently demonstrated between human cases of LCM. and infected mice, together with the facility and persistency with which mice with latent infection spread virulent virus suggests that mouse contaminated food or dust is the most likely means of human infection. It follows that prevention would be favored if mice be removed or eliminated from quarters frequented by man.

Several investigators have developed killed virus vaccines which are capable of inducing immunity in experimental animals but they are not available for human use.

ISOLATION OF THE VIRUS

Isolation of LCM. virus is usually readily accomplished by the inoculation of blood, spinal fluid or emulsified liver, spleen or kidneys intracerebrally into mice or intraperitoneally into guniea pigs. Guinea pigs are preferable to mice for primary inoculation.

SYMPTOMS IN MAN

Since LCM. infection may exert its major and variable effect upon different portions of the central nervous system as well as upon various other organs of the body, the disease has a great potential for producing clinical variations.

Grippal and Asymptomatic Types

Cases of choriomeningitis simulating "grippe" or uncomplicated influenza have been encountered in laboratory workers, experimental volunteers (Kreis 1937) or in nature. The flushed features, absence of stiff neck or of altered reflexes combined with a relative lymphocytosis and low white counts, together with moderate fever, backache and marked prostration are surely suggestive of uncomplicated influenza. It is moreover probable that infection with the virus may be entirely asymptomatic.

Meningeal Type

Recovery from the influenza-like symptoms may terminate the attack, but in others, after a few days of more or less complete remission, there is a reappearance of fever with meningeal symptoms, such as fever, headache, stiff neck, vomiting and with positive Kernig and

Brudzinski's signs. In some instances the meningeal symptoms may usher in the attack. In meningeal cases, the spinal fluid is clear, sterile to bacterial culture, and may contain up to 3,000 cells per cmm., mainly lymphocytes.

Meningoencephalitic Type

In addition to such purely meningeal symptoms, as above described, somnolence, paralysis, anesthesia and altered deep reflexes as well as symptoms of transverse myelitis and of hydrocephalis may be observed.

DIFFERENTIAL DIAGNOSIS

There are many different viruses and other agents capable of simulating LCM. in some of its forms, such as influenza, mumps, poliomyelitis, tuberculosis (meningeal), torula histolytica, Coxsackie, Echo viruses, etc. A differential diagnosis from many of these conditions is not possible on clinical findings alone but must depend upon laboratory assistance. Such assistance includes isolation and identification of the virus together with the demonstration of an increase in complement fixing or virus neutralizing antibodies in convalescent as compared to acute phase serums.

PATHOLOGY

The pathology in experimental animals varies with the virus and route of administration as well as with the animal. A detailed organ by organ report of the findings in experimental animals and man would be unprofitable here. Suffice it to say that in three laboratory-confirmed fatal cases of LCM. contracted in studies on canine distemper, there was some cerebral edema and congestion, but very little was noted in the way of meningeal or choroid plexus involvement.

Blood vessel changes were indicated by the presence of skin rash in one case and by the presence of focal hemorrhages in two cases. These hemorrhages were observed beneath the dura, in the lungs, the kidneys and walls of the small intestines. There was peritoneal and pleaural fluid in at least two cases.

While studying the virus from these three patients, there occurred three spontaneous cases among monkeys at the National Institutes of Health. In one of these, there was a well pronounced generalized macular eruption which faded after three or four days, except in those lesions into which blood had escaped. The lungs of this animal were studded with hemorrhagic spots and there was free virus-rich fluid in both chest and abdominal cavities. Virus was isolated from every organ and tissue tested, 16 in all. Furthermore, microscopic evidence of the presence of virus in these tissues was indicated by the presence of perivascular and focal lymphocytic infiltration and by scattered areas of focal hemorrhage. But the most striking lesion, as reported by R. D. Lillie was a marked destruction of liver tissue beyond any seen with the mouse strains of virus which we had studied.

It appears therefore that this virus, apparently originating from dogs (Dalldorf and Douglass 1938) differs from mouse strains in its virulence for man and monkeys. There is some indication that dogs may in nature convey the infection. For instance Farmer and Janeway (1942) cite the case of a twenty-three year old girl, living in a mouse free home, whose dog became ill, supposedly with canine distemper. Nineteen days from the beginning of the dog's illness, she developed meningeal symptoms and was subsequently found immune to choriomeningitis.

INCUBATION PERIOD

The time from exposure to onset of the systemic symptoms is in the neighborhood of six to ten days while the central nervous symptoms are slower in developing, usually thirteen to twenty-one days.

TREATMENT

Rosenthal (1937) found that Prontosil in large doses afforded slight protection against small doses of virus in mice but Toomey and Takacs (1944) could not demonstrate any benefit against fatal doses of virus. Haas, Stewart and Briggs (1957) found that amethopterin had some sparing effect in mice though the virus was not destroyed by the drug. Panov and Remezov (1960) found that exposure to O_2 under pressure of one atmosphere for five to ten hours tended to be beneficial to infected mice. More of the treated mice survived and their immunity to reinfection was less marked than in the controls.

Since there is no specific or other treatment of proven value for choriomeningitis in man, the treatment must at present be symptomatic. Spinal tap gradually to relieve increased pressure may often reduce headache in cases involving the central nervous system. Due to the tendency for cases to relapse patients should not be allowed to return to normal activities until the spinal fluid cell count has returned to normal, which may be a matter of weeks.

ITEMS OF NOTE

1) Lymphocytic choriomeningitis is caused by a virus.

2) The virus in mice is a model for the study of latent infections.

3) The virus is found in mice, dogs and occasionally in other animals.

4) There is no indication that the disease is transmitted from person to person.

5) Dust and food contaminated by infected mice seem to be the most likely means of transmission to man.

6) Inactivated vaccines capable of inducing immunity in experimental animals have been prepared but are not available for human use.

7) There is no specific treatment.

REFERENCES

ARMSTRONG, CHARLES, and LILLIE, R. D.: Experimental lymphocytic choriomeningitis of monkeys and mice produced by a virus encountered in studies of the 1933 St. Louis encephalitis epidemic. *Pub. Health Rep., 49:*1019, 1934.

ARMSTRONG, CHARLES, WALLACE, J. J., and ROSS, L.: Lymphocytic choriomeningitis: gray mice, *Mus musculus,* a reservoir for the infection. *Pub. Health Rep., 55:*1222, 1940.

BENGTSON, IDA M., and WOOLEY, J. G.: Cultivation of the virus of lymphocytic choriomeningitis in the developing chick embryo. *Pub. Health Rep., 51:*29-41, 1936.

DALLDORF, GILBERT, and DOUGLASS, MARGARET: Simultaneous distemper and lymphocytic choriomeningitis in dog spleen and the sparing effect on poliomyelitis. *Proc. Soc. Exper. Biol. & Med., 39:*294-297, 1938.

DALLDORF, GILBERT, JUNGEBLUT, C. W., and UMPHLET, M. J.: Multiple cases of choriomeningitis in an apartment harboring infected mice. *J.A.M.A., 131:*25, 1946.

FARMER, T. W. and JANEWAY, C. A.: Infections with the virus of lymphocytic choriomeningitis. *Medicine, 21:*1, 1942.

HAAS, VICTOR H., STEWART, S. E., and BRIGGS, G. M.: Folic acid deficiency and the sparing of mice infected with the virus of lymphocytic choriomeningitis. *Virology, 3:*15-21, 1957.

KREIS, BORIS: La maladie d' Armstrong. Chorio-meningite lymphocytaire-une nouvelle entite morbid? *Paris Univ. Thesis, Bailliere,* Paris 1937.

MacCallum, F. O., Findley, G. M., and Scott, T. McNair: Pseudolymphocytic chorio-meningitis. *Brit. J. Exper. Path.*, *20:*260, 1939.

MacCallum, F. O., Scott, T. McNair, Dalldorf, G., and Gifford, Rebecca: Pseudo-lymphocytic choriomeningitis: A correction. *Brit. J. Exper. Path.*, *38:*120-121, 1957.

Panov, A. G., and Remezov, P. I.: The influence of oxygen under pressure on the course of certain experimental neurovirus infections in white mice. *Vopr. Virusol.*, *3:*267-272, 1960. (Russian Text) cited from *Excerpta Medica, 14:* section 4: 265, abstract 1088.

Rosenthal, S. M., Wooley, J. G., and Bauer, H.: Studies in chemotherapy VI. The chemotherapy of infections in mice with sulphonamide compounds. *Pub. Health Rep.*, *52:*1211, 1937.

Scott, T. F. McNair and Rivers, T. M.: Meningitis in man caused by a filterable virus. *J. Exper. Med.*, *63:*397, 1936.

Toomey, J. A. and Takacs, Wm. S.: Chemotherapy of lymphocytic choriomeningitis in mice and guinea pigs. *J. Immunol., Virus Res. & Exper. Chemother.*, *48:*49-55, 1944.

Traub, Erich: Persistence of lymphocytic choriomeningitis virus in immune animals and its relation to immunity. *J. Exper. Med.*, *63:*847-861, 1936.

Traub, Erich: Factors influencing the persistence of choriomeningitis virus in the blood of mice after clinical recovery. *J. Exper. Med.*, *68:*229, 1938.

Traub, Erich: Epidemiology of lymphocytic choriomeningitis in a mouse stock observed for 4 years. *J. Exper. Med.*, *69:*801-817, 1939.

Traub, Erich: The influence of latent lymphocytic choriomeningitis infection on the appearance of lymphomatosis in white mice. *Zentralbl. Bakt.*, *147:*16-25, 1941.

Verlinde, J. D., van der Werff, J., and W. Briet: An encephalitis epidemic caused by virus closely related to choriomeningitis of Armstrong. *Nederland Tijdschr. Geneesk.*, *92:*2802-2809, 1948. Cited from *Biol. Absts.*, 1950, *24:*426, Abst. #4530.

Chapter 33

ARTHROPOD-BORNE VIRAL ENCEPHALITIDES

D. L. COLLINS, PH.D., SC. D.

B<small>Y DEFINITION</small>, the diseases which are discussed in this chapter have in common the fact that they are encephalitides the pathogenic agents of which are viruses carried by arthropods. Since the last edition of this book there has been a vast increase in clinical, biological, serological and geographic knowledge of arthoropod-borne viruses, including those which cause encephalitis, and a number of new ones have been identified and classified. As the details have become better known, different and sometimes more characteristic or distinctive clinical and serological manifestations have been defined, as well as more specific vector relationships. Therefore, it seemed that it would be preferable in the present edition to treat each disease separately, while following for each one in so far as practicable the same headings used by Dr. W. McD Hammon in the previous edition in order to preserve the continuity which featured his presentation. It is a pleasure and a duty to acknowledge that although the arrangement here used is mine, the chapter is built around the framework constructed by Dr. Hammon, and that where no changes have been required because of new information or changed points of view, certain paragraphs from the previous edition have been included verbatim, or paraphrased as seemed desirable.

Attention is called also to the detailed information included by Rivers and Horsfall in *Viral and Rickettsial Infections of Man,* (3rd Edition, 1959) particularly, for our purposes, Chapters 12, 13, and 14, by Casals and Reeves, Olitsky and Casals, and Olitsky and Clarke, respectively. This book has rendered it immeasurably easier for all subsequent workers to assemble material for special purposes, since the same sources must be used. For the present summary, the original sources listed in Rivers and Horsfall, and many others were consulted, and in addition, I have been able to discuss certain points with some of the authors, including Doctors Hammon, Reeves, Chamberlain, Sudia, Work, Hess, Hayes, Jobbins, Wallis, Hoogstraal, Trapido and others. The experiments, observations and thinking of these men, to mention but a few, have been so comprehensive and forward-looking that they constitute the background and foundation of any subsequent general consideration such as this review. Rather than interrupt the text by repetitious references, it is intended that these remarks will be taken as an acknowledgement to these workers and that interested persons will refer to appropriate titles in the bibliography for confirmations, details and more specific information.

CLASSIFICATION

The viruses discussed here may be classified in several ways, but whatever criterion is used there is an overlap in terms of the other criteria. A widely accepted classification on the basis of serology places those that are best known at present in two groups, *A* and *B*, with hitherto unclassified viruses either being added from time to time to the defined groups or remaining temporarily unassigned. On the basis of vector relationships all of those treated here may be classified as mosquito-borne or tick-borne so far as is known at present. There are mosquito-borne viruses in both groups A and B, and group B also includes some that are tick-borne.

Another classification could be made according to geographical distribution, but distinctions on this basis are becoming less significant as records of identification on the serological basis accumulate from all parts of the world.

The accompanying tabular view of the diseases discussed in this chapter is set up on the basis of vector relationships, since the fact of being arthropod-borne is a primary requisite for inclusion. The other classifications are also indicated so that they may be rearranged as desired according to the other criteria. (Table 69)

In the following pages the viruses and the diseases associated with them are discussed in the order listed in the table. Western encephalitis is probably the best known, at least in this country. It is here used as a prototype, with the various subtopics treated in greater detail than with the others. The latter can then be characterized in

TABLE 69
ARTHROPOD-BORNE VIRAL ENCEPHALITIDES

	Name of Disease or Virus	Geographic Range	Serological Group	Presumed or Known Vector Species**
Mosquito-Borne	Western	Throughout Western Hemisphere	A	Culex tarsalis, especially, where it occurs; Culiseta melanura, and species of Aedes, Culex and others, elsewhere.
	Eastern	Eastern and Central U. S. A., Central America, South America, Southeast Philippines	A	Culiseta melanura among birds, presumably Aedes and Culex spp. to man and other mammals.
	Venezuelan	South America, Trinidad	A	Mansonia titillans, Aedes taeniorhynchus
	St. Louis	U. S. A., probably throughout, but especially in Mississippi Valley and West; also in Central America, Caribbean and Northern South America	B	Culex tarsalis where it occurs; elsewhere Culex pipiens complex and others.
	Japanese B	Japan, ESE Asia, Australia, New Guinea	B	Culex tritaeniorhynchus and others.
	Murray Valley	Australia, New Guinea	B	Culex annulorostris Others?
	Ilheus	Northern S. America, Central America, Trinidad	B	Psorophora ferox; other Psorophora spp.; Aedes spp.
	California	California, Montana and possibly other states, U. S. A.	Unclassified	Aedes dorsalis, Culex tarsalis
Tick-Borne	Russian Spring-Summer Russian (Asiatic)	Siberia, E. Asia	B	Ixodes persulcatus; also other Ixodes spp. and spp. of Dermacentor and Haemaphysalis
	Russian (European)	European Russia	B	Ixodes ricinus; other Ixodidae
	Central European	Central Europe	B	Ixodes ricinus; other Ixodidae
	Diphasic Meningo-Encephalitis	Central Europe	B	Ixodes ricinus; other Ixodidae
	Louping Ill	British Isles	B	Ixodes ricinus; other Ixodidae
	Powassan*	Ontario, Canada	B	Ixodidae, possibly Dermacentor andersoni and D. variabilis

*Very little information, but has characteristics that suggest relationship to Russian Spring-Summer Complex.

**Here are included: (1) species that are generally accepted as vectors on the basis of all evidence at hand, and (2) species that appear to be vectors on the basis of strong circumstantial evidence, such as recovery of virus from them in nature, and/or proven ability to become infected and to transmit, in the laboratory.

terms of differences from or similarities to Western Encephalitis. First, however, a few general remarks may be in order.

THE PROBLEMS OF OVERWINTERING

One of the most elusive facts to establish has been how the viruses overwinter in the temperate zones. Much work has been done and more is under way to shed light on this important aspect of the ecology of viruses. For instance, Western and Eastern Encephalitis (WE and EE) are primarily disease of birds, only secondarily or "accidentally" of man and other mammals, but whether the viruses can overwinter as latent infections in birds in temperate areas, with viremias high enough and persistent enough to result in transmission in the spring is uncertain. It has been suggested that migratory birds, returning in the spring from wintering in endemic areas may re-introduce the virus locally, but this has not been proven.

Another possibility is overwintering in the arthropod vector.

WE virus has been isolated from *Culex tarsalis* collected in natural, sheltered hibernation sites during the winter. This virus was also found to persist through the winter in specimens of this species which had been infected, in the laboratory, in the fall. Viremia of long duration and high titer occurs in reptiles, and in experiments with garter snakes inoculated with WE virus in the fall, the virus persisted through the winter and normal mosquitoes fed on these snakes became infected and were able to transmit the virus to 1-day-old chicks.

Studies similar to those cited with *Culex tarsalis* and WE virus have been made with other mosquitoes and EE virus, but to date, the natural or usual method of overwintering of these and other viruses remains unknown. Studies in Europe have even indicated the possibility of an "Eastern-type" virus overwintering in ticks, and although the data are inconclusive, the possibility merits further investigation.

MOSQUITO-BORNE ENCEPHALITIDES:

WESTERN ENCEPHALITIS (WE)

History and Geographic Distribution

The virus of Western [Equine] Encephalitis was the first of the viral agents of the arthropod-borne viral encephalitides of the Western Hemisphere to be isolated and recognized. Although it was isolated from horses in 1930, in California, it was not recovered from the central nervous system of man until 1938. For many years previous to the identification of the virus, typical encephalitis symptoms had been observed in horses in the western states, and enzootics had occurred. Since its recognition in man, epidemics have been confirmed in North Dakota, Minnesota, the prairie provinces of Canada, and, more recently, in the Central Valley of California. In the latter area, as well as in others, the disease appears to be endemic. Antibodies have been found in vertebrate hosts, and virus has been recovered from wild birds and mosquitoes in the eastern, central and southern states, as well as in the west. There is also evidence of the occurrence of the disease in Mexico, in northern South America, and in Argentina, so that it is probably safe to say that it exists throughout the western hemisphere, presumably wherever the potential reservoirs (birds) and vectors (mosquitoes) occur.

Animal Hosts

The intensive study applied to WE on many fronts during the past thirty years has produced a considerable body of information on its animal hosts, reservoirs and arthropod vectors. WE, like EE and SLE and probably others, appears to be primarily a disease of birds rather than of horses, so that the term "equine" is of historic rather than epidemiological significance. In horses there is a comparatively short period (a few hours) of viremia, of a low level, whereas in certain experiments with birds viremia was found to last as long as six days, with four days for the majority of individuals. In other tests, virus was recovered from birds as long as ten days after inoculation. Wild birds appear to maintain higher virus levels in the blood than domestic fowls. Among the birds that have developed viremia after inoculation are English sparrow, house finch, tricolored and red-winged blackbird, white crowned sparrow, towhee, cardinal, white throated sparrow, blue jay, purple finch, domestic fowl, and others. Isolations have been made from some twenty species in nature, as well as from domestic fowls.

Garter snakes are easily infected in the laboratory and, as with EE, reptiles probably have the highest viremias for the longest periods.

Arthropod Vectors

It has been thoroughly established that in the Western United States, where WE is endemic and occasionally epidemic, the principal vector is the locally abundant mosquito *Culex tarsalis*. Other mosquitoes, mostly of the genus *Culex*, but also including especially species of *Aedes, Anopheles* and *Culiseta*, either have been found naturally infected, or have been infected experimentally by feeding, and some of them are presumed to be the natural vectors in areas where *Culex tarsalis* does not occur. Within its range, *C. tarsalis* is ideally suited to be both an endemic and an epidemic vector. It appears to prefer birds, but it feeds readily on man, horses and many other vertebrates. It is easily infected, and it breeds in large numbers in both natural and irrigation overflow water in sites frequented by its avian and mammalian hosts, and in close proximity to man.

The virus has been recovered frequently from naturally infected *C. tarsalis* throughout the western half of the United States, often in the same areas and during the same period where epidemics occurred. Under experimental conditions, the virus is easily acquired and transmitted by these mosquitoes.

Outside the range of *C. tarsalis* it is at present impossible to name a "principal" vector, but not at all difficult to point the finger of suspicion at local species on the basis of such circumstantial evidence as the finding of naturally infected specimens in areas where virus has been isolated from birds. For instance, in eastern states the western virus has been recovered from *Culiseta melanura*, the chief suspect in the transmission of Eastern encephalitis among birds, and also from *Aedes canadensis*, and it was recovered from both wild and domestic birds in the same area. Other mosquitoes that may be considered possible vectors, either on the basis of field or laboratory evidence, or both, include *Culex pipiens quinquefasciatus*, and *Aedes infirmatus, Aedes aegypti, C. restuans, C. stigmatosoma, Aedes melanimon (dorsalis), A. nigromaculis, A. infirmatus, A. vexans, Anopheles freeborni*, and *Culiseta inornata*.

WE virus has also been isolated from the bug *Triatoma sanguisuga*, and from bird mites, but the circumstances were such as to make it rather doubtful that these arthropods could be effective vectors.

Seasonal Prevalence

In the western United States, the epidemics have reached their heights in late summer, i. e., August and early September.

Etiologic Agents; Serology

Both because of its historic role in the group of encephalitides here considered, and because of the comparatively voluminous data on it, the etiology and serology of western encephalitis are here described in detail as a prototype of the others.

The diameter of the WE virus particle appears to be in the median range, measurements varying according to method from about 25 mμ to 50 or more mμ. The electron microscope shows irregularly rounded particles. Chemical studies have not yet yielded a pure material with present techniques, but it has been indicated that a high percentage of components may be extracted with fat solvents, and another high percentage is ribonuclear protein; the remaining small percentage consists of carbohydrates. The virus is most stable in the cold at pH between 6.5 and 8.5. In suspension it withstands room temperature for two hours but titers decrease significantly with longer exposure. It can be preserved indefinitely at low temperatures (below freezing) by several standard methods. It is readily inactivated by ether, so that care must be exercised in the choice of methods in studying suspected vectors, hosts and reservoirs.

The Disease in Animals

Classically, the western virus involved horses, and its first isolation from that animal as well as the occurrence of severe and widely publicised epizootics among horses give point to the use of the term "equine" in referring to the disease. However, the virus, like the others, occurs in several host animals, only a few of which (e. g., horses, mules, man) suffer acute illness from it. Others such as squirrels, pigs, deer and birds, show no clinical symptoms, although the virus can be recovered from them and antibodies may be present. Experimentally, most of the common laboratory animals, except cats, can be infected by intracerebral inoculation, and show some symptoms. Sheep are also resistant. Birds, as a group, may be considered the primary hosts of the virus. They demonstrate viremia and develop antibodies but do not show the disease symptoms characteristic of WE infection in the more susceptible mammalian hosts. White mice are easily infected, as are chick embryos, which makes them favorite subjects for laboratory studies.

The disease as it occurs in horses is described below. This description is designed to serve for reference and comparison, not only for symptoms as they occur in other animals, but also for the other encephalitides described in their respective sections.

Horses of all ages may be affected, but in endemic areas all but the younger horses may be shown to be immune, from previous apparent or inapparent infection. Passive protection from the mare is likely to afford complete protection during the first season's exposure; therefore, one-year-olds have the highest morbidity rates. After an incubation period of a few days to three weeks symptoms appear. The onset may be quite sudden with high fever, staggering, then rapid progressive paralysis and death within two to four days. In the less severe cases several types of clinical manifestations may be observed according to the portion of the central nervous system most involved or the order of involvement of different parts. Fever, incoordination, paralysis of the lips, lassitude, circling, leaning against a fence, standing with hanging head and wide stance, or even with front legs crossed, inability to swallow, falling and inability to rise, grinding of teeth, and spastic or flaccid paralysis of legs are commonly observed signs of the disease. Case fatality rates in the western type disease average 20 to 25 per cent and 80 to 90 per cent in the eastern equine disease. Some surviving animals have permanent damage of some part of the central nervous system. No specific therapy has been shown to have any value.

Specific diagnosis in diseased animals may be made by isolation of virus from the brain, or by neutralization and complement fixation tests made on a series of blood serum specimens, the first one collected during the early acute phase of illness. A rising titer of WE antibody in this series of sera must be demonstrated before a diagnosis can be made.

In smaller mammals such as laboratory mice, the disease runs a faster, more intense course. When they are inoculated with the virus intracerebrally, symptoms appear after two to six days, with indications of meningo-encephalomyelitis, such as generalized spastic muscular contractions, spastic paralyses, wild or uncoordinated movements, torpor, prostration and death. Death may occur within two hours after the onset of symptoms, or at any time up to two days later. Although mice of all ages appear to be equally susceptible to the virus given by the intracerebral or intranasal route, the older animals are less susceptible when the virus is introduced intraperitoneally or subcutaneously, the latter method being more similar to a natural inoculation of a host by a biting arthropod.

The Disease in Man

Specific etiologic diagnosis of human cases is made on the same basis as that mentioned for horses, with the increased application of improved techniques for hemaglutination-inhibition tests. Clinically, western encephalitis and the other arthropod-borne encephalitides are similar, and from inapparent cases, the symptoms range from simple fever and headache, to combinations of these with drowsiness, and gastro-intestinal disturbances, followed by muscular pains, lethargy, speech difficulties and mental confusion, tremor, convulsions and other symptoms. The acute phase, if it occurs, may continue for a week or ten days. In children there is grave danger of serious permanent damage to the central nervous system, with impairment of locomotion, coordination and bodily functions. Older patients are more likely to recover completely.

Pathological indications include, typically, extensive lesions in the grey matter with less extensive indication of inflammation in the white matter. The cord may or may not be involved.

EASTERN ENCEPHALITIS (EE)

History and Geographic Distribution

First isolated from horses and recognized as a new virus in 1933, the Eastern virus was not isolated from human central nervous system tissue until 1938, from fatal cases in the Massachusetts epidemic of that year. The 1938 epidemic and epizootic in Massachusetts focused national attention not only on that disease specifically, but on the arthropod-borne viral encephalitides as a group, with a resultant multiplication of research efforts in all the related fields involved, —serology, epidemiology, host relationships, ecology, vectors and vector control.

From the first, the mortality rate in both humans and horses has been high. In the 1938 Massachusetts epidemic, which was the first on record, there were thirty-four human cases, with a mortality of 74 per cent, and 248 equine cases with a 90 per cent mortality. In Louisiana, in 1947, there was an epizootic in horses which involved some 14,000 cases, with a 90 per cent mortality and there were fifteen human cases, with a 60 per cent mortality. More recently, in 1959, an outbreak occurred in New Jersey in which thirty-three humans were affected. Twenty-one deaths occurred, the mortality thus being 64 per cent. Virus and antibody surveys have revealed, with clinical confirmations, evidence of the disease in all the east coast and Gulf states from New Hampshire to Texas, and in the central states as far west as Kansas, in Central America, and South America, the Philippines and southeast Asia.

Animal Hosts

Like the WE virus, the EE agent seems to have a special affinity for birds, which appear to be uniformly susceptible. It differs from WE in causing a much more severe infection in some of them, as well as in laboratory animals (see below). In a long list of birds that have been tested, all that were free of antibodies developed viremia after inoculation. Gregarious species that inhabit swamps are probably most important under endemic conditions, the smaller wild birds possibly being more efficient natural endemic hosts than the larger ones. During epidemics, thrushes, catbirds, grackles, English sparrows, pigeons, pheasants (wild), sandpipers and other birds have yielded the virus. In serological surveys of birds made in Massachusetts in 1953, 1956 and 1957, neutralization tests were positive in catbird, chickadee, bluejay, robin, sapsucker, sparrow, towhee, kingbird, phoebe, thrush, bluebird, dove, duck, flicker, flycatcher, starling, swallow, vireo, warbler, and waxwing. This list, which is constantly being augmented in other areas, is cited as giving some idea of the intensive surveys that have been made and are being made, especially in areas where epidemics or outbreaks have occurred. The susceptibility of pheasants and turkeys to infection by EE virus has been amply demonstrated in several states, and infection in White Pekin ducks in New York has also occurred, with considerable mortality in young birds. Even with all this information, however, we still cannot name a principal or definitive host, and we do not know how the virus overwinters in the northeast.

After inoculation with EE virus, viremia occurred in crows, rabbits, leopard frog, garter snakes, black snakes, water snakes, and several turtles. The longest period of viremia was three hours, in the spotted turtle. In Panama, viremia from EE virus lasted for as long as seven days in lizards.

Arthropod Vectors

At the time of this writing, close to twenty species of mosquitoes have been found either to be carrying the virus in nature or to be able to carry and transmit it in the laboratory. These include several species each of *Aedes, Culex, Psorophora,* and representatives of several other genera. Because of the number of isolations of EE virus from wild caught *Culiseta melanura,* and from considerable experimental as well as circumstantial evidence, this species is presumed to be the principal enzootic vector, responsible for the perpetuation of the virus in nature. However, since *C. melanura* has a preference for birds and seldom bites man, other species also may be involved in transmission to man.

In the two widely publicised epidemics in recent years, those of 1938 in Massachusetts and 1959 in New Jersey, *Aedes vexans* might have been involved as a vector species in the former and *A. sollicitans* in the latter. EE virus has been isolated from both species, also from *C. restuans* in New Jersey. Isolation of the virus has been made from wild *Culex pipiens quinquefasciatus* and *C. nigripalpus.*

Although the preponderance of evidence is in favor of mosquitoes as the principal, if not the only important vector of the virus from animal hosts (presumably birds) to man, other arthropods may enter the picture either directly or indirectly. EE virus isolations have been made from Simuliidae, including *Eusimulium johannseni* (Hart), and nonengorged *Simulium meridionale* Riley. Isolation from a pool of *Culicoides* species has also been made, and laboratory work by Russian workers with an "Eastern type" virus indicates at least the possibility that ticks (Ixodidae) may be reservoir-vectors in which the virus can overwinter.

Seasonal Prevalence

Late summer and early fall have been the periods of highest incidence of the disease, not only in pheasants and ducks, but also in man.

The Disease in Animals

Since pheasants have been especially prominent in the EE picture, observations on these birds are cited below as showing in general what may be expected in birds, at least domestic birds or birds in confinement. In studies in Connecticut the clinical experiences were divided into systemic and neurologic signs. The former included droopiness, ruffled feathers, soiled vent region and occasional gasping. Neurologic signs varied from simple incoordination to unilateral or bilateral paresis of the legs, and droopy wings, to coarse tremor and torticollis. All of the symptoms did not, of course, occur in all the birds.

The first report of the disease in ducks described symptoms similar to those mentioned for pheasants. The natural disease was not seen in ducklings older than eighteen days. In experiments where ducklings were inoculated with virus the blood virus levels reached a peak in from four to eight hours in one-week-old ducklings, and fell to zero from forty-eight to fifty-four hours after injection.

In pheasants and probably also in ducks, the virus can be transmitted directly from bird to bird by picking by the beak, and can be acquired by healthy birds through cannibalism.

The manifestations of the disease in horses are similar to those caused by the Western virus, and the disease runs a similar course, except that the EE virus produces more severe symptoms and a higher rate of fatality than either WE or St. Louis.

The Disease in Man

In man, as in horses and birds, the disease produced by the EE virus is more serious than that resulting from either WE or St. Louis virus. The average fatality rate has been about sixty per cent. Approximately two-thirds of the human cases have been children under ten years of age. Most of the survivors experience serious permanent after-effects. However, there have been only about 100 cases of EE reported, as against several thousand persons affected in one epidemic of WE.

VENEZUELAN ENCEPHALITIS (VE)

History and Geographic Distribution

The virus was recovered in 1938 and 1939 from equine animals in Venezuela where there was a severe epizootic. It was presumably the same agent that had caused a disease with similar symptoms in horses and mules in Colombia in 1935. It has since been reported in Argentina, Brazil, Ecuador, Trinidad and Panama. Although antibodies have been found in the Seminoles of Florida, U. S. A., there have been no known overt infections in the U. S. A.

Animal Hosts

This virus is another of the "A" group that was first found in horses, and therefore received the name "equine." The extent to which it may affect other animals in nature is not known. Wild birds can become infected through the bites of mosquitoes, but the infection is usually inapparent or silent, and the level of viremia is so low that the role of birds in the epidemiology of the disease is uncertain.

Arthropod Vectors

The mosquitoes *Mansonia titillans* and *Aedes taeniorhynchus* may transmit the disease to horses and to man. Transmission to wild birds (English sparrow) by the bite of infected *Aedes triseriatus* has been accomplished. In experiments with animals, the Venezuelan virus appeared to be particularly virulent in adult animals which were infected by other than neural routes, and it would seem to be reasonable that epidemics could occur without arthropod vectors.

The Disease in Animals

In guinea pigs, rabbits, and mice there is a lymphomyelopoietic necrosis. In mice and also in monkeys, there are central nervous system lesions similar to those caused by other arthropod-borne viruses. Horses usually show pancreatic lesions. They are susceptible to intranasal instillation of the virus, and since the virus may be recovered from the nose, mouth, eyes, urine and milk of infected animals it is not surprising that infection occurs by contact. Infection by the intra-cerebral route has been demonstrated in equines, mice, guinea pigs, rabbits, cats, dogs, sheep and goats, but cattle are resistant. Chick embryos are susceptible.

The Disease in Man

The incubation period is unknown. Laboratory acquired infections have been characteristically mild, without neurologic or other typical encephalitic manifestations. They have appeared more like influenza, with headache, fever, and gastro-intestinal disturbances, rarely with tremor or muscular involvement. These symptoms occurred for three to five days in mild cases, up to eight days in more severe attacks, and were followed by prompt and complete recovery.

In two cases in Trinidad, presumably due to the Venezuela virus, the onset was rapid, definite encephalitis symptoms occurred, followed by coma and death. In Colombia, in an epidemic in 1952, patients complained of muscle and bone pains.

In the disease occurring naturally in man (i.e., infection not incurred in the laboratory) virus has been recovered from the central nervous system and the blood. It was also recovered from the nasopharynx of humans infected in the laboratory. This was to be expected since a characteristic feature of the disease has been that the virus infects man as well as animals by contact exposure. Specific NT, CF and HI antibodies develop during convalescence, one to two weeks after infection.

Diagnosis can be made only by laboratory procedures such as identification of the virus isolated from central nervous system tissue, from the blood, from nasopharyngeal washings, or by finding HI, NT or CT antibodies during convalescence. The finding of neutralizing antibodies in a high per cent or sera from healthy persons in both Trinidad and the Amazon Valley indicates many inapparent infections.

ST. LOUIS ENCEPHALITIS (SLE)

History and Geographic Distribution

The virus of St. Louis encephalitis was first identified in 1933 from human brain tissue, in an epidemic which occurred in St. Louis and Kansas City, Missouri. An epidemic of encephalitis similar to the Missouri outbreak had occurred previously in the summer of 1932, in Southern Illinois. Other epidemics or outbreaks have occurred not only in the Midwest, but in California and Texas. The disease appears to be endemic in certain restricted areas in all the states west of the Mississippi River, in the central states as far east as and including Ohio, Kentucky and Tennessee, and serologic surveys indicate the possibility of its presence in Atlantic coast states (e.g., Florida, New Jersey, New York and Massachusetts). It also occurs in Northern South America, the Caribbean Islands and in Central America.

Animal Hosts and Reservoirs

Extensive investigation of local fauna have failed to yield any appreciable number of SLE virus isolations. As late as 1957 only two birds in nature (a mourning dove in California and a flicker in Kentucky) had yielded SLE virus. Experimental inoculations have produced viremias in a number of species of birds, including finches, English sparrows, pigeons and cowbirds. In Panama, where the virus was found in mosquitoes *(Sabethes chloropterus)* and in the blood of two persons, it was not recovered from the many wild animals and birds included in the surveys. The antibody tests were complicated by the presence of Ilheus encephalitis (q. v.) in the same areas. In Minnesota, St. Louis antibodies have been found in sentinel pigeons. From the meagre data available it is thought that wild birds are the most likely host reservoirs for the St. Louis virus. Chickens may also be important, since they develop a viremia of a level similar to that in wild birds, with especially high titers in young birds. SLE virus does not multiply to such high levels as does WE in birds, nor does it cause clinical symptoms in as many species of mammals.

Arthropod Vectors

In Western United States, the principal vector is generally considered to be the mosquito *Culex tarsalis* but since the disease occurs over a very wide area beyond the range of this species, it seems obvious that other vectors also must be involved. In outbreaks in Texas and Kentucky, *C. pipiens quinquefasciatus* and *Culex pipiens pipiens,* respectively, appear to have been the most likely suspects. Recent work indicates that although the virus multiplies in both forms, multiplication is more rapid in *pipiens.* In Panama, as we have noted above, *Sabethes chloropterus* was incriminated. In the United States, the virus has been isolated from wild-caught *Culex stigmatosoma, Aedes dorsalis* and *Prorophora* (probably *confinnis*); in Trinidad from *Culex coronator, C. candelli* and *Psorophora ferox.* Several other species, including some in genera other than the above, have been shown experimentally to be able to become infected and to transmit the virus. Among these is *Culiseta,* which is so strongly suspect in the epidemiology of EE in the Eastern United States.

Transmission of SLE virus from fourth instar larvae of *Aedes aegypti* mosquitoes to the adults, with infection of baby chicks from them has been reported. But although the technique showed that larval, pupal and adult mosquito tissues could support the virus, the possibility would seem to be rather remote that larval habitats would be contaminated in such a way that the larvae could acquire it to transmit.

Seasonal Prevalence

As might be expected, the seasonal prevalence is correlated with abundance of mosquitoes, and like most of the other arthropod-borne encephalitides, the incidence is highest in the late summer and early fall. All of the recent epidemics have occurred at times when mosquito breeding conditions were unusually favorable.

The Disease in Animals.

White mice, wild mice, young rats, hamsters, horses and rhesus monkeys are susceptible to intracerebral inoculation with some strains, whereas Cebus monkeys, adult rats, sheep, kittens and ferrets are not susceptible. Some animals, e.g., guinea pigs and rabbits, develop inapparent infection after inoculation by any route, and the infection is also inapparent in monkeys, horses and adult mice after small doses of virus injected subcutaneously. The resistance of horses to infection by SLE is evidence of a striking difference between the SLE virus and WE and EE.

The typical response of monkeys is a fever and indication of central nervous involvement with subsequent recovery, whereas in white mice, after an incubation period of three or four days, convulsions and paralysis occur, with ataxia and ruffled fur. Death occurs in from one to five days afterward.

Experiments with different animals indicate that SLE virus produces a comparatively low level of viremia, and often without clinical symptoms.

The Disease in Man

The St. Louis encephalitis virus is apparently not so virulent as either the Western, Eastern or Japanese B. In man, as well as in animals, the disease characteristically runs a short course followed by complete recovery. In the few severe cases, there is sudden onset, with high fever, headache, stiff neck and a feeling of chilliness and malaise. Other signs of an encephalitic infection, such as tremors, speech difficulties and so forth, may also occur. In spite of the sometimes lengthy period of symptoms and a correspondingly slow convalescence the expectation of a complete recovery is high. It is interesting to note that, in contrast to the condition in EE and WE, in many epidemics of SLE the incidence has been highest in individuals over fifty years of age. Mortality has ranged from less than 2 per cent to 11 per cent.

JAPANESE B ENCEPHALITIS (JBE)

History and Geographic Distribution

Although a disease which was probably Japanese B encephalitis has been known in Eastern Asia since the latter part of the 19th century, and has been recognized as a distinct clinical entity in Japan since 1924, the virus which causes it was not isolated until 1935. Epidemics have occurred more or less regularly, almost yearly, in Japan, although the incidence has varied from a few cases to six to eight thousand cases per year. There have also been epidemics in China, Okinawa, and Korea and it is probable that it is this variety of encephalitis that has occurred in other parts of the Far East, as for instance, in India where antibodies have been found and virus isolations have been made. There has been great variability in the incidence of antibodies in different regions. In Korea, some workers have concluded that there have been inapparent infections in virtually the entire population, although clinical cases were rare. In Japan and elsewhere, studies indicate that there may be hundreds of inapparent infections for every case that is clinically evident, and there appears to be a high rate of immunity in endemic areas.

Animal Hosts and Reservoirs; Arthropod Vectors

The JBE virus was first isolated from mosquitoes collected in Okayama prefecture in Japan in 1938. Since that time it has been recovered many time from naturally infected mosquitoes of several species, including *Culex tritaeniorhynchus* (Japan and elsewhere), *C. gelidus* (Malaya) and *C. vishnui* (India). The chief vector, possibly the only vector to man in Japan, where so much of the research has been done, is almost certainly *Culex tritaeniorhynchus.* This species breeds extensively in rice paddies and feeds both on marsh-inhabiting birds such as the black-crowned night heron and on pigs, as well on man. Both the herons and pigs are easily and frequently infected. Infected mosquitoes have been found regularly from late June to early October, and vertebrate infection, e.g., in herons and pigs, occurs most often during the period of highest incidence of infected mosquitoes. The highest incidence of the disease in man is also in the late summer and early fall.

It is not known definitely how the virus survives the winter in nature but it seems quite possible that it could do so in hibernating female *Culex tritaeniorhynchus,* since it has been shown that experimentally infected mosquitoes can transmit the virus after exposure to low temperatures for more than two and one-half months. Migrating birds might also be responsible for renewing the virus in an area each season.

The virus has been experimentally transmitted by seven species of North American mosquitoes, representing three genera, comprising the following: *Culex pipiens (molestus and pipiens), C. quinquefaciatus, C. tarsalis, Aedes dorsalis, Ae. nigromaculis, Culiseta incidens* and *Culiseta inornata.* It would seem not improbable, therefore, that the JBE virus might be spread to and within the Western Hemisphere, where, to date, it has not been identified.

Etiologic Agents; Serology

The etiology and serology are similar in several characteristics to those already described. The techniques used, in the hands of different workers, have produced different views on the speed with which NT, HI and CF antibodies develop, but it has been concluded that NT antibody may endure for life, while CF antibody declines to very low levels by five months, even though it may then persist for several years. HI antibody, also, drops sharply after five or six months but may persist at a low level for several years.

The Disease in Animals

Certain laboratory animals (mice, monkeys, hamsters) are easily infected by intracerebral inoculation, often with fatal results. In others (guinea pigs, rabbits) the disease is inapparent. In mice thus inoculated, paralysis, trembling and convulsions begin three to eight days after inoculation. Inoculation by routes other than through the central nervous system even in susceptible animals ordinarily produces only inapparent infections.

Many if not most domestic animals, including horses, can be infected followed by viremia, and the same is true of wild birds. Although the domestic chicken is easily infected experimentally it appears to be resistant to infection in natural circumstances.

The Disease in Man

Studies indicate that the disease in its milder form may often go unnoticed or unrecorded. A generalized malaise accompanied by headache and low grade fever may be the only clinical symptoms. More severe manifestations which lead to an accurate diagnosis by serological tests may follow these abortive symptoms, or the disease in its severe form may appear rather suddenly. Speech disturbance and lethargy are characteristic. Convulsions are common in children but not in adults. Both children and adults may have high fever but chills are said to occur commonly only in adults. Other disturbances characteristic of central nervous involvement are common and may be severe. The duration of the illness as expressed in the symptoms mentioned is variable, and convalescence may be very slow. The disease is rated as more serious than St. Louis encephalitis, with a higher incidence of serious sequelae such as mental impairment, personality change and paralyses.

MURRAY VALLEY ENCEPHALITIS (MVE)

History and Georgraphic Distribution

Although the virus of this disease was not isolated and recognized until 1951, it is clinically so similar to an encephalitis known as "Australian X disease," epidemics of which occurred in the summers of 1917-18, 1922, 1925 and 1926, that the two are considered synonymous. The Murray River valley in northern Victoria, Australia, was the scene of forty severe clinical cases during the first fifteen weeks of 1951. The virus was isolated from the brains of several fatal cases. Surveys made later showed that inapparent infections were fairly common. The present known distribution of MVE includes only Australia and New Guinea.

Animal Hosts and Reservoirs

In a survey in northern Victoria, antibodies were found in a high percentage of horses and dogs; also in foxes and opossums. Infection in birds appeared to be common, antibodies being found in fifteen species of water birds and seven species of land birds. Herons were among the birds that were positive, one of several similarities to Japanese B encephalitis. A high percentage of domestic fowls were also positive. It seems reasonable to postulate that MVE is primarily an endemic disease of native birds, spread from bird to bird by mosquitoes. It has been suggested also that the virus may be spread by bird mites, which carry it over from season to season. Among the birds studied, viremia occurred between the second and fifth day. Domestic fowls circulated virus for three days following infection.

Arthropod Vectors

Experimental infection and transmission by several species of mosquitoes has been accomplished, and there is circumstantial evidence that the principal vector may be *Culex annulirostris*. Isolations have not yet been made from naturally infected mosquitoes.

Seasonal Prevalence

The first four months of the year (late summer in Australia) appear to be the period of greatest seasonal prevalence. For example, there were 40 severe clinical cases during the first 15 weeks of 1951.

Etiologic Agents; Serology

The disease is closely related to Japanese B encephalitis, but is considered distinct.

The Disease in Animals

There are noticeable differences in reaction among laboratory animals to inoculation with MVE virus. A severe infection in mice, produced by the intracerebral route is characterized by convulsions, incoordination, tremor and paralysis of the hind limbs. The Rhesus monkey, while highly susceptible to intracerebral inoculation, appears immune to subcutaneous inoculation. Rabbits and guinea pigs become immune, but show little reaction to inoculation. Hamsters readily succumb to both cerebral and peripheral inoculation, a different reaction from that produced by Japanese B and St. Louis virus. Although various domestic animals and birds are susceptible to intracerebral inoculation, the more "normal," i.e., natural inoculation peripherally produces only viremia and antibodies. Not much is known about naturally acquired infection among animals.

The Disease in Man

In man the disease resembles Japanese B encephalitis. The original observations, in the epidemics of 1951, recorded malaise, anorexia, headache, fever, lethargy and drowsiness, irritability, vomiting, giddiness, convulsions, semi-consciousness and cervical rigidity. Improvement might begin at any stage, followed by complete recovery, or the disease may become progressively worse, leading to severe sequelae, especially in infants and young children; the patient may become blind, deaf, vegetative and more or less completely incapacitated.

ILHÉUS ENCEPHALITIS (IE)

History and Geographic Distribution

This virus was first isolated from *Aedes* and *Psorophora* mosquitoes, captured in the vicinity of Ilhéus, State of Bahia, Brazil in 1946, but it was not until 1960, in the Belém area, that isolation was made from man. It is now known to occur widely in Central America and the West Indies. Regions from which the virus has been isolated, besides the States of Bahia and Pará in Brazil include Honduras, Guatemala, Panama and Trinidad.

Animal Hosts; Reservoirs

Data from both the laboratory and the field suggest that this virus may be maintained in nature in much the same way as sylvatic yellow fever, in this case by alternate passages between marmosets, for instance, and mosquito vectors, with occasional passages of virus to marsupials or rodents, depending on the locality.

In Panama this virus has been isolated from wild birds (the little blue heron, *Florida caerulea* and the red billed toucan, *Ramphastos sulfuratus*).

Arthropod Vectors

The Ilhéus virus has been isolated from wild caught mosquitoes in Trinidad (pools of *Psorophora* spp. including *ferox, albipes* and *cingulata*); in Honduras from a pool of fifty specimens of *Psorophora,* including mostly *ferox, lutzii* and *varipes;* in Panama from *Haemagogus spegazzinii falco* and from *Trichoprosopon* spp.; in Brazil from a pool of *Aedes* spp. (mostly *serratus,* but including one or two specimens each of *sexlineatus, argyrothorax* and *fulvus*) and from a pool of sixty-seven *Psorophora ferox;* in Honduras from *Sabethes chloropterus. Psorophora ferox* appears to be the species most strongly implicated in several regions, and transmission has been obtained with this species in laboratory experiments. Transmission has also been obtained experimentally with *Aedes aegypti* and *A. serratus.*

Etiologic Agents; Serology

At the time it was first isolated, the virus was shown to be serologically distinct from all other known viruses except Semliki Forest virus which was not available at the time for comparison; later it was found to be distinct from that also. It was classified as a group B virus.

The Disease in Animals

The disease is lethal to mice, in which typical encephalitic lesions develop. In tests with various animals, canaries were found to be more susceptible than chickens or pigeons. Vampire bats and house bats have proven relatively unsusceptible. The virus evidently does not persist as long in Rhesus monkeys or Cebus monkeys as in marmosets and certain marsupials. Young green turtles (*Pseudemys elegans*) have been recorded as not susceptible. No illness was observed in white rabbits, guinea pigs, Rhesus monkeys, chickens, albino hamsters or white rats.

The Disease in Man

Surveys at the time the virus was discovered showed neutralizing antibodies to be present in man in northeastern Brazil. Later, in Trinidad, a high percentage of human cases in certain areas also showed antibodies. Two virus isolations (the first isolations from man) were made in 1960 in the Belém area of Northeastern Brazil. Both patients had fever (100° and 100.2°) which subsided after the fifth day, headache and dizziness. One also had nausea, backache, muscle and joint pain, and photophobia. The other had muscular weakness in the arms and legs.

CALIFORNIA ENCEPHALITIS (CE)

History and Geography

The virus of this disease was first isolated by Hammon and Reeves in 1934-44 from naturally infected mosquitoes (see below) in the San Joaquin valley in California, U.S.A. The same workers described three human cases (see below) in 1952 and suggested that there might be many more inapparent, unrecognized human infections, since surveys showed as high as 11 per cent incidence of antibody in certain hot valleys. The virus was recorded from Montana in 1961 and antibodies have been found in Michigan.

Animal Hosts and Reservoirs

There is little published information on hosts and reservoirs beyond that originally presented by Hammon and Reeves in 1940 and 1952. They reported a high incidence of neutralizing antibody in the sera of horse, cow, rabbit and ground squirrel in California. The viral agent itself was isolated from the blood of a snowshoe hare in Montana and antibodies were found in snowshoe hare from Michigan. There is no evidence that birds can become infected. Although rabbits and ground squirrels do not show obvious signs of infection the virus circulates and multiplies in them after peripheral inoculation and these animals may be an endemic reservoir.

Arthropod Vectors

The virus has been isolated from wild caught *Aedes dorsalis* and *Culex tarsalis* mosquitoes. In transmission experiments with artificially infected *Aedes dorsalis,* rabbit infection occurred, with viremia after eight hours. Other mosquitoes that have been infected experimentally are *Aedes varipalpus, Culiseta melanura* and *Aedes aegypti.*

Seasonal Prevalence

The isolation of virus from snowshoe hare in Montana occurred in August. The human cases cited showed their clinical symptoms in August and early September. The naturally infected mosquito isolations were made in mid-June and late July. We can assume that this disease, like the other encephalitides in the same areas, would have its highest incidence in the late summer and fall when mosquitoes are abundant.

Etiologic Agent; Serology

The virus does not fit into the A, B or C groups as now understood. It multiplies in chick embryos but is lethal in only a few cases. Viremia in rabbits and ground squirrels has followed inoculation, and immunization resulted.

The Disease in Animals

The virus is pathogenic for mice, cotton rats and hamsters when inoculated intracerebrally. The snowshoe hare from which the virus was isolated was ill when observed, presumably from the virus. Clinical symptoms in laboratory animals are the same as for WE and SLE.

The Disease in Man

In three encephalitis cases in man in California, serologic evidence indicated infection with this "California" virus. One patient was a two-months-old boy, one a seven-year old boy, and one, a twenty-two-year old man. The illness was serious only in the infant, with convulsions, twitching, rigidity and continuing sequelae, such as mild convulsion, and inability to sit up. The child died at the age of eleven months.

TICK BORNE ENCEPHALITIDES:

RUSSIAN SPRING-SUMMER, CENTRAL EUROPEAN, LOUPING ILL AND DIPHASIC MENINGO-ENCEPHALITIS

History and Georgraphic Distribution

Several viruses that antigenically are closely related, although they have different geographic manifestations, have in common the fact that they are, or can be, tick-borne. Russian Spring-Summer Encephalitis was recognized as clinically distinct in 1934, and serologically in 1937. After it was found to be more severe in Siberia (i.e., Asiatic Russia) with distinctly milder forms in European Russia and Central Europe, the "typical" or eastern form continued to be known as Russian Spring-Summer Encephalitis, whereas the milder forms became known as West Russian Encephalitis, Central European Encephalitis, Diphasic Meningo-Encephalitis and Louping Ill. One or more of these viruses occur in Russia, in Central Europe, from Sweden and Finland on the north to the Balkan countries on the south; the British Isles; and, in Asia, in Siberia, India and possibly in Malaya. The group as originally limited has not yet been diagnosed in the Western Hemisphere, Africa or Australia, although the Powassan virus, q.v., isolated from man in Powassan, Ontario, Canada, N. A. has been described as "related" to Russian spring-summer encephalitis.

Animal Hosts

Most important host-reservoirs from an epidemiological standpoint would seem to be sheep and goats, from which the disease can be transmitted by infected milk. Hosts of the tick vectors (see below) include goats, cattle, sheep, elk, fox, mice and roe deer *(Capriolus capriolus)*. Virus or antibodies have been found in squirrels, chipmunks, hares, field mice, forest mice, wild rats, moles, hamsters, hedgehogs, porcupines, moles, grouse and various Passerine birds.

The virus has been isolated from the brains of teals *(Querquedula querquedula)* captured in E. Slovakia, and neutralizing antibodies have been found in the blood of several other birds, including *Turdus, Euberiza, Citrinella, Frangilla* and *Anthus silvestris,* and in bats. Migrating birds, like *Querquedula* which migrates from Russia to the Danube, and in which there is a considerable interchange of blood-sucking parasites, may play an important part in spreading the virus.

Arthropod Vectors

The eastern strain or typical Russian spring summer enephalitis is transmitted by ticks *Ixodes persulcatus, Dermacentor silvarum* and *Haemaphysalis concinna,* while the central European forms appear to have *Ixodes ricinus* as the principal vector. Short-term survival of virus (one to two days) also has been demonstrated in mosquitoes (species of *Culex, Aedes* and *Anopheles,* although they are not considered vectors in any practical epidemiological sense.

The ability of ticks to act as both vectors and reservoirs has undoubtedly been an especially important factor in the increase of the disease in central Europe in recent years in view of the instability of the human population, with extensive dislocations and relocations of both people and their domestic animals. Ticks can retain at least some of the viruses in transmissible form over the winter, and can transmit in both immature and adult stages, as well as transtadially, and transovarially to their progeny.

Seasonal Prevalence

The seasonal prevalence of the diseases is correlated with the activities of the tick vectors. Ticks undergo their changes from larva to nymph to adult during the spring, summer and early fall, and most if not all of the species involved change hosts for each successive stage, thus providing new opportunities for infection in these periods.

Etiologic Agent; Serology

Immunologically placed in group B, the viruses in this complex show relatively minor antigenic differences indicating the close relationships among the several strains. In areas where the Japanese B virus also occurs, differentiation between the viruses of the RSS Complex and that of JB can be made by NT and CF tests, except where a current infection with one of them occurs in an individual previously infected with the other.

The Disease in Animals

Louping ill, caused by one of the RSS Complex strains has been a recognized disease of sheep in the British Isles for many years, although, of course the knowledge of its serologic relationship to other viruses in the Group and Complex has been more recent. The infection in sheep typically runs a diphasic course, with the meningo-encephalitis manifestations in the second phase only, as in man.

The term "diphasic milk fever" has arisen from the fact that human infections from certain strains of the RSS Complex can result from drinking raw milk from infected goats and sheep. Infections with some strains, including louping ill also occur from close association with tick-infected animals, cases having occurred in laboratory workers as well as in farm workers and in slaughter-house workers.

Experimentally, many kinds of animals have been infected with one or another of the strains of the RSS Complex. In sheep, intracerebral inoculation with both louping ill and other strains are likely to prove fatal, but the picture is variable when the infective agents are introduced by other routes. The effects of infection also vary in other animals, from inapparent to fatal. Rodents and wild birds as well as sheep and goats have shown viremias lasting several days, a fact which is of epidemiological significance especially in view of the long periods of attachment of ticks to their hosts and the ability of ticks to transmit the virus from one generation to the next.

The Disease in Man

Infections with viruses of this complex may be so mild as to be inapparent or, especially in the East Russian form, they may be severe, with permanent after-effects, and may be fatal. In the "di"- or "bi"-phasic forms there are two periods of illness separated by a short interval during which the symptoms of the first phase disappear to a greater or lesser extent. The first phase is characterized by gastrointestinal disturbances, headache, fever, pains and general malaise, often accompanied by a leukopenia, and meningeal symptoms may also be observed. Although it is the second stage, with central nervous system involvement which determines the classification of the disease as an encephalitis, this second stage either may not occur or may not be recognized. The clinical picture from this point is similar to that of other arthropod-borne encephalitides. Louping-ill in man may cause only the first phase symptoms, or the second phase also may occur, with meningo-encephalitis. Recovery, without sequelae, is usual.

The diphasic aspect of the disease is more marked but not always present, in the Central European or West Russian form. The usual duration of the first phase is five to ten days; of the second, eight to twelve days; and the interphase period from four to ten days. Although there may be such central nervous system involvements as spinal, bulbospinal and ascending types of paralysis and of encephalitis, the most frequent type is serous meningitis of varying severity, preceded by severe headache and high fever.

Convalescence is prolonged and residual paralyses are the most common sequelae, although their incidence is said not to be high.

The "Far Eastern" form, the one originally described as Russian Spring-Summer encephalitis, is similar to the Central European type, except that it is more severe, and is not diphasic.

POWASSAN ENCEPHALITIS

History and Geography

The virus of the disease which has come to be known as Powassan Encephalitis was first isolated in September, 1958, from the brain of a five-year old boy who had lived at Powassan, Ontario, Canada. Powassan is about 200 miles north of Toronto. The recently intensified interest in virus diseases which has stimulated search for new viruses and more complete information on old ones throughout the world has resulted in several isolations which may or may not be the same as Powassan, but if not, are closely related to it. Such a virus has been isolated from a pool of twenty ticks *(Dermacentor andersoni)* (out of thousands tested) in northern Colorado.

Hosts, Reservoirs, Vectors

Very little is known with certainty of the possible hosts, reservoirs and vectors of the Powassan virus. The nature of the clinical symptoms and the resemblance of the histopathological findings to those of the Russian Spring-Summer complex, suggest that the vectors and perhaps the reservoirs may be ixodid ticks. However, even though ticks may spread a virus among animals they may not be vectors to man.

Etiologic Agents; Serology

The virus behaves as a typical Group B virus. Although it has a remote relationship to the Russian spring-summer complex, it appears to be serologically distinct from other described arthropod-borne viruses in North America.

Seasonal Prevalence

The original case occurred in September.

The Disease in Man

The type case from Powassan was characterized by the same abrupt onset and rapid decline which occur in acute infections with Russian spring-summer encephalitis. The victim died on the sixth day after onset of the disease. At autopsy, lesions were found which were indistinguishable from those described in published accounts of St. Louis, Murray Valley or Japanese B encephalitis.

ITEMS OF NOTE

1. Various closely related viruses, carried by arthropods from birds and animals, cause encephalitis in man.
2. Birds, both wild and domestic, are hosts of the viruses of western encephalitis, eastern encephalitis, St. Louis encephalitis, Japanese B encephalitis, Murray Valley encephalitis, and Ilhéus encephalitis. Mosquitoes are vectors, infecting the horse (equine encephalomyelitis) and other animals as well as man.
3. Sheep and goats are among the principal hosts of the viruses of Russian spring-summer encephalitis, Central European encephalitis, louping ill and diphasic meningo-encephalitis, although many wild animals and birds are also implicated. Ticks are vectors of these viruses.
4. Hosts are uncertain for the viruses of Venzuelan encephalitis, California encephalitis and Powassan encephalitis. Mosquitoes are vectors of the first two of the above, while ticks are quite possibly vectors of the Powassan virus.
5. Geographic distribution is wide, one or another of the viruses prevailing in different localities.
6. Mortality in man is high for eastern encephalitis, as high as sixty per cent. Western encephalitis, Japanese B encephalitis and Murray Valley encephalitis have a slightly lower mortality, although serious. St. Louis encephalitis mortality ranges from two to eleven per cent. Other viruses in this group are also sometimes fatal.
7. Progress is being made toward better immunization techniques for several of the diseases described in this chapter, but general

immunization programs are not recommended. It is a common practice for laboratory and field workers to be immunized by vaccination when possible. However, opinions on the value of vaccination vary, and vaccines, even when available, are not uniformly reliable.

8. Vector abatement is still the ultimate aim, where it is feasible, in the control of the arthropod-borne encephalitides. Improvements in vector control techniques have been rapid and spectacular during recent years in most parts of the world. The World Health Organization, The American Mosquito Control Association, The Communicable Disease Center of the U. S. Department of Health, Education and Welfare, and local and state control organizations, especially in the United States, are among the agencies which can supply reliable information on vector control.

REFERENCES

Special References

Rivers, T. M. and Horsfall, F. L., Jr. (Editors): *Viral and Rickettsial Infections of Man.* 3rd Ed. (1959); J. B. Lippincott, Philadelphia and Montreal; Chapters as follows:

Ch. 12. Casals, J. and Reeves, W. C.: Arthropod-borne animal viruses (pp. 269-285) .

Ch. 13. Olitsky, P. K. and Casals, J.: Arthropod-borne group A virus infections of man (p. 286-304).

Ch. 14. Olitsky, P. K. and Clarke, D. H.: Arthropod-borne group B virus infections of man (pp. 305-342) .

General References

1. BEADLE, L. D.: An appraisal of the arthropod-borne viral encephalitides and their possible significance to New Jersey, *N. J. Mosq. Exterm. A. Proc., 47:*59-64, 1960.

2. BOND, J. O.: The status of arthropod-borne encephalitis viruses in Florida. *Fla. Anti-Mosquito A. Ann. Rep., 32:*14-19, 1961.

3. CASALS, J.: The arthropod-borne group of animal viruses. *Tr. N. Y. Acad. Sc., 2* (19):219-235, 1957.

4. CAUSEY, O. R. and THEILER, M.: Virus antibody survey on sera of residents of the Amazon Valley in Brazil. *Am. J. Trop. Med., 7:*36-41, 1958.

5. CHAMBERLAIN, R. W.: Vector relationships of the arthropod-borne encephalitides in North America. *Ann. N. Y. Acad. Sc., 70* (4):312-319, 1958.

6. CHAMBERLAIN, R. W., SIKES, R. K., NELSON, D. B. and SUDIA, W. D.: Studies on the North American arthropod-borne encephalitides. *Am. J. Hyg., 60* (3):278-285, 1954.

7. CHAMRERLAIN, R. W., SUDIA, W. D., BURBUTIS, P. P. and BOGUE, M. D.: Recent isolations of arthropod-borne viruses from mosquitoes in eastern United States. *Mosq. News, 18* (4):305-308, 1958.

8. DONALDSON, A. W.: Arthropod-borne encephalitis in the United States of America. *Am. J. Pub. Health, 48* (10):1307-1314, 1958.

9. EKLUND, C. M.: Mosquito-transmitted encephalitis viruses, a review of their insect hosts and the mechanism for survival and dipersion. *Exper. Parasitol., 3:*285-305, 1954.

10. FERGUSON, F. F.: Biological factors in the transmission of American arthropod-borne encephalitides, a summary. *Public Health Monograph No. 23,* Washington D. C. Government Printing Office, 1954, 37 pp.

11. FRANKHAUSER, R.: Neuropathologic observations in wild animals. *World Neurol., 2:*2-12, 1961.

12. HAMMON, W. McD.: The Arthropod-Borne Virus Encephalitides. The Charles Franklin Craig Lecture, 1947. *Am. J. Trop. Med., 28:*515-525, (July) 1948.

13. HAMMON, W. McD.: Chapter on Encephalitis, Diagnostic Procedures for Virus and Rickettsial Diseases, Publication of the *Am. Pub. Health Assoc.,* New York, 1948, 187-217.

14. HAMMON, W. McD.: Arthropod-borne viral encephalitis (in "Symposium on World Medicine"). *Pub. Health Rep., 76* (9):806-810. U. S. Dept. Hlth. Educ. and Welfare, Washington, D. C., 1961.

15. HAYMAKER, W. and SMADEL, J.: The Pathology of the Viral Encephalitides. *The Army Medical Museum,* (June) 1943.

16. HESS, A. D. and HOLDEN, P.: The natural history of the arthropod-borne encephalitides in the U. S. *Ann. N. Y. Acad. Sc., 70:*294-311, 1958.

17. HOOGSTRAAL, HARRY: Ticks and tick-borne diseases; Some international problems and cooperation in their study. *Intern. Rev. Trop. Med., 1:*247-267, 1960.

18. JETTMAR, H. M.: Arthropoden als Überträger virus bedingtes Krankheiten des Menschen. *Wiener Klinische Wochenshrift., 73* (2):21-26, 1961.

19. KISSLING, R. E.: Host relationships of the arthropod-borne encephalitides. *Ann. N. Y. Acad. Sc., 70:*320-7, 1958.

20. PHILIP, C. B. and BURGDORFER, W.: Arthropod vectors as reservoirs of microbial disease agents. Ann. Rev. of Entomology, pp. 391-412. *Ann. Reviews Inc.,* Palo Alto, Calif., 1961.

21. REEVES, W. C.: The encephalitis problem in the United States. *Am. J. Pub. Health, 41:*678-686, (June) 1951.

22. REEVES, W. C., BELLAMY, R. E. and SCRIVANI, R. P.: Differentiation of encephalitis virus infection rates from transmission rates in mosquito vector populations. *Am. J. Hyg. 73* (3) :303-315, 1961.

23. SANNA, A.: I Virus encephalitici da artropodi. *Igiene Moderna, 51:*234-342, 1958.

24. SCHAEFFER, M., KISSLING, R. E. and CHAMBERLAIN, R. W.: Current views on the North American arthropod-borne virus problem. *Am. J. Pub. Health, 48* (3):336-343, 1958.

25. SCHLESINGER, R. W.: Viral diseases of the central nervous system. Scope and limitations of specific diagnostic methods. *Pediatrics,* 625-633, 1948.

26. THEILER, M. and CASALS, J.: Durch arthropoden übertragene viruskrankungen des menschen. *Klin. Wochs., 37:*59-68, 1959.

27. *WHO Chron:* Ecology of Arthropod-borne viruses. *WHO Chron., 15:*222-6. May-June 1961.

Western Type

28. BARNETT, H. C.: The transmission of western equine encephalomyelitis virus by the mosquito *Culex tarsalis* Coq. *Am. J. Trop. Med., 5:*86-98, 1956.

29. BLACKMORE, J. S. and WINN, J. F.: A winter isolation of western equine encephalitis virus from hibernating *Culex tarsalis* Coq. *Proc. Soc. Exper. Biol. & Med., 91*:146-148, 1956.

30. BURTON, A. N., CONNELL, R., REMPEL, J. G. and GOLLOP, J. B.: Studies on western equine encephalitis associated with wild ducks in Saskatchewan. *Canad. J. Microbiol., 7* (3):295-302, 1961.

31. COX, R. H., JELLISON, W. L. and HUGHES, L. E.: Isolation of Western equine encephalomyelitis virus from a naturally infected prairie chicken. *Pub. Health Reports, 56*:1905-1906, (Sept. 26) 1941.

32. DOW, R. P., REEVES, W. C. and BELLAMY, R. E.: Field tests of avian host preference of *Culex tarsalis* (Coq.). *Am. J. Trop. Med. & Hyg., 6* (2):294-303, 1957.

33. EKLUND, C. M.: Human encephalitis of the Western equine type in Minnesota in 1941; Clinical and epidemiological study of serologically positive cases. *Am. J. Hyg., 43*:171-193, (March) 1946.

34. HAMMON, W. McD. and REEVES, W. C.: Laboratory transmission of Western equine encephalomyelitis virus by mosquitoes of the Genera *Culex* and *Culiseta*. *J. Exper. Med., 78*:425-434, (Dec.) 1943.

35. HAMMON, W. McD. and REEVES, W. C.: Western equine encephalitis control studies in Kern County, California, 1945 II. An evaluation of the effectiveness of certain types of mosquito control including residual DDT on virus infection rates in *Culex* mosquitoes and in chickens. *Am. J. Hyg., 47*:93-102, 1948.

36. HAMMON, W. McD. and REEVES, W. C.: Western equine encephalomyelitis virus in the blood of experimentally inoculated chickens. *J. Exper. Med., 83*:163-173, 1946.

37. HAMMON, W. McD. and REEVES, W. C.: Interepidemic studies on arthropod-borne virus encephalitides and poliomyelitis in Kern County, California, and the Yakima Valley, Washington. 1944 *Am. J. Hyg., 46*:326-335, 1947.

38. HAMMON, W. McD., REEVES, W. C. and GALINDO, P.: Epizoology of Western equine type encephalomyelitis: Eastern Nebraska field survey of 1943 with isolation of the virus from mosquitoes. *Am. J. Vet. Res., 6*:145-148, 1945.

39. HOLDEN, P.: Recovery of western equine encephalomyelitis virus from naturally infected English sparrows in New Jersey, 1953. *Proc. Soc. Exper. Biol. & Med., 88*:490-492, 1955.

40. HOWITT, B. F. and BUSS, W. C.: Human equine encephalomyelitis in Kern County, California 1938, 1939 and 1940. *Am. J. Pub. Health, 31*:935-944, (Sept.) 1941.

41. HOWITT, B. F.: Recovery of the virus of equine encephalomyelitis from the brain of a child. *Science, 88*:455-456, 1938.

42. KELSER, R. A.: Mosquitoes as vectors of the virus of equine encephalomyelitis. *J.A.V.M.A., 82*:767-771, 1933.

43. KITSELMAN, C. H. and GRUNDMANN, A. W.: Equine encephalomyelitis virus isolated from naturally infected *Triatomoe sanguisuga* Le Conte. *Agric. Exp. Sta. Kans. State. Col. Agric. Tech. Bull., 50*:5-15, (Oct.) 1940.

44. MEYER, K. F., HARING, C. M. and HOWITT, B.: The etiology of epizootic encephalomyelitis of horses in the San Joaquin Valley, 1930. *Science, 74*:227-228, (Aug. 28) 1931.

45. MILES, V. I., HOWITT, B. F., CORRIE, R. and COCKBURN, T. A.: Encephalitis in Midwest. V. Western equine encephalomyelitis virus recovered from mites *Dermanyssus americanus* Ewing. *Proc. Soc. Exper. Biol. & Med., 77*:395-396, 1951.

46. NORRIS, MARJORIE: Recovery of a strain of Western equine encephalitis virus from *Culex restuans* (Theo.) (Diptera:Culicidae). *Canad. J. Res., 24:*63-70, 1946.

47. REEVES, W. C. and HAMMON, W. McD.: Feeding habits of the proven and possible mosquito vectors of western equine and St. Louis encephalitis in the Yakima Valley, Washington. *Am. J. Trop. Med., 24:*131-134, 1944.

48. REEVES, W. C.: Observations on the natural history of Western equine encephalomyelitis. *Proc. 49th Annual Meeting U. S. Livestock San. A.,* 1945.

49. REEVES, W. C., HAMMON, W. McD., FURMAN, D. P., McCLURE, H. E. and BROOKMAN, B.: Recovery of Western equine encephalomyelitis virus from wild bird mites *(Liponyssus sylviarum)*, in Kern County, California. *Science, 105:*411-412, (April 18) 1947.

50. REEVES, W. C., HUTSON, G. A., BELLAMY, R. E. and SCRIVANI, R. P.: Chronic latent infections of birds with western equine encephalomyelitis virus. *Proc. Soc. Exper. Biol. & Med., 97:*733-736, 1958.

51. SOOTER, C. A., HOWITT, B. F., GORRIE, R. and COCKBURN, T. A.: Encephalitis in Midwest. IV. Western equine encephalitis virus recovered from nestling wild birds in nature. *Proc. Soc. Exper. Biol. & Med., 77:*393-394, 1951.

52. SULKIN, S. E. and IZUMI, E. M.: Isolation of Western equine encephalomyelitis virus from tropical fowl mites *Liponyssus bursa* (Berlese). *Proc. Soc. Exper. Biol. & Med., 66:*249-250, 1947.

53. SULKIN, S. E.: Recovery of equine encephalomyelitis virus (Western Type) from chicken mites. *Science, 101:*381-383, (April 13) 1945.

54. SYVERTON, J. and BERRY, G.: Hereditary transmission of the Western type of equine encephalomyelitis virus in the wood tick, *Dermacentor andersoni* Stiles. *J. Exper. Med., 73:*507-530, 1941.

55. THOMAS, L. A. and EKLUND, C. M.: Overwintering of western equine encephalomyelitis virus in experimentally infected garter snakes and transmission to mosquitoes. *Proc. Soc. Exper. Biol & Med., 105:*52-55, 1960.

56. THOMAS, L. A., EKLUND, C. M., and RUSH, W. A.: Susceptibility of garter snakes *(Thamnophis* spp.) to western equine encephalomyelitis virus. *Proc. Soc. Exper. Biol. & Med., 99:*698-700, 1958.

57. THOMPSON, G. A., HOWITT, B. F., GORRIE, R. and COCKBURN, T. A.: Encephalitis in Midwest. VI. Western equine encephalomyelitis virus isolated from *Aedes dorsalis* Meigen. *Proc. Soc. Exper. Biol. & Med., 78:*289-290, 1951.

Eastern Type

58. ANDERSON, J. R., LEE, V. H., VADLAMUDI, S., HANSON, R. P. and DeFOLIART, G. R.: Isolation of eastern encephalitis virus from Diptera in Wisconsin. *Mosquito News, 21* (3):244-248, 1961.

59. BEAUDETTE, F. R.: Equine encephalomyelitis in avian hosts. *Proc. 43rd Annual Meeting U. S. Livestock San. A., Chicago,* Dec. 6, 1939.

60. BEAUDETTE, F. R. and BLACK, J. J.: Equine encephalomyelitis in New Jersey pheasants in 1945 and 1946. *J.A.V.M.A., 112:*140-147, 1948.

61. BEAUDETTE, F. R., HOLDEN, P., BLACK, J. J., BIVENS, J. A., HUDSON, C. B. and TUDOR, D. C.: Equine encephalomyelitis in pheasants in 1952-1953. *Proc. 58th. Ann. Meet. U. S. Livestock San. Assn.,* Omaha, pp. 309-321, 1955.

62. BROWN, G. C.: Studies on equine encephalomyelitis in Michigan. *J. Bact., 51:*615, (May) 1946.

63. CAUSEY, O. R., CAUSEY, C. E., MAROJA, O. M. and MACEDO, D. G.: The isolation of arthropod-borne viruses including members of two hitherto undescribed sero-

logical groups in the Amazon region of Brazil. *Am. J. Trop. Med. & Hyg. 10* (2) :227-249, 1961.

64. CHAMBERLAIN, R. W., CORRISTAN, E. C. and SIKES, R. K.: Studies on the North American arthropod-borne encephalitides. V. The extrinsic incubation of EE and WE in mosquitoes. *Am. J. Hyg., 60* (3):269-277, 1954.

65. CHAMBERLAIN, R. W., KISSLING, R. E. and SIKES, R. K.: Studies on the North American arthropod-borne encephalitides. VII. Estimation of amount of Eastern equine encephalitis virus inoculated by infected *Aedes aegypti*. *Am. J. Hyg. 60* (3):286-291, 1954.

66. CHAMBERLAIN, R. W., RUBIN, H., KISSLING, R. E. and EIDSON, M. E.: Recovery of virus of Eastern equine encephalomyelitis from a mosquito, *Culiseta melanura* (Coquillett). *Proc. Soc. Exper. Biol. & Med., 77:*396-397, 1951.

67. CHAMBERLAIN, R. W., SIKES, R. K., NELSON, D. B. and SUDIA, W. D.: Studies on the North American arthropod-borne encephalitides. VI. Quantitative determination of virus-vector relationships. *Am. J. Hyg., 60* (3) :278-285, 1954.

68. CLARKE, D. H.: Two nonfatal human infections with the virus of eastern encephalitis. *Am. J. Trop. Med. & Hyg., 10* (1):67-70, 1961.

69. DAVIS, W. A.: A study of birds and mosquitoes as hosts for the virus of Eastern encephalomyelitis. *Am. J. Hyg., 32:*45-59, 1940.

70. DOUGHERTY, E., 3RD. and PRICE, J. I.: Eastern encephalitis in white Pekin ducklings on Long Island. *Avian Diseases, IV* (3): 248-258, 1960.

71. FEEMSTER, R. F., WHEELER, R. E., DANIELS, J. B., ROSE, H. D., SCHAEFFER, M., KISSLING, R. E., HAYES, R. O., ALEXANDER, E. R. and MURRAY, W. A.: Field and laboratory studies on equine encephalitis. *New England J. Med., 259:*107-113, 1958.

72. FOTHERGILL, L. and DINGLE, J. A fatal disease of pigeons caused by the virus of the Eastern variety of equine encephalomyelitis. *Science, 88:*549-550, (Dec. 9) 1938.

73. FOTHERGILL, L., DINGLE, J., FARBER, S. and CONNERLEY, M.: Human encephalitis caused by the virus of the Eastern variety of equine encephalomyelitis. *New England J. Med., 219:*411, (Sept. 22) 1938.

74. GETTING, V.: Equine encephalomyelitis in Massachusetts. *New England J. Med., 224:*999-1006, 1941.

75. GILTNER, L. and SHAHAN, M. P.: The 1933 outbreak of infectious equine encephalomyelitis in the Eastern states. *North Am. Vet., 14:*25-27, (Nov.) 1933.

76. HAYES, R. O., LAMOTTE, L. C., WHITE, L. A. and BEADLE, L. D.: Isolation of eastern encephalitis from the mosquito *Culex restuans* collected in New Jersey during 1959. *Mosq. News, 20* (2):190, 1960.

77. HOWITT, B. F., BISHOP, L. K., GORRIE, R. H., KISSLING, R. E., HAUSER, G. H. and TRUETLING, W. L.: An outbreak of equine encephalomyelitis, Eastern Type in Southwestern Louisiana. *Proc. Soc. Exper. Biol & Med., 68:*70-72, 1948.

78. HOWITT, B. F., DODGE, H. R., BISHOP, L. K. and GORRIE, R. H.: Recovery of the virus of Eastern equine encephalomyelitis from mosquitoes *(Mansonia perturbans)* collected in Georgia. *Science, 110:*141-142, (Aug. 5) 1949.

79. HOWITT, B. F., DODGE, H. R., BISHOP, L. K. and GORRIE, R. H.: Virus of Eastern equine encephalomyelitis isolated from chicken mites *(Dermanyssus gallinae)* and chicken lice *(Eomenacanthus stramineus)*. *Proc. Soc. Exper. Biol. & Med., 68:*622-625, 1948.

80. KARSTAD, L. H., FLETCHER, O. K., SPALATIN, J., ROBERTS, R. and HANSON, R. P.:

Eastern equine encephalomyelitis virus isolated from three species of Diptera, *Science, 125* (3244):395-396, 1957.

81. KISSLING, R. E., CHAMBERLAIN, R. W., EIDSON, M. E., SIKES, R. K. and BUCCA, M. A.: Studies on the North American arthropod-borne encephalitides. II. Eastern encephalitis in horses. *Am. J. Hyg., 60* (3):237-250, 1954.

82. KISSLING, R. E., CHAMBERLAIN, R. W., SIKES, R. K., and EIDSON, M. E.: Studies on the North American arthropod-borne encephalitides. III. Eastern equine encephalitis in wild birds. *Am. J. Hyg., 60* (3):251-265, 1954.

83. KISSLING, R. E., RUBIN, H., CHAMBERLAIN, R. W. and EIDSON, M. E.: Recovery of virus of Eastern equine encephalitis from blood of a purple grackle. *Proc. Soc. Exper. Biol. & Med., 77:*398-399, 1951.

84. KITSELMAN, C. H. and GRUNDMANN, A. W.: Equine encephalomyelitis virus isolated from naturally infected *Triatoma sanguisuga* Le Conte. *Tech. Bull. Kansas Agric. Exp. Sta., 50:*15, 1940.

85. LUGINBUHL, R. E., SATRIANO, S. F., HELMBOLDT, C. F., LAMSON, A. L. and JUNGHERR, E. L.: Investigation of eastern equine encephalomyelitis. II. Outbreaks in Connecticut pheasants. *Am. J. Hyg., 67* (1):4-9, 1958.

86. PRICE, J. I. and DOUGHERTY, E. 3RD.: Studies with eastern encephalitis in white Pekin ducklings. *Avian Diseases, IV* (4):444-449. (Nov.) 1960.

87. RANDALL, R. and EICHHORN, E. A.: Westward spread of Eastern type equine encephalomyelitis virus. *Science, 93:*595 (June 20) 1941.

88. SCHAEFFER, M. and ARNOLD, E. H.: Studies on the North American arthropod-borne encephalitides. I. Introduction. Contributions of newer field-laboratory approaches. *Am. J. Hyg., 60* (3):231-236, 1954.

89. SCHAEFFER, M., KISSLING, R. E., and CHAMBERLAIN, R. W.: Current views on the North American arthropod-borne virus problems. *Am. J. Pub. Health, 48* (3):336-343, March 1958.

90. SCHAEFFER, M., KISSLING, R. E., CHAMBERLAIN, R. W. and VANELLA, J. M.: Studies on the North American arthropod-born encephalitides. IV. Antibody in human beings to the North American arthropod-born encephalitides. *Am. J. Hyg. 60* (3):266-268, 1954.

91. SELLARDS, A. W., TYZZER, E. E. and BENNETT, B. L.: The infection of birds with virus of equine encephalomyelitis. *Am. J. Hyg., 33:*63-68, 1941.

92. SHAFFER, M. F.: Human infection with virus of equine encephalomyelitis, Eastern type in Louisiana. *New Orleans M. & S. J., 100:*270-273, 1947.

93. STAMM, D. D.: Studies on the ecology of equine encephalomyelitis. *Am. J. Public Hlth., 48* (3):328-335, 1958.

94. TEN BROECK, C. and MERRILL, M. H.: A serologic difference between Eastern and Western equine encephalomyelitis virus. *Proc. Soc. Exper. Biol. & Med., 31:*217-220, 1933.

95. TYZZER, E. E., SELLARDS, A. W. and BENNETT, B. L.: The occurrence in nature of "equine encephalomyelitis" in the ring-necked pheasant. *Science, 88:*505-506, (Nov. 25) 1938.

96. WALLIS, R. C.: *Culiseta melanura* (Coquillett) and eastern equine encephalitis in Connecticut. *Mosquito News, 19* (3):157-158, 1959.

97. WALLIS, R. C., TAYLOR, R. M. and HENDERSON, J. R.: Isolation of eastern equine encephalomyelitis virus from *Aedes vexans* in Connecticut. *Proc. Soc. Exper. Biol. & Med., 103:*442-444, 1960.

98. WEBSTER, L. and WRIGHT, F. H.: Recovery of Eastern equine encephalomyelitis virus from brain tissue of human cases of encephalitis in Massachusetts. *Science, 88:*305-306, 1938.

Venezuelan Type

99. Beck, C. E. and Wyckoff, R. W. G.: Venezuelan equine encephalomyelitis. *Science* *88:*530, (Dec. 2) 1938.

100. Berge, T. O., Banks, I. S. and Tigrett, W. D.: Attenuation of Venezuelan equine encephalomyelitis virus by *in vitro* cultivation of guinea-pig heart cells. *Am. J. Hyg., 73* (2):209-218, 1961.

101. Chamberlain, R. W., Kissling, R. E., Stamm, D. D., Nelson, D. B. and Sikes, R. K.: Venezuelan equine enchephalomyelitis in wild birds. *Am. J. Hyg., 63:*261-273, 1956.

102. Gilyard, R. T.: A clinical study of Venezuelan virus equine encephalomyelitis in Trinidad, B. W. I. *J.A.V.M.A., 106:*267-277, (May) 1945.

103. Gilyard, R. T.: Mosquito transmission of Venezuelan virus equine encephalomyelitis in Trinidad. *Bull. U. S. Army Med. Dept., 75:*96-107, 1944.

104. Kubes, V.: Venezuelan type equine encephalomyelitis virus in Trinidad. *Science, 99:*41-42, (Jan. 14) 1944.

105. Kubes, V. and Rios, F. A.: The causative agent of infectious equine encephalomyelitis in Venezuela. *Science, 90:*20-21, (July 7) 1939.

106. Randall, R. and Mills, J.: Fatal encephalitis in man due to the Venezuelan virus of equine encephalomyelitis in Trinidad. *Science, 99:*225-226, (March 17) 1944.

107. Sanmartin-Barberi, C., Groot, H. and Osborno-Mesa, E.: Human epidemic in Colombia caused by the Venezuelan equine encephalomyelitis virus. *Am. J. Trop. Med., 3:*283-293, 1954.

St. Louis Type

108. Blattner, R. J. and Heys, F. M.: Experimental transmission of St. Louis encephalitis to white Swiss mice by *Dermacentor variabilis. Proc. Soc. Exper. Biol. & Med., 48:*707-710, 1941.

109. Blattner, R. J. and Heys, F. M.: Blood sucking vectors of encephalitis: Experimental transmission of St. Louis encephalitis (Hubbard Strain) to white Swiss mice by the American dog tick. *D. variabilis* Say. *J. Exper. Med., 29:*439-454, 1944.

110. Cox, H. R., Philip, C. B. and Kilpatrick, J. W.: Susceptibility of horses to St. Louis encephalitis virus. *Pub. Health Rep., 56:*1391-1392, (July 4) 1941.

111. Galindo, P., Rodaniche, E. de and Johnson, C. M.: St. Louis encephalitis in Panama. I. Isolation of the virus from forest mosquitoes and human blood. *Am. J. Trop. Med. & Hyg., 8:*557-560, 1959.

112. Hammon, W. McD., Carle, B. N. and Izumi, E. M.: Infection of horses with St. Louis encephalitis virus, experimental and natural. *Proc. Soc. Exper. Biol. & Med., 49:*335, 1942.

113. Hammon, W. McD. and Reeves, W. C.: *Culex tarsalis* Coquillett as a proven vector of St. Louis encephalitis. *Proc. Soc. Exper. Biol. & Med., 51:*142-143, 1943.

114. Hammon, W. McD. and Reeves, W. C.: Laboratory transmission of St. Louis encephalitis virus by three genera of mosquitoes. *J. Exper. Med., 78:*241-253, (Oct.) 1943.

115. Hammon, W. McD., Reeves, W. C. and Izumi, E. M.: St. Louis encephalitis virus in the blood of experimentally inoculated fowls and mammals. *J. Exper. Med., 83:*175-183, 1946.

116. Holden, P., Solomon, G. C. and Blackmore, J. S.: Use of chicks for detecting

western equine and St. Louis encephalitis viruses in mosquitoes. *Am. J. Vet. Res., 21* (85):1078-1093, 1960.

117. KOKERNOT, R. H., SHINEFIELD, H. R. and LONGSHORE, W. A., JR.: The 1952 outbreak of encephalitis in California. Differential diagnosis. *Calif. Med., 79:*73-77, 1953.

118. LENNETTE, E. H.: Isolation of St. Louis encephalitis virus from a fatal human case in California. *Proc. Soc. Exper. Biol. & Med., 61:*206-210, 1946.

119. MEIKLEJOHN, G. and HAMMON, W. McD.: Epidemic of encephalitis predominantly St. Louis type in Pinal County, Arizona. *J.A.M.A., 118:*961-964, (March 21) 1942.

120. MUCKENFUSS, R. S., ARMSTRONG, C. and WEBSTER, L. T.: Etiology of the 1933 epidemic of encephalitis. *J.A.M.A., 103:*731-733, 1934.

121. OLSON, T. A., KENNEDY, R. C., RUEGER, M. E., PRICE, R. D. and SCHLOTTMAN, L. L.: Evaluation of activity of viral encephalitides in Minnesota through measurement of pigeon antibody response. *Am. J. Trop. Med. & Hyg., 10* (2):266-270, 1961.

122. PHILIP, C. B., COX, H. R. and FOUNTAIN, J. H.: Protective antibodies against St. Louis encephalitis virus in the serum of horses and man. *Pub. Health Rep., 56:*1388-1390, (July 4) 1941.

123. RANZENHOFER, E. R., ALEXANDER, E. R., BEADLE, L. D., BERNSTEIN, A. and PICKARD, R. C.: St. Louis encephalitis in Calvert City, Ky., in 1955. An epidemiologic study. *Am. J. Hyg., 65:*147-161, 1957.

124. REEVES, W. C., HAMMON, W. McD. and IZUMI, E. M.: Experimental transmission of St. Louis encephalitis virus by *Culex pipiens* Linnaeus. *Proc. Soc. Exper. Biol. & Med., 50:*125, 1942.

125. Report on the St. Louis Outbreak of Encephalitis. *U. S. Pub. Health Ser., Pub. Health Bull.,* (Jan.) 1935, No. 214.

126. RODANICHE, E. DE and JOHNSON, C. M.: St. Louis encephalitis in Panama. II. Survey of human blood for antibodies against St. Louis and two related Group B viruses, Ilhéus and yellow fever. *Am. J. Trop. Med. & Hyg., 10* (3):387-389, 1961.

127. RODANICHE, E. DE and GALINDO, P.: St. Louis encephalitis in Panama. III. Investigation of local mammals and birds as possible reservoir hosts. *Am. J. Trop. Med. & Hyg., 10* (3):390-394, 1961.

128. SHAHAN, M. D., MOTT, L. O., KNUDSON, R. L., OSTEEN, O. L. and GILTNER, L. T.: The relationship of St. Louis encephalitis virus to the equine encephalitis problem. *Vet. Med., 37:* (Aug.) 1942.

129. SMITH, M. G., BLATTNER, R. J. and HEYS, F. M.: Further isolation of St. Louis encephalitis virus: Congenital transfer of virus in chicken mites *(Dermanyssus gallinae). Proc. Soc. Exper. Biol. & Med., 59:*136-138, (June) 1945.

130. SMITH, M. G., BLATTNER, R. J. and HEYS, F. M.: The isolation of the St. Louis encephalitis virus from chicken mites *(Dermanyssus gallinae)* in nature. *Science, 100:*362-363, (Oct. 20) 1944.

131. SMITH, M. G., BLATTNER, R. J. and HEYS, F. M.: St. Louis encephalitis infection of chicken mites, *Dermanyssus gallinae,* by feeding on chickens with viremia; transovarian passage of virus into the second generation. *J. Exper. Med., 84:*1-6, (July) 1946.

132. SMITH, M. B., BLATTNER, R. J. and HEYS, F. M.: St. Louis encephalitis. Transmission of virus to chickens by infected mites *Dermanyssus gallinae* and resulting viremia as source of virus for infection of mites. *J. Exper. Med., 86:*229-237, 1947.

133. WEBSTER, L. T. and FITE, G. L.: A virus encountered in the study of material from cases of encephalitis in the St. Louis and Kansas City Epidemics of 1933. *Science, 78:*463-465, (Nov. 17) 1933.

Western and St. Louis Types

134. HAMMON, W. McD.: Encephalitis in the Yakima Valley, mixed St. Louis and Western equine types. *J.A.M.A., 117:*161-167, (July 19) 1941.

135. HAMMON, W. McD.: Encephalitis, Eastern and Western equine and St. Louis types, as observed in 1941 in Washington, Arizona, New Mexico and Texas. *J.A.M.A., 121:*560-564, (Feb. 20) 1943.

136. HAMMON, W. McD., LUNDY, H. W., GRAY, J. A., EVANS, F. C., BANG, F. and IZUMI, E. M.: A large-scale serum neutralization survey of certain vertebrates as part of an epidemiological study of encephalitis of the Western equine and St. Louis types. *J. Immunol., 44:*75-85, (May) 1942.

137. HAMMON, W. McD. and REEVES, W. C.: Interepidemic studies on arthropod-borne virus encephalitides and poliomyelitis in Kern County, California and the Yakima Valley, Washington, 1944. *Am. J. Hyg., 46:*326-335, (Nov.) 1947.

138. HAMMON, W. McD., REEVES, W. C., BENNER, S. F. and BROOKMAN, B.: Human encephalitis in the Yakima Valley, Washington, 1942, with 49 virus isolations (Western equine and St. Louis types) from mosquitoes. *J.A.M.A., 128:*1133-1139, (Aug. 18) 1945.

139. HAMMON, W. McD., REEVES, W. C., BROOKMAN, B. and GJULLIN, C. M.: Mosquitoes and encephalitis in the Yakima Valley, Washington. V. Summary of case against *Culex tarsalis* Coquillett as a vector of the St. Louis and Western equine viruses. *J. Infect. Dis., 70:*278-283, 1942.

140. HAMMON, W. McD., REEVES, W. C., BROOKMAN, B. and IZUMI, E. M.: Mosquitoes and encephalitis in the Yakima Valley, Washington: I. Arthropods tested and recovery of Western equine and St. Louis viruses from *Culex tarsalis,* Coq. *J. Infect. Dis., 70:*263-266, 1942.

141. HAMMON, W. McD., REEVES, W. C., BROOKMAN, B., IZUMI, E. M. and GJULLIN, C. M.: Isolation of the viruses of Western equine and St. Louis encephalitis from *Culex tarsalis* mosquitoes. *Science, 94:*328-330, (Oct. 3) 1941.

142. HAMMON, W. McD., REEVES, W. C., CUNHA, R., ESPANA, C. and SATHER, G.: Isolation from wild bird mites *(Liponyssus sylviarum)* of a virus or mixture of viruses from which St. Louis and Western equine encephalitis viruses have been obtained. *Science, 107:*92-93, (Jan. 23) 1948.

143. HAMMON, W. McD., REEVES, W. C. and GALINDO, P.: Epidemiologic studies of encephalitis in the San Joaquin Valley of California, 1943, with the isolation of viruses from mosquitoes. *Am. J. Hyg., 42:*299-306, 1945.

144. HAMMON, W. McD., REEVES, W. C. and GRAY, M.: Mosquito vectors and inapparent animal reservoirs of St. Louis and Western equine encephalitis viruses. *Am. J. Pub. Health, 33:*201-207, (March) 1943.

145. HAMMON, W. McD., REEVES, W. C. and IRONS, J. V.: Survey of the arthropod-borne virus encephalitides in Texas with particular reference to the lower Rio Grande Valley in 1942. *Texas Rep. Biol. & Med., 4,* 2:366-375, (Winter) 1944.

146. HAMMON, W. McD., REEVES, W. C. and SATHER, G. E.: Western equine and St. Louis encephalitis viruses in the blood of experimentally infected wild birds and epidemiological implications of findings. *J. Immunol., 67:*357-367, 1951.

147. HOWITT, B. F. and VAN HERICK, W.: Relationship of the St. Louis and Western

equine encephalitis viruses to fowl and mammals in California. *J. Infect. Dis., 71:*179-191, (Sept.-Oct.) 1942.

148. REEVES, W. C. and HAMMON, W. McD.: Feeding habits of the proven and possible mosquito vectors of Western equine and St. Louis encephalitis in the Yakima Valley, Washington. *Am. J. Trop. Med., 24:*131-134, 1943.

149. REEVES, W. C., MACK, W. N. and HAMMON, W. McD.: Epidemiological studies on Western equine encephalomyelitis and St. Louis encephalitis in Oklahoma, 1944. *J. Infect. Dis., 81:*191-196, 1947.

Japanese B Type

150. BAWELL, M. B., DEUEL, R. E. JR., MATUMOTO, M. and SABIN, A. B.: Status and significance of inapparent infections with virus of Japanese B encephalitis in Japan in 1946. *Am. J. Hyg., 51* (1):1-13, 1950.

151. BUESCHER, E. L., SCHERER, W. F., GROSSBERG, S. E., CHANNOCK, R. M. and PHILPOT, VAN B., JR.: Immunologic studies of Japanese encephalitis virus in Japan. I. Antibody responses following overt infection in man. *J. Immunol., 83* (6):582-593, 1959.

152. BUESCHER, E. L., SCHERER, W. F., ROSENBERG, M. Z., GRESSES, I., HARDY, J. L. and BULLOCK, H. R.: Ecologic studies of Japanese encephalitis virus in Japan. II. Mosquito infection. *Am. J. Trop. Med. & Hyg., 8* (6):651-664, 1959.

153. BUESCHER, E. L., SCHERER, W. F., ROSENBERG, M. Z., KUTNER, L. J. and McCLURE, H. E.: Immunologic studies of Japanese encephalitis virus in Japan: IV. Maternal antibody in birds. *J. Immunol., 83* (6):614-619, 1959.

154. BUESCHER, E. L., SCHERER, W. F., ROSENBERG, M. Z. and McCLURE, H. E.: Immunologic studies of Japanese encephalitis virus in Japan: III. Infection and antibody responses of birds. *J. Immunol., 83* (6):605-613, 1959.

155. DEUEL, R. E., JR., BAWELL, M. B., MATUMOTO, M. and SABIN, A. B.: Status and significance of inapparent infections with virus of Japanese B encephalitis in Korea and Okinawa in 1946. *Am. J. Hyg., 51* (1):13-21, 1950.

156. BURNS, K. F. and MATUMOTO, M.: Japanese equine encephalomyelitis: 1947 Epizootic. I. Epizootiology. *J.A.V.M.A., 115:*167-170, 1949.

157. HAMMON, W. McD.: Japanese B encephalitis. *Proc. Fourth Internat. Congr. Trop. Med. & Malar.,* Washington, D.C., 1948, 568-575.

158. HAMMON, W. McD., REES, D. M., CASALS, J. and MEIKLEJOHN, G.: Experimental transmission of Japanese B encephalitis virus by *Culex tritaeniorhynchus* and *Culex pipiens* Var. *pallens,* suspected natural vectors. *Am. J. Hyg., 50:*46-50, 1949.

159. HAMMON, W. McD., REEVES, W. C. and BURROUGHS, R.: *Japanese B encephalitis* virus in the blood of experimentally inoculated chickens. *Proc. Soc. Exper. Biol. & Med., 61:*304-308, 1946.

160. HAMMON, W. McD., REEVES, W. C. and SATHER, G. E.: Japanese B encephalitis virus in the blood of experimentally inoculated birds: Epidemiological implications. *Am. J. Hyg., 53:*249-261, (May) 1951.

161. HAMMON, W. McD., TIGERTT, W. D., SATHER, G. and SCHENKER, H.: Isolation of Japanese B encephalitis virus from naturally infected *Culex tritaeniorhynchus* collected in Japan. *Am. J. Hyg., 50:*51-56, 1949.

162. HURLBUT, H. S.: The transmission of Japanese B encephalitis by mosquitoes after experimental hibernation. *Am. J. Hyg., 51:*265-268, 1950.

163. HURLBUT, H. S. and THOMAS, J. I.: Observations on the experimental transmission of Japanese encephalitis by mosquitoes. *Am. J. Trop. Med., 5:*30, (Sept.) 1950.

164. KASAHARA, S., UEDA, M., OKAMOTO, Y., YOSHIDA, S., HAMANO, R. and YAMADA, R.: Experimental studies on epidemic encephalitis. I. Transmission test of the Japanese encephalitis in 1935 and some characteristics of infectious agent. *Kitasato Arch. Exper. Med., 13:*48-65, 1936.

165. KAWAMURA, R., KODAMA, M., ITO, T., YASAKA, T., and KOBAYAKAWA, Y.: Studies concerning the virus of epidemic encephalitis, Japanese type. *Kitasato Arch. Exper. Med., 13:*281-323, 1936.

166. KOBAYASHI, R., ANDO, K., TOYANA, Y., KURATSUKA, K., ARIMA, S., SAITO, K., TAKAYAMA, Y., HIRONAKA, N., ISHI, K., HONDA, Y. and KONDO, K.: Susceptibility of Japanese wildbirds for Japanese B encephalitis. *Jap. M. J., 1:*282-288, 1948.

167. LAMOTTE, L. C., JR.: Japanese B encephalitis virus in the organs of infected mosquitoes. *Am. J. Hyg., 72* (1):73-87, 1960.

168. LEWIS, L., TAYLOR, H. G., SOREM, M. B., NORCROSS, J. W. and KINDSVATTER, V. H.: Japanese B encephalitis. Report of clinical data from 1945 Okinawa outbreak. *Arch. Neurol. & Psychiat., 57:*430-463, (April) 1947.

169. MITAMURA, T., KITAOKA, M., MORI, K. and OKUBO, K.: Isolation of the virus of Japanese epidemic encephalitis from mosquitoes caught in nature. *Report of the Ninth Meeting of the Committee on Encephalitis,* Tokyo Iji Shinshi, *62:*820-824, 1938.

170. MITAMURA, T., MORI, K., KITAOKA, M. and TENJIN, S.: Experimental transmission of Japanese B virus by artificially infected mosquitoes. A compilation of reports of the ninth meeting of the third subcommittee (on epidemic encephalitis) of the Japanese Association for the Advancement of Science. *Tenth Report Tokyo Iji Shinshi, 3076:*812-819, (Nov. 25) 1947.

171. MITAMURA, T., MORI, K., KITAOKA, M. and TENJIN, S.: Reports to the Ninth Meeting of the Committee on Encephalitis: Experiments on the transmission of virus by various species of mosquitoes artificially infected with the virus of Japanese epidemic encephalitis. *Tokyo Iji Shinshi, 62:*812-819, (March) 1938.

172. REEVES, W. C. and HAMMON, W. McD.: Laboratory transmission of Japanese B encephalitis virus by seven species (three genera) of North American mosquitoes. *J. Exper. Med., 83:*185-194, (March) 1946.

173. SABIN, A. B.: Epidemic encephalitis in military personnel. Isolation of Japanese B virus on Okinawa in 1945, serologic diagnosis, clinical manifestations, epidemiologic aspects and use of mouse brain vaccine. *J.A.M.A., 133:*281-293, (Feb.) 1947.

174. SABIN, A. B.: Search for virus of Japanese B encephalitis in various arthropods collected in Japan in 1946-1947. *Am. J. Hyg., 51:*36-62, 1950.

175. SABIN, A. B., GINDER, D. R. and MATUMOTO, M.: Difference in dissemination of the virus of Japanese B encephalitis among domestic animals and human beings in Japan. *Am. J. Hyg., 46:*341-355, 1947.

176. SABIN, A. B., SCHLESINGER, R. W., GINDER, D. R. and MATUMOTO, M.: Japanese B encephalitis in American soldiers in Korea. *Am. J. Hyg., 46:*356-375, 1947.

177. SARA, M. and SABIN, A. B.: Ecological studies on the mosquitoes of Okayama in relation to the epidemiology of Japanese B encephalitis. *Am. J. Hyg., 51* (1):21-36, 1950.

178. SCHERER, W. F. and BUESCHER, E. L.: Ecologic studies of Japanese encephalitis virus in Japan. I. Introduction. *Am. J. Trop. Med. & Hyg., 8* (6):644-650, 1959.

179. SCHERER, W. F., BUESCHER, E. L., FLEMINGS, M. B., NOGUCHI, A. and SCANLON, J.:

Ecologic studies of Japanese encephalitis virus in Japan. III. Mosquito factors. Zootropism and vertical flight of *Culex tritaeniorhynchus* with observations on variations in collections from animal-baited traps in different habitats. *Am. J. Trop. Med. & Hyg., 8* (6):665-677, 1959.

180. SCHERER, W. F., KITAOKA, M., GROSSBERG, S. E., OKUNO, T., OGATA, T. and CHANNOCK, R. M.: Immunologic studies of Japanese encephalitis virus in Japan. II. Antibody responses following inapparent human infection. *J. Immunol., 83* (6):596-604, 1959.

181. SCHERER, W. F., KITAOKA, M., OKUNO, T. and OGATA, T.: Ecologic studies of Japanese encephalitis virus in Japan. VII. Human infection. *Am. J. Trop. Med. & Hyg., 8* (6):707-715, 1959.

182. SCHERER, W. F., MOYER, J. T. and TOSHIAKI, IZUMI: Immunologic studies of Japanese encephalitis virus in Japan. V. Maternal antibodies, antibody responses and viremia following infection in swine. *J. Immunol., 83* (6):620-626, 1959.

183. TANIGUCHI, T., HOSOKAWA, N. and KUGA, S.: A virus isolated in 1935 epidemic of summer encephalitis of Japan. *Jap. J. Exper. Med., 14*:185-196, 1936.

184. TIGERTT, W. D. and HAMMON, W. McD.: Japanese B encephalitis. A complete review of experience on Okinawa 1945-1949. *Am. J. Trop. Med., 30*:689-722, (Sept.) 1950.

California Type

185. BURGDORFER, W., NEWHOUSE, V. F. and THOMAS, L. A.: Isolation of California encephalitis virus from the blood of a snowshoe hare *(Lepus americanus)* in western Montana. *Am. J. Hyg., 37* (3):344-349, 1961.

186. HAMMON, W. McD. and REEVES, W. C.: California encephalitis virus, a newly described agent: I. Evidence of natural infection and disease of man and other animals. *Calif. Med., 77*:303-309, (Nov.) 1952.

187. HAMMON, W. McD., REEVES, W. C. and SATHER, G.: California encephalitis virus, A newly described agent. II. Isolations and attempts to identify and characterize. *J. Immunol., 69*:493-510, (Nov.) 1952.

188. REEVES, W. C. and HAMMON, W. McD.: California encephalitis virus, a newly described agent. III. Mosquito infection and transmission. *J. Immunol., 69*:511-514, (Nov.) 1952.

Russian Spring-Summer Type

189. ALEKREYEV, B. P. and GULAMOVA, V. P.: Natural immunity of the population in foci of tick-borne encephalitis. Smorodintsev, A. A., Neurotropic virus infections (Engl. Transl.) pp. 186-189—*Medgiz.,* Leningrad, 1954.

190. BEDJANIC, M., RUS, S., KMET, J. and VESENJAK-ZMIJANAC, J.: Virus meningo-encephalitis in Slovania. 2. Clinical observations. *Bull. World Health Organ., 12*:503-512, 1955.

191. BLASKOVIC, D.: Tick-borne encephalitis in Europe; some aspects of the epidemiology and control of the disease. *Ann. Soc. Belge. Med. Trop., 38*:867-883, 1958.

192. BREWIS, E. G., NEUBAUER, C. and HURST, E. W.: Another case of louping-ill in men. Isolation of the virus. *Lancet, 256*:689-691, 1949.

193. GRINSCHGL, G.: Virus meningo-encephalitis in Austria. 2. Clinical features, pathology and diagnosis. *Bull. World Health Org., 12*:535-564, 1955.

194. LAWSON, J. H., MANDERSON, W. G. and HURST, E. W.: Louping-ill meningo-encephalitis. A further case and serological survey. *Lancet, 257:*696-699, 1949.

195. NOSEK, J., GRERIKOV, M. and REHACEK, J.: Persistence of tick-borne encephalitis virus in hibernating bats. *Acta Virol.,* (Eng.) *5:*112-116, 1961.

196. SMORODINTSEFF, A. A.: The spring-summer tick-borne encephalitis. *Arch. & Ges. Virusforsch., 1:*468-480, 1940.

197. SMORODINTSEV, A. A., DROBYSHEVSKAYA, A. I., ILYENKO, V. I., ALEKSEYEV, B. P., GULAMOVA, V. P. and FEDORTSCHUK, L. V.: Etiology and epidemiology of a new neurotropic virus infection, biundulant meningo-encephalitis; in *Smorodintsev, A. A.: Neurotropic Virus infections.* Leningrad, *Medgiz.,* pp 4-37, 1954. (English translation).

198. SILBER, L. A. and SOLOVIEV, V. D.: Far Eastern tick-borne spring-summer (spring) encephalitis. *Am. Rev. Sov. Med.* 5-74, (Spec. Suppl.) 1946.

199. VON ZEIPEL, G., SVEDMYR, A., HOLMGREN, B. and LINDHAL, J.: Tick-borne meningo-encephalitis in Sweden. *Lancet,* 7011, 104, 1958.

200. WARREN, J.: Epidemic encephalitis in the Far East. *Am. J. Trop. Med., 26:*417-435, (July) 1946.

Louping Ill Type

201. POOL, W. A., BROWNLEE, A. and WILSON, D. R.: The etiology of "Louping Ill." *J. Comp. Path. & Therap., 43:*253-290, 1930.

202. CASALS, J. and WEBSTER, L. T.: Relationship of the virus of Louping Ill in sheep and the virus of Russian spring-summer encephalitis in man. *J. Exper. Med., 79:*45-63, (Jan.) 1944.

203. GORDON, W. S., BROWNLEE, A., WILSON, D. R. and MACLEOD, J.: Studies in Louping Ill. *J. Comp. Path. & Therap., 45:*106-140, 1932.

204. SILBER, L. A. and SCHUBLADZE, A. K.: Louping Ill in the U.S.S.R. *Am. Rev. Sov. Med., 2:*332-338, (April) 1945.

Murray Valley Type

205. FRENCH, E. L.: Murray Valley encephalitis: Isolation and characterization of the aetiological agent. *Med. J. Australia, 1* (39th yr.): 100-103, Jan. 26, 1952.

206. DOHERTY, B. L. and CARLY, J. G.: Studies of arthropod-borne virus infections in Queensland. II. Serological investigation of antibodies of Dengue and Murray Valley encephalitis in Eastern Queensland. *Austral. J. Exper. Biol. & Med. Sc., 38:*427-39, 1950.

207. ANDERSON, S. G., DONNELLEY, M., STEVENSON, W. J., CALDWELL, M. J. and EAGLE, M.: Murray Valley encephalitis: Surveys of human and animal sera. *Med. J. Australia, 1* (39th yr.): 110-114, Jan. 26, 1952.

208. FRENCH, E. L., ANDERSON, S. G., PRICE, A. V. G. and RHODES, F. A.: Murray valley encephalitis in New Guinea. I. Isolation of Murray valley encephalitis virus from the brain of a fatal case of encephalitis occurring in a Papuan native. *Am. J. Trop. Med. & Hyg., 6:*827-834, 1957.

209. MCLEAN, D. M.: Transmission of Murray Valley encephalitis virus by mosquitoes. *Austral. J. Exper. Biol. & Med. Sc., 31:*481-490, 1953.

210. MCLEAN, D. M.: Vectors of Murray Valley encephalitis. *J. Infect. Dis., 100:*223-227, 1957.

Ilhéus Type

211. ANDERSON, C. R., AITKEN, T. H. G. and DOWNS, W. G.: Isolation of Ilhéus virus from wild caught forest mosquitoes in Trinidad. *Am. J. Trop. Med. & Hyg.,* 5 (4):621-625, 1956.

212. *Animal Disease Eradication Division,* ARS, U.S.D.A.: Reported incidence of infectious equine encephalomyelitis and related encephalitides in the U.S., 1961.

213. CAUSEY, O. R., CAUSEY, C. E., MAROJA, O. M. and MACEDO, D. G.: The Isolation of arthropod-borne viruses, including members of two hitherto undescribed serological groups in the Amazon region of Brazil. *Am. J. Trop. Med. & Hyg.,* 10 (2):227-249, 1961.

214. DOWNES, W. G., ANDERSON, C. R., AITKEN, T. H. G. and DELPECHE, K. A.: Notes on epidemiology of Ilhéus virus infection in Trinidad, B. W. I. *Caribbean M. J.,* 18:74-79, 1956.

215. DOWNES, W. G., ANDERSON, C. R. and THEILE, M.: Neutralizing antibodies against certain viruses in the sera of residents of Trinidad, B.W.I. *Am. J. Trop. Med. & Hyg.,* 5 (4):626-641, 1956.

216. GALINDO, P., RODANICHE, E.DE.: Birds as hosts of Ilhéus encephalitis virus in Panama. *Am. J. Trop. Med. & Hyg.,* 10 (3):395-396, 1961.

217. KOPROWSKI, H. and HUGHES, T. P.: The virus of Ilhéus encephalitis. Physical properties, pathogenicity and cultivation. *J. Immunol.,* 54:371-385, 1946.

218. LAEMMERT, H. W., JR., and HUGHES, T. P.: The virus of Ilhéus encephalitis. Isolation, serological specificity and transmission. *J. Immunol.,* 55:61-67, 1947.

219. RODANICHE, E. DE: Isolation of the virus of Ilhéus encephalitis from mosquitoes of the genus *Psorophora* captured in Honduras. *Am. J. Trop. Med. & Hyg.,* 5:797-801, 1956.

220. RODANICHE, E. DE, and GALINDO, P.: Isolation of Ilhéus virus from *Sabethes chloropterus* captured in Guatemala in 1956. *Am. J. Trop. Med. & Hyg.,* 6:686-687, 1957.

221. RODANICHE, E. DE, GALINDO, P.: Isolation of the virus of Ilhéus encephalitis from mosquitoes captured in Panama. *Am. J. Trop. Med. & Hyg.,* 10:393-394, 1961.

222. SOUTHAM, C. M. and MOORE, A. E.: West Nile, Ilhéus and Bunyamwera virus infections in man. *Am. J. Trop. Med., 31* (6):724-741, 1951.

Powassan Type

223. CASALS, J.: Antigenic relationship between Powassan and Russian spring-summer encephalitis viruses. *Canad. M. A. J.,* 82:355-358, 1960.

224. MCLEAN, D. M. and DONAHUE, W. L.: Powassan virus: Isolation of virus from a fatal case of encephalitis. *Canad. M. A. J.,* 80:708, 1959.

225. THOMAS, L. A., KENNEDY, R. C. and EKLUND, C. M.: Isolation of a virus closely related to Powassan virus from *Dermacentor andersoni* collected along North Cache la Poudre River, Colo. *Proc. Exper. Biol. & Med.,* 104:355-359, 1960.

Chapter 34

RIFT VALLEY FEVER

J. H. S. Gear, M.D.

Rift Valley fever, or enzootic hepatitis, is an infection primarily of forest animals, but often involves sheep and cattle. It is transmitted by mosquitoes and caused by a virus with a selective affinity for the parenchymal cells of the liver which undergo characteristic eosinophilic degeneration. The infection causes a short but severe sometimes fatal disease in sheep and cattle. Most pregnant ewes and cows abort, and there is a very high death rate among newborn lambs. Man may be infected by direct contact with the tissues of diseased animals. His illness is clinically characterized by an incubation period of three to six days, by a sudden onset with painful stiffness of the limbs, backache, headache and photophobia, and by nausea, occassionally vomiting, and abdominal discomfort. The fever lasts up to one week and typically shows a bi-phasic temperature chart. The disease in man is rarely fatal and is followed by a long lasting immunity.

HISTORY

Rift Valley fever has probably occurred for many years in East Africa. In 1912, there was an epidemic of unknown etiology that carried off large numbers of newborn lambs on the farms in the Rift Valley in Kenya. In 1913, Montgomery[1] in his *Annual Report,* recorded the first description of the disease. After remaining apparently free from infection during the intervening years, this area in 1930 again suffered another severe epizootic which destroyed 3,600 ewes and 1,200 newborn lambs in seven weeks. Daubney, Hudson and Garnham[2] studied this epizootic among the sheep on a farm on the shores of Lake Naivasha. They proved that the causal agent was a filtrable virus which they suspected was transmitted by mosquitoes and then showed that animals protected by screens did not contract the disease under natural conditions. They also showed that the virus survived in certain species of *Mansonia* mosquitoes for several days. In 1944, Smithburn and his co-workers[3] isolated Rift Valley fever virus from mosquitoes caught in the Semliki Forest in Western Uganda, and later proved that *Eretmapodites chrysogaster* was able to transmit the infection under experimental conditions.

GEOGRAPHIC DISTRIBUTION AND PREVALENCE

The infection is widespread and endemic in many regions of tropical Africa,[4] including Uganda, the Sudan, and the territories which once constituted French Equatorial Africa. Recent work[5] has also revealed that the infection is endemic in the "tropical corridor" running from Central Africa through Mozambique into Northern Natal, South Africa. Epizootics involving the domestic animals have been recognized in the Rift Valley in Kenya, and have also occurred in South Africa[6] affecting sheep and cattle and wild antelopes in the sheep farming districts of the Orange Free State, Transvaal and Cape Province, and later in South-West Africa. As far as is known, Rift Valley fever does not occur under natural conditions outside Africa. Several laboratory infections have been contracted in England[7] and the United States.[8]

THE ETIOLOGIC AGENT

Rift Valley fever is caused by a filtrable virus. The fully formed elementary bodies are spherical and have a particle size of about 50 m/μ.[9] This virus is not resistant to ether and is readily destroyed by heat. Infective blood is inactivated in fourteen minutes at 56° C. When stored in an ordinary refrigerator or at $-10°$C., it loses its activity in two to three months. It can be preserved indefinitely if stored on dry ice at $-70°$ or in lyophilized form. The virus grows well in tissue culture and in the tissues of the developing chick embryo.

INSECT VECTORS

The infection is transmitted by mosquitoes or by direct contact with the infected tissue. Smithburn and his co-workers[3] isolated Rift Valley fever virus from batches of mosquitoes which included six species of the genus *Eretmapodites* and three of the genus *Aedes*. They found that *Eretmapodites chrysogaster* twenty days after an infecting feed, but not before, is able to transmit the infection under experimental conditions. It is probable that this species plays some part in the transmission of infection in the forests of Central Africa. However, *Eretmapodites chrysogaster,* a forest-dwelling mosquito, does not occur in the regions of South Africa where Rift Valley fever broke out in 1951 and 1953. Study[10] in these epizootics proved that *Aedes caballus* is an efficient vector and that *Culex theileri* may also harbour the virus, but it has not yet been shown to be an effective transmitter.

THE DISEASE IN ANIMALS

The disease in animals runs an extremely rapid course. Infected sheep, after an incubation period of two to six days, become listless and do not feed. Many become progressively weaker and often die within twenty-four hours of the first sign of illness. They often have blood-stained discharges. If pregnant, the ewes almost invariably abort. The mortality rate in ewes may be as high as 50 per cent and in newborn lambs it may be over 90 per cent. In cattle, the disease is not so severe, and most animals recover, but pregnant cows abort. It has been noted that at the time of an epizootic of Rift Valley fever the wild buck and antelopes also aborted.

Findlay[11] made a detailed study of this infection in experimental animals. A febrile non-fatal illness is produced in monkeys. The rabbit, guinea-pig, mongoose, hedgehog, tortoise, frog, hen, pigeon, canary and parakeet were found to be insusceptible. The virus is highly pathogenic for mice, field voles, wood mice, dormice and golden hamsters. Death occurs in from 98 to 100 per cent of these animals thirty-six to ninety-six hours after inoculation. Rats, especially young rats, are also extremely susceptible to the virus.

So far, no veld or forest rodent has been clearly implicated as a reservoir of the infection, but presumably such a reservoir does exist. Weinbren and others[12] have suggested that an African wild rodent, *Arvicanthis niloticus,* is a possible natural host of Rift Valley fever and McIntosh[13] has shown that a number of the common veld rodents develop viremia after experimental inoculation and thus would be capable of infecting mosquitoes.

The characteristic pathological change is a focal necrosis of the liver. The foci may be discrete as in adult sheep, goats or monkeys, or tend to coalesce so as to involve the whole liver as in rats, mice and other small rodents. The parenchymal cells of the liver show a characteristic eosinophilic hyaline degeneration of the cytoplasm and eosinophilic intranuclear inclusions. These pathological changes are somewhat similar to those seen in the livers of human beings and rhesus monkeys dying of yellow fever but Weinbren has noted that monkeys immune to yellow fever are susceptible to Rift Valley fever and human immune yellow fever serum does not protect mice against the virus.

THE DISEASE IN MAN

Man seems to be very susceptible to Rift Valley fever. During the 1930 epizootic in Kenya every native herder engaged with sick sheep became infected. Four Europeans studying the disease likewise all developed the disease. In South Africa[14] the experience was similar. Many of the farmers, and the farm hands, and all of the veterinary medical officers in the affected area were ill. In every case the infection was contracted by direct contact with the infected tissues of dead animals. This virus is extremely infectious to laboratory personnel. These laboratory infections have revealed the typical picture of the illness in man.

The incubation period is from three to six days. The onset is sudden with chills or rigors, painful stiffness of the muscles and joints of the back and limbs, anorexia and slight nausea, marked photophobia and severe headache and fever.

On examination it is noted that the face is flushed, the eyes congested, and the tongue furred. There may be slight epigastric tenderness, the spleen is not palpable, the pulse rate is raised but is relatively slow in relation to the temperature. Many patients become delirious and may have hallucinations. The urinary findings are usually normal. The blood may show a neutrophil leucocytosis on the first day of illness, but this is followed by a leucopenia.

After two to four days the temperature returns to normal and the symptoms subside. In some patients after one day's normal temperature, the fever and the other symptoms return. This recrudescence lasts two or three days, when the symptoms again subside. Most patients then make a rapid and uneventful recovery. However, in one case in Kenya and in several associated with the epizootic in South Africa[15,16] the patients complained of blurred vision or even blindness which developed several days after the end of the fever.

This visual defect was due to a white macular exudate. It persisted for several months but gradually improved during this time. Only one fatal case has been recorded. Death was due to thrombophlebitis and occurred some weeks after the acute phase of illness and so can only be indirectly attributed to Rift Valley fever.

The diagnosis is suggested when human beings suffer from an acute severe but short febrile illness at the same time as an epizootic with a high mortality occurs among sheep. The diagnosis can be established during the acute febrile phase of the illness by the intraperitoneal inoculation of mice. If the patient has Rift Valley fever the mice will die within a week, showing characteristic changes in the liver. This procedure clearly differentiates Rift Valley fever from dengue, sandfly fever, yellow fever and influenza, which may resemble Rift Valley fever clinically but the viruses of which are not pathogenic to mice when inoculated intraperitoneally.

In the convalescent phase a retrospective diagnosis can be made by detecting serum antibodies by applying the complement-fixation test, using antigen prepared from infected mouse liver. The virus neutralization or mouse protection test is a more delicate and more specific test for detecting antibodies. In both tests, however, it is necessary to compare an acute and convalescent phase serum and to note the development of antibodies in the latter. Both tests may still detect antibodies in the patient's serum as long as 20 years after his acute infection.

Treatment is entirely symptomatic as no specific treatment is yet available.

PREVENTION

Eradication of mosquitoes may be attempted by the application of DDT or BHC or similar long lasting insecticides, but the area involved may be so extensive that the cost may be prohibitive.

As most human infections are acquired by direct contact with the tissues of infected sheep or cattle, the disease can be avoided by wearing post-mortem gloves, and protective masks and goggles. Previous experience has shown that almost all laboratory workers engaged in the study of this virus contract the disease. Stringent precautions are therefore necessary in the laboratory. These include the wearing of gloves and protective clothing, and working under hoods fitted with ultraviolet lamps.

Neurotropic strains of the virus have been deveolped (Mackenzie[17] *et al.*, Smithburn,[18] Kitchen[19]). The strain developed by Smithburn after further passage in egg culture has been used successfully for the vaccination of large numbers of sheep and cattle in South Africa (Alexander[20]). The immunity conferred by this vaccine like that conferred by the disease lasts many years, perhaps a life-time.

Randall and his co-workers[21] have developed a killed vaccine from virus grown in tissue cultures of monkey kidney cells. After 3 appropriately spaced inoculations of this vaccine, a high proportion of individuals develop serological immunity and also apparently an immunity to laboratory infections.

ITEMS OF NOTE

1) Rift Valley fever, presumably transmitted by mosquitoes, is primarily a disease of sheep and cattle in Tropical Africa.

2) Man is exceedingly susceptible when exposed to infection by direct contact with diseased animals or in the laboratory.

3) The disease is caused by a filtrable virus which produces characteristic degeneration of the parenchymal cells of the liver.

4) The death rate in newborn lambs and in small laboratory animals is over 90 per cent.

5) Man suffers a short but severe febrile illness with a characteristic bi-phasic temperature chart. It is rarely fatal, but some cases develop visual defects associated with a macular exudate.

6) It is possible to protect animals by vaccination with a relatively non-virulent neurotropic strain of the virus, and to protect man with a formalin inactivated vaccine prepared from tissue culture suspensions.

REFERENCES

1. MONTGOMERY, R. E.: *Ann. Rep. Dept. Agri.*, Kenya Colony, 1912-13.
2. DAUBNEY, R., HUDSON, J. R. and CARNHAM, P. C.: *J. Path. Bact.*, *34*:545, 1931.
3. SMITHBURN, K. C., HADDOW, A. J. and LUMSDEN, W. H. R.: *Brit. J. Exper. Path.*, *30*:35, 1949.
4. FINDLAY, G. M., STEFANOPOULO, G. M. and MacCALLUM, F. O.: *Bull. Soc. Path. Exot.*, *29*:986, 1936.
5. SMITHBURN, K. C., KOKERNOT, R. H., HEYMAN, C. S., WEINBREN, M. P. and ZENTKOWSKY, D.: *South African M. J.*, *33*:555, 1959.
6. GEAR, J., DE MEILLON, B., MEASROCH, V. and DAVIS, D. H. S.: *South African M. J.*, *25*:908, 1951.
7. FINDLAY, G. M.: *Trans. Roy. Soc. Trop. Med. Hyg.*, *25*:229, 1931.

8. SCHWENTKER, F. F. and RIVERS, T. M.: *J. Exper. Med., 59:*305, 1934.

9. DU. T. NAUDE, W., MADSEN, T. and POLSON, A.: *Nature, 173:*1051, 1954.

10. GEAR, J., DE MEILLON, B., LE ROUX, A. F., KOFSKY, R., ROSE-INNES, R., STEYN, J. J., OLIFF, W. D. and SCHULZ, K. H.: *South African M. J., 29:*54, 1955.

11. FINDLAY, G. M.: *Brit. J. Exper. Path., 14:*207, 1933.

12. WEINBREN, M. P. and MASON, P. J.: *South African M. J., 31:*427, 1957.

13. McINTOSH, B.: *Trans. Roy. Soc. Trop. Med. Hyg., 55:*63, 1961.

14. JOUBERT, J. D. S., FERGUSON, A. L. and GEAR, J.: *South African M. J., 25:*890, 1951.

15. SCHRIRE, L.: *South African M. J., 25:*926, 1951.

16. FREED, L.: *South African M. J., 25:*930, 1951.

17. MACKENZIE, R. D., FINDLAY, G. M. and STERN, R. O.: *Brit. J. Exper. Path., 17:*352, 1936.

18. SMITHBURN, K. C.: *Brit. J. Exper. Path., 30:*1, 1949.

19. KITCHEN, S. F.: *Ann. Trop. Med., 44:*132, 1950.

20. ALEXANDER, R.: Personal communication.

21. RANDALL, R., GIBBS, C. G., AULISIO, C. G., and BINN, L.: *Fed. Proc., 19:*219, 1960.

Chapter 35

CHIKUNGUNYA FEVER

J. H. S. GEAR, M.D.

CHIKUNGUNYA FEVER is caused by a virus transmitted by mosquitoes and in man gives rise to a dengue-like illness, with an incubation period of from two to six days, most commonly three to four, and clincally characterized by sudden onset with joint pains, followed by fever, headache, photophobia, and general muscular pains associated with painful stiffness involving particular joints, and in many cases a morbilliform rash. The feverish illness lasts 3 to 6 days, but is followed characteristically by prolonged convalescence, during which the patient develops recrudescences of the painful stiffness of joints, and often suffers from neuritic pains and weakness.

HISTORY

The virus causing chikungunya fever was first isolated in an outbreak of this illness which occurred in the Newala district of the Southern Province of Tanganyika in 1952 and 1953.[1,2] The disease was given its African native name of chikungunya fever which means, "painful stiff joints." A similar virus was isolated from an outbreak which occurred in the north-eastern, sub-tropical part of South Africa, in which a number of visitors to this area, as well as recently arrived residents, contracted the infection. In both outbreaks, it was presumed that the disease was transmitted by mosquitoes. Since then, similar or closely related viruses have been isolated from a number of other countries in the tropical and sub-tropical regions of the world.

GEOGRAPHIC DISTRIBUTION AND PREVALENCE

Since its first isolation in Tanganyika, chikungunya fever has been one of the most frequently recognized arthropod-borne virus infections of man. Outbreaks of this, or closely related infections, have been seen in South Africa,[3] Rhodesia,[4] Uganda[5,6,7] and a virus possibly identical with chikungunya fever virus has been isolated from cases in Thailand.[8] A closely related virus, Mayaro virus, has been identified in Brazil,[9] Columbia[10] and Trinidad, and another related virus has been isolated from human beings suffering from a feverish illness resembling chikungunya fever in the Murray Valley[11] and Queensland[12] in Australia.

THE ETIOLOGICAL AGENT

Chikungunya fever is caused by a filterable virus. This virus is pathogenic, after intracerebral or intraperitoneal inoculation, for suckling mice which, after an incubation period of two to five days, die of an acute illness. It is relatively nonpathogenic for adult mice, guinea-pigs and rabbits. It is immunologically related to Mayaro and Semliki Forest viruses, and together, these three viruses constitute a sub-group of the group A arthropod-borne viruses.[13] O'nyong-nyong fever responsible for an extensive outbreak of illness in Kenya and Uganda in 1959-1960, is caused by a virus closely related to chikungunya virus.

INSECT VECTORS

Chikungunya virus has been isolated from *Aedes aegypti* and *Culex fatigans* caught in huts in Tanganyika; from *Aedes africanus* caught in the Zika Forest of Uganda. A closely related virus was isolated from *Anopheles gambiae* and *Anopheles funestus* in the recent outbreak of o'nyong-nyong fever. *Aedes aeqypti* has been shown experimentally to be an efficient vector.

THE DISEASES IN ANIMALS

It is presumed that there is an animal reservoir of this virus. Serological surveys carried out in Southern Africa have indicated that blood from monkeys in the region of Lumbo in Mozambique,[14] have antibodies against this infection. In Tongaland, the sera of 13 per cent of donkeys tested were found to be protective.[14] However, sera from cattle, goats, sheep and birds were not protective. Attempts to transmit the infection to several varieties of birds by inoculation of the virus also gave negative results, and antibodies were not formed subsequently, suggesting that these species were resistant to the infection. Infection of rodents results in a viraemia and a subsequent development of antibodies.[15]

Although the evidence of the role of animals is meagre, it seems almost certain that there is some cycle of the virus occurring, apart from man, in animals of forest and bush countries, as several of these outbreaks have affected human beings soon after their invasion of primeval bush to undertake farming and various industrial enterprises.

DISEASE IN MAN

The incubation period is from two to six days, most commonly three to four days. The onset of the illness is sudden, with acute incapacitating pain involving one or more joints, followed by fever, headache, photophobia, muscular pains and painful stiffness of one or more joints. The fever lasts from three to six days and often shows a diphasic course, the first bout lasting from one to six days, followed by an apyrexial period of one to three days, followed, in most patients, by another shorter episode of fever. Many patients develop a maculopapular morbilliform rash on the trunk and extensor surfaces of the limbs which may become haemorrhagic. The rash may occur during the first bout, but most often is seen at the time of recrudescence of the fever. Few deaths have occurred in Africa. In south-east Asia the death rate of the haemorrhagic fevers was relatively high, but the role of chikungunya fever in these fatal cases is not yet clear. Convalescence is prolonged and is characterized by recrudescences of painful stiffness of the joints and the patient may suffer from neuritic pains and weakness.

The diagnosis is suggested when human beings, after coming into contact with bush or forest country, acquire a feverish illness with a sudden onset of severe pain in the joints, followed by fever with a diphasic course, and in many by the development of a maculo-papular rash, sometimes haemorrhagic, and by a prolonged convalescence with painful stiffness of the joints. It can be confirmed by the isolation of the virus from the patient's blood during the acute phase. This is usually done by the inoculation of the blood into a litter of baby mice. If the virus is present in the blood, the mice develop weakness and paralysis after an incubation period of two to six days. On pathological examination, they show focal encephalitis, but few other lesions. The virus may be identified by neutralization tests with specific antiserum. Diagnosis can also be determined by antibody tests, contrasting the acute and convalescent phases of blood, the former showing no antibodies either by neutralization, complement-fixation or hemagglutination-inhibition tests, whereas the latter will show a development of these. The neutralization test being more specific, will differentiate chikungunya virus from other closely related members of the A group.

Treatment is entirely symptomatic, but is of considerable importance in alleviating the joint pains and incapacity.

The infection may be avoided by avoiding contact with forested or bush areas where the infected mosquitoes occur. When outbreaks occur, presumably they could be controlled to some extent by use of DDT and other long-acting insecticides, in houses and huts where people sleep.

So far, no vaccine has been produced, although, should this prove a desirable means of prevention, such a vaccine could be developed.

ITEMS OF NOTE

1) Chikungunya fever virus infection has been recognized in East Central Africa and in South Africa, and similar or closely related virus infections in South East Asia, Australia and South America.

2) The virus is transmitted by mosquitoes and presumably is primarily an infection of forest animals.

3) The illness in man is characterized by sudden onset with joint pains and by a fever often showing a biphasic course and in some cases by the appearance of a morbilliform rash. Convalescence is often prolonged and the patient may experience painful stiffness of his joints.

REFERENCES

1. ROBINSON, M. C.: *Trans. Roy. Soc. Trop. Med. Hyg., 49*:28, 1955.
2. LUMSDEN, W. H. R.: *Trans. Roy. Soc. Trop. Med. Hyg., 49*:33, 1955.
3. GEAR, J. and REID, F. P.: *South African M. J., 31*:253, 1957.
4. RODGER, L. M.: *South African M. J., 35*:126, 1961.
5. HADDOW, A. J., DAVIES, C. W. and WALKER, A. J.: *Trans. Roy. Soc. Trop. Med. Hyg., 54*:517, 1960.
6. WILLIAMS, M. C. and WOODALL, J. P.: *Trans. Roy. Soc. Trop. Med. Hyg., 55*:135, 1961.
7. SHORE, H.: *Trans. Roy. Soc. Trop. Med. Hyg., 55*:361, 1961.

8. HAMMON, W. M., RUDNICK, A. and SATHER, G. E.: Viruses associated with epidemic haemorrhagic fevers of the Philippines and Thailand. *Science, 131*:1102, 1960.

9. CAUSEY, O. R. and MAROJA, O. M.: *Am. J. Trop. Med. Hyg., 6*:1017, 1957.

10. ANDERSON, C. R., DOWNS, W. G., WATTLEY, G. H., AHIN, N. W. and REESE, A. A.: *Am. J. Trop. Med. Hyg., 6*:1012, 1957.

11. ANDERSON, S. G. and FRENCH, E. L.: *M. J. Austr., 2*:113, 1957.

12. DOHERTY, R. L., ANDERSON, S. G., AARON, K., FARNWORTH, J. K., KNYVETT, A. F. and NIMMO, D.: *M. J. Austr., 1*:276, 1961.

13. CASALS, J.: *Bull. World Health Org., 24*:723, 1961.

14. McINTOSH, B. M.: Personal communication, 1961.

15. McINTOSH. B. M.: *Trans. Roy. Soc. Trop. Med. Hyg., 55*:63, 1961.

Chapter 36

COLORADO TICK FEVER

CARL M. EKLUND

COLORADO tick fever (CTF), acute febrile disease, occurs four to five days after bite of infected *Dermacentor andersoni*. The etiologic agent is a virus maintained in nature by the immature stages of *D. andersoni* and their small mammalian hosts.

HISTORY

Apparently, the first mention in medical literature of a disease entity which was probably CTF was made by Wilson and Chowning in 1902.[1] In discussing spotted fever as it occurred in the Bitter Root Valley, Montana, they stated that some physicians recognized a mild type of disease without rash but the relationship of this entity to spotted fever was unknown. Becker, in 1926,[2] in discussing disease in Colorado following tick bite, stated that physicians recognized a febrile disease in which no rash occurred and which they called "tick fever." He gave a brief account of the clinical picture in three of these cases but was unable to demonstrate spotted fever rickettsiae as the cause of illness by inoculation of patient's blood into guinea pigs, although he was able to do this with blood from typical cases of spotted fever. In 1930, Becker[3] used the term "Colorado tick fever" and stated that some Colorado physicians saw as many as ten to twenty cases during a tick season.

Toomey, in 1931[4,5] presented a review of the literature concerning the "mountain fevers" of the West since their first settlement by white people. He was able to distinguish a clinical entity characterized by intermittent fever and the absence of rash which he considered on both clinical and epidemiological grounds to be distinct from spotted fever. The "mountain fever" he discussed appears to be the same as the disease described by Becker. Topping *et al.*[6] were the first to present a good clinical description of CTF and to point out that leucopenia was characteristic of this disease. In 1944 Florio *et al.*[7] transmitted the disease serially in human volunteers by the inoculation of blood. They showed that volunteers immunized against spotted fever were not resistant to infection by CTF infected blood. He also showed that inoculation of such blood into hamsters produced a leucopenia. In subsequent papers, Florio *et al.*[8,9] reported that the infective agent passed through a 181 mμ gradacol membrane and was, therefore, a virus. Virus was isolated from *D. andersoni* collected in an endemic area in Colorado. They[10] also reported the isolation of CTF virus from *Dermacentor variabilis* collected on Long Island. In 1946, Koprowski and Cox[11] reported the adaptation of one of Florio's hamster strains of CTF virus to dba and Swiss mice by intracerebral inoculation. In subsequent papers[12,13] they reported the direct isolation in dba mice of virus from a patient's serum. In laboratory studies they showed that viremia could be produced in opposums, hamsters, and eastern cotton rats following intraperitoneal inoculations of virus. Also, the virus was not related to the agents of Venezuelan equine encephalitis, Western equine encephalitis, Eastern equine encephalitis, Japanese B encephalitis, St. Louis encephalitis, lymphocytic choriomeningitis, yellow fever, dengue, BFS 283, tick-borne fever, louping ill, and Russian spring-summer encephalitis. They showed that suckling mice were much more susceptible to infection by intraperitoneal inoculation than were weaned mice. Their mouse adapted virus passed a gradacol membrane of an average pore size of 160 mμ but was retained by membranes with an average pore diameter of 110 mμ. They were able to demonstrate both neutralizing and complement fixing antibodies in patients recovered from CTF infection. In 1949[14] Oliphant and Tibbs finally reported that virus could be readily isolated from the blood of patients by intraperitoneal inoculation into three to four day-old mice. This simple method of isolating virus made detailed studies of the geographical distribution of human disease and the ecology of the virus possible.

EPIDEMIOLOGY

The accompanying map shows the distribution of patients in whom a diagnosis has been established by the isolation of virus at the Rocky Mountain Laboratory. (Figure 131) As indicated in this map, all patients from whom virus has been isolated have been exposed to ticks within the distribution of *D. andersoni*. Cases have been recognized in Washington, Montana, South Dakota, Wyoming, Idaho, Oregon, California, Nevada, Colorado, and Utah. Virus has also been isolated from ticks in New Mexico and in southern British Columbia and Alberta, so cases may be expected from these areas. The majority of cases have been recognized in Colorado, Idaho, and Nevada.

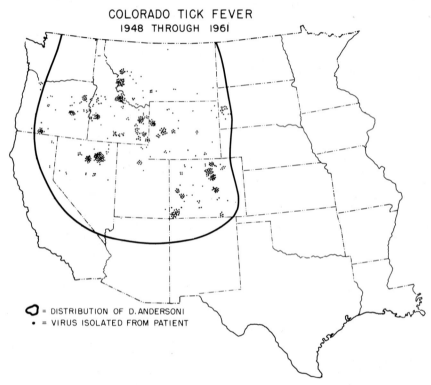

COLORADO TICK FEVER
1948 THROUGH 1961

⬮ = DISTRIBUTION OF D. ANDERSONI
• = VIRUS ISOLATED FROM PATIENT

Fig. 131. Revised from the illustration which appeared in the June 1961 issue of the *Rocky Mountain Med. J.* and reproduced with their permission.

Cases have been recognized from March 1 up to October 14 but the majority occur during May and June and the usual months in which disease is to be expected are April to July.

Adult males are most commonly affected, since they are the persons who are most often exposed to *D. andersoni* during occupational and recreational activities. Disease, however, has been recognized in both sexes and all age groups.

ETIOLOGIC AGENTS

The best method of demonstrating the presence of the etiologic agent in infected ticks, blood of patients, or animal hosts is by intracerebral or intraperitoneal inoculation of three to four-day-old mice. Illness appears in the mice within six to nine days and death occurs one or two days later. Freshly isolated strains can only be adapted to adult mice with some difficulty. Koprowski and Cox[15] showed that following inoculation of virus into the yolk-sac of seven-day-old embryos, virus grew in the central nervous system. The titers reported, however, were low. In an egg-adapted strain, the maximum titer reached was $10^{-4.85}$. Since titers as high as 10^{-8} are reached in the brain of suckling mice, it is evident that growth in the central nervous system of the chick embryo is relatively poor.

Hamsters, mice, and human beings develop both neutralizing and complement fixing (CF) antibodies following infection. To date, it has not been possible to obtain hemagglutination with CTF virus. CF antigens are readily prepared from infected suckling mouse brain with Casals and Brown's acetone-ether extraction method.[16] Neutralizing antibodies can be demonstrated by the standard intracerebral neutralization test in adult white mice by use of the Florio strain which was originally adapted to adult mice by Koprowski and Cox. The inoculation of hamsters, both adult and suckling, generally does not produce any symptoms and infection must be detected by the demonstration of a leucopenia. Virus may be demonstrated in tissue culture of KB cells.[17]

VECTORS

D. andersoni is the only arthropod with the geographical distribution, feeding habits, and seasonal activity which can account for the occurrence of the human disease. Virus is readily isolated from the adult population of this tick and infection rates of 10-15 per cent are common in drag collections. Infection rates are higher in well-watered mountainous areas than in dry, sagebrush covered plains areas. Virus has also been isolated from engorged larvae and from nymphs collected from small mammals. Virus has been isolated from *Dermacentor occidentalis*, *Dermacentor parumapertus*, *Dermacentor albipictus*, *Otobius lagophilus*,[18] and *Haemaphysalis leporispalustris* (unpublished data, Rocky Mountain Laboratory), but these species do not have the feeding habits or the geographical distribution necessary to account for the occurrence of human disease.

ANIMAL RESERVOIRS

Virus has been isolated from the golden mantled ground squirrels *(Citellus lateralis lateralis, Citellus lateralis tescorum)*, Columbian ground squirrel *(Citellus columbianus columbianus)*, porcupine *(Erethizon dorsatum)*, deer mouse *(Peromyscus maniculatus)*, chipmunk *(Eutamias amoenus)*, pine squirrel *(Tamisasciurus hudsonicus richardsoni)*[19,20] and field mouse *(Microtus pennsylvanicus*, unpublished data, Rocky Mountain Laboratory). In the laboratory, viremia of several days duration has been demonstrated in several of these animals.[21] In these animals no illness is observed following inoculation of virus. At present the evidence obtained from field and laboratory studies indicates that the virus is maintained by a cycle of infection between larval and nymphal *D. andersoni* and their small mammalian hosts. An infected nymph carries the virus through the winter months and in the early summer or spring when it feeds on one of the small mammals, viremia results and any larvae or nymphs also feeding at this time become infected. The larvae molt to infected nymphs and, in their turn, carry the virus through the winter. Infected adults play some role in the maintenance of the virus from year to year since all three stages of *D. andersoni* may feed simultaneously on animals the size of porcupines. The adult can infect such an animal and larvae and nymphs feeding at the same time may become infected.

DISEASE IN MAN

The usual clinical picture observed following infection with CTF virus is a febrile illness resembling dengue. Four to five days after tick bite there is sudden onset with a chilly sensation, headache, general aching, and fever which rises rapidly to 102° to 104° F. For two or three days there is severe aching, especially pronounced in the lower back, followed by a marked lessening of symptoms and a drop in temperature for twenty-four to forty-eight hours. Then the same symptoms recur and persist one to three days. There are no significant physical findings. In a young adult there is rapid convalescence; in an older person there may be a rather prolonged period of weakness. Marked leucopenia is usual and is especially marked during the second febrile period when counts of 4000 or less are common.

In children, more serious disease syndromes may occur. Some children have central nervous system involvement, as revealed in the milder cases by a stiff neck and increased spinal fluid cell counts; in others there is, in addition, further evidence of involvement of the central nervous system, such as disorientation, mental confusion, delirium, drowsiness, stupor or semicoma. Occasionally, children have such severe bleeding from the nose and mouth and into the gastro-intestinal tract that they require blood transfusions. The evidence to date suggests that severe bleeding is due to thrombo-cytopenia.

The pathology of the disease in human beings is unknown because the disease is rarely fatal.

PREVENTION

The best method is the avoidance of tick-infested areas. If this is impossible, exposure to ticks should be minimized as much as possible by the use of suitable clothing and the use of repellents; the body should be examined frequently for ticks.

REFERENCES

1. WILSON, L. B. and CHOWNING, WM.: *J. A. M. A., 39*:131, 1902.
2. BECKER, F. E.: *J. Infect. Dis., 39*:81, 1926.
3. BECKER, F. E.: *Colo. Med.*, March, 1930.
4. TOOMEY, N.: *Ann. Int. Med., 5*:585, 1931.
5. TOOMEY, N.: *Ann. Int. Med., 5*:601, 1931.
6. TOPPING, N. H., CULLYFORD, J. S. and DAVIS, G. E.: *Pub. Health Rep., 55*:2224, 1940.
7. FLORIO, L., STEWART, M. O., and MUGRAGE, E. R.: *J. Exper. Med., 80*:165, 1944.
8. FLORIO, L., STEWART, M. O., and MUGRAGE, E. R.: *J. Exper. Med., 83*:1, 1946.
9. FLORIO, L., MILLER, M. S., and MUGRAGE, E. R.: *J. Immunol., 64*:257, 1950.
10. FLORIO, L., and MILLER, M. S.: *Am. J. Pub. Health. 38*:211, 1948.
11. KOPROWSKI, H. and COX, H. R.: *Proc. Soc. Exper. Biol. & Med., 62*:320, 1946.
12. KOPROWSKI, H. and COX, H. R.: *J. Immunol., 57*:239, 1947.
13. KOPROWSKI, H., COX, H. R., MILLER, M. S., and FLORIO, L.: *Proc. Soc. Exper. Biol. & Med., 74*:126, 1950.
14. OLIPHANT, J. W., and TIBBS, R. O.: *Pub. Health Rep., 65*:521, 1950.
15. KOPROWSKI, H., and COX, H. R.: *J. Immunol., 57*:255, 1947.
16. CASALS, J., and BROWN, L. V.: *J. Exper. Med., 99*:429, 1954.
17. PICKENS, E., and LUOTO, L.: *J. Infect. Dis., 103*:102, 1958.
18. EKLUND, C. M., KOHLS, G. M., and BRENNAN, J. M.: *J. A. M. A., 157*:335, 1955.
19. BURGDORFER, W., and EKLUND, C. M.: *Am. J. Hyg., 69*:127, 1959.
20. EKLUND, C. M., KOHLS, G. M., JELLISON, W. L.: *Science, 128*:413, 1958.
21. BURGDORFER, W.: *J. Infect. Dis., 107*:384, 1960.

Chapter 37

JUNGLE YELLOW FEVER

CARROLL L. BIRCH, M.D.

Yᴇʟʟᴏᴡ ꜰᴇᴠᴇʀ is a specific virus infection of vertebrates, transmitted by blood-sucking invertebrates. Long known as a human urban and maritime disease, it has since 1932 been shown to be basically a disease of forest-inhabiting primates, man, apes, monkeys, marmosets and lemurs with evidence implicating marsupials as a factor in certain areas. Among blood-sucking arthropods, evidence of ability to transmit the yellow fever virus has been found only in the case of certain mosquitoes. Infected mosquitoes carry the infection for life but do not pass it to the next generation. The infection in vertebrates is never chronic, nor does a carrier state occur. The persistence of the virus in a region apparently depends on an unbroken chain of self-limited infections in vertebrates infecting successive generations of vectors.

Epidemiologically yellow fever may be considered as being:

1) A human disease, with transmission occurring in or near the house and with man-to-man transference responsible for maintaining the virus.

2) A jungle disease with transmission to man occurring in or near the forest and with animal-to-animal transference responsible for maintaining the infection.

Because the *Aedes (Stegomyia) aegypti* mosquito is the traditional vector of urban yellow fever, the human disease has, in the Americas, been called aegypti-transmitted yellow fever to distinguish it from jungle yellow fever; a more general term should be used, however, since in Africa the *Aedes aegypti mosquito* is often present, at least in small numbers, in forests where the jungle disease exists, and im-

---

Note. This chapter was originally prepared by Fred L. Soper, M.D., in 1955. It has been reviewed and brought up-to-date by Carroll L. Birch, M.D.

792

portant outbreaks of the human disease with transmission from man-to-man, in or near the house, may occur in which aegypti is not necessarily the only or even the principal vector.

HISTORY

Yellow fever was the first disease in man shown to be caused by an ultra-microscopic filterable virus. It was also the first virus disease in which the mosquito was demonstrated to be the vector.

Yellow fever, according to Nogueira, probably existed in the Americas before the coming of the white man. In 1790, Benjamin Rush noted that persons who lived and worked in smoky houses escaped the disease. The same year Crawford suggested an insect as the carrier. Cathrall (1799) and Ffirth (1802) both submitted evidence that yellow fever was probably insect-borne.

In 1881, Finlay suggested, and in 1900 Reed and his co-workers proved, that the traditional urban and maritime yellow fever is mosquito borne, *Aedes (Stegomyia) aegypti* being the vector. Anti-mosquito campaigns in Cuba, Brazil, Panama, Mexico and the United States were followed by the spectacular disappearance of yellow fever not only in the cities but also in the smaller communities of the surrounding regions. By 1927, yellow fever was apparently limited, in the Americas, to a small section of northeastern Brazil. But the appearance of the disease during the next few years at widely separated points in South America which had no easy means of communication with one another or with the known infected districts of northeastern Brazil, showed that there were still unknown elements in its epidemiology.

Rio de Janeiro, the beautiful former capital of Brazil, which had been free of yellow fever for twenty years after having paid heavy tribute to the disease from 1850 to 1908, was the first of these points to suffer in 1928. In 1929 yellow fever was confirmed at Socorro, Colombia, and at Guasapati, Venezuela, and in 1932 at Santa Cruz de la Sierra, Bolivia, buried in the center of the continent. The traditional vector, *Aedes aegypti,* was found in all these places and was undoubtedly responsible for the recorded urban outbreaks, but the source of the virus which initiated the outbreaks could not be determined.

In the meantime, yellow fever virus had been established in laboratory animals *(Macacus sinicus* and *Macaca mulatta)* in 1927, and various monkeys and certain mosquitoes of both Africa and South America had served in the laboratory as vertebrate and invertebrate elements in the yellow fever infection cycle.

In 1932, a rural outbreak of yellow fever occurred in the Vale do Canaan in the State of Espirito Santo, Brazil, in the absence of *Aedes aegypti*. This outbreak has been followed by others in Argentina, Bolivia, Brazil, Colombia, Costa Rica, Ecuador, the Guianas, Panama, Paraguay, Peru and Venezuela, in which *aegypti* could not be incriminated. In 1934, field studies indicated that cases were almost entirely limited to persons having close contact with the forest; neutralization tests on wild monkeys showed that the disease was present in the forest. In 1935, *Haemagogus capricornii* later identified as *H. spegazzini* was incriminated, by epidemiological investigations, as being a probable mosquito vector. Attempts to capture infected mosquitoes, oriented by the occurrence of human cases, were unsuccessful until 1938, when infected *Haemagogus spegazzini, Aedes (Finlaya) leucocelaenus* and an unidentified sabethine were captured in the forests of the State of Rio de Janerio, Brazil. In 1944 virus was isolated from naturally infected marmosets captured at Ilheos, Bahia, Brazil. Positive diagnoses of yellow fever were made on liver tissues taken from naturally infected monkeys in Costa Rica in 1951.

On the other hand, continued observation in northeastern Brazil, the only area where yellow fever was known to persist in 1927, has failed to implicate vertebrates other than man or any vector other the the aegypti mosquito in the transmission of yellow fever in this region. The infection disappeared in 1934 following an intensive rural anti-aegypti campaign. Yellow fever in the Americas has during the succeeding years been limited to the jungle disease and an occasional small aegypti-transmitted outbreak secondary to the jungle infection. Between 1942 and 1954, no aegypti-transmitted outbreaks have occurred in the Americas.

There were 1606 cases of yellow fever in fourteen countries from 1948 to 1957, according to a recent report from Soper, occurring in Guatemala, Honduras, Nicaragua, Costa Rica, Panama, Colombia, Venezuela, British Guiana, Trinidad, Ecuador, Peru, Boliva, Brazil and Argentina, without the occurrence of any aegypti-transmitted outbreak. From Argentina to Guatemala *Aedes aegypti* has been eradicated or is under heavy attack.

In Africa renewed interest, stimulated by the findings in South America, has resulted in observations indicating that there also yellow fever is basically a disease of the forest, although it seems probable that man-to-man transmission by mosquitoes other than aegypti may be more frequent than in America.

GEOGRAPHIC DISTRIBUTION

While at one time or another during the 18th and 19th centuries, every county in the Americas suffered inroads of urban yellow fever, this form of the disease has been brought under control through anti-*Aedes aegypti* measures and no important outbreaks have occurred in the cities of the Americas since 1929. "Since 1932, evidence has been gradually brought together by microscopic examination of liver tissue from fatal human cases of the existence of jungle yellow fever in all of the countries of South America, except Chile and Uruguay. Studies on the sera of wild monkeys caught in Mexico in 1951 have given evidence of the animal infection in the southern part of that country and suitable conditions are known to exist in Nicaragua, Honduras and Guatemala."

In Africa, the line has not been so closely drawn between aegypti-transmitted and jungle yellow fever. Before 1930 yellow fever in Africa was apparently limited to the west coast, extending for an unknown distance into the interior. Neutralization tests indicate that the disease has existed in recent times in Anglo-Egyptian Sudan, Angola, Bechuanaland, the Belgian Congo, the Cameroons, Eritrea, Ethiopia, French Equatorial Africa, French British and Italian Somaliland, French West Africa, Gambia, Ghanna, Kenya, Liberia, Nigeria, Northern Rhodesia, Nyasland, Portuguese Guinea, Sierra Leone, Spanish Guinea, Tanganyika, Togoland and Uganda. Cases have been observed clinically and confirmed by laboratory methods as far east as Kenya and the Anglo-Egyptian Sudan.

PREVALENCE

The prevalence of yellow fever is most difficult to determine, and available official statistics are often misleading. In the absence of dramatic epidemics, only routine viscerotomy can be expected to reveal the presence of the disease. There have been no important urban outbreaks of yellow fever in the Americas since the one occurring in Rio de Janeiro in 1928-29; and most of the jungle yellow fever occurs in rural areas, many of which are isolated and without medical services. That even jungle yellow fever may be an important disease in its own right is shown by the 1938 epidemic in southern Brazil, when there were an estimated 15,000 cases in the states of Minas Geraes and Rio de Janeiro. In spite of the fact that yellow fever is undoubtedly much more prevalent in West Africa than in the Anglo-Egyptian Sudan, the largest recorded outbreak in Africa was that in the Nuba Mountains in 1940 with over 20,000 cases. The importance of yellow fever cannot be gauged by the number of reported cases but by the much greater number which are known to occur on the basis of neutralization test surveys and by the threat of epidemics in *aegypti*-infested areas.

The passage from jungle to town has occurred twenty times or more, according to Theiler, before 1955.

THE ETIOLOGIC AGENT

The ultramicroscopic, filtrable nature of the causative agent of yellow fever was reported by Reed and Carroll in 1902 but was not fully accepted previous to 1927, when the virus was established in laboratory animals. Once so established, the virus of yellow fever has been studied intensively The limited geographic distribution of yellow fever, with the consequent availability of definite negative controls, and the high specific antigenicity of the virus have made this agent especially valuable for developing methods and technics applicable to the more general study of viruses.

The virus of yellow fever is one of the smallest of the pathogenic viruses (between 17 and 28 millimicrons). When thoroughly desiccated it can be preserved over long periods at low temperatures. It succumbs readily to a temperature of 55° C. and is very susceptible to chemicals and disinfectants.

The inoculation of yellow fever virus from a human patient subcutaneously into the rhesus monkey and intracerebrally into the white mouse generally produces a severe disease involving the visceral organs of the monkey and the brain of the mouse. The term pantropic is used to designate this unmodified virus containing both viscerotropic and neurotropic properties.

Repeated brain-to-brain transmission of the virus in the mouse causes a decrease in viscerotropism and an increase in neurotropism. The neurotropic virus no longer causes visceral disease in the monkey but does produce encephalitis when inoculated intracerebrally. It has a shortened incubation period in mice, with a mortality approaching 100 per cent. The neurotropic virus has been widely used in the neutralization test.

Yellow fever virus has been grown in special tissues, both *in vitro* an *in vivo*, and has been adapted to chick embryos and even to young chicks. The famous 17D strain, used for vaccination since 1937, became modified while in tissue culture of embryonic chick cells in such a way that it is no longer viscerotropic for the rhesus monkey and has a greatly reduced neurotropism, as shown by the prolonged incubation period in the mouse and the low percentage of rhesus monkeys which develop encephalitis even after direct intracerebral inoculation.

Yellow fever virus has not been grown in the absence of living cells. The essential intracellular nature of the virus is emphasized by the observation that the addition of immune serum to tissue culture does not destroy the virus already present in the cellular elements. There is no evidence of different phases in the life cycle of the virus, and the infected mosquito can be shown to have the virus in active form at all times after the infective meal. The extrinsic incubation period of yellow fever apparently depends on the speed with which the virus is able to multiply within the cells of the mosquito and spread to the salivary glands.

The behavior of the virus in different blood-sucking invertebrates varies. In some there seems to be no persistence of the virus beyond a few hours after the infective meal. In others the virus persists for days and even weeks but apparently never invades the salivary glands, since transmission does not occur. Even among those mosquitoes which can be shown to transmit the virus there are wide variations in the ease with which transmission occurs and in the percentage of each species which becomes infective. Although it is possible to produce infective adult mosquitoes from larvae immersed in high concentrations of serum virus, there is no evidence that the virus ever carries over from one generation to the next.

The infected insect apparently remains infected for life. Virus has been observed to persist three months in a self-propagating protected colony of aegypti mosquitoes. But in nature urban yellow fever routinely disappears some six weeks after the effective curtailment of aegypti production in infected districts.

The behavior of virus in vertebrates varies so widely that it is unsafe to draw conclusions on any form which has not been exposed to the virus under controlled conditions in the laboratory. In man, after an incubation period of two to six days, virus is found circulating in the blood stream in sufficient quantities to infect mosquitoes during the first seventy-two hours after onset of illness. The more sensitive test of animal inoculation has revealed virus as late as the fifth day. In certain forms, especially the lower primates, virus may circulate for several days, after a variable incubation period. But the circulation of virus is always limited and never continues over long periods in the same individual, nor does it recur at intervals. In other forms, such as the canines, inoculation of virus is not followed by circulation of virus in recoverable amounts. In still other vertebrates, circulation is uncertain and in small amounts. Animals which circulate virus in amounts so small that insect infection does not occur can take no part in the epizootiology of the disease.

The vaccine virus 17D can circulate in man and in the rhesus monkey, but it has been impossible to infect mosquitoes by allowing them to feed on vaccinated persons and animals.

The yellow fever virus is highly antigenic, producing specific homologous antibodies in the primates and certain other forms. The antibodies are long enduring and generally persist throughout life. The neutralization test for yellow fever immunity is one of the most specific of all biological tests when applied to the blood of primates and certain other forms susceptible to infection with the production of immunity. The blood of certain groups apparently contains virucidal substances which may give rise to doubtful tests.

Complement-fixing antibodies and precipitins are produced in man and monkeys in yellow fever, but tests based on such production have not been widely used since the development of the neutralization test in white mice. Apparently some information as to the severity of the attack and even of the remoteness of the attack might be obtained by combining such tests with the neutralization test.

Porterfield in 1959 devised a plague technic for the titration of yellow fever virus and antisera which in time may replace mice for arbor-virus work.

VERTEBRATE HOSTS

A vertebrate to be of importance in the natural maintenance of yellow fever must be: 1) relatively numerous; 2) suseceptible to infection, with circulation of large amounts of virus in the peripheral blood stream; and 3) acceptable and accessible to the vectors as a source of blood meals.

The ideal host would be a short-lived and prolific vertebrate, not killed by the infection, since a constant supply of non-immune hosts is required to keep the infection going. Man, the traditional victim of yellow fever, fails to fulfill these conditions, and history is full of instances when yellow fever invaded an area only to die out after a short time in spite of an adequate density of aegypti mosquitoes. Only large cities with a constant influx of non-immunes could maintain the disease constantly in a small area over long periods of time. Through crowding in towns and cities and through trade and immigration, man created conditions which, during the 18th and 19th centuries, permitted yellow fever to become the greatest scourge of the American tropics.

Observations on jungle yellow fever show that the forest infection tends to persist at a given point for a comparatively short time, generally measured in weeks or at most in months. The intervals between sweeps of the virus through a given area vary widely. Certain relatively small districts, such as Muzo in Colombia and Ilheos in Brazil, seem to keep the virus circulating with a short cycle of one to three years; whereas the observed cycle in the Vale do Canaan, where yellow fever without *Aedes aegypti* was first confirmed in 1932, was eight years, and in the states of Mato Grosso (1934-1944-1951) Goias (1935-1945-1951) it was ten years and six years. Since repeated observations in study areas have failed to show important differences in the density of probable vectors during epidemic and interepidemic periods, the dying out of the virus is attributed to the reduction of the susceptible vertebrate population to the point where the local vectors can no longer keep the infection active.

Extensive yellow fever immunity surveys of animal populations in South America and Africa have been made. The known reservoir lies in three money genera—*Cebus, Alomatta* and *Ateles.* Among animals found positive, only the primates, the marsupials and the rodents are present in sufficient numbers to be considered important as vertebrate hosts. The results of laboratory infections suggest that, of these, the primates must be given special consideration in the epizootiology of yellow fever. In certain districts where jungle yellow fever has occurred, however, primates are very scarce and the possibility of other hosts must be considered. Marsupials, some of which can be infected in series, have been reported as an element in the cycle in Colombia. Although some of the large rodents have been found naturally immune, there is little or no evidence incriminating them in the yellow fever cycle.

The observed rapidity of spread of yellow fever in southern Brazil between 1934 and 1940 suggested the intervention of more rapidly moving forms than mosquitoes and primates or marsupials. Studies on a relatively small number of families of birds have failed to reveal any susceptible species. Studies in Brazil with marked insects show that *H. spegazzini* and *A. leucocelaneus* can and do migrate over distances up to ten and twelve kilometers over open country from one bit of forest to another. This may be the normal method of spread for the virus in jungle outbreaks.

INVERTEBRATE VECTORS

An arthropod, to be of importance in the maintence of yellow fever, must be infectible, sufficiently long lived to survive the extrinsic incubation period, numerous and widespread, and must feed on susceptible vertebrates.

The *Aedes (Stegomyia) aegypti* mosquito is probably the only arthropod capable of maintaining yellow fever for long periods as a human disease. This vector, adaptable as it is to completing its life cycle on shipboard, must have been responsible for the trans-Atlantic passage of the yellow fever virus.

Aegypti has occupied its position as the "yellow fever mosquito" not because it is more infectible or transmits the virus more readily than certain other mosquitoes but rather because of its adaptation to the completion of its life cycle in close contact with man in and around human habitations. Thoroughly adapted to passing through the aquatic stages in clean water in containers such as jars, tanks, barrels, tins, roof gutters, cisterns, cocoanut shells, etc., and having a resistant egg, viable for many months when properly matured, aegypti has spread, from its Old-World home, around the globe with man. The tropical forests of the Americas are free of the aegypti mosquito, but those of Africa harbor it in small numbers. Aegypti control measures in the Americas are generally required only in and about human habitations. Aegypti is often most dangerous in regions where there is so little water at certain seasons of the year that supplies have to be conserved by storing, and it has never effectively established itself in many centers of population along the Amazon where water is so constantly accessible that no storage occurs.

Aegypti require about a week, under ideal conditions, to develop from egg to imago. If an aegypti feeds on a vertebrate in whose blood stream the virus of yellow fever is circulating freely it can later, after an incubation period in which the virus multiples in its body, transmit the infection to a non-immune vertebrate by bite. At the usual summer temperature the incubation period of the virus in the mosquito is nine to twelve days. Experimentally this period can be varied by keeping the infected insect at different temperatures, from four days at 37° C. to eighteen days at 21°.

Bradley and Atchley in 1955 reported on the *Aedes aegypti* situation in U.S.A. They found this mosquito throughout southeastern United States. They also found it in Tucson, Arizona; Carlsbad, New Mexico and on the Island of Key West. They are also found in Texas, Alabama, Georgia, and South Carolina.

In Central America the epizootic travelled eight hundred miles in under five years.

Laboratory tests have shown that many mosquitoes other than aegypti can transmit yellow fever virus from animal to animal. The potential vectors include species of several different genera (Table 70).

The first evidence that *Haemagogus* might be involved in the transmission of jungle yellow fever came in 1935 from the State of Goiaz, Brazil, after laboratory tests with this genus had given disappointing results. The natives of districts where yellow fever occurred insisted, and observation confirmed, that the principal blood-sucking insects which molested them as they worked at the edge of the forest was the "little blue mosquito." Three years later *Haemagogus spegazzini* together with *Aedes leucocelaenus* and an unidentified sabethine, was found naturally infected in the forests of Rio de Janeiro, Brazil. In Colombia, in 1940 and 1941 natural infections were found in *A. leucocelaenus* and in mosquitoes then identified as *H. capricornii*. Recently evidence has been presented to show that the most important mosquito vector of yellow fever in Colombia, previously identified as *H. capricornii* Lutz, is really subspecies of *H. spegazzinii* Brèthes, known as *H. spegazzinii falco.*

TABLE 70

POTENTIAL VECTORS OF YELLOW FEVER

FOR AFRICA:

Aedes (Stegomyia) metallicus
Aedes (Aedimorphus) stokesi
Aedes (Stegomyia) africanus
Aedes (Stegomyia) luteocephalus
Aedes (Stegomyia) simpsoni
Aedes (Stegomyia) vittatus
Aedes (Diceromyia) taylori
Eretmapodites chrysogaster
Taeniorhynchus (mansonioides) africanus
Culex thalassius

FOR SOUTH AMERICA:

Aedes (Ochlerotatus) scapularis
Aedes (Finlaya) leucocelaenus
Aedes (Taeniorhynchus) fluviatilis
Haemagogus capricornii
Haemagogus spegazzinii

FOR NORTH AMERICA:

Aedes (Finlaya) triseriatus
Aedes (Taeniorhynchus) taeniorhynchus

FOR EUROPE:

Aedes geniculatus

FOR EAST INDIES:

Aedes (Stegomyia) albopictus

Of these, *Haemagogus spegazzinii* and *Aedes leucocelaenus* in America and *Aedes simpsoni* and *Aedes africanus* in Africa have been found infected in nature.

The accidental observation by Boshell that *Haemagogus* prefers to live considerably above ground level has led to studies in both America and Africa which indicate that jungle yellow fever is largely arboreal. This finding helps to explain the high incidence of jungle yellow fever among wood cutters and lumbermen and among farmers at the time new fields are being cleared.

Theiler suggests that the *Phlebotomus* fly be re-examined as a vector.

YELLOW FEVER IN MAN

The symptoms of yellow fever are those of an acute infection—fever, headache, backache, congestion, pain in the legs, vomiting and severe prostration—followed on the third day by those of a severe intoxication associated with disturbances of renal and hepatic function. These symptoms of intoxication are common to a number of diseases and intoxications involving destruction of liver parenchyma. The classical clinical picture of yellow fever depends not so much on the symptom complex—hemorrhage, jaundice, albuminuria and anuria—as on the timing and sequence of their appearance with relation to onset. In yellow fever the onset is usually abrupt after an incubataion period of two to six days, and both pulse and temperature tend to reach their peaks within a few hours after onset. Both drop on the second and third days, the pulse earlier and more rapidly than the temperature (Faget's sign). The pulse may be expected to be below 100 by the third day and to drop to the fifties or even forties as the disease progresses. Initial headache and facial congestion are constant findings. Although epistaxis, localized hemorrhages, low albuminuria and slight jaundice may be apparent during the first days of illness, the classical symptoms of yellow fever appear characteristically during the period of intoxication.

The periods of infection and intoxication may be separated by a spurious lull in which the patient has a sense of well-being, but often one period shades into the other. In fulminant cases the symptoms of infection are precocious and may blend early with those of the first period. The change generally comes from the third to the fifth day. The active congestion is replaced by venous congestion with low arterial tension. The bradycardia may be extreme and persist in spite of a secondary rise in temperature. Nausea and vomiting become more severe, are associated with marked epigastric pain and are of grave import.

Albuminuria is one of the most constant findings of the second period even in mild cases. A sudden *progressive increase* in the albumin content of the urine in a much great amount than can be explained on the basis of the febrile condition, occurring as early as the second day or as late as the fourth or fifth day, is almost pathognomonic of yellow fever.

Overwhelming intoxication becomes apparent with the appearance of the dreaded triad—jaundice, hemorrhage and anuria.

Hemorrhage may be slight or severe, and jaundice is generally slight during the first four or five days of illness. But some degree of icterus and some tendency to hemorrhage can be found in practically all clinically diagnosable cases. Although hemorrhage, black vomit and melena never fail to impress the patient and the lay observer, the most dreaded symptom for the experienced is anuria. Anuria seems to depend on the destruction of liver parenchyma, and its appearance is not closely correlated with that of albuminuria.

Death may occur as early as the second day but is more common from the fourth to the seventh days. Although late deaths do occur, the disease has generally run its course before the tenth day. Late deaths are generally due to intercurrent infections.

The observation of previous generations of clinicians that numerous mild immunizing infections occur during epidemics of yellow fever has been amply confirmed by the isolation of virus and by immunity surveys before and after known outbreaks. Mortality figures for different outbreaks and different areas vary, but *clinically diagnosable* yellow fever is always a serious disease carrying a mortality ranging from 40 per cent upward. Yellow fever infection on the other hand probably has a mortality of somewhere between 5 and 10 per cent.

Romero and Trejas reported an epidemic of yellow fever in Costa Rica, with a mortality of 37 per cent in the unvaccinated. There is a lower mortality among children (6.2%) while adults have a mortality of 27.4%. An epidemic in Ethiopia in 1959 resulted in ninety-eight deaths among 257 cases, a mortality of 41.3 per cent. The white man suffers a higher mortality than the native. In Antigua, in 1960 Uttley found that among 100 deaths, eighty-four were in white people, although they constituted only 4 per cent of the population.

Downs et al reported an epidemic in Trinidad. Since 1914 there had been no human case until the outbreak in 1954. There were fifteen cases from fourteen of whom the yellow fever virus was isolated. Four cases were fatal.

The differential diagnosis of yellow fever is not difficult when several associated cases with adequate histories can be examined. The clinical diagnosis of a single case on first inspection may be most confusing, since various severe infections and intoxications involving the the liver parenchyma may produce albuminuria, hemorrhage, jaundice and anuria. Fortunately the laboratory can help through:

1) Isolation of virus by inoculation of the rhesus monkey or white mouse with blood from a person suspected of having yellow fever.

2) Neutralization test during the first three days of illness repeated after the fifth day. If the first test is negative and the second positive, the presence of yellow fever is definitely confirmed. If both are negative or if both are positive, yellow fever can be ruled out. A single positive test on the fourth or later is inconclusive, since the date of infection cannot be fixed.

3) Microscopic examination of liver tissue removed post mortem. The pathologic picture in the liver is very characteristic and for practical purposes is almost pathognomonic. Certain intoxications (carbon tetrachloride, tannic acid) may cause confusion in individual cases in which details of the clinical picture are unknown, but no other acute infectious disease has been found to duplicate the yellow fever lesion.

4) Trejas and Romera reported in 1954 the prothrombin levels of fatal cases was 20.25% and cases who recovered were 66.7%. Percentages below 25 were almost always fatal.

Persons with natural infections never lose their immunity for neutralizing antibodies, this having been demonstrated seventy-five years after the attack.

PATHOLOGY OF YELLOW FEVER IN MAN

On post-mortem examination the heart is apt to be found pale and flabby, the kidneys tense and swollen. Hemorrhage may be seen in any of the organs or serous surfaces but is especially common in the stomach and intestines, where partially digested blood is often observed.

From the standpoint of differential diagnosis, the liver is the all-important organ to be examined. In yellow fever it is generally normal in size and of a mottled color and a fatty consistency. The gross appearance often fails to indicate the degree of destruction to be found on microscopical examination.

On microscopic section, the typical yellow fever liver shows fatty degeneration and a widely varying amount of parenchymal necrosis without evidence of inflammation or of connective tissue proliferation. There is a jumbling of the trabeculae, which is more accentuated in the midzone of the lobule. The number and size of the fat globules observed vary greatly. The necrosis of the parenchyma may involve a few or almost all of the cells, but its distribution is always of a "salt-and-pepper" rather than of a focal or massive type. The greatest concentration of necrotic cells is in the midzone of the lobule, and the necrosis of the cells about the periphery and the central vein is never complete.

TREATMENT

No specific therapy of value has been found for yellow fever. Chemical analyses of the blood suggest the use of glucose to combat hypoglycemia and of calcium salts to neutralize the guanadine-like toxins common to destruction of liver parenchyma, but these measures have not been followed by recovery in monkeys showing signs of intoxication nor have striking results in man been demonstrated. Tests of various antibiotics in Costa Rica in 1951 fail to give encouraging results; large doses of Vitamin K seem to have some influence in controlling hemorrhage.

All cases of yellow fever infection merit careful handling, which means handling as little as possible. Unless unavoidable the patient should not be moved from the place of onset of the disease after the first day. Activity during convalescence should be renewed gradually.

The gastro-intestinal tract should be relieved by a saline purge on the first day. Abstinence from food, except fruit juices, is recommended during the initial period and until the temperature returns to normal in the intoxication phase.

For relief of vomiting, cracked ice and codeinehydrochloride may be given by mouth. Antipyretics are containdicated.

EPIDEMIOLOGY

Aegypti-transmitted yellow fever in the Americas tends to attack both sexes and all ages and races when first introduced into a community. In towns where the disease has previously occurred the distribution of cases will depend on the distribution of immunity from previous outbreaks. In highly endemic areas infection is limited to the young age groups. Since the human population is slow to replace one generation with another, the continued presence of yellow fever as a strictly human disease in a region depends on: 1) large population centers where the number of non-immune arrivals from births and immigration is great; and 2) large rural and village populations together with a widespread distribution of the aegypti mosquito able to maintain a wandering endemicity. Human yellow fever tends to die out, through failure of the human host, in towns and villages subject to explosive outbreaks of yellow fever.

Aegypti-transmitted yellow fever tends to spread slowly within the infected community, and its movement from one place to another is along the lines of human travel. In the past, yellow fever has spread through transport of the infected vector, through transport of the infected human during the incubation period of the disease or during the early days of illness and also through the transportation of all the elements of an epidemic—infected humans, infected mosquitoes, non-immunes, and a breeding colony of aegypti on shipboard. Under modern conditions the greatest threat of long-distance transportation of yellow fever virus to clean areas is the air passenger traveling during the incubation period of the disease.

Jungle yellow fever apparently depends on a supply of non-immune animals in the forest and tends to die out rapidly in many places within a matter of weeks after discovery. In other outbreaks the virus persists much longer, the whole picture being remarkably similar to that observed for human yellow fever. The inter-epizootic period for given areas has been observed to vary widely from three to ten years, probably depending on the rapidity with which a large non-immune population of susceptible animals could be established and on the intimacy of contact with areas where the virus was present at the time the non-immune population became established. Much of our knowledge of jungle yellow fever in the past has come from investigation of outbreaks in humans. It is now apparent that jungle yellow fever tends to be arboreal rather than terrestrial and that animal infections may pass through a district without the production of human cases. Field studies indicate that in the jungle, just as in the cities and towns, yellow fever virus lives a wandering existence, passing constantly from place to place even in the most suitable areas.

The distribution of human cases of jungle yellow fever will depend in great part on local conditions and even on local industries. Among Indian tribes living in the forest all ages and both sexes are apt to become infected early in life, and the distribution of immunity resembles that seen in urban populations subject to the aegypti-transmitted disease. In other districts, where the young boys and girls work in the coffee plantations bordering the infested forest, cases tend to occur in young men and in boys and girls. In still other districts, where heavy logging is going on, women and children are of little use and cases are found to be limited to adult men. Man is not an essential factor in the mechanism of jungle yellow fever transmission and often takes no part in maintaining the virus since, if acutely ill, he remains at home. The distribution of immunity in the human population cannot be taken as a measure of the immunity of the susceptible animals in the forests. Jungle yellow fever tends to spread entirely independently of human travel routes. In general, it makes its way through forest areas and along gallery forests bordering streams, but it also appears in isolated bits of forest which have no connection with the main source of infection. It has been difficult to reconcile the observed spread of the disease with what is known of the habits of vertebrate hosts and the spread of the disease is apparently due to the mosquito vectors which may fly long distances.

Cases of jungle yellow fever have been observed to initiate aegypti-transmitted outbreaks in a number of instances in South America and it is probable that the virus causing the outbreak in the Anglo-Egyptian Sudan in 1940 was of such origin.

PROPHYLAXIS OF YELLOW FEVER

In these days of rapid travel, all parts of the world suitable for yellow fever are accessible from known infected areas within the incubation period of the disease in man. The control of yellow fever, then, is important not only to South and Central America, Mexico and Africa, but also to those countries where conditions exist which would permit outbreaks were the virus introduced. The United States and the West Indies have a direct interest in yellow fever of South and Central America. Once introduced into Asia, yellow fever might well become established as an urban and jungle disease.

The discovery of jungle yellow fever first in Brazil and later in several other countries of South America and Africa, the demonstration that this jungle yellow fever in animals constitutes a permanent source of virus for the infection of clean areas, the proof that the jungle yellow fever regions of Africa extend practically across the continent from the Atlantic to the Indian Ocean, and the development of rapid inter-regional aviation with its inherent threat of carrying passengers in the incubation period of infection from endemic to clean areas, have all stimulated, among health workers, a renewed interest in yellow fever control. Fortunately the recognition of the increased threat comes at a time when control methods are vastly superior to those of twenty years ago. The development of an efficient vaccine providing a means of individual protection and the improvement of methods for the eradication of *Aedes aegypti* permit the health worker to face the future with equanimity.

ANTI-AEGYPTI MEASURES

In the early years of this century anti-aegypti measures consisted of fumigation of houses to destroy the adult mosquitoes and of weekly inspections of all premises to prevent aegypti breeding in neglected exposed water in various types of artificial containers. Both measures proved to be very expensive, and fumigation was eventually abandoned following the observation that antibreeding measures alone would cause the disappearance of yellow fever in about the same period as the combined program. In the early 1930's, antibreeding measures were improved to the point that complete species eradication became the standard practice for anti-aegypti campaigns. After eradication, a small survey squad carrying out inspections at long intervals is sufficient to guard against dangerous reinfestation, thus making permanent control possible at low cost. Brazil and Bolivia have led the way in promoting regional eradication of the aegypti mosquito. This measure is very important in preventing the spread of yellow fever away from the jungle area and is also valuable for the control of dengue. With the development of the DDT insecticide with its residual toxic action, the eradication of *Aedes aegypti* became relatively easy, DDT being equally effective when used against the adult and against the aquatic forms.

VACCINATION

Vaccination with modified yellow fever virus was made by Sawyer as early as 1931, but only since 1937 has it been practiced on a large scale. The 17D virus now used in vaccination is apparently free of all tendency toward viscerotropism and possesses a greatly reduced neurotropism. Millions have been vaccinated with this virus and in spite of certain difficulties which have been encountered from time to time it can be considered as one of the most successful immunizing agents known. Inoculation may be followed by slight symptoms of malaise five to seven days later but, in general, persons immunized with this virus feel nothing. Neutralization tests show that most of those inoculated develop demonstrable antibodies, and field observations indicate that adequate protection develops in most cases within a week. Vaccination is recommended for all persons living in or traveling to or through tropical areas of South America and Africa and then proceeding to other parts of the world. It is of primary importance to inhabitants of forest areas, since there is not now any known method of preventing jungle yellow fever except through vaccination. Vaccination apparently gives a long-lasting immunity, and it is probable that the period of six years now officially designated as the proper interval between vaccinations will be lengthened.

In 1956 the World Health Organization issued a monograph in which they drew up international regulations for yellow fever vaccination. 17D vaccine can be given by subcutaneous injection or by scarification.

Many millions of persons in Africa have been vaccinated since 1938 with a neurotropic virus vaccine applied by scarification, often combined with smallpox vaccine. Recent studies indicate that the 17D virus can be used in a similar manner.

Vaccination with yellow fever alone does not cause any local reaction. After yellow fever and small pox vaccination the local reaction is similar to small pox alone. Children under two years of age if possible should not receive yellow fever vaccination especially where mumps, measles and encephalitis have been found. Yellow fever vaccination should precede vaccination for small pox by at least four days. Infants under nine months of age should have an interval of twenty-one days between the two vaccinations.

Encephalitis after yellow fever vaccination occurs occasionally. Feitel (1960) reports such a case in a girl ten weeks old. Combescot de Marsquet *et al.* (1961) encountered twenty-four cases of meningo-encephalitis in Africans after vaccination, twenty-three of whom had received a combined yellow fever-smallpox vaccine. Twenty-one of these occurred in children under five years of age. Meers (1960), however, vaccinated 60,000 children between the ages of five and fifteen years with a combination of yellow fever and smallpox vaccine, with no ill effects. Meers believes that a combination of the two vaccines is not justified, since only 64.5 per cent of cases receive an immunity against yellow fever of a degree sufficiently high for protection.

Vaccination has a great advantage over antilarval measures as a means of controlling unexpected outbreaks of urban yellow fever, in that its protective action begins much earlier than does that of the curtailment of mosquito breeding. Vaccination in mass of the entire population, together with the rapid spraying of all houses with DDT, should be the first-line emergency measure against urban yellow fever.

Passive immunity may be inherited from mother to child in utero, this immunity disappears during the first few months of life.

Since it is the human case which represents the principal threat of the spread of the virus from the jungle to the town or rural settlement infested with mosquitoes capable of effective transmission of the human disease, and since it is the human case which endangers clean regions, the vaccination of native populations in rural endemic regions may be expected not only to reduce the incidence of jungle yellow fever but indirectly to reduce all yellow fever in the future.

QUARANTINE AND TRAVEL RESTRICTIONS

The attempt to delimit dangerous yellow fever areas for the purpose of establishing quarantine and travel restrictions encounters difficulties, and these difficulties should increase rather than decrease with the widespread use of vaccination. Vaccination will prevent the human cases which have heretofore been an indication of the existence of yellow fever in the jungle and will make the neutralization test unreliable, since this test does not differentiate between the immunity produced by an attack of yellow fever and that produced by vaccination. More and more will it be necessary to rely on immunity surveys in animals to follow the movement of yellow fever virus in the forests.

In considering the results of immunity surveys it must be remembered that a highly immune population may be innocuous for the immediate future, whereas one with a low index may be on the eve of becoming dangerous. The region in which yellow fever has previously been present but in which no evidence of its recent existence can be found, may be just awaiting the chance introduction of the virus from contiguous areas to become active. Thus the forest areas of southern Brazil were invaded by a wavelike opizootic between 1934 and 1940. But the disease died out in each forest soon after it appeared, and careful investigations failed to reveal cases in the following years. But in 1944 and 1951 cases were diagnosed in the area first found infected in 1934, and the area of the 1935 epidemic produced numerous cases in 1945 and 1951. It would seem best to consider all areas in which jungle yellow fever has once been found and all areas in which immune primates have been captured as potentially dangerous. In the same way all cities and ports in close proximity to such areas should be considered dangerous if infested with aegypti whenever epizootics occur.

ITEMS OF NOTE

1) Yellow fever is a disease of man and animals.

2) It is caused by a filtrable virus.

3) In the jungle, primates and marsupials are sources of infection.

4) The vectors of the disease are *Aedes* and *Haemagogus* mosquitoes.

5) Persons living in the forest, or working in areas adjacent to the forest, are liable to become infected.

6) The disease may be introduced into towns and cities, resulting in large epidemics.

7) Jungle yellow fever occurs in extensive areas of South America and Africa.

8) Rapid means of communication has increased the possibility of spreading the disease to other parts of the world.

9) An efficient vaccine is available for the protection of man.

10) Only the complete eradication of the *Aedes aegypti* mosquito can permanently guarantee the cites of the Americas against the reintroduction of yellow fever.

Chapter 38

KOREAN HEMORRHAGIC FEVER

WILLIAM L. JELLISON, PH.D.

AND

CORA R. OWEN, PHD.

Korean hemorrhagic fever (KHF) or Korean epidemic hemorrhagic fever is an acute febrile disease first encountered by the Armed Forces of the United Nations in central Korea in 1951. For that year, 988 cases and ninety-one deaths were recorded. This is generally accepted to be the same disease the Japanese and Russian military forces encountered in Manchuria from 1932 to 1945. It is still present in Korea but the number of cases probably does not exceed fifty per year.

For this discussion it is assumed: 1) that KHF is a disease entity and that it is closely related to or identical with Far Eastern hemorrhagic fever of Manchuria as referred to in Japanese and Russian literature; 2) that it is an infectious disease in the usual sense of the term; and 3) that it probably has a cycle or reservoir in wild rodents in nature.

KHF is well described in a Department of the Army Technical Bulletin (various authors) and by Smadel. It is characterized clinically by signs and symptoms of a mild to very severe febrile illness with changes in capillary permeability, evidence of renal damage, hypotension and hemorrhagic phenomena. About one-fourth of the patients are so severely affected that they show signs of shock. The illness in most cases follows a course which may be divided for convenience into the following phases: febrile, hypotensive, oliguric, diuretic, and convalescent. Well defined second attacks were not recorded and no characteristic sequelae have been recognized.

An estimate of the number of cases that were experienced by the United Nations troops in Korea can be compiled from reports of the 406th Medical General Laboratory (various authors). Approximately

813

3,110 cases with 194 deaths occurred through 1957 (see Table 71). It should be emphasized that this includes only frank clinical cases, most of them serious. There was no way to diagnose with certainty the mild, abortive or suspected cases which never developed the degree of severity that clinicians set as a criterion for hemorrhagic fever, and it is possible that many subclinical infections also occurred. No figures appear to be available on the experience of the Northern Korean armies with this disease.

TABLE 71

CASE INCIDENCE AND FATALITIES FROM KOREAN HEMORRHAGIC FEVER

Year	Number of Cases	Number of Deaths
1951 (June through December)	988	91
1952	1,041	47
1953	607	41
1954	359	10
1955	43	2
1956	44	2
1957	28	1
Total	3,110	194

RELATED DISEASES

There are at least eighteen hemorrhagic fever-like diseases in Europe and Asia which are difficult to classify because of our limited knowledge of the etiologic agent or agents involved. These diseases have been reviewed by Gajdusek and by Smorodintsev *et al.* A division of these diseases into two quite definite groups is made by the latter, namely: 1) hemorrhagic nephroso-nephritis, and 2) hemorrhagic fever. Both are accepted as being virus diseases but claims of tick transmission and tick association pertain almost exclusively to the second group and claims for virus isolation are also more common in this group. By this classification, Far Eastern hemorrhagic fever, and thus KHF, belong to the hemorrhagic nephroso-nephritis group.

A disease which appeared in epidemic proportions in France in World War I has been referred to by the Germans (Arnold; and others) as "feld-nephritis" and by the British (Bandford; Abercrombie; and others) as "trench nephritis." Over 2000 cases occurred among British soldiers in 1915. The whole history of the disease is reminiscent of the experience in Korea although "trench nephritis" was not as highly fatal as KHF.

The several kinds of mosquito-associated hemorrhagic diseases which have been recently discovered are not considered here.

ETIOLOGY

Russian and Japanese scientists claimed the Manchurian disease was caused by a filterable virus and that they were able to transmit the disease to human beings by inoculation of tissue and fluid filtrates. American scientists working in Korea and elsewhere on materials from Korea were unable to demonstrate a virus or even an infective agent.

When the first few cases were seen in 1951, it was suggested that these men had been accidentally poisoned by Warfarin which was being used in rodent control. This diagnosis was not sustained by epidemiological study or by the rapid rise in case incidence.

Leptospirosis appeared to be a reasonable tentative diagnosis but intensive study did not support this. It was also suspected in other areas where acute epidemic nephritis appeared, as in Finland, Germany and Russia.

The disease had some of the characteristics of rickettsial infections, but this diagnosis could not be confirmed. Failure of the disease to respond to any of the therapeutic agents effective against rickettsiae also discounted this theory. Rickettsial etiology was not considered seriously in the several treatises on Russian work until the studies of Korshunova who described a new agent, *Rickettsia pavlovskii,* as the cause of some types of infectious nephroso-nephritis.

Some features of KHF are suggestive of enterotoxemia in domestic animals caused by *Clostridium perfringens.* Marshall and Anslow tested a number of sera from convalescent patients for the presence of antitoxins to *Cl. perfringens.* Their findings are summarized as follows: "Hemorrhagic fever sera contained a significantly higher quantity of neutralizing antibodies than did the control sera." Further studies along this line have not been conclusive.

A widespread and devastating disease of muskrats, *Ondatra zibethica* in the United States is commonly referred to as hemorrhagic disease or Errington's disease. Lord *et al.* found a *Clostridium* associated with the disease and it is believed to be the etiologic agent. These findings are of interest because emphasis is placed on the muskrat as the reservoir of Omsk hemorrhagic fever in Russia (Gajdusek).

Allergy, including sensitivity to plant pollens, or to nonpathogenic fungus spores, and mycotoxicosis were not seriously considered in the epidemiology of KHF although there are diseases in each of these categories that have some parallel in epidemiology and clinical symptoms to KHF.

The high seasonal incidence in both spring and fall does not suggest allergy to a specific pollen unless a long blooming plant is involved. A person once affected with pollinosis should be more susceptible to a second attack, but this was not the case. While relapses were noted when patients resumed active duty too soon after convalescence, frank unquestionable second attacks were never reported. One type of pollinosis, "inhalation favism," has some clinical similarity to hemorrhagic fever but the etiologic diagnosis of this condition is based on association only. There is no specific laboratory test for "inhalation favism" and it may really be some type of hemorrhagic fever. This does not apply to favism from eating fava beans.

Epidemiologically, KHF is in many ways comparable to the systemic fungal diseases, histoplasmosis and coccidioidomycosis. A fungal agent, later named *Emmonsia crescens* Emmons and Jellison, was found to be prevalent in Korean rodents but attempts to further associate this organism with the disease have been unsuccessful.

It has been suggested that KHF is an idiopathic disease ("A morbid state of spontaneous origin") brought on by stress and not dependent on any specific etiologic or especially on any infectious agent. The concentration of cases near the front lines or in the advanced sections supports this theory but the continued occurrence of cases without much decrease in incidence during the first season after the truce would weigh against it. In France (1915), and in Lapland (1942), epidemic nephritis was once attributed to exposure to severe weather conditions in winter months, but this theory had to be abandoned when the case incidence increased in May and June in mild weather.

Partly by the process of elimination, but probably more because both the Japanese and Russians claimed they had demonstrated a virus in Far Eastern hemorrhagic fever, much of the laboratory work in Korea was devoted to attempts at virus isolation. It seemed impossible to test the claims of the Russians and Japanese without experimentation on human beings, which was not done. Despite accumulated negative results from numerous skilled virologists over a period of several years, the virus theory was accepted as a fact by many. No better theory has been advanced and the virus theory is still dominant (November 1961). It should be emphasized that the etiologic agent is entirely unknown and that there is not even any proof that KHF is an infectious disease.

VECTOR

Once the virus theory of etiology for KHF was accepted, transmission by an arthropod seemed essential.

An analysis of the epidemiological features of KHF seemed to eliminate all possible arthropod vectors but chiggers, the minute larvae of mites of the family Trombiculidae. Intensive study of chiggers gave some support to this theory. Two periods of seasonal abundance were found that corresponded closely with the incidence of cases. Some chiggers were found on wild rodents in the winter. Scrub typhus, which is transmitted by chiggers, occurred in Korea. The chigger theory of transmission was developed through logical elimination or exclusion of other possible vectors, and not as a result of direct observation or experiment. If a vector is involved, it is probably a chigger.

Two points especially militate against the chigger theory: 1) No outbreaks followed combat or training maneuvers in chigger infested areas. Outbreaks during such activity were characteristic of scrub typhus during World War II and shorty thereafter, whereas all group outbreaks of KHF were tent or camp outbreaks. 2) The failure of an intensive miticidal program to control the disease. The year following introduction of most intensive control measures, 1954, the disease incidence was about one-half of that in previous years.

Miticidal treatment of clothing was accompanied by other control measures aimed at rodents and mites in particular, but these were so general they would be partially effective against almost any vector, reservoir or etiologic agent.

Numerous references to the mite, *Laelaps jettmari* (Vitz.), as a possible vector of hemorrhagic fever seem to be based on one report of a Japanese scientist who claimed that in a single experiment he induced hemorrhagic fever in a human volunteer by the injection of

an inoculum composed of 200 mites. Traub, *et al*, studied host relationships and seasonal abundance of this mite in Korea and the
seasonal abundance did not correspond with the seasonal incidence
of disease. It is entirely possible that an arthropod vector is not involved in the ecology of KHF.

RESERVOIR OR RESERVOIRS OF DISEASE

KHF probably, though not certainly, has its reservoir in rodents.
This view was supported by most epidemiologists, ecologists and
others associated with the problem. Some of the reasons are as
follows:

There was no indication of transmission from man to man, directly or indirectly, or through human pollution of the environment.
Domestic animals were scarce in the endemic area and birds did not
not seem to fit the qualifications of a reservoir. The only other
numerous warm-blooded vertebrates inhabiting the diverse ecological situations, i.e., mountain tops, grass covered hillsides and
fertile valleys, that were recognized as endemic areas were several
species of rodents and small insectivores. Some of them invaded the
camps. Conversely, in the course of military activities, men invaded
every habitat of rodents by trenching, digging foxholes and gun emplacements, bonification operations and sleeping on the ground.
Contact with rodent habitats was intimate, frequent and prolonged.
Small insectivores, mainly shrews, were also abundant in the area
concerned and should not be dismissed from consideration. However, rodents have an especially bad and well-earned reputation as
reservoirs of agents causing human disease.

Some of the small mammals that were present in the endemic areas
of Korea were: *Apodemus agrarius, Apodemus speciosus, Mus musculus, Clethrionomys rufocanus, Microtus fortis, Cricetulus triton,*
and *Micromys minutus,* all of which are rodents, and *Sorex* spp. and
Crocidura lasiura which are insectivores.

If the relationship of the live rodent reservoir to man had been
immediate with direct transmission as in the case of rat-bite fever
from the bite of a rodent, or of ulceroglandular tularemia by gross
contamination of the skin or wounds with infected tissue, this relationship would have been discovered promptly. It is probably not as
close as in plague with transmission by a single arthropod after a
short extrinsic incubation period. The reservoir relationship is

distant and implies a stage-to-stage development and passage in a vector, as is postulated in part for spotted fever, or a generation-to-generation passage and development, as is accepted for scrub typhus in chiggers. If an arthropod vector is not involved, an organism or parasite with an essential life cycle outside the rodent reservoir is postulated.

If a reservoir does exist among rodents it probably is in wild rodents rather than in the semi-domestic forms, *Mus* and *Rattus*. There are frank statements and subtle suggestions that Microtine rodents are especially important in several of the hemorrhagic diseases. The possibility must be considered, however, that animal reservoirs are not involved in the maintenance of KHF in nature.

EPIDEMIOLOGY

Seasonal Incidence

For four or five consecutive years there was a regular cycle of two marked epidemic seasons per year, spring and fall; however, a substantial number of cases were reported every month of the year. These epidemics were anticipated and appeared with remarkable regularity. They could not be associated with increased troop movement or deployment but seemed to be dependent on natural phenomena which affected either the vector or the etiologic agent. If any one adjective can be applied to both epidemic seasons, it is *dry*, as has been mentioned by several writers. The winter is cold and damp and mid-summer is a rainy or monsoon season. Under these circumstances, many biological phenomena would be accentuated in the spring and fall.

Incubation Period

The incubation period has been fairly accurately established as 8 days minimum and about forty-two days maximum: some soldiers became ill 8 days after entering the known endemic area, while others became ill as late as forty-two days after leaving it. Probably the usual incubation period is twelve to twenty-four days. While the onset was often sudden, disease did not appear abruptly in new arrivals, as would a sudden allergic or toxic response to something in the environment. The incubation period suggested an infectious process.

Age and Sex Distribution

Hemorrhagic fever was largely a disease of young able-bodied men because this was the largest group in the endemic area. There was no indication that it was selective for the youngest or oldest within the age groups represented. When Koreans moved back into the area, the incidence of cases among civilian men and women was about the same.

Sources of Infection

The disease was not considered to be contagious. When patients were removed from the endemic environment e.g., to hospitals, man-to-man transmission did not occur.

Epidemiological studies did not indicate either food or water as the source of infection. Group outbreaks were limited to one or a few adjacent tents in a camp with a common mess hall and water supply serving the entire camp. Individual cases, sporadic in time and place, were the rule; group outbreaks were rare and involved less than 10 per cent of all cases. The same rations were issued to advance and base units or to units north and south of Seoul, yet the disease appeared only in troops north of Seoul. Local foods or beverages never came under suspicion. There is no apparent reason to reconsider this epidemiological conclusion.

Since 1953, the dominant theory on mode of infection has been by bites of chiggers. This theory presupposes close contact with the soil as a factor in infection because these mites live in litter top soil, and low vegetation when not attached to vertebrate hosts. There was practically unanimous agreement that intimate contact with the soil was an essenial factor for infection.

Domiciliary or Group Outbreaks

It was often stated that group outbreaks involved single tents or a small group of adjacent tents, usually on the corner or periphery of a camp. Two authors (i.e., Ley and McClure) disagree with this and have stated that in most camps all tents were on the periphery. In one group outbreak in officers, their tent was isolated from the remainder of the camp.

Occupational Incidence

Within the military organization there appeared to be no definite association of the disease with any particular type of service except that the men were in close contact with nature in their work or camp life.

The highest incidence was in artillery units a few miles behind the front lines, but the morbidity rate in infantry units was also considerable. These men were living in tents, bunkers or trenches in close contact with the soil. Digging trenches and artillery emplacements and constructing roads gave abundant opportunity for contact with soil organisms of all types.

Treatment

No specific treatment has been found although various antibiotics, steriods and other pharmaceutical agents were tried. Transfusions of blood or serum from convalescent patients did not give encouraging results.

Prompt hospitalization at the first suspicion of onset of disease was recommended and patients were evacuated to base hospitals by helicopter rather than by ambulance over rough roads. Symptomatic treatment with special attention to saline balance during the diuretic phase was employed.

Prevention and Control

Application of chemicals, toxic or repellent to mites, to the clothing of soldiers was recommended. Camp areas were cleaned of surface litter and top soil. Soldiers were advised to avoid contact with brush and grassy areas. After intensive application of these measures early in 1954, the case incidence dropped about 50 per cent. Much of this decrease was attributed to the measures employed.

ITEMS OF NOTE

1) Much has been learned of the epidemiology, physiology and treatment of Korean hemorrhagic fever since its discovery in 1951.

2) The etiology, mode of transmission, vector and reservoir in nature (if they exist) remain unknown.

3) There is no specific diagnostic test for the disease and no specific treatment has been found.

REFERENCES

ABERCROMBIE, R. G.: *J. Roy. Army Med. Corps, 27:*131-157, 1916.

ARNOLD, O. H.: Die Sogenannte Feldnephritis. Schrift. zur Deut. Med. Wochen., George Thieme, Verlag, Leipzig, 1944, pp. 1-154.

BRADFORD, J. R.: *J. Roy. Army Med. Corps, 27:*445-459, 1916.

GAJDUSEK, D. C.: Acute infectious hemorrhagic fevers and mycotoxicosis in the Union of Soviet Socialist Republics. Med. Sci. Pub. 2, Army Med. Service Graduate School, Walter Reed Army Medical Center, Washington, D. C., 1953, pp. 1-140.

KORSHUNOVA, O. S.: *Natural nidus of human disease.* Medgis, Leningrad, 1955, pp. 239-243. (Translation from Russian.)

LEY, H. L. and McCLURE, W. W. (presented by GAULD, R. L.): Second Ann. Report Comm. on Hemorrhagic Fever, Armed Forces Epidemiological Board, 1954 (mimeographed).

LORD, G. H., TODD, A. C., KABAT, C. and MATHIAK, H.: *Am. J. Vet. Res., 17:*307-310, 1956.

MARSHALL, J. D., JR. and ANSLOW, R. O.: *Proc. Soc. Exp. Biol. & Med., 90:*265-267, 1955.

MAYER, C. F.: *Military Med., 110:*226-284, 1952.

SMADEL, J. E.: Hemorrhagic fever. In *Viral and Rickettsial Diseases of Man,* Third Edition. Philadelphia, J. B. Lippincott Co., 1959, pp. 400-404.

SMORODINTSEV, A. A., CHUDAKOV, V. G. and CHURILOV, A. V.: *Hemorrhagic nephroso-nephritis.* London, Pergamon Press, 1959, pp. 1-124.

TRAUB, R., HERTIG, M., LAWRENCE, W. H. and HARRIS, T. T.: *Am. J. Hyg., 59:*291-305, 1954.

VARIOUS AUTHORS: Epidemic hemorrhagic fever. Dept. of the Army Tech. Bull., February 1953 (mimeographed).

VARIOUS AUTHORS: 406th Med. Gen. Lab. Ann. Hist. Reports, 1951, 1952, 1953, 1954, 1955, 1956, 1957 (mimeographed).

Chapter 39

TICKBORNE VIRAL HEMORRHAGIC FEVERS

Telford H. Work, M.D.

Hemorrhagic fever in man has been reported from localities distributed widely over the face of the earth. While many sporadic cases of unknown etiology occur, a number of outbreaks have been caused by arthropod-borne viruses.[1] Just as almost all of the known arboviruses have been shown to produce encephalitis in some laboratory animal, many of these agents, in their pathogenesis under certain circumstances, also induce hemorrhagic proclivities and manifestations in naturally existing or laboratory vertebrates. This is apparently unassociated with any definable characteristics of antigenic relationship, vector, or natural host of many arboviruses. Thus, some dengue infections resulting from several antigenically distinct mosquito-borne viruses produce hemorrhagic fever in man.[2]

Several other human hemorrhagic fever viruses are transmitted by acarine vectors. Newly described Argentine hemorrhagic fever[3] is thought to be an inapparent infection of small wild mammals transmitted to man by mites.[4] *Dermacentor*-transmitted Colorado tick fever, which occurs widely over western United States, where the reservoir is in small wild mammals, occasionally develops hemorrhagic complications in human patients.[5]

The best known tickborne hemorrhagic fevers have been elucidated in Eurasia. These are Crimean hemorrhagic fever (CHF)[6] and Omsk hemorrhagic fever (OHF)[7] of the Soviet Union and Kyasanur Forest disease (KFD) of India.[8]

HISTORY

Acquisition of knowledge about the tick transmitted hemorrhagic fevers of the Soviet Union results primarily from the investigations by M. P. Chumakov[9] who was initiated into tickborne virus disease research as a young member of the 1937 USSR Academy of Medical

Sciences expedition to the Soviet Far East. This virological expedition isolated the virus of tickborne Russian spring summer (RSS) encephalitis from man and *Ixodes persulcatus* ticks for the first time. It was during the second world war when the Russians again had concentration of military forces in historic Crimea that Chumakov was requested by the Academy of Medical Sciences of the USSR to investigate the etiology and epidemiology of a hemorrhagic disease afflicting widely dispersed agricultural workers.[10] This disease which came to be known as Crimean hemorrhagic fever (CHF) was occurring in an area where an independent Russian military force was potentially exposed during a critical phase of the war as a result of the German invasion of southern USSR. Chumakov's investigations of 1944-46 established the etiology of CHF as a virus transmitted by *Hyalomma marginatum* ticks. Clinical and epidemiological studies of other hemorrhagic fever cases and outbreaks in southern USSR imply that CHF occurs all the way from Bulgaria to Astrakhan. However, no specific antigenic relationship has been established in the laboratory. Absence of reports of recent cases of Crimean hemorrhagic fever and paucity of investigations of the problem indicate that the disease has not been considered of great importance in recent years.

Simultaneous with the 1944 recognition of hemorrhagic fever cases in the Crimea, clinicians in the Omsk region of central Siberia recognized a spring-autumn occurrence of hemorrhagic disease in human inhabitants of rural areas. Professor P. M. Akhremovich of the Omsk Medical Institute began investigation of what is now known as Omsk hemorrhagic fever. These investigations were extensive, oriented toward establishment of a rickettsial, leptospiral or atypical tularemia etiology. Although carried out by a large and competent medical and scientific staff, the etiology remained obscure. The occurrence of increased number of cases in 1945 and 1946 with a 1 to 3 per cent mortality focussed attention of Moscow's Central Ministry of Health on the problem.

Having successfully outlined the tickborne virus etiology of Crimean hemorrhagic fever in 1944-46, Professor Chumakov and his colleagues were invited to undertake hemorrhagic fever investigations in Omsk in collaboration with the staff already there. Commencing work in 1947, first in guinea pigs, Chumakov's group found that OHF virus could be isolated in mice from blood of acute human cases, *Dermacentor pictus* ticks, and rodent hosts. These findings outlined the etiology and epidemiology of Omsk hemorrhagic fever. It was years later that the antigenic relationship of OHF virus, Chumakov's third successful tickborne virus elucidation, was demonstrated to be closely related to RSSE virus, the first tickborne agent with which he had had profitable experience. This close antigenic relationship between encephalitis and hemorrhagic fever virus proved to have far-reaching implications in regard to the discovery of another tickborne RSS complex virus hemorrhagic fever in India, Kyasanur Forest disease.[12]

Rumor of a fatal epizootic in bonnet macaque *(Macaca radiata)* and langur *(Presbytis entellus)* monkeys of forested Shimoga District in western Mysore of peninsular India, in 1957 led to description and elucidation of what was named Kyasanur Forest disease, commemorating the locality from which isolation of the first monkey virus was made. Initial reaction to the first rumor of epizootic monkey deaths, received at the Virus Research Centre in Poona on March 23, 1957, was that yellow fever had finally appeared in India, where a non-immune human population of a half a billion lived in a subcontinent of Asia where yellow fever has never been known to exist.

Field investigations of this "monkey disease" were initiated on March 27 by autopsy of a *Presbytis entellus* monkey captured moribund in Kyasanur Forest. In the following nineteen days the virus isolated from this monkey was characterized as a group B arthropod-borne virus not identical with yellow fever but similar or identical with RSSE virus. The monkey virus was demonstrated to be identical with strains isolated from villagers suffering a hemorrhagic fever which they called the "monkey disease" because it occurred a few days after seeing or smelling dead monkeys in the forest. Serological studies proved that the human patients and wild monkeys were suffering and often dying from infection with the same virus which was later determined to be transmitted in the forest by *Haemaphysalis spingera* ticks.[13] Prior to this event, yellow fever was the only arthropod-borne disease known to naturally afflict wild monkeys.

Kyasanur Forest disease has continued to recur each year since 1957 with human cases and monkey deaths occurring in the Indian "spring-summer" January to June pre-monsoon season. It is the subject of long-term detailed field and virological studies being continued by the Indian Council of Medical Research Virus Research Centre.

GEOGRAPHICAL PREVALENCE

Allusion has been made to several other acarine-transmitted virus diseases of varying relation to hemorrhagic fever. While the three tickborne hemorrhagic fevers described in detail here have geographical localization in the old world, it is important to remember that ticks are among the most ubiquitous arthropods and our knowl-

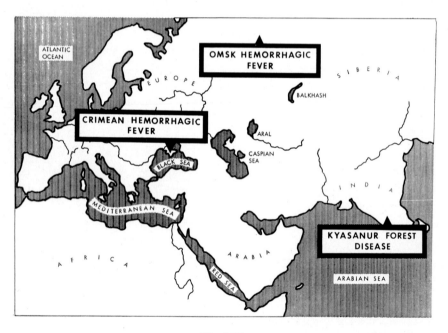

Fig. 132.

edge of tick viruses is in its infancy. Therefore, the principles associated with these three localized tickborne virus hemorrhagic fever problems—CHF in southern European USSR, OHF of subarctic Asiatic Siberian USSR, and KFD of tropical India—are only guides to what should be considered when hemorrhagic or tickborne virus disease comes to attention elsewhere in the world (Fig. 132).

SEASONAL PREVALENCE

As indicated elsewhere, infection and disease resulting from virus transmission by ticks is dependent upon tick activity. Since this varies according to climate and ecological situation, each of the disease problems considered here has a different seasonal occurrence. CHF occurs more or less continuously during the summer months (June to September) because *Hyalomma marginatum* is active during that period. OHF has two peaks of incidence (May and August) which follow shortly after the peak incidence and activity of *Dermacentor pictus* nymphs. KFD occurs in a tropical climate where tick activity continues the year around. Fluctuations in virus activity reflects fluctuations in relative abundance of larvae, nymphal, and adult *Haemaphysalis spinigera* ticks. Greatest activity occurs between January and June although virus is recoverable from acarine and primate sources throughout the year. Human exposure from forest occupation during the January-June spring-summer season of peak nymphal prevalence produces highest incidence of human cases at this time of year.

ETIOLOGIC AGENTS

Considering the refractory response to infection with CHF virus in a variety of laboratory animals, the amount of information reported by the Russians on characterization of this agent is remarkable. It must therefore be assumed that much of it is derived from experimental studies in man much the same way as virological information about hepatitis viruses has been accumulated. CHF virus is relatively small and passes Berkfeld V and N and Seitz SF filters. It is heat labile, losing viability after several days at room temperature. Such inactivated virus, however, appears to produce a specific antibody response after inoculation in man. Reports of its ability to withstand lyophilization and subsequent storage for years in the dry state raises the question that if this is so, it should have become available for comparative studies with other arboviruses in the past fifteen years. There is no information available on its chemical sensitivity to ether or desoxycholic acid.

Serum from early acute human infections with CHF virus contains a complement fixing antigen which has been used in cross CF tests with OHF virus antigen and antisera which demonstrates no antigenic relationship. Cross neutralization tests in mice and cross challenge tests in rhesus monkeys, using a febrile response and anti-body production as criteria of infection, confirms the antigenic in-dependence of CHF virus from OHF and other agents of the RSS complex.

OHF and KFD are both members of the tickborne RSS virus com-plex of Casals' arbovirus antigenic Group B and therefore possess characteristics common to this complex and group. In this regard, they are filterable through systems of small pore diameter and with-stand lyophilization and long-term storage in the frozen state well. OHF and KFD viruses are antigenically very closely related but can be distinguished by definitive HI, CF, and agar gel diffusion tests with group absorbed hyperimmune mouse sera reacting with highly concentrated mouse brain antigen.[14]

Viremia is produced by experimental infection of a number of ex-perimental animals with stimulation of specific antibody response. Experimental studies of KFD virus in *Haemaphysalis spinigera* shows that virus propagates and passes transtadially in these vectors.[15]

ARTHROPOD VECTORS

The three different genera of tick vectors of the three tickborne hemorrhagic fever viruses reflect the diversity of ecological and zoogeographical situations in which natural foci of the viruses exist. The recognized primary vector for CHF virus is *Hyalomma margi-natum,* for OHF virus it is *Dermacentor pictus,* and for KFD virus, *Haemaphysalis spinigera.* This does not conclude that these species are involved exclusively. However, the major proportion of virus isolations and implicated vertebrate host infestations are associated with these acarine species. They are therefore considered to be the vectors and long-term reservoirs essential for transmission and main-tenance of the respective viruses in their natural foci.

The generic differences of the tick vectors also reflect the diver-gent faunal complexes available to prey upon in such different zo-ogeographical areas where the evolutionary durability of the tick fauna provides the common denominator in the parasitic cycles of virus persistence. In the Crimea, the hare *Lepus europaeus trans-sylvanicus,* is considered the definitive vertebrate host for *H. mar-ginatum* in the CHF virus cycle. In the central Siberian oblast of Omsk, *Microtus (Stenocranius) gregalis,* a mouselike rodent of the

TABLE 72

<small>Arthropod-Borne Viral Fevers and Hemorrhagic Fevers</small>

	Geographic Range	*Serologic Group*	*Presumed or Known Vector Species*
Mosquito-Borne			
Rift Valley fever	Africa from central Africa to Union of South Africa	Ungrouped	*Eretmapodites* 6 species, *Aedes* 3 species, *Culex theileri* possibly
Chikungunya fever	East Africa, South Africa	A	*Aedes aegypti* *Aedes africanus* *Culex fatigans*
Tick-Borne			
Colorado tick fever	United States, Rocky Mountain area, Colorado north	Ungrouped	*Dermacentor andersoni* possibly other *Dermacentor* and *Haemaphysalis* species
	Hemorrhagic Fevers		
Mosquito-Borne			
Jungle yellow fever	Tropical Africa, Tropical South America	B	*Aedes aegypti, A. leucocelaenus, A. africanus, A. simpsoni*, other *Aedes*, and *Haemogogus* species
Tick-Borne			
Crimean hemorrhagic fever	Southern European Russia	Ungrouped	*Hyalomma marginatum*, probably others
Omsk hemorrhagic fever	Omsk area, Siberia	B	*Dermacentor pictus*, probably others
Kyasanur forest disease	Mysore state India	B	*Haemaphysalis spinigera*, perhaps others
Mite-Borne			
Korean hemorrhagic fever	Korea Manchuria		Mite suspected, possibly *Laelaps jettmaro*

Note: One hundred and twenty-five aethropod-borne viruses have been identified with a known or suspected animal host, of which 51 cause a febrile or more severe disease in man (Work, 1961).

Baraba Steppe, has been implicated as the primary host of *Dermacentor pictus* in the perpetuation of the OHF virus focus.

In the tropical evergreen and deciduous forest focus of KFD virus in Mysore, *Haemaphysalis spinigera* excels in a complex of three dozen species of ticks in transmitting the virus not only between forest rodents such as the three-striped palm squirrel, *Funambulus t. tristriatus,* but apparently among many avian species as well as primates *Presbytis entellus, Macaca radiata,* and man.

Most virus isolations and vertebrate host infestations have been derived from nymphal stages of these tick species. This is of epidemiological significance because maximum evidence of virus transmission to man has been observed to occur simultaneous with seasonal peak appearance and activity of nymphs.

Only occasionally have isolations been made from unengorged larvae. This raises the question of transovarial transmission of these viruses which has been reported experimentally achieved by Russian workers. Although this proposition is a popular concept among many investigators, the great rarity of such isolations from larvae, relative to the number which have been collected and examined, would appear to diminish the epidemiological significance of such a phenomenon to a non-essential in the mainstream of tickborne virus circulation in a natural focus.

TICKBORNE HF VIRUS INFECTION IN NON-HUMAN VERTEBRATE HOSTS

Such serious difficulties have been encountered in attempts to induce CHF disease in experimental animals that no source of CHF virus harvest material has been available for study by western virologists. The Russians have reported that the virus infection has been established in cats, mice, guinea pigs, and monkeys but without production of hemorrhagic manifestations which are characteristic of the human infection. It is thought unlikely that overt disease occurs in wild hares which have been implicated as the probable sylvan vertebrate reservoir host in the Crimea. However, it was reported that a widespread dieoff of rodents occurred in 1945 when remains of many dead animals were found in their burrows. This followed a year or so of rodent abundance which, in turn, was considered by some investigators to be associated with greater incidence of disease in man.

Russian studies in volunteers and mental patients requiring induction of high fever therapy have demonstrated that man suffers high susceptibility to disease within an incubation period of two to three days following inoculation of acute blood containing CHF virus. CHF virus has been established in mice only after blind passage, while the laboratory animal of choice for isolation and study of OHF and KFD viruses is the suckling or weanling mouse which suffers encephalitic manifestations typical of the more neurotropic viruses of the RSS complex.

Evidence of OHF infection of guinea pigs is confined to transient febrile episodes lasting 24-72 hours, three to twelve days following inoculation. The muskrat (ondatra), which was imported from Karelia into Omsk Oblast in 1936 and 1938 is the only animal experimentally infected with OHF virus by the Russians which develops hemorrhagic manifestations. In contemplating genetic development of resistance to disease by other rodent species indigenous to the Omsk natural focus, there are those who consider that a refractory disease response of indigenous vertebrate species substantiates prolonged existence of the virus in the area. The muskrat, being a recent immigrant into the focus, suffers overt disease to which it has no genetically selected constitutional resistance.

Reports vary as to the importance of the muskrat as a sentinel animal in signaling exposure to or extension of the OHF virus infected area. Some observers report recognition of the disease in man following an epizootic in the muskrats while others claim that the disease is rare or non-existent in these animals because their habits confine them to water courses which are not intimately associated with the forest habitat of *Dermacentor pictus* ticks. This may not allow for periodic migrations or foraging sorties during periods of food scarcity which are known to take water dwelling mammals long distances over dry land and through forests where exposure may occur.

Whatever the cause of infection producing hemorrhagic disease in muskrats, it is well established that human exposure to infected tissues and blood during skinning or autopsy is hazardous. Numerous human infections have occurred from such exposure. Kyasanur Forest disease virus is also highly infectious to laboratory workers, more than forty such infections having already occurred in several laboratories where it has been studied since it was discovered in 1957.

It was an epizootic of KFD in wild monkeys which led to isolation of this virus and discovery of the associated hemorrhagic disease in man. As has been observed in sylvan yellow fever, there is a species difference in severity of disease resulting from natural infection. The langur appears to suffer most with higher mortality than the bonnet macaque. *Macaca radiata,* in turn, suffers overt disease from which they occasionally die while its close relative the rhesus *(Macaca mulatta)* from North India, where the natural monkey disease is not known, appears refractory to disease after experimental peripheral inoculation which, however, does produce a viremia and antibody response. Disease proclivity in other mammalian and avian vertebrate species possessing antibodies by natural exposure to KFD virus has not been evaluated.

HEMORRHAGIC DISEASE IN MAN

CHF, OHF, and KFD virus infection of man results in essentially the same disease. The incubation periods differ. The Crimean disease, which is usually more severe with higher incidence of hemorrhagic complications and higher mortality rate (8-15%) is characterized by skin manifestations ranging from scattered petechiae to widespread hemorrhagic purpura. Lymphadenopathy is rare in Crimean hemorrhagic fever but common in Omsk hemorrhagic fever and Kyasanur Forest disease.

These tickborne virus hemorrhagic diseases begin with sudden onset of a headache and high fever, soon followed by prostration associated with severe pains in the neck, which becomes stiff, and pain in the back and extremities. There is marked inflammation of the scleral and palpebral conjunctivae which continues for the duration of fever that lasts from five to fourteen days. Lesions ranging from a maculopapular eruption to hemorrhagic sloughing may appear on the mucous membranes of the oropharynx. There is marked leucopenia down to 1500 WBC/mm^3 with relative lymphocytosis accompanied usually by a thrombocytopenia which contributes to the hemorrhagic tendency.

There is severe anorexia and by the third day there is frequently vomiting and diarrhea which may consist of digested coffee ground vomitus and/or tarry stools, and occasionally discharge of frank red blood by both orifices. In such cases, the prognosis is grave. Those who die expire in the second week of disease from exsanguination into the gastrointestinal tract or lungs or due to secondary bacterial pneumonia.

Convalescence is prolonged over many weeks before the patient can fully resume pre-illness activity. In Omsk and Kyasanur Forest disease there may be a second febrile episode beginning in the third week after initial onset, lasting for one to seven days, occasionally accompanied by pleocytosis in the spinal fluid which is routinely normal during the acute phase of the disease. Although recovery is slow, it is complete with no permanent sequelae, no neurological manifestations having been observed as consistent with these diseases.

Details of viral hemorrhagic fever pathogenesis are obscure. At autopsy, the picture is of a generalized toxemia ranging from brain changes consistent with hepatic coma to focal necrosis in the liver, inflammatory lesions in the myocardium, depletion of malpighian follicles in the spleen and sloughing of the tubular epithelium in the kidney. Besides the massive exudation of blood into visci reflecting increased capillary permeability without focal vascular lesions, oozing of erythrocytes into interstitial spaces, tissues and organs are common, diffuse, and widespread.

Histologic evidence of encephalitis which is invariable in experimental infection in mice has been found rarely in wild monkeys killed by KFD. However no such lesions have been seen in man. Considering histological evidence of kidney damage, it is surprising that abnormal urine findings appear so rarely and then consist only of a few red cells and casts.

PREVENTION AND CONTROL

Lack of a laboratory animal or tissue culture cell adapted strain of CHF virus has inhibited development of a killed virus prophylactic vaccine such as have been produced on an investigational basis for OHF and KFD virus infections. These consist of formalin-inactivated mouse brain suspensions of virus given in three 1 cc subcutaneous injections, the first two a week apart and the third five weeks after the second. Experience with these vaccines in protecting against infection with homologous viruses has not been extensive enough for definitive evaluation. It is known that a formalin-killed high passage RSSE virus vaccine which did initiate a homologous neutralizing antibody response in a substantial percentage of recipients, failed to provide significant protection against natural KFD virus infection in India, or against laboratory infection with this virus in several institutions in the U.S. and abroad. The Russian clinicians value homologous convalescent serum in treatment of acutely ill patients.

Control of the disease still calls for immunoprophylaxis by means of formalin-inactivated virus vaccines previously described and effective means of preventing exposure to tickbite in infected areas. Protective clothing and organic repellants which avoid tick infestation have been used to a limited degree of success in the Soviet Union where activity of rural people brings them into contact with infected forest and other natural foci. Insecticide control of ticks has been widely applied with enthusiastic reports of success. This has not yet been objectively evaluated in regard to anything more than temporary control by limited extermination of an infected tick population.

In the subarctic climate of Siberia, cold and snow are elements which aid in control through many months of the year by immobilizing vector ticks. These elements also aid in reinforcing insecticide control by allowing slow insecticide penetration by permeating seepage during the spring thaw of snow to which chemical has been applied during colder months. Protective clothing and benefits of climatic extremes are not applicable to KFD virus transmission control in tropical India.

Because of the wide and irregular dispersal of infected foci of tick-borne viruses, the definitive means of hemorrhagic disease prevention rests on immunoprophylaxis which still awaits development of effective vaccines.

REFERENCES

1. WORK, T. H. (1961a): The Expanding Role of Arthropod-borne Viruses in Tropical Medicine. *Proceedings of the Fourth Conference Industrial Council for Tropical Health,* Harvard School of Public Health, Boston, 1961, 225-248.
2. HAMMON, W. M., RUDNICK, A. and SATHER, G. E. (1960): Viruses associated with epidemic hemorrhagic fevers of the Philippines and Thailand. *Science, 131:* 1102-1103.
3. PIROSKY, I., ZUCCARINI, J., MOLINELLI, E. A., DI PIETRO, A., BARRERA ORO, J. G., MARTINI, P. and COPELLO, A. R. (1959): Virosis hemorragica del Noroeste Bonaerense. Ministerio de Asistencia Social y Salud Publica, Instituto Nacional de Microbiologia, Republica Argentina, Buenos Aires.
4. PARODI, A. S., RUGIERO, H. R., GREENWAY, D. J., METTLER, N., MARTINEZ, A., BOXACA, M. and DE LA BARRERA, J. M. (1959): Isolation of the Junin virus (Hemorrhagic fever) from Acaros *(Echinolaelaps echidninus)* of the epidemic zone. *La Prensa Medica Argentina, 46:*2242-2244.
5. EKLUND, CARL M. (1960): Insect-Borne and Animal-Borne Virus Diseases of Man *Minnesota Medicine, 43:*184-189.
6. CHUMAKOV, M. P. (1948): Crimean Hemorrhagic Fever. In *Encyclopedia of Military Medicine, 3:*268-271. State Publishing House of Medical Literature, Moscow.
7. CHUMAKOV, M. P. (1948): K Itogam Ekspeditsii Instituta Nevrologii Po Izucheniiu Omskoi Gemorragichskoi Likhoradki (OL) (Results of the study made of Omsk)

Hemorrhagic Fever (OL) by an expedition of the Institute of Neurology). *Vestn. Akad. Med. Nauk.*, No. 2, 19-28.

8. Work, T. H. (1958): Russian Spring-Summer Virus in India—Kyasanur Forest Disease. *Prog. Med. Virol.*, 1:248-279.

9. Chumakov, M. P. (1957): Etiology, epidemiology, and prophylaxis of hemorrhagic fevers. In United States-U.S.S.R. Medical Exchange Mission, 1956. Microbiology and epidemiology. Public Health Monograph No. 50. U.S. Public Health Service Publication No. 536, Washington, D.C. U.S. Government Printing Office, 1957.

10. Chumakov, M. P. (1948): K Itogam Ekspeditsii Instituta Nevrologii Po Izucheniiu Omskoi Gemorragichskoi Likhoradki (OL) (Results of the Study Made of Omsk Hemorrhagic Fever (OL) by an Expedition of the Institute of Neurology). *Vestn. Akad. Med. Nauk.*, No. 2, 19-28.

11. Zeitlenock, N. A., Vanag, K. A., and Pille, E. R. (1957): Cases of illness of the Crimean hemorrhagic fever type observed in the Astrakhan oblast. *Problems of Virology*, 2:90-96.

12. Work, T. H., Trapido, H,. Murthy, D. P. N., Rao, R. L., Bhatt, P. N., and Kulkarni, K. G. (1957): Kyasanur Forest disease. III. A preliminary report on the nature of the infection and clinical manifestations in human beings, *Indian J. M. Sc. 11*:619-645.

13. Trapido, H., Rajagopalan, P. K., Work, T. H., and Varma, M. G. R. (1959): Kyasanur Forest Disease, VIII. Isolation of Kyasanur Forest disease virus from naturally infected ticks of the genus *Haemaphysalis*. *Indian J. M. Res., 47:* 133-138.

14. Clarke, D. H. (1961): Antigenic relationships between viruses of the tickborne encephalitis complex as studied by antibody absorption and agar gel precipitin techniques. *Proceedings of the Symposium on the Biology of Viruses of the Tick-borne Encephalitis Complex, Smolenice, Czechoslovakia, October 10-14, 1960.*

15. Varma, M. G. R., Webb, H. E., and Pavri, K. M. (1960): Studies on the Transmission of Kyasanur Forest disease virus by the tick *Haemaphysalis spinigera* Newman. *Trans. Roy. Soc. Trop. Med. Hyg., 54:*509-516.

SECTION THREE

THE RELATION OF HUMAN AND
ANIMAL DISEASES

Chapter 40

ANIMAL DISEASES OF MINOR PUBLIC HEALTH SIGNIFICANCE

Thomas G. Hull, Ph.D.

THE AMERICAN PUBLIC HEALTH ASSOCIATION lists 134 diseases of major public health significance. Of this number, eighty-six diseases find a reservoir in animals or birds and may be transmitted to man (Table 73). They are discussed elsewhere in this book.

In addition to the diseases mentioned above, there are 85 infections of minor public health significance, which create problems of lesser proportions (Table 74). Animal parasites, responsible for forty-five of this number, may occur only occasionally in man, and often in other parts of the world than the United States. (See Chapter 17). Wright has listed 120 animal parasites which are found in both man and animals, of which number seventy-six occur rarely in man and some with only a single case on record. Many of the latter have been omitted in these discussions.

In other chapters of the book most of the infections of minor public health importance are discussed. Among the fungus diseases of lesser importance are included adiaspiromycosis, aspergillosis, epizootic lymphangitis, cutaneous streptococcosis, nocardiosis and rhinosporidiosia (see Chapter 18). Vibriosis, a disease of cattle and sheep, has on record only a few human infections (see Chapter 4). Swine erysipelas, a disease primarily of swine and poultry, is not uncommon in man, but the causative organism is often found in dead matter of plant or animal origin. So called "sealers finger" is probably caused by one of the *Erysipelothrix* group (see Chapter 5). Listeriosis is widely disseminated among many animals and birds, with occasional human-infections (see Chapter 7). Vesicular stomatitis, as

TABLE 73

Actinomycosis
African tick-borne fever, rickettsial (Boutennense fever, South Africian tick-bite fever,
   African tick typhus fever, Kenya dog fever)
Amebiasis (amebic dysentery)
Anthrax
Blastomycosis, North American
Botulism
Brucellosis (undulant fever, Malta fever, Mediterranean fever)
Bunyamwera fever (animal reservoir suspected)
Bwamba fever (animal resevoir suspected)
Cat scratch disease (cat fever, benign inoculation lymphoreticulosis)
Chickenpox (varicella)
Chikungunya fever (animal reservoir suspected)
Clonorchiasis (Chinese liver fluke disease)
Coccidioidomycosis (valley fever, coccidioidal granuloma)
Colorado tick fever
Common cold
Crimean hemorrhagic fever
Cryptococcosis (European blastomycosis, torulosis)
Dengue (breakbone fever, (animal) reservoir suspected)
Diphasic meningoencephalitis
Diphtheria
Diphyllobothriasis (broad tapeworm infection, fish tapeworm infection)
Dracontiasis (Guinea worm disease)
Eastern encephalitis
Echinococcosis (echinococciasis, hydatid disease)
Endemic relapsing fever, tick borne.
Fasciolopsiasis
Glanders
Histoplasmosis
Influenza
Japanese B encephalitis
Jungle yellow fever
Korean hemorrhagic fever (epidemic hemorrhagic fever) (suspected)
Kyasanur forest disease
Larva migrus, visceral
Leishmaniasis, cutaneous (oriental sore, espundia)
Leishmaniasis, visceral (kala azar)
Leptospirosis (Weils disease, canicola fever, swineherd disease, mud fever, Fort Bragg
   fever, hemorrhagic jaundice, rice field fever, cane field fever)
Loaiasis
Louping ill
Lymphocytic choriomeningitis
Malaria, quartan
Measles (rubeola, morbilli)
Mumps (infectious parotitis)
Murine typhus fever, flea borne
Murray Valley encephalitis
Omsk hemorrhagic fever
Ornithosis (psittacosis)
Paragonimiasis (Oriental lung fluke disease, pulmonary distomiasis, endemic hemoptysis)
Phlebotomus fever, (sandfly fever, three-day fever, Pappataci fever, Naples strain and
   Sicilian strain, animal reservoir suspected)
Plague
Philippine hemorragic fever (animal reservoir suspected)
Q fever
Rabies

TABLE 73—(cond't.)

Rat-bite fever (Haverill fever, *Streptobacillus moniliformis* infection)
Rat-bite fever (sodoku, *Spirillum minus* infection)
Rickettsial pox
Rift Valley fever
Ringworm, scalp tinea capitis
Ringworm, body tinea corporis
Rocky Mountain spotted fever
Russian spring-summer encephalitis
Salmonellosis
Schistosomiasis (Bilharziasis)
Sporotrichosis
St. Louis encephalitis
Staphylococcal infection
Streptococcal infections, hemolytic
   A. Scarlet fever
   B. Streptococcal sore throat
Strongyloidiasis
Taeniasis and cysticercosis
   A. bovine (*Taenia saginata*)
   B. porcine (*Taenia solium*)
Tetanus
Thailand hemorrhagic fever (animal reservoir suspected)
Toxoplasmosis
Trichinosis
Trypanosomiasis, African (African sleeping sickness)
Trypanosomiasis, American (Chagas' disease)
Tsutsugamushi disease (scrub typhus, mite typhus)
Tuberculosis, avian
Tuberculosis, bovine
Tuberculosis, human
Tularemia
Venezuelan encephalitis
West Nile fever
Western encephalitis

*Diseases of major public health significance are those listed in *Control of Communicable Diseases in Man* Ninth Edition, 1960, American Public Health Association.

virus infection of cattle and horses resembling foot and mouth disease, is sometimes found in man as a disease resembling influenza (see Chapter 11). Contagious ecthyma is a virus disease of sheep and goats, man being infected at rare intervals (see Chapter 14). Newcastle disease, a virus affliction primarily of poultry and other birds is occasionally found in man (see Chapter 15). Pseudotuberculosis is a relatively rare disease of many mammals and birds, with human infections being uncommon (see Chapter 23). Milk sickness in cattle, horses and sheep is due to a chemical poison found in white snakeroot and the rayless goldenrod, man being poisoned by ingesting milk or milk products from affected cows (see Chapter 20). Other chemicals, including anthelmintics, antibiotics, sulfonamides, pesticides and certain other agricultural chemicals are stored in the mus-

TABLE 74

DISEASES OF MINOR PUBLIC HEALTH SIGNIFICANCE WHICH MAY BE TRANSMITTED FROM
ANIMALS TO MAN

Acanthocheilonemiasis
Adiaspiromycosis (haplomycosis)
Amebiasis, porcine
Ancylostomiasis, canine
Anthelmintics in animal products
Antibiotics in animal products
Ascariasis, porcine
Aspergillosis
Balantidiasis
Bertiella infection
Brazilian spotted fever
Brugia infection
California encephalitis
Central European encephalitis
Chigger mite dermatitis
Chigoe (jigger flea) dermatitis
Colombian spotted fever
Contagious ecthyma of sheep and goats
Cowpox
Cutaneous streptothricosis
Dog mite dermatitis
Dog tapeworm infection
Duck tapeworm infection
Dwarf tapeworm infection
Echinochasmus infection
Echinococcosis (*E. multilocularis*)
Echinostomiasis
Encephalomyocarditis
Epizootic lymphangitis
Equine infectious anemia
Fascioliasis
Foot-and-mouth disease
Fowl mite dermatitis
Gas gangrene
Gastrodiscoides infection
Giardiasis
Gnathostomiasis (*G. hispidum*)
Gnathostomiasis (*G. spinegerum*)
Gongylonemiasis
Hemorrhagic septicemia
Herpesvirus simae infection
Heterophyiasis
Ilheus encephalitis
Insecticides in animal products
Larva migrans, bovine
Larva migrans, cutaneous
Larva migrans, filarial
Listeriosis
Malaria, simiam
Mange mite dermatitis
Melioidosis
Metagonimiasis
Metastrongyliasis
Milk sickness
Milkers nodules
Newcastle disease
Nocardiosis
Oesophagostomum infection

TABLE 74—(*cont'd.*)

Oestrus ovis conjunctivitis (sheep bot)
Opisthorchiasis
Ostertagia infection
Ox bot
Paragonomiasis (*P. kellicoti*)
Powassan encephalitis
Pseudotuberculosis
Rat mite dermatitis
Rat tapeworm infection
Rhinosporodiosis
Salivary gland virus infection
Sarcocystitis
Schistosomiasis, bovine
Sealers finger
Sheep wireworm infection
South African tick fever
Streptothricosis cutaneous
Sulfonamides in animal products
Swine erysipelas
Syngamus infection
Ternidens infection
Thelaziasis (*Th. californiensis*)
           (*Th. callipaeda*)
Trichostrongylosis
Tumor, mammalian
Vesicular stomatitis
Vibriosis (Vibrio abortion)

cles of meat animals or secreted in the milk of milk animals and are thus a menace to man (see Chapter 19). Gas gangrene in man is caused by anaerobic spore-forming organisms found in the intestinal canal of various normal animals (see Chapter 42). Milkers nodules occur on persons who have milked cows affected with a disease closely allied to cowpox (see Chapter 13). Mention should be made of cowpox which, in the form of vaccine virus, certainly is not of minor significance (see Chapter 12).

Other diseases of animals that are found occasionally in man are discussed in the following pages.

EQUINE INFECTIOUS ANEMIA

Equine infectious anemia is a disease of horses, mules and donkeys, of world wide distribution. The causative virus has not been cultivated to date (1961). It may be transmitted from animal to animal by the common stable fly, *Stomoxys calcitrans* (and possibly by mosquitoes in Germany), although direct contact is often the manner of spread. No other animals except members of the equine family are of importance in the epidemiology of the disease. Human infection is in doubt. Stein and his associates, as well as Dregruss and Lombard, have presented evidence against infection in man. However, both Peters and Karl reported human cases with fever, anemia, diarrhea, renal pain and viremia. The blood of one person was reported infective for horses over a period of three years.

FOOT-AND-MOUTH DISEASE

Foot-and-mouth disease, an exceedingly contagious disease of cattle and other cloven-footed animals, is world wide in distribution. In the United States it has appeared from time to time (at least nine outbreaks to 1961) but each time it has been eliminated. The causative virus—one of the smallest known in size—is quite resistant to cold and remains alive in meat and milk over long periods of time. Cattle and hogs are most susceptable, but other cloven-footed animals, especially sheep and goats, are affected. Outbreaks have also occurred in deer and other wild ruminants. In England hedgehogs were found naturally infected. Human cases have been reported in the past, but they are probaby quite rare. However, the disease in man is usually very mild and it is possible that infection is overlooked.

HEMORRHAGIC SEPTICEMIA
(Pasteurella multocida infection)

Hemorrhagic septicemia is caused by any one of a group of organisms belonging to the *Pastuerella multocida* group, which, for practical purposes, are indistinguishable. It was formerly believed that these organisms were responsible for "shipping fever" in cattle, but more recent work would indicate a virus as the etiologic agent. However, *Pasteurella* organisms are wide spread in the animal kingdom, being found in normal horses, cattle, hogs, sheep, poultry, dogs, cats and rats, usually in the upper respiratory tract but sometimes the intestinal tract. Apparently saprophytic strains acquire a marked virulence on animal passage, causing severe losses in livestock, among which may be mentioned the following:

Hemorrhagic septicemia of cattle, sheep and goats, a pneumonia that often occurs after exposure or shipping (hence shipping fever, *Past. boviseptica.*

Swine plague, a pneumonia of hogs that is often found in association with hog cholera.—*Past. suiseptica*

Fowl cholera, a disease of hens, ducks, geese, turkeys and wild
birds—*Past. aviseptica*

Rabbit septicemia, pneumonia of rabbits that is often described
as snuffles—*Past. leptiseptica.*

Sheep pneumonia—*Past. oviseptica.*

Human infections have been reported from countries in Europe
and North and South America. They are of two types—those resulting from animal bites or other animal contact and those not connected with any known direct cause.

The cat has been responsible for many cases of the disease in man.
In an incomplete survey, Meyer reported ninety-five cases of which
twenty-nine were due to animal bites. There were twenty-three cat
bites, four dog bites, one rabbit bite and one panther bite. Miscellaneous animal contact include a case resulting from the consumption of infected chicken, a case where rabbit muscle was used as a
hemostat and a patient which was kicked in the face by a horse.
Exposure to the carcasses of cattle, hogs or rabbits has likewise resulted in infection.

The symptoms from animal bite are quite similar. There is a
local inflammatory process, with an ulcer at the point of the abscess,
from which *Pasteurella* organisms may be isolated. The pain is severe, but there is little or no rise in temperature and no swelling of
the lymph nodes. Osteomyelitis may be a complicating factor. The
duration of illness may last from a few weeks to several months.

Cases arising from causes other than animal contact often show no
direct cause. The symptoms vary widely and may be severe, with
sinusitis, pleuritis or meningitis. When the infection is generalized,
death may result—five deaths reported in 1951 (Meyer).

Diagnosis depends upon isolation and identification of *Past. multocida* by cultural and serological means and animal pathogenicity
tests. Organisms isolated from infected tissues will agglutinate in the
serum of the same patient in a high titer.

MELIOIDOSIS

Melioidosis is a disease of rodents, cats, dogs, swine, sheep, goats
and horses. It is of extensive geographic distribution, having been

encountered in Asia, Europe, North America and Australia. The causative agent is *Malleomyces pseudomallei*.

Rats are natural hosts, the infection being transmitted by biting insects such as mosquitoes *(Aedes aegypti)* and fleas *(Xenopsylla cheopsis)*. Swine, sheep and goats were naturally infected in Australia. Infection has been found in the cow. Horses develop the disease, which resembles glanders in the clinical manifestations, but is more acute.

The first infection in man was reported in 1912, but there is little more of record until 1946 when the disease was encountered in man in Guam. A number of cases occurred in military personel that had been stationed in the Far East following World War II. In 1951, cases in man appeared that apparently were contracted in the United States. The disesase in man has a fatality rate of about 95 per cent, following an acute or subacute septicemia. Chronic forms may last for months or years. Apparently the infection is not passed directly from person to person. It is uncertain how they occur, but probably from biting insects.

HERPESVIRUS SIMIAE INFECTION
(B virus Infection)

Herpesvirus simiae infection is caused by a virus found in many apparently normal monkeys. The disease is acquired by man from a monkey-bite or through skin abrasions contaminated with monkey saliva. Sabin and Wright, in 1934, were the first to isolate the virus from the brain of a laboratory worker who had been bitten eighteen days previously by a monkey. Sabin reported a similar fatal case in 1949. Love and Jungherr describe another case in a laboratory worker, describing the infection as an occupational hazard. To date (1962) eighteen cases in humans are on record, and probably others have taken place.

The clinical features in man are variable—an acute encephalitis, myelitis or encephalomyelitis. The disease in man is almost invariably fatal. No vaccine is available.

SALIVARY GLAND VIRUS INFECTION

Salivary gland virus infection is caused by a virus found in the monkey, rat, mouse and probably other animals more or less commonly. In man, the disease is rare in adults but may cause various symptoms in children such as diarrhea, pneumonia, cerebral lesions and liver damage. The virus has been isolated from human adenoids and from liver biopsies by both Rowe, *et al.* and Weller *et al.* There is no known therapy.

ENCEPHALOMYOCARDITIS

Encephalomyocarditis is a virus disease that has been recognized since 1940. The disease is widespread having been recognized in Germany, Holland, Uganda, the Philippines and the United States (Florida and New York State).

Animals which have been found to harbor the virus include the monkey, baboon, chimpanzee, mongoose, squirrel and cotton rat. The host range is apparently very wide, most laboratory animals being susceptible.

Warren lists seven human cases, with a possible epidemic among United States troops in the Philippines. The clinical symptoms were of short duration, two to four days, usually with a sudden onset, high fever, vomiting and headache. The recovery was rapid. There are no known control measures and no specific treatment. No human deaths have been reported.

BOT FLY INFESTATION

Oestrus ovis conjunctivitis in man is caused by the sheep nasal fly (sheep bot fly) *Oestrus ovis*. Sheep, goats and game animals are the natural habitats of the larvae, the eggs being deposited inside the nose, after which the larvae crawl upwards to the nasal sinuses where they remain six or eight months or longer before they mature. They cause great discomfort, resulting in emaciation and sometimes death of the animal. In India, the Sahara and Caucasus the fly may lay its eggs on the conjunctival and nasal mucosa of man, causing much trouble. In the Western Hemisphere, the investation has been reported on Catalina Island off the coast of California. Goats that roam the hillsides of the island are afflicted, as are summer visitors to the island. One physician reported the removal of fourteen *Oestrus ovis* larvae from a single conjunctivitis patient.

Hypoderma creeping eruption in man is caused by the ox warble (bot fly) *Hypoderma bovis* or *Hypoderma lineatum*. The former is widely prevalent in Europe while the latter is more common in the

United States and Asia, afflicting cattle, goats, game animals and sometimes horses. The flies lay their eggs on hairs of the animal's leg usually. The larvae hatch in about four days, crawling up the hair and penetrating the skin. After traveling through the subcutaneous connective tissue towards the diaphragm, the larvae migrate to the back of the animal, from where they wriggle out of their cysts and fall to the ground. The parasite causes much loss in milk production and damage to hides. In man, the larvae migrate from one place to another in the subcutaneous tissue, causing "creeping eruption" or swellings first in one part of the body than in another. The larvae may be excised before they reach maturity.

MAMMALIAN TUMOR VIRUSES

The first report of a tumor-inducing virus was made by Ellerman and Bang, in 1908, since when there have been many occasions where viruses have been encountered capable of causing cancer in the chicken, dog, mouse, rabbit, frog and monkey. Bearcroft and Jamieson in 1958 reported a spontaneous outbreak of subcutaneous tumors in rhesus monkeys in Yaba, Nigeria. Grace and Feltz showed that the virus can multiply and induce localized benign tumors in man. The instance is cited of a laboratory worker that accidently infected himself through the broken skin while working with the virus. He developed antibodies to the virus within a week's time and a typical lesion about four months later.

There is no cross infection of monkeys through contact, and normal animals placed in the same cage with infected animals do not contract the disease. It has been suggested that possibly mosquitoes or other arthropods might be responsible for spontaneous outbreaks in wild life. The case of infection in man through the broken skin would substantiate this possibility.

ITEMS OF NOTE

1) In addition to the 87 diseases of major public health importance there are 84 other diseases of minor significance, (discussed in other chapters).

2) Equine infections anemia is a virus disease of horses, mules and donkeys, with human cases rare.

3) Foot-and-mouth disease is an exceedingly contagious disease of

cloven-footed animals. The virus is only slightly infectious for man, but human cases have been reported.

4) Hemorrhagic septicemia (associated with shipping fever of cattle) is caused by a variety of closely related organisms. Many different animals are susceptible. Man is infected by association or by an animal bite.

5) Melioidosis is found in rodents, cats, dogs and domestic animals. In the horse it resembles glanders. In man it is highly fatal.

6) Herpes virus simae infection is caused by a virus which is found in many apparently normal monkeys. Man is infected by a monkey bite through the abraded skin.

7) Salivary gland infection of monkeys and rodents may cause a disturbance in children.

8) Encephalomyocarditis is a virus disease with a wide host range over many parts of the world. Several human infections have occurred.

9) The sheep bot fly, *Oestrus ovis,* carried by sheep and goats, may cause a conjunctivtis in man, while the ox warble *Hypoderma bovis* and *H. lineatrim* of cattle, goats and other animals produces "creeping eruption" in man.

10) Spontaneous outbreaks of tumors in monkeys are caused by a virus which is capable of causing tumors in man. Arthropods are suspected of conveying the disease.

REFERENCES

AMERICAN PUBLIC HEALTH ASSOCIATION: *Control of Communicable Diseases in Man,* Ninth Edition. New York, 1960.

BEAMER, P. R., VARNEY, P. L., BROWN, W. G.: *Am. J. Clin. Path.,* 24:1231, 1954.

BEARCROFT, W. C. G. and JAMIESON, H. F.: *Nature, 182*:195, 1958.

DREGUSS, M. and LOMBARD, L. S.: *Experimental Studies in Equine Infectious Anemia.* University of Pennsylvania Press, 1954.

FELTZ, E.: *Proc. Cancer Res.,* 1961, *3*:224.

GARRY, M. W. and KOCH, M. L.: *J. Lab. & Clin. Med.,* 38:374, 1951.

GRACE, J. T.: Scientific Exhibit, American Medical Association, New York Meeting. June, 1961.

KARL, F.: *Vet. Ext. Quart.,* University of Pennsylvania, *116*:14-55, 1949.

LOVE, F. M. and JUNGHERR, E.: *J.A.M.A., 179*:804, 1962.

MIRICK, G. S., ZIMMERMAN, H. M., MAUER, G. D. and HUMPHREY, A. A.: *J.A.M.A., 130*: 1063, 1946.

PETER, J. T.: *Ann. Int. Med., 23*:271-274, 1945.

ROWE, W. P., HARTLEY, J. W., WATERMANN, S., TURNER, H. C. and HUEBNER, P. J.: *Proc. Soc. Exper. Biol. & Med., 92*:418-424, 1956.

SABIN, A. B.: *J. Clin. Invest., 28:*808, 1949.

STEIN, C. F., OSTEEN, O. L., MOTT, L. O. and SHAHAN, M. S.: *Vet. Med., 39:*46-52, 1944.

WARREN, JOEL: *Virus and Rickettsial Infections of Man,* 3rd. Edition, 1959.

WELLER, T. H., MACAULEY, J. C., CRAIG, J. M., and WIRTH, P.: *Proc. Soc. Exper. Biol. & Med., 94:*4-12, 1957.

WRIGHT, W. H.: *Ann. New York Acad. Sc., 48:*553-576, 1947.

Chapter 41

HUMAN DISEASES SPREAD BY ANIMALS

Thomas G. Hull, Ph.D.

Animals are responsible for transmitting certain diseases which are primarily of human origin, the infection being acquired from man and passed again back to him. Among diseases of major public health significance more than a dozen are in this category. Tuberculosis of the human type is acquired by both the hog and the dog (discussed in Chapter 1). Several of the animal parasites are also passed from man to animal to man, including amebic dysentery (rat, dog, cat, monkey), cutaneous leishmaniasis (dog, jackal and gerbil in the old world and the dog, cat and wild rodents in the Americas), visceral leishmaniasis (dog, cat, jackal and gerbil), and schistosomiasis (dog, hog, cow, horse, water buffalo, rat and mouse), all of which are discussed in the chapter on Animal Parasites (Chapter 17). The place of cowpox in the man-animal-man chain is discussed in the chapter on Pox Diseases (Chapter 12). On occasion, cows have been infected by persons recently vaccinated against smallpox.

DIPHTHERIA

There have been reported in the past a considerable number of instances of infection of dogs, cats, and fowls with *Corynebacterium diphtheriae*. Bacteriologic evidence, however, is either entirely lacking or is faulty, with diphtheroid organisms often mistaken for true diphtheria bacilli.

Cats have been found by several investigators to be susceptible to diphtheria toxin as well as to the bacilli. When injected subcutaneously either with toxin or with live cultures such animals exhibit definite symptoms and often die (Klein, Brodie, Yabe).

Klein rubbed cultures into the cornea of cats as well as injected intratracheally with definite results. Infection by feeding the organisms in milk was unsuccessful, however. Intratracheal inoculations were successfully made by Welch and Abbott with the production of membranes from which the organisms could be recovered. Henke was unsuccessful in the production of membranes.

Savage sought to determine experimentally whether cats were capable of harboring diphtheria bacilli. The implantation of large numbers of virulent organisms into the nasal cavities were ineffective in setting up any general or local lesion. The same was true when massive doses were applied to the throat by swabs. The organisms survived but a short period of time, usually disappearing within twenty-four hours. Savage believes that the mucous membranes of cats are unfavorable for the growth or persistence of the diphtheria bacillus, and that cats do not serve as carriers of diphtheritic infection. He analyzes the epidemiologic evidence of previous cases reported, concluding that the view that cats can acquire the disease naturally is entirely without foundation.

Simmons, on the other hand, found two cats harboring true diphtheria bacilli, one in the nasal fossa and the other in lesions of the vocal cords. The first animal developed a croupy cough, was unable to swallow, and cried continually. About a week after the cat developed this condition, a woman with whom the cat slept, developed a typical case of diphtheria which proved fatal. The organisms isolated from both the woman and the cat were virulent for guinea pigs as proved by the injection of two animals, one of which was protected by antitoxin.

Domestic fowls were found by Litterer capable of not only harboring diphtheria bacilli, but of transmitting the disease to man. Two hundred and fifty-six human cases suffering from acute or carrier diphtheritic infection were investigated, where the family owned fowls suffering from roup, fowl diphtheria, cholera, etc. A total of 1,126 sick fowls were examined; in two flocks several fowls were found harboring virulent diphtheria bacilli as proved by morphologic and virulence tests. In each instance a child in the family owning the fowls showed similar virulent organisms. Successful inoculations of the virulent diphtheria organisms isolated from both the fowls and the children were made into other fowls suffering from roup; later the infection in the experimental fowls was cured with diphtheria antitoxin.

Horses are quite susceptible to diphtheria toxin when injected for the purpose of producing antitoxin, and consequently considerable care must be used on initial injections. True diphtheria occurs but rarely, however. Corbett reports such a case in a pony infected by its rider. Minett likewise recorded several cases of ulcerative lymphangitis in horses infected with diphtheria bacilli probably from human cases.

Other animals exhibit some susceptibility to toxin but apparently do not contract the disease naturally. Sheep have been used to some extent for the production of antitoxin and may succumb from overdoses of toxin as noted by Roux and Yersin in 1889. Wernicke in 1893 likewise killed a sheep by gradually increasing the doses of diphtheria culture. Goats have been used for the production of diphtheria antitoxin for toxin-antitoxin mixtures. Ledingham found that goats would succumb to large injections of toxin (250 cc.). Wladimiroff injected diphtheria cultures into the teats of three lactating goats. Only one of them exhibited any constitutional symptoms. Diphtheria bacilli were found in the milk for a period of six days, but they rapidly diminished in numbers. Dogs have been utilized by various workers in experimental investigations. They are susceptible to injections of both toxins and cultures. Unconfirmed reports of natural diphtheria infection in dogs have been recorded. Brandt in 1908 obtained from a dog a culture which he considered true diphtheria, but it did not kill guinea pigs when injected. Hull had cases reported of diphtheria infection in dogs, but complete laboratory confirmation was lacking.

The laboratory animals vary in susceptibility. Rats and mice are quite immune. Guinea pigs are very constant in susceptibility and hence are the animals of choice in experimental work. The standardization of both diphtheria toxin and diphtheria antitoxin is based upon the amount of toxin required to kill a guinea pig weighing 250 grams in four days.

Monkeys were found by Burnet, in 1910, rather resistant to infection. Seventeen experiments were made by rubbing virulent cultures into the abraded mucous membranes of young animals. Eleven experiments were entirely negative, in five the results were slight, while in one animal which was ill at the time of inoculation, the lesions were extensive.

Eels were shown susceptible to diphtheria toxin by Pettit on two occasions, while alligators were found highly susceptible by Metchnikoff. Frogs, when injected with toxin, remained well at low temperatures, but developed paralysis when maintained at 37° C.

Cows are quite susceptible to diphtheria toxin. They have been recommended from time to time as a substitute for the horse in the production of antitoxin, but they are not altogether saisfactory. Diphtheria bacilli, when injected under the skin, were found by Klein to kill cows in as short a period as eleven days. Fifteen animals so treated either died or showed marked reactions. Wladimiroff had a similar experience but Abbott could not confirm Klein's findings on two cows with which he worked.

Cows fed diphtheria bacilli by mouth exhibited no ill effects (Klein). Diphtheria bacilli injected into the udder through the teat by Wladimiroff killed a cow in ten days, although diphtheria toxin administered in the same way caused no trouble.

Dean and Todd in 1902 found two cows with scabby teats from which diphtheria bacilli were isolated. The animals were implicated in a diphtheria epidemic. The authors concluded that the cows were infected by the milker. Ashby in 1906 similarly found diphtheria bacilli in ulcers on the teats of a cow implicated in an epidemic. The milker of the cow, however, was probably responsible for this condition since he lived in the house where the first case of the epidemic originated.

Henry describes an epidemic of thirty-two cases where a cow was involved. A girl who did the milking had a lesion on the finger which proved to be harboring diphtheria bacilli. With her removal the epidemic ceased, only to flare up again two weeks later. It was found that one of the cows had developed a sore on its teat which harbored diphtheria bacilli. The organisms isolated were virulent by the usual protection tests.

Graham and Golaz reported a cow with sores on the teats, covered with thick, black scabs. When the scabs were removed a ragged, ulcerated surface was left that exuded a mucopurulent fluid. The teats were tender and the sores did not heal. Cultures showed virulent diphtheria bacilli present. An investigation revealed that the cow had been infected by a milker who was a diphtheria carrier. This cow was responsible for fifty-two cases of diphtheria mostly among adults.

Pfeiffer and Viljoen, in South Africa, have reported diphtheria mastitis in two cows which caused several human cases.

Numerous epidemics of diphtheria spread by cow's milk have been reported. In 1908, Trask collected fifty-one such records which had occurred up to that time and Armstrong and Parron added twenty-five more from 1908 to 1926 in the United States. In the latter study pasteurized milk was implicated once, certified milk once, ice cream once, and butter once. The epidemics were mostly in the northern states, although one epidemic occurred at Austin, Texas, and one at Charlottesville, Virginia. In England, from 1857 to 1929 there were forty-two such epidemics recorded, with 3,433 cases.

Milk in such instances has been commonly thought to receive its contamination with virulent diphtheria bacilli directly from a human carrier or case either on the farm where the milk is produced or en route to consumer. The cow was not implicated in all of the epidemics due to milk. In some instances contamination of the milk occurred after it left the cow, from a human case of diphtheria, or from a carrier.

In the United States during the years 1918 to 1948 there were only eleven milk-borne epidemics of diphtheria on record. Since 1948 none have been reported.

STREPTOCOCCAL SORE THROAT

Streptococcal sore throat due to infected milk has been recognized in Great Britain for many years. In 1875, there occurred at South Kensington, England, several cases of sore throat and scarlet fever among twenty persons who had used cream coming from a district where there had been 119 cases of sore throat. It is impossible to determine from the evidence presented whether this was a scarlet fever outbreak or a mixed infection of scarlet fever and septic sore throat.

The first authentic record of an epidemic of the tonsillitis or quinsy type is that at Aberdeen in 1881. Among 110 families supplied by a single dairy, ninety families were affected, with 300 cases. During the following years similar epidemics occurred with considerable regularity, the milk supply being incriminated by circumstantial evidence only.

The first outbreak of Streptococcal sore throat recognized in the United States occurred in Boston, Massachusetts, in May, 1911. Winslow made a careful epidemiological study of the 1,400 cases involved, finding that 70 per cent were supplied with milk from one dairy, the cases exactly coinciding with the two main delivery routes of that dairy. The symptoms all pointed to a streptococcus as the infecting agent but there was little definite information available on this point. In the laboratory of the Boston Board of Health as well as other laboratories no constant organism was found. Theobald Smith, however, isolated streptococci from four cases at autopsy.

The relationship of streptococci to udder infections of cows was suspected as early as 1884 by Nocard and Mollerau. In 1889 Bang produced inflammation of the udder of a cow by injecting into the milk duct a streptococcus isolated from a case of mastitis in another cow.

Davis, in 1915, distinguished *Streptococcus epidemicus* from the ordinary bovine streptococci. This organism is included in the *Streptococcus pyogenes* group.

The incidence of mastitis in cows is high and is of considerable economic significance. In only a small proportion of the cases, however, is the trouble caused by a human pathogen. Davis and Capps applied a hemolytic streptococcus directly to an abrasion on the udder of a cow, causing an infection as evidenced by the enormous number of streptococci found in milk, but no external sign of inflammation, caking, or "gargety" milk. In another experiment streptococci directly from a case of tonsillitis were introduced into the milk duct, causing an infection of several weeks' duration with numerous streptococci in the milk. Their conclusions, that streptococci of human origin may cause mastitis without external evidence of infection, were soon corroborated by other investigators (Mathers).

Smith and Brown, as well as Krumwiede and Valentine showed that streptococci commonly associated with bovine mastitis could be differentiated from those causing human tonsillitis.

Frost and his associates noted that not all animals harboring *Streptococcus epidemicus* may cause epidemics. Only two cows out of seventeen in which the organisms were found were associated with epidemics; the other fifteen cows apparently caused no human cases. The streptococci from all of them showed typical virulence when cultured. Brooks believed that while the types of streptococci which were common incidents of mastitis in dairy cattle apparently were not infective for man, they might sometimes produce severe toxic disturbances, especially in children, when the organisms were present in milk in large numbers, together with their toxins.

The usual source of infection of the cow is an infected person.

Frost and Carr recite their experience with an epidemic arising from a very high grade milk supply. Laboratory examinations revealed enormous numbers of *Streptococcus epidemicus* — 36,000,000 per cubic centimeter — in the milk of one animal. A few days later a second cow was found infected and a little later still a third cow. Cultures from the nose and throat of each person in the dairy revealed that two were carrying *Streptococcus epidemicus*. One was a woman in the house who had no part in handling the milk; the other was the hired man, whose chief duties were the care of the cows and the milk. After he left the dairy, there was no more trouble.

One quarter of the udder may be infected with streptococci without the other quarters becoming involved. It is necessary therefore, to examine milk from each quarter when looking for infection. Cows once infected with *Streptococcus epidemicus* are likely to remain sources of danger over long periods of time and probably never should be returned to the milking line.

Hadley and Frost found that cows could be quite easily infected by the simple process of smearing the teats with *Streptococcus epidemicus,* and that mastitis subsequently developed. The infected quarter usually lost its function of secretion because of the severity of the disease.

Since udder infection with *Streptococcus epidemicus* often produces no apparent evidence of its presence, cases of mammitis often go unrecognized till a considerable amount of damage has been done. Even in certified dairies with regular examination of both employees and cattle, Frost, Gumm, and Thomas found by laboratory examination four cows infected with *Streptococcus epidemicus*. Brooks has emphasized the necessity, in an extensive outbreak of Streptococcal sore throat lasting several days, of looking for the cow which is causing the trouble. A person who is a carrier of *Streptococcus epidemicus* may contaminate the milk once, but not usually several days in succession. After the cow which is harboring virulent streptococci has been found, then it is necessary to find the person who is harboring the germs in his throat that infected the cow.

The United States Public Health Service tabulated 105 epidemics of milk-borne streptococcus sore throat in the United States between 1920 and 1952, almost all of which were associated with raw milk. There have been no milk-borne epidemics reported in this country since 1952.

SCARLET FEVER

The responsibility of the cow for scarlet fever epidemics was suggested from time to time in the absence of other evidence. Power, in 1882, attributed an outbreak to contamination by a cow suffering with puerperal fever. Klein at the same time showed that cows inoculated subcutaneously with material from a human case of scarlet fever developed an abscess at the site of inoculation and material from such an abscess could produce a similar lesion when injected into another cow.

In 1885, Power, Cameron, and Klein encountered another epidemic which they attributed to bovine origin, lacking any human sources. A vesicular eruption on the udder and buttocks of several animals accompanied by constitutional symptoms and discharge from the eyes and nose, with sore throat (Hendon disease) was thought to be the cause. Russell, in 1888, Hill, in 1890, and Jones, in 1909, all reported similar instances where a milk epidemic of scarlet fever occurred and cows in the responsible herd were found suffering from a condition similar to that described by Power, Klein, and Cameron. Bacteriologic evidence was, of course, entirely lacking.

In 1923, Dick, as well as Dochey, differentiated the scarlet fever streptococcus from other organisms in the group, making bacteriologic evidence possible. Jones and others isolated a typical scarlet fever streptococci of human origin from the udder of a cow.

Jones and Little were the first to furnish bacteriologic evidence that cows could be infected with scarlet fever streptococci. In a scarlet fever outbreak of 200 cases studied by the New Jersey State Department of Health, the usual relation of a case of scarlet fever on one of the farms supplying the milk was found. More careful observations indicated that one of the cows was suffering from an acute injury of the teat. An investigation by Jones and Little of the milk from this cow indicated that as many as 345,000,000 streptococci per cubic centimeter were being eliminated. The organisms answered all the necessary requirements of scarlet fever streptococci of human origin.

Jones claimed that usually milk-borne epidemics of scarlet fever are not due to a human case or carrier on the farm or in the dairy. Milk is not only an inhibitive agent in which such organisms fail to grow, but it contains an active principle which greatly diminishes the number of streptococci at room temperature. He concluded that "the opinion that severe outbreaks of scarlet fever result from human contamination of milk must be viewed with considerable doubt." It is possible that a few individuals may contract the disease through direct human contamination of the milk, but the occurrence of epidemics would imply a much heavier inoculation of the milk than would be probable by this means. The enormous numbers of streptococci shed from the udder of a single cow infected with this organism may contaminate a large bulk of milk and even after some of the streptococci have perished, still show sufficient numbers of living organisms to infect man. This is a reasonable explanation of milk-borne epidemics.

Many outbreaks of scarlet fever have been attributed to contaminated milk supplies in the past. In England, Wahby reported eighty-eight epidemics with 7,650 cases from 1857 to 1929. In Canada Murray tabulated seven epidemics embracing 192 cases that occurred between 1906 and 1935; there were no deaths. In the United States Trask listed 125 milk-borne epidemics which occurred prior to 1908. Armstrong and Parron added forty more outbreaks between 1908 and 1926. During the years 1927 to 1944 there were eighty-one milk-borne epidemics in this country according to the United States Public Health Service. No such milk-borne epidemics have been reported in the United States since 1944.

Animals other than the cow are probably of small importance in the spread of scarlet fever. Reports have been made from time to time concerning infection of dogs in contact with human cases, but all lack bacteriologic confirmation. Numerous attempts were made before the discovery of *Streptococcus scarlatinae* to induce infection in laboratory animals with material direct from human cases, but all were unsuccessful. Several workers were able to produce lesions in monkeys and chimpanzees with human material while others failed. The failure of Hektoen and Weaver in producing the disease in monkeys fed on milk to which had been added material from the throats of scarlet fever patients, is explained by the work of Jones.

Since 1923, experimental infection has indicated the susceptibility of certain animals. The dog is highly susceptible to the infection of a living culture of the organism, succumbing in three to five days from an acute hemorrhagic nephritis. Killed cultures and culture lysates are also highly toxic for dogs (Duvall and Hibbard). Goats are quite susceptible to scarlet fever toxin and have been used to a certain extent as a substitute for human subjects in standardizing such toxin. Mice, rats, guinea pigs, cats, chickens, pigeons, monkeys, calves, and sheep have been found entirely unsusceptible to toxin while rabbits and pigs give conflicting results (Kirkbride and Wheeler).

STAPHYLOCOCCAL INFECTIONS

Man has been considered the principal host of *Staphylococcus aureus,* according to Rountree and his associates. Animals suffer from staphylococcus infections, however, from one source or another. Attempts have been made to classify human strains and animal strains, but lines of demarcation are not always constant. Recent problems of hospital-acquired infections in man have been sufficiently serious to include them among communicable diseases of major public health importance. With improved methods of typing, it is possible to identify certain strains when encountered in epidemics.

Gastroenteritis from milk and other food products contaminated with staphylococci has been long recognized, but the source and type of the offending organism was seldom established. In 1954, Steede and Smith reported an instance in which a cow was infected with staphylococci by the milker—with a subsequent epidemic of "food-poisoning." The milker was suffering from a staphylococcic infection of the anterior nares. The same strain was in the milk.

Skaggs *et al.,* encountered an instance where two different herds of dairy cattle were infected by the same attendants. The first herd developed furunculosis with lesions so severe that they interfered with milking. The entire herd was sold and replaced by a new herd free from any signs of disease. A new dairy barn was built to ensure further precautions. However, in a few months lesions began to appear on mammary glands of the new animals. Extensive bacteriological studies of the cows, family pets and members of the family showed that two of the dairy attendants were found to harbor staphylococci in the anterior nares of the same type that infected the cows. The authors concluded "the bovine species may thus serve as an additional host for antibiotic-resistant staphylococci which are currently a major problem in human hospitals".

MUMPS

The chief reservoir of the virus of mumps is man himself. Other animals, however, may be a factor in the spread of the disease from time to time.

Wollstein (1916) found that young cats were susceptible to infection and displayed typical symptoms of the disease. The results were confirmed by further experiments two years later. Other investigators, however, were not successful in their attempts to transmit the disease to cats. Johnson and Goodpasture (1935) passed the virus of mumps through eleven generations of monkeys, producing symptoms of the disease. At the end of the period the virus was still infective for susceptible persons.

Dogs also may acquire the disease. Morris, Blount and McCown (1956) showed the presence of complement-fixing bodies in the serums of normal dogs, thus suggesting the possible susceptibility of this animal. Noice, Bolin and Eveleth (1959) reported two instances of mumps in dogs. A six-month old dachshund was allowed the freedom of the sickroom, even the bed, during the illness and convalesence of the patients with mumps. The dog became ill, with swollen parotid glands, difficulty in swallowing and mumps virus in the saliva. After a few days the animal died. The second case was that of a Boston terrier three months old. This animal likewise was allowed free contact with the family when there were three cases of mumps. The dog became ill with the usual symptoms, including mumps virus in the saliva, and a positive complement-fixation test. After fourteen days the animal recovered.

CHICKENPOX (VARICELLA)

Chickenpox is an almost universal affliction of children. Transmission of the virus occurs through secretions of the respiratory tract from an infected person to a healthy subject. Man was long considered the only host, with animals of no importance.

Heuschele has reported the disease in three apes—a chimpanzee, an orangutan and a gorilla. These animals were exhibited in a Children's Zoo, in close contact with the public. They participated in children's parties and attended luncheons, dinners, charity shows and other functions. At the time there was a high incidence of chicken pox among children of the community. The signs, course of disease and lesions in the animals were typical of human chickenpox. The chimpanzee, a three and a half year old animal, was the most severely affected with rash, high temperature and scabs. After nineteen days the animal was free of all signs of the disease. The orangutan, two and a half years old, exhibited similar but less severe symptoms. Both animals were examined by a pediatrician who confirmed the diagnosis. The gorilla, 20 months old, developed papules in the axilla, which lasted only one day.

MEASLES

Measles is a highly communicable disease caused by a virus. Man is the chief reservoir of infection, the disease being spread by droplet transmission of secretions from the nose and throat of an infected person. The role of animals in the spread of the disease has not been considered of importance.

A possible relationship between canine distemper and measles virus was suggested by Adams (1953). Skaggs (1960) has shown that the viruses of the two diseases share identical antigenic components and stimulate closely related antibodies. Similar clinical syndromes and histopathologic changes occur in the respective hosts.

Enders (1957) and his associates infected forty-eight dogs with measles virus. Fever was present in 50 per cent of the animals while coryza and rash occurred in 28 per cent. There was viremia for two to eight days following inoculation. The virus was isolated and passed to a second group of pups where it produced similar effects.

Warren *et al.* (1960) found that dogs infected with measles virus (Edmonston strain) uniformly developed subclinical infection with a subsequent appearance of antibodies for both measles and distemper. Further investigation is required to determine whether measles infection in man is associated with canine distemper in dogs and whether canine distemper vaccine will provide protection against measles.

THE COMMON COLD

The common cold is an acute catarrhal infection of the upper respiratory tract caused probably by more than one filter-passing agent. Attempts to infect animals with any of the viruses have been unsuccessful, except for the chimpanzee. Many investigators have transmitted the infection experimentally to the chimpanzee, both in the United States and elsewhere.

Morris, Blount and Savage studied an outbreak of coryza in a colony of chimpanzees. The virus was recovered from one of the animals, for which antibody reactions were obtained with the serums of the other animals as well as an attendant who experienced a respiratory infection while working with the animals.

Chanock and his associates recovered a virus from a child that was indestinguishable from the chimpanzee coryza agent. In testing a large group of children four years of age they found that 80 per cent showed antibody reaction for this agent.

Chimpanzees are apparently quite susceptible to the virus causing the common cold and are capable of passing the infection back to man.

INFLUENZA

Shope has shown that the virus causing the influenza pandemic of 1918 was probably the same virus as that causing influenza in swine (Type A influenza). It was thought that man originally transmitted the infection to the hog. There was also epidemological evidence that influenza of horses belonged to the same type. The ferrett was shown susceptible to human influenza type A by Smith et al in 1933. Anderson in Australia suggested the possibility of sheep acting as a reservoir of influenza virus. Rasmussen suggests that the Asian influenza epidemic of 1957 may have had its source in a hog or a hen or a duck in some Chinese barnyard.

Similarity of human and animal types of influenza has long been recognized. Rasmussen has given further study to the problem, finding that in southeast Asia and Formosa strains of the virus isolated from the hog, the duck and the horse, as well as a strain of fowl plague from the hen, were all closely related to Asian influenza virus in man.

It must be realized that the viruses of influenza are exceedingly pleomorphic and strains appear and disappear, to be replaced by other strains. The problem is receiving serious attention in several of the virus laboratories of the country.

OTHER DISEASES

Attempts have been made to incriminate animals in the spread of poliomyelitis. The virus has been transmitted through cows milk, but it is not believed the cow had any connection with the contamination of the milk. Work done at the University of Berne, Switzerland would indicate that the cow and the hog might act as reservoirs of poliomyelitis virus. One case of spontaneous poliomyelitis in a heifer was reported in which the microscopic findings were typical of the disease. It is probable however that animals have a small part, if any, in the epidemiology of poliomyelitis.

The typhoid bacillus has been encountered in an animal in one instance. The paratyphoid organisms *(Salmonella paratyphi A* and *Salmonella paratyphi B)* have been found in animals on such rare occasions that animals can be ignored for all practical purposes in the spread of these diseases. The same is true of dysentery bacillus, causing bacillary dysentery.

ITEMS OF NOTE

1) Human diseases may infect animals and be passed back again to man.

2) Several such infections are discussed elsewhere in this book, including tuberculosis (human type) and cowpox, as well as diseases caused by animal parasites—amebic dystentery, leishmaniasis of both the cutaneous and visceral types and schistosomiasis.

3) Diphtheria may infect the cow, dog and cat. Contaminated milk has caused explosive epidemics in years past, but none are on record in the United States since 1948.

4) The streptococcus causing scarlet fever in man has been transmitted to the cow and the dog. There have been numerous milk-borne epidemics, but none in the United States since 1944.

5) The streptococcus causing sore throat in man may infect the cow, resulting in milk-borne epidemics. There have been none in the United States since 1952.

6) Staphylococcal infections of man may be passed to the cow with resulting milk-borne infections in man. The place of animals in perpetuating strains of staphylococci resulting in hospital-acquired infections is still uncertain.

7) Mumps has been found in dogs which had access to the sickroom.

8) Measles virus is closely related to canine distemper and dogs are considered susceptible to measles infection.

9) Chickenpox has been contracted by young apes—chimpanzee, orangutan and gorilla.

10) The common cold may be transmitted to chimpanzees which are capable of infecting people. No other animals have been found susceptible to the common cold.

11) Influenza type A has been found in the hog, which perhaps was infected by man during the influenza pandemic of 1918. Other animals which harbor strains of influenza closely related to human types include the horse, the sheep, the duck and the hen.

12) There is no adequate evidence to implicate animals in the spread of poliomyelitis, typhoid fever, paratyphoid fevers A and B and bacillary dysentery.

REFERENCES

ADAMS, J. M.: *Pediatrics, 11*:15-25, 1953.

CHANOCK, R., ROIZMAN, B. and MYERS, R.: *Am. J. Hyg., 66*:281-290, 1957.

CHANOCK, R. and FINBERG, L.: *Am. J. Hyg., 66*:291-300, 1957.

DAVIS, D. J. and CAPPS, J. A.: *J. Infect. Dis., 15*:135, 1914.

DUVALL, C. W. and HIBBARD, R. J.: *J. Exper. Med., 46*:379-390, 1927.

ENDERS, J. F., PEEBLES, T. C., McCARTHY, K., MILOVANOVIC, M. MITUS, A. and HOLLOWAY, A.: *Am. J. Pub. Health, 47*:275-282, 1957.

FROST, W. D., THOMAS, R. C., GUMM, M. and HADLEY, F. B.: *J. Infect. Dis., 46*:240-252, 1930.

HEUSCHELE, W. P.: *J.A.V.M.A., 136*:256-257, 1960.

JOHNSON, C. D. and GOODPASTURE, E. W.: *Am. J. Hyg., 21*:46, 1935.

JONES, F. S. and LITTLE, R. B.: *J. Exper. Med., 47*:945-956, 1928.

LITTERER, W.: *South. M. J., 18*:577-581, 1925.

MINETT, M. C.: *J. Comp. Path. & Therap., 33*:267, 1920.

MORRIS, J. A., BLOUNT, R. E. and McCOWN, J. M.: *Cornell Vet., 46*:525-531, 1956.

MORRIS, J. A., BLOUNT, R. E., JR. and SAVAGE, R. E.: *Proc. Soc. Exper. Biol. & Med., 92*: 544-549, 1956.

MURRAY, R. H.: *Canad. Pub. Health J., 27*:555-559, 1936.

NOICE, F., BOLIN, F. M. and EVELETH, D. F.: *A.M.A.J. Dis. Child., 98*:350-352, 1959.

PFEIFFER, D. H. and VILJOEN, N. F.: *J. South African Vet. M. A., 14*:148-152, 1946.

ROUNTREE, P. M., FREEMAN, B. M. and JOHNSTON, K. G.: *J. Path. & Bact., 72*:319-321, 1956.

SAVAGE, W. G.: *J. Hyg., 18*:448, 1919-20.

SIMMONS, J. S.: *Am. J. M. Sc., 160*:589, 1920.

SKAGGS, J. W.: *J.A.V.M.A., 138*:8-11, 1960.

SMITH, T. and BROWN, J. T.: *J. M. Res., 31*:455, 1915.

STEEDE, F. D. F. and SMITH, H. W.: *Brit. M. J.,* 576-578, Sept. 4, 1954.

TRASK, J. W.: *Hygienic Lab. Bull., 41*:21-147, 1908.

WARREN, J., NADEL, M. K., SLATER, E. and MILLIAN, S. J.: *Am. J. Vet. Res., 21*:111-119, 1960.

WINSLOW, C. E. A.: *J. Infect. Dis., 10*:73-112, 1912.

WOLLSTEIN, M. J.: *J. Exper. Med., 23*:353, 1916.

WOLLSTEIN, M. J.: *J. Exper. Med., 28*:377, 1918.

ZINN, R. D., ANDERSON, G. R. and SKAGGS, J. W.: *J.A.V.M.A., 138*:382-386, 1961.

Chapter 42

ANIMALS AS PASSIVE CARRIERS OF DISEASE ORGANISMS

Thomas G. Hull, Ph.D.

ANIMALS MAY CARRY in their intestinal tracts, without apparent harm to themselves, the spores of the organism causing tetanus, gas gangrene and botulism.

TETANUS

The natural habitat of the tetanus organism is the intestine of herbivorous animals from where it is spread universally. To a less degree man likewise acts as an intestinal carrier.

Clostridium tetani is an anaerobic spore-bearing organism of considerable resistance. The spores are destroyed by direct sunlight but when protected will remain alive and virulent for years. They are not susceptible to the ordinary disinfectants or to boiling water except when exposed over long periods.

The distribution of the spores is universal. They are present in the soil everywhere, but are especially abundant in soil fertilized with human or animal excreta.

Animals may carry tetanus organisms in their intestines over long periods of time without harm to themselves. Noble found 18 per cent of the horses in the vicinity of New Haven so affected. The presence of the organisms in the intestine is not always due to constant reinfection for Noble found one horse to harbor the organism continuously for four months, although other horses in the same stable were free. Apparently the organisms grow and multiply in the intestine and are eliminated in great numbers with the dejecta.

According to Park, 15 per cent of the horses and calves in the vicinity of New York harbored tetanus bacilli in their intestines. Ninni cultivated the organisms from eight different portions of the stomach and intestine in forty-two rabbits and guinea pigs with very constant results.

Man may carry the organisms in his intestine, likewise, Pizzini found 5 per cent of human feces to harbor tetanus bacilli. Men working around horses and stables, however, were carriers in about 30 per cent of the instances while men in other occupations showed about 2.2 per cent. Tulloch studied the feces of twenty-one men returned from overseas army service in 1919, obtaining positive results in 33 per cent; from 33 civilians in England 16 per cent were positive. Ten Broeck and Bauer in 1921 examined the stools of seventy-eight Chinese in Peking and found 34.7 per cent harboring tetanus bacilli; in 1924 they examined 539 more such specimens from various parts of China, finding 26.5 per cent positive. Buzello and Rahmel in Germany found 20 per cent of the feces from forty individuals positive. Van der Reis found tetanus bacilli in practically pure culture in the large intestine of one of his patients. Bauer and Meyer studied 487 specimens of human dejecta in California of which 24.6 per cent were positive. In addition forty-three specimens from nineteen other states were examined, of which nine showed tetanus bacilli. Sex, age, and occupation played no part in the distribution of carriers. No atoxic strains were found in the 129 cultures isolated.

Although the natural habitat of the tetanus bacillus is the intestine of the herbivorous animal (the horse or the cow), spores of the organisms have been found in numerous locations. McCoy showed them in hay dust, in the mortar of old masonry, in the dust from horse hair, in the dust in houses, barracks, and hospitals, and in court plaster. It is only natural to expect to find such a resistant organism anywhere that the wind might carry the dust of the soil.

Giles studied sixty-three samples of street dust collected over a wide area in Baltimore, as far as possible free from recent contamination with horse manure. Eleven samples yielded tetanus bacillus, nine of which produced toxin and two no toxin. Apparently the elimination of the horse from city streets has not entirely freed street dust from tetanus organisms.

Gelatin sold for human consumption may contain numerous spores. In Rettger's laboratory in New Haven for several years the stock culture of tetanus, for the demonstration of the disease in laboratory animals, was a package of household gelatin.

Tetanus, whether in man or animals, is a wound infection requiring a broken skin for the passage of the organisms. By mouth neither the organism nor its toxin is harmful.

Among domestic animals the horse is most susceptible to the disease, followed by sheep and goats in order. Cattle are only slightly susceptible, although they may develop the disease upon artificial inoculation. Dogs and cats are seldom affected. Among the laboratory animals guinea pigs and mice are extremely susceptible, but rats and rabbits require larger amounts of material. The hen is quite refractory.

The prevalance of the disease in man varies in different localities according to the contamination of the soil with tetanus spores. For instance the Hudson River Valley and Long Island have shown a much higher incidence than other parts of the country—a fact that coincided with the contamination of the soil.

The nature of the wound influences the development of the tetanus organism. Puncture wounds such as those caused by stepping on a nail are bad. Wounds infected with other organisms, such as the Welch bacillus, favor the development of the tetanus bacillus.

GAS GANGRENE

Gas gangrene in man is caused by the invasion into injured tissues of certain anaerobic spore-forming organisms belonging to the group of which the Welch bacillus is a member. These organisms are frequently found in the intestinal canal of normal animals, where they lead a saphrophytic existence.

A large number of anaerobic spore-forming bacilli have been described as the cause of gas gangrene. In some instances, different names have been used for the same organism; at other times the organism was only an incidental invader and was not responsible for the gangrenous condition. Reed and Orr listed twenty-one members of the group associated with the disease.

Clostridium septicum (Vibrion septique, Clostridium edemitismaligni) was discovered by Pasteur in 1877 associated with the infections of animals which were supposed to have died of anthrax. Koch and Gaffkey later isolated the organism and studied it carefully. It is considered that Bacillus III of von Hibler and the bacillus of Gohn and Sachs are identical with it. The bacillus is 0.8 to 1.0 μ

broad by 2 to 10 μ or more long, occurring principally in long chains. The spores are oval and excentric, and are very resistant. The bacillus is motile and does not form a capsule. It produces a powerful exotoxin.

Clostridium perfringens (Clostridium welchii, Bacillus aerogenes capsulatus, Bacillus phlegmonis emphysematosae) is the Welch bacillus, isolated by Welch and Nuttall in 1892, in an autopsy of a cadaver which showed gas bubbles in the blood vessels.

Six toxicogenic types have been encountered and it is entirely possible others will be added.

Type A. The organism is found in the normal ileum and colon of man (where it produces no toxin). It causes many human infections (gas gangrene) when entering the broken skin. In animals, it causes death in suckling lambs (McGowan *et al.*, 1958) and in calves.

Type B. Associated with lamb dysentery; found occasionally in enterotoxemia of calves.

Type C. Cause of "struck" in sheep, produces enteritis in young pigs (Field *et al.*) and enterotoxemia in calves (Grimer *et al.*, 1956).

Type D. Associated with enterotoxemia of sheep and lambs; probably also cause of enterotoxemia of calves and goats.

Type E. Cause of dysentery in lambs and calves.

Type F. Cause of necrotic inflamation of the small intestine in men with high mortality rate (Zeissler *et al.*). Organism produces much beta toxin.

Besides certain cultural differences, all six types produce powerful toxins which are distinct from each other. The antitoxins of each type will neutralize the toxin of some of the other types.

Morphologically, all types are similar. They are 1.0 to 1.5μ wide by 4.0 to 8.0 μ long. They occur singly or in pairs and occasionally in long threads or chains. Capsules are present on specimens taken directly from the animal body. They are non-motile. Spores when present are oval, central or excentric; very often specimens from the animal body will not show spores, however.

Clostridium novyi (Clostridium edematiens) was isolated in 1894 by Novy from a guinea pig. Weinberg and Seguin described it as a new species when they isolated it from a human case during the First World War. It is 0.8 by 1.0 broad and 4 to 5 μ long, with rounded ends, occurring singly or in pairs and is somewhat motile. It is a strict anaerobe growing with great difficulty and forming abundant central or subterminal spores. It produces an active soluble toxin which is virulent for all laboratory animals.

All these organisms are found in the soil. Normal animals carry most of them in the intestine. *Clostridium perfringens,* type A, seems to be especially widespread. Taylor and Gordon and others have found it in the intestinal canal of normal cattle, sheep, pigs, dogs, cats, rabbits, guinea pigs, poultry and man. Maes demonstrated that woolen cloth carried large numbers of anaerobic, spore-forming gas-producing bacilli morphologically resembling the *Clostridium* group.

Altemier and Furst collected dust from major street intersections in Cincinnati, Ohio, all of which contained viable *Clostridium welchii.* They quote the experience of Endo who found the dust on a battleship to be contaminated with pathogenic clostridia in 48 per cent to 59 per cent of the samples.

Wound infections of animals with members of the gas gangrene group are known as malignant edema. The horse is most susceptible, the affection appearing as a complication of surgical or accidental wounds. Sheep are often affected after castration or wounds inflicted while shearing. Cattle are not as susceptible to the disease but occasionally develop it following parturition. Dogs are sometimes infected through wounds inflicted while fighting. Guinea pigs, rabbits, mice, etc., are very susceptible to infection of any of these organisms. The affection in animals is characterized by a hot painful, crepitating swelling at the point of inoculation. The outcome is usually fatal. Large numbers of gas bubbles are found on post mortem examination in the subcutaneous tissue surrounding the point of infection. *Cl. novyi* causes "black disease" in sheep in various countries of the world. The sheep liver fluke is probably responsible for the spread of the disease.

Infection by ingestion causes serious damage in sheep and lambs. *Cl. septicum* produces a disease known as "braxy" or "bradsot" in the Scandinavian countries. *Cl. perfringrens,* type B, causes lamb dysentery in the British Isles and northwestern United States. The toxin forms in the intestine. "Struck" is caused by type C of this organism. It is found in England and Wales. Enterotoxemia is a condition of sheep caused by *Cl. perfringens, type D.* It occurs in the United States, Australia and Wales.

Gas gangrene in man is a war-time affliction. Soils heavily fertilized with animal or human excreta contain numerous spores of the offending organisms with which gunshot wounds become contaminated. The depth of the wound as well as the introduction of other organisms influence the extent of the resulting edema. The site of the wound influences to some extent the chances of infection. The buttock and the thigh are more apt to show gas gangrene, when wounded, than other parts of the body. (Maes)

Reports of gas gangrene infections are increasing in civil life, whether actually or from better diagnosis it is difficult to state. Ghormley found that compound fractures produced the largest number of cases of this trouble. Reeves experienced most cases in patients past fifty years of age who were constitutionally below normal, especially those with circulatory failure, arteriosclerosis, thromboangitis obliterans, and diabetes mellitus. Silver reported four cases following intestinal perforation. Koons and Boyden called attention to the potential hazard of gas gangrene in parenteral medication, citing a case following the injection of epinephrine. Roberts and Bassett noted the necessity of early excision of devitalized tissue followed by open treatment of the wound. Wilson noted *Clostridium welchii* in the wounds of sixty-three patients who had received surgical treatment or had been admitted to the hospital for burns or traumatic injuries.

BOTULISM

Botulism is an acute toxemia caused by the toxin of one of the botulinum group of bacteria. The toxin is usually ingested in foods in which this organism has grown.

The first case of botulism to be recorded, according to Dickson occurred in 1735. The disease was given its name by Müllen in 1870, because meat products were supposed to be responsible, hence botulism from the Latin botulus, sausage. Numerous cases and outbreaks occurred in the years that followed, but little was added to the knowledge of the disease. In 1895 van Ermengen studied an outbreak involving thirty-four cases and three deaths. The causative agent was isolated from a ham which the patients had eaten, and was named *Bacillus botulinus*.

There are a number of different organisms, closely related, which cause botulism. Bengston divided them into five types.

Type A. Cause of most American outbreaks from canned foods.

Type B. Cause of a few American outbreaks.

Type C. No human outbreaks. Cause of outbreaks in wild aquatic birds.

Type D. No human outbreaks. Low toxicity for man.

Type E. Cause of a few human outbreaks.

Breed et al. classify the organisms into two groups. *Clostridium botulinum* includes types C, D, and E. They are non-proteolytic. Meyer and Gunnison found fifteen sub-types in this group on the basis of toxicity, agglutination and fermentation. *Clostridium parabotulinum* includes types A and B. They are proteolytic and grow more easily than other types. They are apparently more common in the United States and hence are the cause of more outbreaks of food poisoning.

The toxin formed by the organisms under suitable conditions of anaerobiosis and non-acidity, is one of the most powerful poisons known.

The spores are very resistant to heat. One strain was reported by Easton and Meyer to withstand 212° F. for 330 minutes. Such heat resistance is of significance in food preservation by canning.

The spores are widely distributed in nature. Since the organisms are strict anaerobes, they probably grow symbiotically in soil with aerobes. In view of the wide distribution in nature, the organisms would be expected to be present occasionally in intestinal tracts of man and animals. Dickson and Burke isolated them from the feces of a hog and Easton and Meyer from the feces of three hogs and two cattle. Tanner and Dick isolated them from two of ten specimens of feces from normal individuals. This does not necessarily mean that man is a carrier of the spores but that the organisms may enter and pass through the intestinal tract should they happen to be on green food. The organisms were also found in tannery waste sludge by Greer.

Horses develop botulism from eating moldy or spoiled hay, corn or other feed in which botulism toxin has been produced. The disease is manifested by loss of muscular control, sometimes called "blindstaggers." Bacteriologic confirmation is often lacking, however, and no accurate figures are available on the extent of the disease.

Cattle are rather infrequently infected, although outbreaks have been reported by Graham and Schwarze and others. Spoiled hay and other feed in which the toxin has developed is usually the cause. The disease has been described in cattle in France by Rossi and Vigel, with symptoms in the bovine similar to those occurring in man.

Hogs, sheep and dogs show a marked resistance to botulism and do not develop the disease from natural causes. Goats, however, are susceptible. Among the laboratory animals cats, rabbits, guinea pigs, and mice are extremely susceptible to subcutaneous injections of the toxin; white rats, frogs, and fishes are almost completely resistant.

Various birds are afflicted with botulism. The crop of the bird is supposed to act as an incubator, allowing the ingested *Cl. botulinum* to produce toxin. One cause of limber-neck in chickens is toxin of *Cl. botulinum* type C. Remnants of foods which have caused illness and death among human beings have frequently caused limber-neck and death when thrown to chickens. Such outbreaks among fowls are not uncommon. Two outbreaks occurred in 1910 with 103 outbreaks during the next ten years. In twenty-two instances, the outbreaks in chickens were caused by careless disposition of food which had caused human outbreaks and to which the chickens had access.

Botulism in wild ducks has been described by Quortrup and Holt. In shallow waters which serve as feeding grounds for these birds, the vegetation produces an oxygen-deficient condition which is ideal for the production of botulinum toxin. *Cl. botulinum* type C is the causative agent.

Fish carry *Clostridium botulinum* Type E. Among seven outbreaks in man in the United States where type E was identified, five were associated with fish and one with a whale, according to Meyer. Fish-borne botulism in man in Russia and Germany is more common.

Meyer and Eddie have collected figures on 483 outbreaks of botulism in the United States in man, all traced to food. Home canned food products are the most serious offenders. There also have been several reports of botulism from wound infections. Among three fatal cases Type A was isolated from the wounds of two cases, (Davis et al., Thomas et al.) and type B from one case (Hampson). Hall however, isolated Type A from two wound cases and Type B from one case where no symptoms of botulism appeared, and the patients recovered.

ITEMS OF NOTE

1) Animals may carry in their intestinal tracts, usually without apparent harm to themselves, the spores of several disease producing organisms.

2) The tetanus organism finds its natural habitat in the intestine of herbivorous animals (horse and cow). The spores contained in contaminated soil and dust are responsible for the disease when they enter the broken skin.

3) Gas gangrene organisms are found in the intestines of many animals, infection in man resulting from the introduction of the spores through the broken skin.

4) Botulinum spores are present in the intestinal tract of certain animals, as well as being widely distributed elsewhere in nature. Botulism is caused in man and animals by the ingestion of food in which the organisms have produced toxin, or by wound infections.

BIBLIOGRAPHY

ALTMEIER, W. A. and FURATE, W. L.: *Int. Abs. Surg., 84:*507-523, 1947.
BAUER, J. H. and MEYER, K. F.: *Infect. Dis., 38:*295-305, 1926.
BENGSTON, IDA: *Hygienic Laboratory Bull., 136:*1-96, March 1924.
BREED, R. S., MURRAY, E. G. D. and SMITH, N. R.: *Bergey's Manual of Determinative Bacteriology,* 6th edition. Baltimore, Williams and Wilkins, 1957.
DAVIS, J. B., MATTMAN, L. H. and WILEY, M.: *J.A.M.A., 133:*255-263, 1951.
DICKSON, ERNEST C.: *Rockefeller Inst. Med. Research, monograph, 8:*1-117, 1918.
EASTON, E. J. and MEYER, K. F.: *J. Infect. Dis., 35:*207-212, 1924.
GHORMLEY, R. K.: *Proc. Staff Meet., Mayo Clin., 10:*312-314, 1935.
GILLES, E. C.: *J.A.M.A., 109:*484-486, 1937.
GREER, F. E.: *Am. J. Pub. Health, 15:*860-867, 1925.
GRIMER, L. A. and BRACKEN, F. K.: *J.A.V.M.A., 122:*99-102, 1953.
GRIMER, L. A. and JOHNSON, H. W.: *J.A.V.M.A., 125:*127-129, 1954.
HALL, I. C.: *J. Bact., 50:*213, 1945.
HAMPSON, C. R.: *J. Bact., 61:*647, 1951.
KOONS, T. A. and BOYDEN, G. M.: *J.A.M.A., 175:*46-47, 1961.
LANGLEY, F. H. and WINKELSTEIN, L. B.: *J.A.M.A., 128:*783, 1945.
MAES, URBAN: *Arch. Surg., 41:*393-402, 1940.
McCOY, G. W.: *Pub. Health Rep., 32:*219, 1958.
McGOWAN, B., MOULTON, J. E. and ROOD, S. E.: *J.A.V.M.A., 133:*219, 1958.
MEYER, K. F. and EDDIE, B.: *Zeitschr Hyg., 133:*255-263, 1951.
NINNI, C.: *J.A.M.A., 76:*1617, 1921.
NOBLE, W.: *J. Infect. Dis., 16:*132, 1915.
PIZZINI: *Baumgartens Jahresbericht, 16:*236, 1894.
QUORTRUP, E. R. and HOLT, A. L.: *J. Bact., 41:*363, 1941.
REEVES, J. R.: *J.A.M.A., 104:*526-529, 1935.
ROBERTS, J. M. and BASSETT, F. H. III: *J.A.M.A., 177:*148-149, 1961.

ROE, A. L. and EDGAR, G.: *Australian Vet. J.*, *12*:212-220, 1936.

SILVER, M. D.: *Canad. M. A. J.*, *84*:1418, 1961.

TAYLOR, A. W. and GORDON, W. S.: *J. Path. & Bact.*, *50*:271-277, 1940.

TENBROECK, C. and BAUER, J. H.: *J. Exper. Med.*, *36*:261, 1922.

THOMAS, C. G., KELCHER, M. F. and McKEE, A. P.: *Arch. Path.*, *51*:623, 1951.

TULLOCH, W. J.: *J. Hyg.*, *18*:102-203, 1919.

VAN DER REIS, V.: *Ergebn. inn. Med. Kinderlk.*, *27*:77, 1925.

VAN ERMENGEN, E.: *Zeitschr. Hyg.*, *26*:1-56, 1897.

WILSON, T. S.: *Canad. J. Surg.*, *4:* Oct. 1960.

ZEISSLER, J. and ROSSFELD—STERNBERG, L.: *Brit. M. J.*, *1*:267-269, 1949.

Chapter 43

THE ROLE OF DIFFERENT ANIMALS AND BIRDS IN DISEASES TRANSMITTED TO MAN

Thomas G. Hull, Ph.D.

THE PROGRESS of man, from cave-shelter to pent-house, has been influenced constantly by animals. It is human nature to take credit for all desirable attainments, to refuse responsibility for the undesirable. Man can pride himself therefore on the wisdom of his ancestors, going back as far as the "stoneage," who brought under domestication various animals. But for that, he would be living under conditions which he passed some thousands of years ago, for no people have advanced very far who have not made use of domestic animals. Because of that, his ascent from a savage state was hastened —he was assured both bountiful larder and plentiful labor; the excess food supply not required for home use was a source of barter and the emancipation from the heaviest burdens of labor allowed time and energy for trade, commerce and travel. That was only the beginning, however. Animals proceeded to change the frontiers of nations, to crown and uncrown kings, to dictate religious practices and to cause many a diplomatic headache; they have left a mark on architecture, on landscapes, on styles of clothes; they have sent to death untold millions of people and have saved from death other millions.

THE HORSE

The family *Equidae* of the *Perissodactyla* (odd-toed hoofed mammals) includes some of the most useful of mammals, and among them, the horse and its allies (mule, donkey) lead the rest.

The horse was domesticated at a relatively recent date, but it immediately took a leading role in the destinies of mankind. No other animal has so fired the imagination. There have been demon horses, angel horses, ghost horses, witch horses, fairy horses, sun horses, moon horses, wind horses, sea horses, night horses and headless horses. The centaur of the early Greeks, that weird combination of a horse with a man's body at its head, resulted from impressions formed by the first encounters of Greek worriors with an enemy mounted on horses. The American Indians also believed that horse and rider were one being when they first met mounted Spanish soldiers. Horses have been worshipped in various lands. The Trojan horse was accepted by the people of Troy because they thought the Greeks had built it as a peace offering to the Goddess Athena.

The horse has left a more complete record over the earth, for a longer period of time than any other of the domestic animals. Some millions of years ago it was a dog-like creature with five toes. Fossil remains would indicate that it roamed pretty well over the earth, including America. By the time that man took his place in the scheme of things, perhaps a hundred thousand years ago, it had reached its final state of development, the "equus" form that we know today. Its range by then was confined to the plains of Asia, north of the Caspian sea and eastward to Mongolia. Primitive man used the horse only as a source of food supply. In the late stone-age period, about 25,000 year ago, horses must have been quite plentiful, for one camp-site of less than two acres in France has shown the bones of more than eighty thousand horses. Through the centuries that followed, drawings of horses were made on the walls of caves, but always indicating the animal in a wild state. The strength, the speed and the sagacity of the beast made it difficult to capture and domesticate.

The period known as civilization was ushered in as a "horseless" age. Babylonia in all its wisdom owned no horses; Egypt had no horses with which to build the pyramids and none for several hundred years to come; the Arabs did not use horses until after the Christian era. Horses were first introduced as servants of man by the wild tribes living in the hills of Persia. About 4,000 years ago these tribes descended to the plains of Mesopotamia raiding the settlements and driving out the Sumerians and Babylonians. The progress of the invaders was greatly facilitated by the "asses of the east," so-called by the dismayed Babylonians.

The horse has held a significant place in military operations. At first it was used to draw war-chariots, for it was a small animal. By

750 B.C. breeds had been developed large enough to carry riders. As time went on, horses made it possible for armies to carry with them food supplies, ammunition and even heavy cannon which otherwise would have been left behind.

The horse has had an even more important part to play in the development of civilization from a non-military standpoint. The wagons of commerce, the carriages of society, the messengers of mercy and love all depended upon the horse, man's faithful servant and friend. The flesh of the horse has been used for food by various nations and the hide makes excellent leather.

The horse is an intelligent animal and his friendship for man has often been close. It is usually a docile beast, but it may be easily frightened, and careless or incompetent persons were often kicked or bitten in times past. The run-away horse hitched to a wagon was especially dangerous. It has been estimated that, for miles traveled, there were more fatal accidents with horses in former days than with motor cars today. (There are no comparative statistics.) In fact, the horse was called "the most dangerous animal."

The number of horses has been steadily diminishing during the past forty years. In 1918, there were in the United States 21,550,000 such animals, with 15,270,000 in 1927, and 10,444,000 in 1940. The number of mules has likewise decreased. In 1950, horses and mules together numbered 7,781,000 compared to a total in 1960 of 3,089,-000. It is expected that draft animals will continue to decrease in numbers but light horses and pleasure ponies will probably increase to some extent.

The control of contagion in horses has been made easier not only by their lessened numbers, but by their disappearance from city streets. The animals that are left lead lives more or less isolated and hence have less opportunity than in previous times for contracting diseases from each other (Table 75).

Several virus diseases inflict the horse, although other animals are usually more important in human contagion. The arthropod-borne encephalitedes were formerly attributed to the horse, such as western equine encephalomyelitis, eastern equine encephalomyelitis and Venezuelan equine encephalomyelitis. It was discovered, however, that the horse was not the true host of the virus but an accidental victim. Antibodies of Murray Valley encephalitis and California encephalitis have been found in horses, but the disease may be in-

TABLE 75

DISEASES TRANSMITTED FROM HORSE TO MAN

Virus Diseases

Athropod-borne viral encephalitides
  Eastern encephalitis
  Murray Valley encephalitis
  Western encephalitis
  Venezuelan encephalitis
Equine infectious anemia
Rabies
Vesicular stomatitis

Bacterial Diseases

Anthrax
Brucellosis, *Br. abortus, Br. suis*
Glanders
Hemorrhagic septicemia
Listeriosis
Meliodosis
Tetanus
Tuberculosis, bovine type
Tularemia

Spirochetal Diseases

Endemic relapsing fevers
Leptospirosis

Fungous Diseases

Actinomycosis
Aspergillosis
Blastomycosis
Coccidioidomycosis
Cryptococcosis
Cutaneous streptothricosis
Epizootic lymphangitis
Histoplasmosis
Nocardiosis
Rhinosporidiosis
Ringworm
Sporotrichosis

Protozoan Diseases

Sarcocystitis
Trypanosomiasis

Trematode Diseases

Schistosomiasis, *Schistosoma japonicum*

Arthropod Diseases

Mange, *Sarcoptes* sp.
Ox bot

---

apparent. The horse can be infected with Japanese B encephalitis experimentally but probably plays no part in perpetrating the disease. Equine infectious anemia is found only in horses, mules and donkeys. Rabies infects the horse, but less than two score such cases are reported annually (in 1959 there were 22 rabid horses reported).

The horse suffers from vesicular stomatitis, along with many other animals.

Anthrax is sometimes communicated to man from infected hides or horse hair used in shaving brushes, but such cases are not numerous. Brucellosis (cow and hog strain of the organism) is found in horses, but other animals are more important sources of human infection. Glanders, for all practicel purposes, has been eliminated in the United States and Canada, and closely related melioidosis is rare. There has been a suspicion that influenza found in horses may be in some way related to influenza in man. There have been a few cases of listeriosis, tularemia and hemorrhagic septicemia in horses, along with other animals which are more important in the epidemiology of these diseases. The *Salmonella* group of organisms are found in a wide range of animals and birds and a few human cases have been reported from the consumption of horse meat. The horse is supposed to be immune to swine erysiplas, but human infections have occurred from this source. The horse is susceptible to bovine tuberculosis, but not to human or avian strains. The tetanus organism finds a natural habitat in the intestine of the horse, without apparent harm to the animal.

Two of the spirochetal diseases found in horses are communicated to man. Leptospirosis is occasionally transmitted by both the horse and donkey. The horse is host to both the spirochetes of endemic relapsing fever and the ticks that transmit the disease, but wild rodents and birds are more important.

The horse shares with other animals a dozen fungus infections which from time to time have been transmitted to man. Among the more important ones are actinomycosis, coccioidomycosis, cryptomycosis, histoplasmosis, ringworm of several varieties and sporatrichosis. The horse, mule and donkey alone are afflicted with *Histoplasma farciminosum* causing epizootic lymphangitis. Aspergilliosis, cutaneous streptococcosis, norcardiosis and rhinosporidiasis are of less concern to man, but many human cases do occur. A single case only of blastomycosis in the horse is on record.

Horses suffer from a variety of animal parasites, few of which are of significance to man. *Sarcocystis,* a protozoa of cosmopolitan distribution, is common but with few human cases. African trypanosomiasis, carried by the tsetse fly, is found only in Africa. *Schistosoma japonicum* is occasionally found in the horse in the Orient.

The mange mite, *Sarcoptes,* is carried by the horse, as well as ox-bot, from which source man may be afflicted.

THE COW

The *Artrodactyla,* even-toed hoofed animals, includes several important families of domesticated animals of which cattle are the most numerous.

The number of cattle in the United States has been increasing over the years. In 1960, the total number of cattle and calves was 101,520,000 of which 21,331,000 were dairy animals. In 1920, the figures were 66,639,556 total of which 31,361,456 were dairy animals. The number of dairy animals fell in forty years from 47 to 21 per cent of the total.

More than two score diseases may be transmitted from the cow to man (Table 76).

TABLE 76

DISEASES TRANSMITTED FROM COW TO MAN

Virus Diseases

Arthropod-borne viral encephalitides
   California encephalitis
   Louping ill
   Rift Valley fever
Foot-and-mouth disease
Milkers nodules
Rabies

Rickettsial Diseases

Q fever

Bacterial Diseases

Anthrax
Brucellosis, *Br. abortu, Br. suis, Br.*
  melitensis
Diphtheria
Haverhill fever
Hemorrhagic septicemia
Listeriosis
Melioidosis
Salmonellosis
Scarlet fever
Septic sore throat
Staphylococcus infection
Tuberculosis, bovine type
Tularemia
Vibriosis

Spirochetal Diseases

Endemic relapsing fevers
Leptospirosis

TABLE 76—(*cont'd.*)

Fungous Diseases

Actinonomycosis
Aspergillosis
Coccidioidomycosis
Cryptococcosis
Cutaneous streptothricosis
Histoplasmosis
Nocardiosis
Rhinosporidosis
Ringworm
Sporotrichosis

Protozoan Diseases

Sarcocystis
Toxoplasmosis
Trypanosomiasis (Africian)

Nematode Diseases

Gongylonemiasis
Larva migrans
Metastrongyliasis
Ostertagia infection
Sheep wireworm infection
Syngamosis
Trichostrongylosis

Cestode Diseases

Echniococcosis (hydatid disease)
Taeniasis (beef tapeworm infection)

Trematode Diseases

Fascioliasis
Schistosomiasis, *Sch. bovis*
Schistosomiasis, *Sch. japonicum*

Arthropod Diseases

Mange (*Sarcoptes* species)
Ox bot

Chemical Poisonings

Anthelmintics
Antibiotics
Insecticides
Milk sickness
Radioactive isotopes
Sulfonamides

Several of the virus diseases are of importance. Cowpox is contracted directly from the cow, but in the United States the disease is rare except as the virus may be propogated for vaccine to be used in smallpox immunization. Sometimes cows are infected with cowpox by persons recently vaccinated and pass the infection back to susceptible persons. The virus of smallpox is infective for cattle, but it is so modified by animal passage that it never again produces smallpox in man. Milkers nodules occur in persons who have been associated with cows suffering from this infection. Rabies is a serious disease (in 1960, 700 rabid cattle were reported). Rabies virus is present in the milk several days before symptoms appear in the cow, but human infections from this same source are rare. Foot-and-mouth disease is seldom transmitted to man, but the closely related disease of vesicular stomatitis causes human infections. The arthropod-borne viral encephalitides, especially California encephalitis, louping ill and Rift Valley fever, are found in the cow, but other animal hosts may be more important in the infection of man.

Q fever is the only rickettsial disease from which cattle suffer. Slaughter house workers are especially liable to infection.

Brucellosis is the most serious of the bacterial diseases which man may contract from the cow, all three types of the organism being implicated. Bovine tuberculosis, once so common, has been reduced but not eliminated in the United States. Salmonellosis may be contracted by man from eating infected meat. Melioidosis is occasionally found in the cow. Anthrax in man may arise from handling infected hides. Other bacterial diseases which are sometimes passed from cow to man include listeriosis, hemorrhagic septicemia, tularemia and vibrio abortion. The human diseases of diphtheria, scarlet fever and septic sore throat, which the cow may contract from man, are an ever present threat, but no milk-borne epidemics have been reported for several years. Staphylococci may cause a gastroenteritis in man from milk contaminated with this organism. The cow is sometimes infected by man, passing the infection back to him. A few epidemics of Haverhill fever (rat-bite fever) have been traced to cows milk, but it is not known whether the cow was responsible or the milk contaminated by rats. The cow carries in its intestine the spore-forming organisms of botulism, gas-gangrene and tetanus which occasionally cause an infection in man.

The spirochetal diseases which the cow may transmit to man are few. Leptospirosis, a very serious disease in cattle, is widespread. The spirochetes of endemic relapsing fever have been recovered from the cow, but other animals are probably more important in human infections.

The fungus diseases found in the cow are also found in a variety of other animals. Human infection is usually by contact, the milk apparently not being a serious factor in the epidemiology of these diseases. Among ten fungus diseases, actinomycosis is the most common in the cow, but a variety of *Trichophyton* and *Microsporum,* causing ringworm in man are also found. The other diseases in this group are listed in Table 76.

Three protozoan diseases may infect the cow, none of which are of importance to man in the United States. Sarcocystis is a cosmopolitan parasite frequently found in cattle. Toxoplasmosis is occasionally found in the cow but other animals are more important in the spread of the disease. African trypansomiasis is found only in Africa.

The nematodes (round worms) cause a variety of difficulties, few of which are of importance in cattle in the United States. Tricho-strongylosis and ostertagia infection are encountered more often in Asia and Africa. Gongylonemiasis is occasionally found in the United States. Syngamosis is present in the upper respiratory tract of cattle in certain tropical areas, and man is sometimes infected. The sheep wireworm, *Haemonchus contortus* is found in cattle also. Larva migrans (creeping eruption) of the bovine type is a hookworm of cattle occasionally causing trouble in man.

Two tapeworms among the cestodes are of importance. The beef tapeworm, *Taenia saginata,* is not uncommon in the United States, man being infected by eating insufficiently cooked beef. The related hydatid worm *Echinococcus granulosus* is found in the cow but the dog is a more important factor for the disease in man.

The trematodes (flukes) which may infect man are seldom en-countered in cattle in the United States. Elsewhere several species of *Schistosoma* are carried by cattle, among other animals. Fascioliasis includes the sheep liver fluke, *Fasciola hepatica,* which is harbored occasionally by the cow; only one case of human infection has been reported in the United States. *Fasciola giganticum* the giant cattle liver fluke is widespread and sometimes found in man.

Two arthropods carried by cattle cause trouble in man. One is the mange mite, *Sarcoptes* species, infecting a variety of animals, causes a dermatitis in man. The other is the bot-fly *Hypoderma bovis,* which deposits its eggs or larvae on the skin.

Certain chemicals are imbibed or absorbed by cows and located in the tissues or are secreted in the milk. Milk sickness occurs when the cow eats white snake root, passing the poison trematol in the milk. Chemicals used in the control of pests have created problems with their residues being found in the milk or meat. Sulfonamides, antibiotics and anthelmintics are likewise stored in the muscles or secreted in the milk. Radioactive isotopes, either absorbed or imbibed from contaminated plants, are stored in the tissue of cattle and may be dangerous for man. It has been said however, that "if you can lead a steer to slaughter after the bomb falls, you can eat him," because external radiation probably will kill farm animals before the effects of eating radioactive forage affects their health. Processes have also been developed by the dairy industry to remove from milk as much as 98 per cent of radioactive strontium present from contaminated plants which cows might eat.

THE HOG

Domesticated swine (Family *Suidae,* Order *Artiodactyla*) are important in the human economy. In 1960, in the United States, there were 58,464,000 hogs of all ages, which is about the same number for the past several decades.

Swine have been used for food since early times. In Turkestan, bones of swine were found in camp litter, dating about 6000 B.C.: in China swine were supposed to have been domesticated in 3468 B.C.

Hogs do not have the intimate contact of the home in the United States that they do in some countries, hence the opportunity to transmit infection (as well as to contract it from the household) is lessened. Furthermore, the relatively short life of the pig before it is slaughtered, lessens the opportunity for it to develop many diseases. The hog, however, is an omniverous animal, eating almost anything that it encounters, including rats. Hence they are responsible for a considerable numbers of human diseases. (Table 77).

Few instances of virus infections are attributed to swine. They may acquire encephalitis of the Western type and Japanese B type but are not important in the epidemiology of these diseases. They are susceptible to foot-and-mouth disease but human infections are doubtful. Influenza in swine has been suspected of being the source of influenza epidemics in man, but confirmation is lacking. Rabies is encountered less often than formerly, in 1960 only eight such cases being reported in hogs. Vesicular stomatitis is contracted by hogs along with other animals.

A dozen bacterial diseases are encountered in swine which are of importance to man. Anthrax is acquired usually by handling the hides and bristles. Brucellosis in hogs is usually due to *Brucella suis,*

TABLE 77

DISEASES TRANSMITTED FROM HOG TO MAN

Virus Diseases

Arthropod-borne viral encephalitides
   Murray Valley encephalitis
   Western encephalitis
Foot-and-mouth disease
Influenza (possibly)
Rabies
Vesicular stomatitis

Bacterial Diseases

Anthrax
Brucellosis, *Br. suis, Br. meliteusis.*
Gas gangrene
Hemorrhagic septicemia
Listeriosis
Melioidosis
Pseudotuberculosis
Salmonellosis
Swine erysipelas
Tuberculosis, avian type
Tuberculosis, bovine type
Tuberculosis, human type
Tularemia

Spirochetal Diseases

Leptospirosis (Swineherds disease)

Fungous Diseases

Actinomycosis
Aspergillosis
Coccidioidomycosis
Cryptococcosis
Histoplasmosis
Nocardiosis
Ringworm

Protozoan Diseases

Amebiasis, *Entomoeba polecki*
Ascariasis, porcine
Balantidiasis
Trypanosomiasis, Africian

Nematode Diseases

Gongylomiasis
Metastrongyliasis
Trichinosis

Cestode Diseases

Echniococcosis (Hydatid disease)
Taeniasis, porcine

Trematode Diseases

Fasciolopsiasis
Gastrodiscoides infection
  (amphistomiasis)
Gnathostomiasis, *Gnathostoma
  hispidum*
Paragonimiasis (Oriental lung fluke
  disease)

TABLE 77—(*cont'd.*)

Arthropod Diseases

Chigoe dermatitis

Chemicals

Anthelmintics
Antibotics
Insecticides
Radioactive isotopes
Sulfonamides

sometimes to *Brucella melitensis,* but not often to *Brucella abortus.* Listeriosis, melioidosis and pseudotuberculosis are all found in this animal. Many food infections due to *Salmonella* organisms have been traced to infected pork. The hog is one of the chief sources of swine erysipelas, but human infections may be acquired from other sources also. Human tuberculosis may be contracted by hogs from uncooked garbage, and the pork can be a menace to man. Tuberculous hogs are eliminated by inspection of slaughter houses under federal supervision, but numerous hogs are slaughtered on farms without inspection. The hog is susceptible to all three types of tuberculosis. Normal hogs carry the organism *Pasteurella multocida,* cause of hemorrhagic septicemia. Tularemia is occasionally encountered in hogs and human cases have resulted from hog-bite. The hog carries within its intestine, the spore forming organisms causing gas gangrene in man.

Leptospirosis in hogs, called swineherds diseases, is due to *Leptospira pomona.*

The hog is afflicted with surprisingly few fungus infections. Actinonomycosis and histoplasmosis are not uncommon, but coccidioidomycosis, aspergillosis and nocardiosis are encountered less often. Among the numerous fungi causing ringworm in man, the only one found in the hog is *Trichophyton mentagraphytes.*

The animal parasites found in the hog, because of the nature of the animal, are numerous. The several protozoan diseases include amebiasis *(Entamoeba polecki),* ascariasis of the porcine strain, balantidiasis and African trypanosomiasis.

Trichinosis is by far the most serious. This round worm has probably influenced the course of man's activities for thirty centuries, and was in part responsible for the ancient Jewish prohibition against pork. The hog shares with other animals gongylomiasis and metastrongyliasis.

Two tapeworms are of importance. *Taenia solium,* the pork tapeworm, is very common. *Echinococcus granulosus* causing echinococcosis or hydatid disease is often found in the hog, but the dog is more often implicated in human infection.

The several flukes found both in hog and man include fasciolopsiasis, gastrodiscoides infection, gnathostomiasis *(Gnathostoma hispidium)* and paragonimiasis *(Paragonimus westermani),* but none of them are of importance in the United States.

The chigoe (jigger flea, sand flea) infests the hog and causes a dermatitis in man.

The hog may absorb or imbibe some of the insecticides, sulfonamides, antibiotics, antihelmintis or radioactive isotopes and store them in the muscles. Pork is thus rendered dangerous for man.

THE SHEEP AND GOAT

Sheep and goat raising are among the oldest agricultural pursuits. Sheep furnish not only mutton, but wool and hides. Goats are prized in many regions for their milk, and they furnish meat and hides as well. Special breeds of these animals are often raised, such as karakul sheep for Persian lamb wool and Angora goats for mohair. The number of sheep in the United States in 1903 was reported as 64,000,000; the number had dwindled by 1960 to 29,481,000. Goat raising in the United States has never been extensive, the number of such animals in 1956 being 2,713,000.

Sheep and goats (Order *Artiodactyla,* family *Bovidae)* in relation to public health have less significance than some other animals, yet carry a considerable number of diseases (Table 78). Sore-mouth of sheep and goats (contagious ecythma) causes a few human infections, but foot-and-mouth disease is of small importance in man. Rabies is not uncommon (in 1959 only 8 rabid sheep were reported, compared to 164 in 1938). Sheep have been suspected of being responsible for human influenza but confirmation is lacking. Several of the arthropod encephalitides are found in sheep or goats. They are the chief hosts of louping ill in Scotland and England, the virus being carried in the milk as well as by ticks. Rift Valley fever is serious in sheep and goats in Africa, but wild rodents are probably the main

TABLE 78

DISEASES TRANSMITTED FROM SHEEP AND GOATS TO MAN

Virus Diseases

Arthropod-borne encephalitides
   Central European encephalitis
   Diphasic meningo-enchephalitis
   Louping ill
   Rift Valley fever
   Russian spring-summer cencphalitis
Foot-and-mouth disease
Influenza (suspected)
Rabies
Sore mouth of sheep and goats
   (contageous ecthyma)

Rickettsial Diseases

Q fever
Rocky Mountain spotted fever

Bacterial Diseases

Anthrax
Brucellosis, *Br. melitensis, Br. abortus,*
   Br. suis
Hemorrhagic septicemia
Listeriosis
Melioidosis
Plague
Pseudotuberculosis
Salmonellosis
Swine erysipelas
Tuberculosis, avian type (sheep)
Tuberculosis, bovine type
Tularemia
Vibriosis

Spirochetal Diseases

Leptospirosis

Fungous Diseases

Actinomycosis
Aspergillosis
Coccidioidomycosis
Cryptococcosis
Cutaneous streptothricosis
Histoplasmosis
Nocardiosis
Ringworm

Protozoan Diseases

Sarcocystiasis
Trypanosomiasis

Nematode Diseases

Metastrongyliasis
Ostertagia infection
Sheep wireworm infection
Syngamosis
Trichostrongylosis

Cestode Diseases

Echinococcois (hydatid disease)
   Echinococcus granulosus

TABLE 78—(*cont'd.*)

Trematide Diseases

Fascoioliasis
Schistosomiasis, *Schistosoma bovis*

Arthropod Diseases

Mange, *Sarcoptes species*
Ox bot, *Hypoderma bovis*
Sheep bot, *Oestrus ovia* conjunctivitis

Chemicals

Anthelmintics
Antibiotics
Insecticides
Radioactive isotopes
Sulfonamides

hosts. Russian spring-summer encephalitis, Central European encephalitis and diphasic meningoencephalitis infect sheep and goats but other animals and birds are more important.

The rickettsial diseases include Q fever and Rocky Mountain spotted fever, sheep and goats carrying the causative agents, but not being the chief hosts.

Several bacterial diseases are on the list. Anthrax is important and not uncommon. The goat is susceptible to brucellosis, especially *Brucella melitensis,* with sheep to a lesser extent. Other diseases include listeriosis and occasionally melioidosis, avian and bovine tuberculosis, hemorrhagic septicemia, swine erysipelas and *Salmonella* food infections. Sheep have been incriminated with plague, but the disease in them is rare. Vibriosis is a communicable disease of sheep, but human infections are rare. The Welch bacillus, causing gas gangrene in man, is a normal inhabitant in the intestines of sheep and goats. Goats are rather susceptible to bovine tuberculosis and in the past have caused trouble by passing the infection back to the cow, or infecting man directly through goats milk.

Leptospirosis is found in both the sheep and goat.

Sheep and goats are afflicted with various fungous infections, along with other animals. Actinomycosis occurs, but is rare, in both of them. Goats are hosts of nocardiosis, cryptococcosis, and cutaneous streptothricosis. Sheep have been found with coccidioidomycosis, histoplasmosis and, in young lambs aspergillosis. Ringworm due to *Microsporum canis* and *Trichophyton mentagrophytes* is carried by sheep while *Trichophyton verrucosum* is found in both animals.

Animal parasites are not of great importance to man from sheep and goats. Among the protozoan diseases are rare cases of sarcocystiasis and African trypanosomiasis. The nematode diseases include metastrongyliasis, ostertagia, syngamosis and trichostrongylosis. The only tapeworm in sheep and goats which might infect man is *Echinococcus granulosus*. The fluke diseases are fascioliasis and schistosomiasis *(Schistosoma bovis)*. Sheep and goats carry the mange mite and are subject to infestation with two bot flies causing sheep bot and ox bot. Animals that imbibe or absorb radio-active materials, insecticides, sulfonamides, antibiotics or antihelmintics will store the material in the muscles, or secrete them in the milk.

THE CAMEL

The camel, a representative of the *Artiodactyla* (Family *Camelidae*), was domesticated in very ancient times. These "ships of the desert" have been indispensable animals in certain desert regions of Asia and Africa, furnishing not only labor, but meat, milk, leather, hair for weaving and fuel for fires.

Camels were pronounced "unclean" by the Law of Moses and the eating of their flesh was forbidden. However, at the present time very few human infections can be attributed to them. They carry the hydatid worm causing echinococcosis but other animals are more important in transmitting the disease to man. Among the fungous diseases are sporotrichosis and ringworm *(Trichophyton verrucosum)*. Plague has been encountered in camels in Russia and elsewhere.

Other members of this family include the llama and the alpaca, long ago domesticated in South America. The llama furnishes labor, meat, milk and hair for the manufacture of cloth, while the alpaca is bred for its long wooly hair so useful in making blankets and other articles.

There is little information available on diseases which either of these animals contribute to mankind. The llama has been found afflicted with actinomycosis and coccidioidomycosis.

THE DOG

The carnivores—flesh eating animals—are a large group, most of which are wild. The family *Canidae* contains, besides the dog, the coyote, fox, wolf and jackal (see Wild Animals, page 907).

The dog was the first animal to become domesticated, probably some 60,000 years ago by savage cave-men, and for the same reason that the society matron of today owns a dog—namely, the desire of the human being for a pet. The early dogs were half-wild wolves or jackals, which developed rather rapidly through domestication and crossbreeding. They adapted themselves quite readily to purposes of economic usefulness. They were natural hunters, assisting in procurement of food supply; they were trained to protect other domestic animals, tending the flocks and herds in agricultural communities; they were hitched to harness, pulling wagon or sled, even as they do today; they were put into treadmills, turning the wheels of industry; they were sources of entertainment, baiting the bull and the bear or fighting with each other in the pit.

The American Indians owned dogs before the coming of the white man. The flesh of the dog in times past was used for food by the American Indians as well as by peoples in other parts of the world. To fulfill the requirements of the numerous activities assigned to dogs, different breeds have been established.

The number of dogs in the United States in 1957 was estimated at 25,000,000. Accurate figures are difficult to obtain, however, because some owners fail to register their animals. There are also dogs which can boast no master, but live on scraps of the street and the garbage pail, a menace not only to mankind, but to other dogs as well. The number of dogs in Great Britain was approximately 3,000,000 in 1961.

The dog enjoys a more intimate contact with man than any other animal, sharing not only his dwelling, but sometimes even his bed and his board. Candlin suggests that there is a correlation between the emotional manifestation of the dog and his owner. Many dogs become a mirror image of their masters emotions and if the master does not adjust well to society, neither does the dog.

Dogs have been a source of danger under some conditions. They have occasionally been a problem as sheep killers in rural areas. In 1961, it was estimated that more than 600,000 Americans were bitten by dogs annually. Very often this was because the animal was startled or irritated, or became excited in the course of play. Small children may gouge the eyes, pull the tail, try to ride piggyback or otherwise annoy a dog, and while the dog usually accepts these insults, sometime it retaliates. Persons who attempt to separate two

TABLE 79

Diseases Transmitted from Dog to Man

Virus Diseases

Lymphocytic choriomeningitis
Measles
Mumps
Rabies

Rickettsial Diseases

African tick fever
Boutonneuse fever
Brazilian typhus
Colombian typhus
Kenya typhus

Bacterial Diseases

Anthrax
Brucellosis, *Br. abortus*, *Br. melitensis*,
   Br. suis
Diphtheria
Gas gangrene
Hemorrhagic septicemia
Listeriosis
Melioidosis
Plague
Salmonellosis
Scarlet fever
Tuberculosis, bovine type
Tuberculosis, human type
Tularemia

Spirochetal Diseases

Leptospirosis
Rat-bite fever (sodoku)

Fungous Diseases

Actinomycosis
Blastomycosis
Coccidiodyomycosis
Cryptococcosis
Cutaneous streptothricosis
Histoplasmosis
Nocardiosis
Ringworm
Sporotrichichosis

Protozoan Diseases

Amebiasis
Leishmaniasis, Espundia
Leishmaniasis, Kala azar
Leishmaniasis, Oriental sore
Toxoplasmosis
Trypanosomiasis, American

Nematode Diseases

Ancylostomiasis
Dirofilaria infection (heatworm)
Dracontiasis
Gnathostomiasis
Larva migrans, filarial

TABLE 79—(*cont'd.*)

Nematode Diseases—(cont'd)

Larva migrans, cutaneous
Larva migrans, visceral
Strongylodiasis
Thelaziasis, *Th. californicus*
Thelaziasis, *Th. callipaeda*
Trichinosis

Cestode Diseases

Diphyllobothriasis
Dog tapeworm infection
Echinococcosis
Trematode Diseases
Clonorchiasis
Echinochasmus infection
Fasciolopsiasis
Heterophydiasis
Opisthorchiasis *Opis. felineus*
Opisthorchiasis *Opis. sinensis*
Opisthorchiasis *Opis, viverrini*
Paragonomiasis, *P. westermani*
Schistosomiasis, *Sch. japonicum*

Arthropod Diseases

Chigoe dermatitis
Dog mite dermatitis

fighting dogs may be turned upon by one or both animals and be severely injured.

Rabies has long been a serious affliction of the dog, but there are other animal hosts of the virus which perhaps are equally, if not more important, in the perpetuation of the disease. The dog is still the most usual source of rabies in man, but effective immunization has helped in its control. In the fifteen years from 1944 to 1959 the number of rabid dogs in the United States decreased from 9,067 to 1,124, while human cases of rabies fell from fifty-three to six per year. Lymphocytic choriomeningitis is another virus disease that occurs spontaneously in the dog, as well as other animals, but human infections are not numerous. The virus of measles and mumps may afflict the dog on occasion and such animals should be kept out of the room where a human case exists.

The dog is the chief host of the rickettsia which cause tick-borne Boutonneuse fever, Brazilian typhus, Colombian typhus and Kenya typhus in other parts of the world. This animal may also harbor ticks that cause Rocky Mountain spotted fever and Q fever in the United States, but it probably is not a factor in spreading these diseases.

Many of the bacterial diseases inflict the dog, but other animals are often more important in human infections. Dogs, however, are assuming an increasingly important place in the epidemiology of leptospirosis, especially the disease due to *Leptospira canicola* and *Leptospira icterohaemorrhagiae*. Other diseases from which dogs may suffer from time to time include anthrax, brucellosis *(abortus, melitensis* and *suis* types), hemorrhagic septicemia, listeriosis, salmonellosis, tularemia and the bovine type of tuberculosis. Dogs are susceptible to melioidosis and they have been known to pass plague bacilli directly to man.

Among human infections besides measles and mumps that may be acquired by the dog and passed back to man, are the human type of tuberculosis, diphtheria and scarlet fever. Dogs should not be allowed close contact, therefore, with persons suffering from those diseases. Dogs, as well as many other animals, harbor in their intestines *Clostridium* that causes gas gangrene in humans.

The dog shares with other animals responsibility for transmitting fungous diseases to man. Ringworm is the most common, the dog being afflicted with several of the organisms causing this disease -*Microsporum canis, M. distortum, M. cookii, Karatinomyces ajello, Trichophyton mentagrophytes* and occasionally *T. gallinae.* Blastomycosis is found chiefly in dogs, rarely in other animals. Histoplasmosis has been found in 38 per cent of dogs tested. Actinomycosis and cryptococcosis are rare but are sometimes found, sporotrichosis occurs sporadically, while nocardiosis, coccidioidomycosis and cutaneous streptothricosis are encountered from time to time.

Dogs are afflicted with a large number of animal parasites, more than a score of which infect man. Dogs are the chief host of *Leishmania* of both the cutaneous and visceral forms (oriental sore, espundia and kala azar). Amebiasis *(Entamoeba histolytica)* and American trypanosomias (Chagas disease) are both found in dogs in the United States, but other sources of human infection are more important. Toxoplasmosis is an affliction which the dog shares with many other animals.

The nematodes (round worms) are of interest. The dog is the chief host of organisms causing larva migrans (creeping eruption) of the cutaneous, filarral and visceral types. In southeastern United States the cutaneous type is caused by *Ancylostoma braziliense* which passes directly through the skin—hence dogs should be kept from bathing beaches where people go barefoot. A closely related organism, *Ancylostoma ceylonicum,* the dog hookworm, is occasionally found in man but is rare. Dirofilariasis (heartworm infection) and strongylodiasis are not uncommon in the United States. Trichinosis is acquired by dogs, but hogs are the source of the disease in man. Thelaziasis is rare in the United States and other nematodes—dracontiasis and gnathostomiasis—are not found there. There are three tapeworms *(Cestodes)* which are of interest. The dog tapeworm is acquired by man from dogs through swallowing infected fleas. The fish tapeworm comes from eating fish that were taken from lakes or streams contaminated by dog feces. Hydatid disease (echinococcosis) is acquired by man directly through swollowing the parasite eggs from dog feces.

The trematodes, or flukes, are not of great importance in the United States. Elsewhere in the world they infect dogs, incidently in the same manner as man is infected. Dogs are of importance, however, in passing the parasite back again to fish and crabs. The liver flukes *Clonorchis sinensis* and the several *Opisthorchis* group, as well as the intestinal flukes *Heterophyes heterophyes* and *Fasciolopsis buski* are acquired from eating infected fish, while the intestinal fluke *Echinostoma ilocanum* comes from the snail. The lung flukes *Paragonimus westermani* is carried by crayfish and crabs. The blood fluke *Schistosoma japonicum* passes directly through the skin from water in which it is swimming. The echinostamate fluke, *Echinochasmus perfoliatus,* is acquired by eating infected fresh water fish.

Two mites, the chigoe and the dog mite, infest the dog and cause a dermatitis in man.

THE HOUSE CAT

The cat family *(Felidae)* is one of the larger groups of carnivores, including the lion, tiger, leopard, jaguar, cheetah, mountain lion (congar, puma, panther) lynx, bob-cat and wild-cat, among others. The house cat is the only member of the family that has been domesticated to any extent.

The house cat has enjoyed an intimate contact with the human family for many centuries. The number of cats in the United States was estimated as 26,700,000 in 1957, slightly exceeding the number of dogs. It must be remembered, however, that most communities

TABLE 80

DISEASES TRANSMITTED FROM CAT TO MAN

Virsus Diseases

Cat scratch disease
Mumps
Rabies

Bacterial Diseases

Anthrax
Brucellosis (*Br. melitensis*)
Hemorrhagic septicemia
Melioidosis
Plague
Pseudotuberculosis
Salmonellosis
Tuberculosis, bovine type
Tularemia

Spirochetal Diseases

Leptospirosis
Rat-bite fever (Sodoku)

Fungous Diseases

Actinomycosis
Aspergillosis
Cryptococcosis
Histoplasmosis
Nocardiosis
Ringworm

Protozoan Diseases

Amebiasis
Toxoplasmosis
Trypanosomosis

Nematode Diseases

Ancylostmiasis (dog hookworm)
Brugia infection
Gnathostomiasis
Larva migrans, cutaneous
Larva migrans, filarial
Larva migrans, visceral
Thelaziasis
Trichinosis

Cestode Diseases

Diphyllobothriasis (fish tapeworm)
Taeniasis, canine (dog tapeworm)

Trematode Diseases

Clonorchiasis
Heterophydiasis
Opisthorchiasis, *Opisthorchis* sp.
Paragonomiasis
Schistosomiasis

Athropod Diseases

Dog mite dermatitis

have restrictive legislation concerning dogs while very few communities restrict cats in any manner. There are large numbers of cats that wander homelessly, due to prolific breeding and the mistaken sympathy of some persons in not destroying unwanted animals. In Great Britain the number of cats is estimated at six to twelve million, exceeding the number of dogs as pets two to four times.

The economic status of the house cat has long been a matter of discussion. The animal is independently selfish, usually placing its own comfort first, with allegiance to the family second. It catches some mice, but is not a natural "mouser." It catches very few rats, many cats being actually afraid of the house rat. It is a natural bird catcher, destroying several million birds in the United States every year. "On the whole it probably does at least as much harm as good, in the destruction of useful birds and otherwise" (Henderson and Craig).

Rabies, a widespread virus affliction, is not uncommon in cats. The reported incidence in 1959 in the United States was 310 which is about the yearly average during the previous twenty years. The rabid cat is a serious menace, especially to children. Catscratch disease is being recognized more and more frequently, caused either by the bite or the scratch of a cat. Mumps has been found in the cat occasionally and the animal should be excluded from the sickroom.

The cat is not important in the rickettsial diseases. The animal is susceptible to murine typhus fever, but the rat is the more important host, from which the cat may be infected. The cat also is infested with the mite which causes tsutsugamushi disease but field rats and mice are the important hosts.

Cats are fairly resistant to most bacterial diseases. Farm cats have contracted anthrax from feeding on infected carcasses. Brucella organisms (*Brucella melitensis*) have been isolated from the mesenteric glands of cats and the animals have given positive agglutination tests. Leptospirosis is acquired from contact with dogs or eating infected rodents, but the cat is not usually considered a factor in human infections. Spontaneous infection with plague is rare in the cat, but does occur occasionally, probably from eating infected rats. The organisms of rat-bite fever are carried mechanically on the teeth of cats which have fed on infected animals and human cases have been reported following cat-bite. Tularemia has been reported following a scratch by a cat with contaminated claws. A survey of 625 cats showed 3.0 per cent to be carriers of *Salmonella* organisms. Likewise normal cats are carriers of *Pasteurella multocida* and infect man by cat-bite. Melioidosis and pseudotuberculosis have been encountered in cats, but other animals are more important in the epidemiology of these diseases. On rare occasions cats have been found suffering from bovine tuberculosis, from infected meat or milk. The relation of diphtheria to cats is in doubt, but Simmons reported two cats from which he isolated diphtheria bacilli—probably cats should be prevented from contact with human cases of the disease.

Fungus infections in the cat are not uncommon, especially ringworm, *Microsporum canis, M. gypseum,* and *Trichophyton mentagrophytes* being the chief members of the group for this disease. The cat, along with other animals, is responsible for human infections with nocardiosis, cryptococcosis, aspergillosis, histoplamosis and a rare case of actinomycosis.

The protozoan parasite, *Entamoeba histolytica,* has been found in the cat, but other sources of human infection are more important. Toxoplasmosis is found in many animals of which the cat is one. American trypanosomiasis (Chagas' disease) is transmitted to the cat by the cone-nosed big *Triatoma.*

Larva migrans or creeping eruption is the most serious nematode disease found in the cat. The organism causing the cutaneous form, *Ancylostoma brazilliense,* passes directly through the skin. Cats therefore should be kept from bathing beaches where people go barefoot. The filarial form, caused by *Dirofilaria* species, is carried by a mosquito bite, while the visceral form is acquired by man through parasite eggs being in the feces of the cat. Another filarial worm acquired by the cat is *Brugia malayi.* Ancylostomiasis (*Ancylostoma ceylonicum*), the dog hookworm, is occasionally an affliction of the cat. *Gnathostoma spinigerum* and *Thelazia californiensis* are other round worms harbored by the cat. Trichinosis is acquired by the cat from eating infected pork, or perhaps an infected rat, but the cat is not considered an important factor in the spread of the disease.

Two tapeworms are of importance. The dog tapeworm (*Dipylidium caninum*) is acquired by man through swallowing a flea from the cat that is carrying the tapeworm egg. The fish tapeworm

(Diphylobothrium latum) is carried by the cat but man is infected through eating fish.

The trematodes, or flukes, which infect the cat are not found in the United States. Heterophydiasis (Egypt), clonorchiasis (Far East) and opisthorchiasis (Europe and Asia) are acquired by man from eating infected fish, and the cat acquires the disease in the same way, but may be a factor in passing the parasite back to the fish. The blood fluke, *Schistosoma japonicum,* (Orient), passes directly through the human skin. The Oriental lung fluke, *Paragonimus westermani,* is acquired by both man and cat from eating crayfish and crabs.

The dog mite is carried by the cat, causing a dermatitis in man.

THE RAT AND MOUSE

The rat and the mouse belong to the order *Rodentia*—gnawing animals. Among the more than 12,000 species of mammals the rodents are much the largest order, including in individuals more than all the other orders combined. Most rodents are prolific breeders. The house rat averages from three to six litters a year with an average of ten young to each litter. It has been estimated that, if all lived, at the end of three years the number of rats would total more than twenty million on a three-litter per annum basis and more than 350,000,000 million on a six-litter per annum basis. The house mouse with a gestation period of twenty-one days, might increase to more than a million at the end of a year. Fortunately there are limiting factors such as food supply, weather conditions and natural enemies which prevent these enormous increases. (For a discussion of other rodents, see Wild Animals, page 907.)

There are hundreds of different species of rats and mice in different parts of the world. Some are found in human dwellings and others in the field or forest. In different parts of the globe different types of house-rats are encountered, and in most countries more than one type is present. Their importance as disease-carriers varies according to the morphologic and biologic type.

The domestic rat—domestic in the sense that it makes its abode with man—is the most useless of all animals. There is nothing to say in its favor; there are numerous reasons why it should be exterminated. As a marauder it has taken heavy toll of farmer and merchant and householder; as a murderer it has destroyed millions of innocent

TABLE 81

DISEASES TRANSMITTED FROM RATS AND MICE TO MAN

Virus Diseases

Lymphocytic choriomeningitis
Rift Valley fever
Rabies

Rickettsial Diseases

Murine typhus fever
Rickettsialpox
Rocky Mountain spotted fever
Tsutsugamushi disease

Bacterial Diseases

Anthrax
Hemorrhagic septicemia
Melioidosis
Plague
Pseudotuberculosis
Rat-bite fever (Haverhill fever)
Salmonellosis
Swine erysipelas

Spirochetal Diseases

Endemic relapsing fevers
Leptospirosis
Rat-bite fever (sodoku)

Fungous Diseases

Adiaspiromycosis
Histoplasmosis
Sporotrichosis

Protozoan Diseases

Amebiasis, *Entamaeba histolytica*
Sacrocystiasis
Toxoplasmosis
Trypanosomiasis, American

Nematode Diseases

Trichinosis

Cestode Diseases

Dwarf tapeworm infection
Echinococcosis (hydatid disease)
Rat tapeworm infection

Trematode Diseases

Paragonimiasis (Oriental lung fluke
    disease)
Schistosomiasis, (*Sch. japonicum*)

Arthropod Diseases

Rat mite dermatitis (*Bdellonyssus
    bacoti*)

persons. Among the animals, it is man's public enemy number one. Rats were present in Europe in the Pliocene period, as indicated by fossil remains; the "lake dwellers" during the glacial period in Europe knew it; the Philistines made golden images of them; the Romans pictured them on coins; Greek, Roman and Etruscan works of art show them at various occupations, such as gnawing the ropes of ships or feeding on mussel beds; from Palestine and Italy ancient bronze and terra cotta works indicate the presence of rats.

The brown rat, *Rattus norvegicus,* also called the Norway rat, sewer rat, wharf rat, and barn rat, is supposed to be of Asiatic origin. It appeared in Europe early in the eighteenth century and reached North America about the time of the American Revolution, probably being brought from England as an accidental passenger (it is not a natural inhabitant of ships as are the black rat and the roof rat). It is now the most common species in the United States. It is larger and more ferocious than the black rat or roof rat and has driven out those species in many places. It has made its home in houses and farms in the country and in warehouses and about markets and wharfs in the city. It lacks ability to climb to any extent and lives in the ground, in excavations or under floors. It often uses the seweres in cities for highways, hence the name "sewer rat." It breeds prolifically, the female, after gestation period of twenty-one days, giving birth to a dozen or more young. From three to five litters a year occur, usually during the warm months of the year. Some females, however, may produce more litters, and it is not uncommon to find young rats in cold weather. It is a great traveler, migrating from building to building and from farm to farm. Sometimes these migrations include hundreds of rats traveling together.

The black rat or English rat, *Rattus rattus rattus,* has been known in Europe since the twelfth century. It appeared in North America in the sixteenth century, where it was the common rat among the early settlers. Later it was supplanted to a large degree by the more ferocious and more prolific brown rat. At the present time its range in this country is confined to certain areas in the southern states, where it finds a warmer climate more to its liking. The black rat is a great sea-traveler, breeding in the walls of cargo vessels. In some instances as many as 99.5 per cent of rats on a ship are black rats. It is a good climber and finds its habitat in the upper stories of buildings. The black rat was the cause of plague in the middle ages.

The roof rat or Alexandrian rat, *Rattus rattus alexandrinus,* was supposed to have originated in Egypt. It is closely related to the black rat, the chief difference being that of color (tawny black or gray). It is not numerous in the United States, but may be found in the semitropical portions of the southern states. Like the black rat, the roof rat is a great climber and often nests in trees. It may be found on ships also.

The common house mouse, *Mus musculus,* found its way to America with the earliest settlers. It has been able to hold its own with the brown rat because of its ability to escape into retreats too small for the rat to follow. The distinction between rats and mice is arbitrary, the main point of difference being size.

Field rats and field mice in the United States are numerous and are of importance from the economic standpoint in destroying crops. They are of lesser significance as far as disease is concerned, although potential sources of danger.

The number of rats in the United States was formerly estimated to equal the human population. Better control methods have reduced this ratio. Davis reported surveys in 1947, showing that in New York city there was one rat for every thirty-six persons and in Baltimore, with a warmer climate one rat for every fifteen persons.

More than a score of diseases are carried by domestic rats and mice which can be transmitted to man. Lymphocytic choriomeningitis is a virus disease carried by mice. Rats are not responsible for Rift Valley fever, but are susceptible, especially young rats. Rabies in rats is not unusual.

Several of the rickettsial group of diseases are found in rats and mice—rickettsial pox in the mouse and murine typhus fever in the rat. Domestic rats are susceptible to Rocky Mountain spotted fever and tsutsugamushi disease, but other animals are more important hosts.

Plague is by far the most serious disease carried by rats, and while it does not exist in rats in the United States at present, it is always a potential danger (sylvatic plague is found in ground squirrels in many western states). Salmonella food infections have been traced to rats and mice on numerous occasions. Tularemia has occurred in house mice but wild rodents and other animals and birds are responsible agents in the spread of the disease. Anthrax sometimes occurs in a house mice, hemorrhagic septicemia *(Pasteurella mul-*

tocida infection) is found in both rats and mice without causing any apparent symptoms, and pseudotuberculosis is occasionally found in rats. Swine erysipelas occurs in rats and the infection may be passed back to hogs that eat such rats. The streptobacillus causing Haverhill fever (rat-bite fever) finds its principal reservoir in the rat.

Rats and mice likewise are reservoirs of the spirillum causing sodoku, the common form of rat-bite fever. Leptospirosis is a common infection of rats and mice, the animals seemingly being not at all inconvenienced. Endemic relapsing fever is occasionally found in house mice, but they are unimportant factors.

Fungous diseases in rats and mice are not numerous. Sporotrichosis occurs sporadically, especially in Norway rats. Histoplasmosis has also been found in the Norway rat as well as the roof rat. Adiaspiromycosis is possibly an infection of rats and mice along with other rodents, but human infections are rare.

The several animal parasites which afflict both rats and man are sometimes important. Amebiasis and American trypanosomiasis are usually transmitted to man from other sources while sarcocystiasis and toxoplasmosis find reservoirs in numerous animals and are somewhat rare in man. Trichinosis is common in the rat, but the hog is the usual source of human infection. However, rats are important because hogs eat them and may thus be infected. The rat tapeworm is acquired by man from swallowing insects that carry the tapeworm eggs. The dwarf tapeworm is transmitted through food contaminated with rat droppings. Echinococcosis may be found in rats along with many other animals. Lung fluke disease (paragonomiasis) and schistosomiasis do not occur in man in the United States.

The rat mite, *(Bdellonyssus bactoi),* causes dermatitis in man.

THE DOMESTIC FOWL AND OTHER POULTRY

Poultry is the most numerous of all livestock on the farm. The domestic fowl, the "barnyard fowl," has been decreasing in numbers in the United States, due to the decrease in the number of farms. In 1930, there were 378,878,281 hens and chickens on 5,372,397 farms, twenty five years later there were 340,489,127 such birds on 2,406,338 farms. However, during this time there was a large increase in the number of commercial poultry farms which raised most of the poultry for broilers as well as produced most of the eggs for human consumption.

Turkeys have become increasingly important over the last forty years. In 1910, there were less than four million turkeys raised on 870,000 farms, mostly four or five birds to a farm. Turkey raising since that time has become a highly commercial industry with 63,000,000 birds in 1954, mostly on commercial farms some of which include as many as 20,000 in a single flock.

The extent of duck raising in the United States has not changed much in the last quarter century. About 11,000,000 ducks are found on farms, the only change being a larger number of birds on fewer farms.

Geese are comparatively unimportant in the poultry industry in the United States. In 1929, there were nearly 4,000,000 such birds on farms while the number dropped to less than 2,000,000 in 1954. Most of the geese were confined to a few areas in the country.

The diseases of poultry are numerous, some of which afflict man. The hen is assuming an increasing importance as a carrier of human disease (Table 82).

The viruses of some of the arthropod-borne encephalitides find natural reservoirs in poultry and other birds. The hen is implicated in western encephalitis, St. Louis encephalitis and Murray Valley encephalitis and, with the duck and turkey eastern encephalitis. The virus of Newcastle disease is present in the domestic fowl, turkey, duck, goose and guinea fowl—in fact, all avian species. Ornithosis, once considered strictly a disease of psittacine birds, is now much more widespread, the hen and the turkey being important hosts.

Several bacterial diseases are carried by poultry. Brucellosis of all three types occurs in the fowl and the turkey. Listeriosis and pseudotuberculosis are found in the hen, duck, goose and turkey. *Pasteurella multocida* infection (hemorrhagic septicemia) occurs in both the fowl and the duck. Many *Salmonella* types have been isolated from poultry and egg products and the domestic fowl has been considered the main reservoir of these organisms. The turkey, duck and goose also are responsible for human infections. Swine erysipelas has been encountered in both the fowl and the turkey. Tuberculosis of the avian type is common in all poultry but fortunately man is not very susceptible. The organisms of avian tuberculosis are found in the fowl, turkey, duck and goose. The hen has been charged with being a carrier of diphtheria bacilli. Ducks and geese are subject to anthrax but the fowl seems to be immune; however, live anthrax

TABLE 82

DISEASES TRANSMITTED FROM THE DOMESTIC FOWL AND OTHER POULTRY TO MAN

Virus Diseases

Arthropod-Borne Viral Encephalitides
    Eastern encephalitis—fowl, turkey,
      duck
    Murray Valley encephalitis—fowl
    St. Louis encephalitis—fowl
    Western encephalitis—fowl
Newcastle disease—fowl, turkey, duck,
    goose
Ornithosis—fowl, turkey, duck

Bacterial Diseases

Anthrax—duck, goose
Botulism—fowl
Brucellosis, *Br. abortus*—fowl, turkey
Brucellosis, *Br. melitensis*—fowl, turkey
Brucellosis, *Br. suis*—fowl, turkey
Diphtheria—fowl
Gas gangrene—duck, fowl
Hemorrhagic septicemia—fowl, duck
Listeriosis—fowl, duck, goose
Pseudotuberculosis—fowl, turkey, duck,
    goose
Salmonellosis—fowl, turkey, duck,
    goose
Swine erysipelas—fowl, turkey
Tuberculosis, avian type—fowl, turkey,
    duck, goose

Fungous Diseases

Aspergillosis—young poultry, (chicks,
    ducklings, poults)
Cryptococcosis—fowl
Histoplasmosis—fowl
Ringworm (*Trichophyton gallinae*)—
    fowl

Cestode Diseases

Duck tapeworm infection—duck

Tremode Diseases

Echinostomiasis (*Echinostomia revolutum*)—fowl, duck, goose

Arthropod Diseases

Fowl mite dermatitis—fowl

bacilli or spores may be carried on the beak of the fowl that has feed on the carcass of an animal dead of anthrax. The fowl carries in its intestine the spores of gas gangrene and the duck botulinum spores.

Among the fungous diseases cryptococcus and histoplasmosis are probably carried by the normal hen because both *Cryptococcus neo-formans* and *Histoplasma capsulatum* are often isolated from areas inhabited by them. Aspergillosis is an infection of domestic birds often assuming epizootic proportions, young chickens, ducklings and turkeys being especially susceptible. Fowls are the chief reservoir of *Trichophyton gallinae,* the cause of favus in birds and occasionally ringworm in man, *Microsporum gypseum* has occasionally found in fowls.

The animal parasites of poultry are not a great menace to man. The duck tapeworm is not often found in persons. Echinostomiasis *(Echinostoma revolutum)* of the duck, goose and fowl does not occur in the United States.

The fowl mite, *Dermanyssus gallinae,* causes an itchy dermatitis in persons who come in contact with poultry carrying this mite.

WILD ANIMALS AND BIRDS

Many wild animals harbor agents of disease with which man might become infected, but contact with man is so remote that comparatively few infections take place (Table 83).

TABLE 83

DISEASES TRANSMITTED FROM WILD ANIMALS AND BIRDS TO MAN

Virus Diseases

Arthropod-Borne Viral Encephalitides
  California encephalitis—ground squirrel and rabbit (probably)
  Central European encephalitis—mole, hedgehog, porcupine, ground squirrel, chipmunk, wild rats and mice, grouse, passerine birds
  Chikungunya fever—forest animals suspected
  Colorado tick fever—porcupine, ground squirrel, pine squirrel, chipmunk, field mice
  Crimean hemorrhagic fever—hares
  Diphasic meningo-encephalitis—mole, hedgehog, porcupine, chipmunk, ground squirrels, wild rats and mice, passerine birds
  Eastern encephalitis—swamp birds, pheasant, ground squirrels.
  Ilheus encephalitis—monkey, marmoset, other wild rodents and marsupials
  Japanese B encephalitis—marsh birds
  Jungle yellow fever—monkey, marsupials, wild rodents
  Korean hemorrhagic fever—insectivores and wild rodents suspected
  Kyasanur forest disease—monkey
  Louping ill—ground squirrels, chipmunk, porcupine, wild rats and mice, passerine birds
  Murray Valley encephalitis—swamp birds (15 species), land birds (7 species), opossum, fox.
  Omsk hemorrhagic fever—wild rodents.
  Powassan encephalitis—wild animal hosts suspected.
  Rift Valley fever—Veld and forest rodents probably.
  Russian spring-summer encephalitis—mole, hedgehog, ground squirrel, chipmunk, porcupine, wild rats and mice, grouse.
  St. Louis encephalitis—wild birds.
  Venezuelan encephalitis—wild host suspected.
  Western encephalitis—wild birds, squirrel, deer.

TABLE 83—*(cont'd)*

Virus Diseases—*cont'd*

Chickenpox—chimpanzee, gorilla, orangutan.
Common cold—chimpanzee.
Encephalomyocarditis—squirrels, mongoose, monkey, baboon, chimpanzee.
Foot-and-mouth disease—deer, hedgehog, others.
Herpesvirus simiae infection—monkey.
Lymphocytic choriomeningitis—monkey, fox, cotton rat, chinchilla.
Measles—monkey.
Mumps—monkey.
Newcastle disease—quail, partridge, English sparrow, osprey, swan, crow, marten, starling, owl, dove, others.
Ornithosis—wild parrots, parakeets, English sparrow, tern, gull, pheasant.
Rabies—bat, wolf and other wild canines, skunk, squirrel, other animals.
Salivary gland virus infection—monkey, others.

Rickettsial Diseases

Murine typhus fever—cotton rat, rice rat, meadow mouse, whitefooted mouse, golden mouse, dwarf mouse, garden mouse, cotton mouse, squirrels, rabbit, opossum, hedgehog, chimpanzee, monkey.
Q fever—bandicoot, brush animals, wild rodents, wild birds.
Rickettsial pox—wild rodents.
Rocky Mountain spotted fever—squirrels, woodchuck, cotton tail rabbit, others.
Tsutsugamushi disease—field rats and mice, vole, swamp hen, and other swamp birds, bush hen, parrot, and other wild birds, monkey, buffalo.

Bacterial Diseases

Anthrax—bear, civet cat, badger, tiger, jaguar, fox, lion, leopard, puma, bob-cat, raccoon, mink, coypu, rabbit, deer, antelope, buffalo, elephant, and on feet and bill of buzzard, owl, vulture, other birds.
Botulism—wild birds; organisms are intestinal inhabitants of many animals.
Brucellosis—deer, American buffalo, European hare, jack rabbit.
Gas gangrene—wild birds; organisms found in intestines of many animals.
Glanders—ferret, mole, field mice.
Listeriosis—raccoon, fox, chinchilla, gerbille, rabbit, eagle, capercallie.
Melioidosis—rabbit, guinea pig (in captivity).
Plague—rodents and lagamorpha, 227 species; occasional case in owl, shrew, badger, ferret, suricate, yellow mongoose, monkey.
Salmonellosis—skunk, monkey, baboon, rabbit, pigeon, quail and other birds.
Swine erysipelas—mouse, pigeon.
Tetanus—spores found in the intestines of many animals.
Tularemia—rabbit, beaver, muskrat, prairie dog, woodchuck, water rat, field mouse, deer mouse, tree squirrel, chipmunk, quail, grouse, pheasant, sage hen, gull, horned owl.
Tuberculosis, avian—wild birds in captivity.
Tuberculosis, bovine—monkeys, apes, other wild animals in captivity.
Tuberculosis, human—monkey and apes in captivity.

Spirochetal Diseases

Endemic relapsing fevers—armadillo, opossum, bat, weasel, tree squirrel, chipmunk, woodchuck, chimpanzee, wild birds.
Leptospirosis—chimpanzee, deer, jackal, fox, wildcat, raccoon, mongoose, skunk, opossum, bandicoot, hedgehog, muskrat, nutria, bat, field rats and mice.
Rat-bite fever (Sodoku)—wild rodents, bite of weasel, ferret, other carnivores.

Fungous Diseases

Actinomycosis—deer, bear, tapir, antelope, muskrat.
Adiaspiromycosis—rabbit, carnivores, insectivores, rodents.
Aspergillosis—wild birds in captivity.
Coccidioidomycosis—chinchilla, coyote, gorilla, monkey.
Cryptococcosis—cheetah, monkey, civet cat, ferret, pigeon.

TABLE 83—*(cont'd)*

Funguous Diseases—(cont'd)

Cutaneous streptothricosis—deer, eland.
Histoplasmosis—fox, skunk, opossum, marmot, bat, wild birds.
Nocardiosis—rabbit, kangaroo, wallaby.
Ringworm—monkey, chinchilla, muskrat, squirrel, fox, rabbit, tiger.

Protozoan Diseases

Amebiasis (*E. histolytica*)—monkey.
Balantidiasis—monkey.
Giardiasis—chinchilla.
Leishmaniasis, cutaneous—wild rodents, wild canines.
Leishmaniasis, visceral—wild rodents, wild canines.
Malaria, quartan and simian—monkey and other apes.
Sarcocystiasis—rabbit, other animals.
Toxoplasmosis—wild rodents, mink, wild birds.
Trypanosomiasis, African—antelope, wild game.
Trypanosomiasis, American—monkey, bat, opossum, armadillo, ferret, squirrels and
  other wild rodents.

Nematode Diseases

Acanthocheilonemiasis—monkey, chimpanzee.
Brugia infection—wild felines.
Dracuntiasis—fur bearing animals.
Gongylonemiasis—bear, monkey, hedgehog.
Larva migrans, cutaneous—fox.
Larva migrans, filarial—fox, wolf.
Loaiasis—chimpanzee.
Oesophagostomum infection—monkey.
Strongylodiasis—chimpanzee.
Ternidens infection—monkey.
Trichinosis—walrus, bear, other carnivores.

Cestode Diseases

Ancylostomiasis—wild carnivores.
Bertiella infection—monkey.
Diphyllobothriasis—bear, fish eating mammals.
Echinococcosis (*E. granulosus*)—fox, wolf, dingo, moose, caribou, reindeer, wild rodents.
Echinococcosis (*E. multilocularis*)—fox, wild mice.

Trematode Diseases

Clonorchiasis—wildcat, marten, badger, mink.
Heterophydiasis—fox, other wild animals and birds.
Metagonomiasis—wild birds, fish eating mammals.
Paragonomiasis (*P. kellicoti*)—mink, muskrat, wildcat, fox.
Paragonomiasis (*P. westermani*)—wildcat, tiger, panther, wolf, wild rats.
Schistosomiasis (*Sch. japonicum*)—skunk, mole, wild rats and mice, deer, water buffalo.
Schistosomiasis (*Sch. haemotobium*)—monkey.
Schistosomiasis (*Sch. mansoni*)—monkey.

Arthropod Diseases

Chigger mite dermatitis (*Trombucula irritans*)—wild birds and rodents, other animals.
Chigoe or jigger flea dermatitis (*Tunga penetrams*)—many wild animals.
Dog mite dermatitis (*Demodex folliculorum*)—wild canines and felines.
Oestrus ovis conjunctivitis—wild sheep and goats, game animals.
Ox bot (*Hypoderma bovis*)—deer, game animals.
Rat mite dermatitis (*Bdellonyssus bacoti*)—wild rats and mice.

Neoplastic Diseases

Mammalian virus tumor—monkey.

The marsupials are relatively not very important. The opossum is a host of histoplasmosis, leptospirosis, murine typhus fever, American trypanosomiasis and endemic relapsing fever in the United States and Murray Valley fever in Australia, while the bandicoot carries Q fever and leptospirosis. In Trinidad marsupials are a host of Ilheus fever. The kangaroo is subject to nocardiosis.

Insectivores are suspected hosts of Korean hemorrhagic fever and adiaspiromycosis. The shrew sometimes carries plague. The mole is subject to glanders, and together with the hedgehog is a factor in the spread of Russian spring-summer encephalitis, Central European encephalitis and diphasic meningo-encephalitis. In addition the hedgehog spreads leptospirosis and carries the round worm causing gongylonemiasis as well as being implicated in murine typhus fever.

The *Chiroptera* includes bats and flying foxes (fruit bats). In the United States bats are an important source of rabies and a lesser menace in American tryponosomias (Chagas' disease), pseudotuberculosis, endemic relapsing fever, leptospirosis and histoplasmosis.

The carnivores are a very large group of animals of world-wide distribution. (The dog and the cat are discussed elsewhere, pages 891). The bear has caused trichinosis when the flesh has been eaten without sufficient cooking. It also carries the tapeworm *Diphyllobothriam latum* and the round worm *Gongylonema pulchrum*. Actinomycosis is occasionally found. The bear likewise may spread anthrax along with the civet cat, badger, tiger, jaguar, leopard and puma. The badger is involved also in a rare case of plague. The raccoon is susceptible to listeriosis, and the raccoon and the bobcat are both implicated in the spread of anthrax, vesicular stomatitis and leptospirosis. The weasel is a host of adiaspiromycosis and endemic relapsing fever, the mink of adiaspiromycosis, anthrax, pseudotuberculosis, toxoplasmosis and cryptococcosis, the otter of pseudotuberculosis, the skunk of histoplasmosis, adiaspiromycosis, salmonellosis, leptospirosis and vesicular stomatitis, and the ferret of listeriosis and plague. The fox is sometimes a factor in the spread of rabies, anthrax, listeriosis, pseudotuberculosis, leptospirosis, histoplasmosis, ringworm *(Trichophyton mentagrophytes)*, echinococcosis and both cutaneous and filarial larva migrans. The wolf has been implicated in rabies, echinococcosis and filarial larva migrans, while the lion may carry anthrax and pseudotuberculosis the dingo of Australia echinococcosis, the coyotte rabies and coccidioidomycosis and the cheetah, the civet cat and the ferret cryptococcosis. The jackal and the mongoose are infected with leptospirosis.

The *Pinnipedia* are of small importance in the spread of disease to man. The walrus sometimes is infected with trichinosis. One case of blastomycosis was found in the sea lion.

The primates, other than man, suffer from numerous diseases many of which may be passed on to man. The monkey is the chief offender, the list including more than a score of infections. They are encephalomyocarditis, endemic relapsing fever, Ilheus encephalitis, jungle yellow fever, Herpres virus simiae infection, lymphocytic choriomeningitis, murine typhus fever, pseudotuberculosis, plague, malaria of both the quartan and simian types, salmonellosis, salivary gland virus infection, tsutsugamushi disease and rabies. Fungous diseases found in the monkey include actomomycosis, cryptococcosis, coccidioidomycosis and ringworm *(Microsporum canis, M. distortum and M. gypseum)*. Among the animal parasites carried by the monkey are those of acanthocheilonemiasis, ambiasis, balantidiasis, bertiella infection, gongylonemiasis, oesophagostomum infection, schistosomiasis *(Sch. mansoni* and *Sch. haematobium)*, ternidens infection and American trypanosomiasis (Chagas' disease). Subcutaneous tumors, caused by a virus, are epidemic in some monkeys and may be transmitted to man through the broken skin. Human diseases which the monkey may acquire and pass back to man include measles, mumps and tuberculosis (monkeys only in captivity). Other apes which acquire human infections are the gorilla which may be infected with coccidioidomycosis and chickenpox, the orangutan which suffers from chickenpox, and the chimpanzee which has been known to acquire both chickenpox and the common cold. Other diseases with which the chimpanzee is afflicted are encephalomyocarditis, murine typhus fever and endemic relapsing fever, together with the intestinal parasites of acanthocheilonemiasis, loaiasis and strongylodiasis. The baboon has been implicated with encephalomyocarditis. An epidemic in baboons due to *Salmonella typhimurium* was reported by Scott. An epidemic in chimpanzees, studied by Wilbert, showed spirochetes similar to *Leptospira icterhemorrhagiae*.

Wild rodents vary in size from tiny mice weighing a few ounces to the capybara weighing 220 pounds. (The latter is easily domesticated.) Over 200 wild representatives of *Rodentia* are naturally infected with plague and are capable of transmitting the disease to man. Domestic rats *(R. norvegicus, R. rattus rattus* and *R. rattus alexandrinus)* however, have been responsible for most of the epidemics in man. Various rodents are hosts (or suspected hosts) of Rift Valley fever, Ilheus encephalitis, Korean hemorrhagic fever, Omsk hemorrhagic fever, Q fever, rickettsialpox, jungle yellow fever, pseudotuberculosis, American trypansomiasis, both the cutaneous and visceral forms of leishmaniasis, toxoplasmosis and adiaspiromycosis. Wild rats carry Russian spring-summer encephalitis, Central European encephalitis, louping ill, diaphasic meningoencephalitis, tsutsugamushe disease and schistosomiasis *(Sch. japonicum)*. The cotton rat harbors the organisms of encephalomyocarditis, lymphocytic choriomeningitis and murine typhus fever. The rice rat also carries murine typhus fever, while the water rat carries tularemia and adiaspiromycosis.

Field mice and forest mice may be infected with Russian spring-summer encephalitis, Central European encephalitis, louping ill and diphasic meningo-encephalitis. Field mice also may be carriers of Colorado tick fever, tularemia, murine typhus fever and schistosomiasis *(Sch. japonicum)*. Murine typhus fever has been found in the garden mouse, dwarf mouse, cotton mouse, golden mouse, meadow mouse and white footed mouse. The deer mouse has been responsible for tularemia. Wild rats and mice are hosts of the rat mite, *Bdellonyssus bacoti,* that causes an itchy dermatitis in man. More than a score of wild rats, mice and other rodents are infected with leptospirosis.

Squirrels of various species may carry American trypanosomiasis, adiaspiromycosis, encephalomyocarditis, murine typhus fever, Rocky Mountain spotted fever, rabies, western encephalitis and ringworm *(Trichophyton mentagrophytes* and *Keratinomyces ajello)*. Ground squirrels in different parts of the world are susceptible also to eastern encephalitis, Russian spring-summer encephalitis, Central European encephalitis, louping ill, diphasic meningoencephalitis and Colorado tick fever. Tree squirrels may carry endemic relapsing fever and tularemia. Pine squirrels carry Colorado tick fever. Other small rodents which from time to time are infected include the vole with adiaspiromycosis and tsutsugamushi disease, the chinchilla with pseudotuberculosis, listeriosis, lymphocytic choriomeningitis, giardiasis, coccidioidomycosis and ringworm *(Microspirum canis* and *Trichopphyton mentagrophytes)*. The chipmunk carries tularemia, endemic relapsing fever, Colorado tick fever, Russian spring-summer encephalitis, Central European encephalitis, louping ill and diphasic meningoencephalitis. The shrew is suspected of being host to Korean hemorrhagic fever.

The beaver and muskrat both carry tularemia and adiaspiromycosis, while the latter may be infected as well with leptospirosis, Omsk hemorrhagic fever, actinomycosis and ringworm *(Trichophyton mentagraphytes)*. The prairie dog is infected with plague and tularemia and the wood chuck with histoplasmosis, murine typhus fever, tularemia, Rocky Mountain spotted fever and endemic relapsing fever. The porcupine may be the host of Colorado tick fever, louping ill, diphasic meningo-encephalitis, Central European encephalitis and Russian spring-summer encephalitis. The nutria (coypu) carries anthrax, leptospirosis and pseudotuberculosis while the gerbille carries listeriosis.

The guinea pig, domesticated from the wild cony (cony pig) of South America, is a natural subject to a variety of infections, including salmonellosis, listeriosis, melioidosis, murine typhus fever, actinomycosis, histoplasmosis and ringworm *(Trichophyton mentagrophytes* and *Keratinomyces ajello)*.

Rabbits and hares *(Lagomorpha)* are subject to a considerable number of diseases which man may acquire. Most common is tularemia, but also sometimes listeriosis, salmonellosis, anthrax, pseudotuberculosis and brucellosis. Plague is a serious disease in these animals. Antibodies of California encephalitis have been found in rabbits and they are suspected of being implicated in Crimean hemorrhagic fever. Rabbits share with many other animals the responsibility of perpetuating Rocky Mountain spotted fever and murine typhus fever. Fungous diseases include adiaspiromycosis, nocardiosis and ringworm *(Trichophyton mentagrophytes)*. They carry in their intestines, without damage to themselves, tetanus spores. Rabbits domesticated for laboratory use are subject to natural infection with melioidosis and numerous other diseases.

The even-toed hoofed wild animals are not responsible for as many diseases as are domestic members of this order (cow, sheep, goat, hog), probably because of their relative isolation from each other and from man. Deer suffer from anthrax, brucellosis, pseudotuberculosis, actinomycosis and vesicular stomatitis. They acquire foot-and-mouth disease on occasion and western encephalitis in the same way that man is infected, by mosquito bite. Ox bot also afflicts them as well as other game animals. The moose, caribou and rein-deer carry echinococcosis and the latter suffer from pseudotuberculosis as well. Antelope may be infected with actinomycosis and anthrax and, in Africa, with African trypanosomiasis. The wild hog suffers from the virus of vesicular stomatitis. Buffalo in different parts of the world carry anthrax, brucellosis, tsutsugamushi disease and schistosomiasis *(Sch. japonicum)*.

Other wild animals are of little significance in human disease. Wild horses and wild asses *(Perissodactyla)* probably are subject to the same afflictions as their domestic relatives. The tapir may be infected with actinomycosis. The armadillo *(Edentata)* is infected with endemic relapsing fever and American trypanosomiasis. The elephant *(Probiscidea)* is subject to anthrax and actinomycosis.

Wild birds carry a variety of ailments that may be transmitted to man, although contact is not as intimate as with domestic poultry. Hoogstrall has called attention to migrating birds as a factor in the spread of disease, especially by ticks. The process, however,—the migration of tick infected birds,—has been going on "from time immemorial," and present migrations can not do much more harm than reinforce an already infested area. The problem is a serious one, on the other hand, for new diseases appear from time to time, and old diseases develop new characteristics, or a geographical area changes climatic conditions favorable to ticks that could not previously exist here.

Afflictions charged to various wild birds include Newcastle disease, endemic relapsing fever, tsutsugamushi disease, heterophydiasis, toxoplasmosis and metagonimus infection. A long list of birds are responsible for western encephalitis while others carrly Ilheus encephalitis. Various swamp birds carry eastern encephalitis and fifteen species of water birds and seven species of land birds carry Murray Valley encephalitis. The heron is infected with Murray Valley fever and Japanese B encephalitis, the mourning dove and flicker with St. Louis encephalitis, the grouse and many passerines (perching birds) with Russian spring-summer encephalitis, Central European encepaalitis, louping ill and diphasic meningo-encephalitis. Three kinds of grouse are naturally infected with tularemia. The pheasant carries eastern encephalitis, tularemia, psittacosis and pseudotuberculosis. The swan, blackbird and partridge may be afflicted with pseudotuberculosis and Newcastle disease. The sage hen and horned owl can be infected with tularemia and the eagle and capercaille with listeriosis. The buzzard, vulture and owl may carry anthrax spores on feet and beak while the owl also may be infected with pseudo-tuberculosis, Newcastle disease and occasionally plague. Quail are infected with tularemia, salmonellosis and Newcastle disease. Wild parrots are responsible for ornithosis and may carry tsutsuganmushi disease. The gull can be infected with tularemia and ornithosis and English sparrows with ornithosis and Newcastle disease. The osprey, crow, martin and starling are all subject to Newcastle disease. Wild birds are hosts of numberous ectoparasites, among them the chigger mite and the fowl mite. The pigeon, a pest of barnyard and city street alike, usually has allegiance to no master and therefore can be considered "wild." Besides ornithosis, salmonellosis, swine erysipelas and Newcastle disease, it probably carries the organisms of crypto-coccosis. Even though not infected with the disease, *Cryptococcus neoformans* is found in the excreta of the bird. Wild birds in zoos and as pets in the home are afflicted with aspergillosis.

Wild birds and animals are often taken into the home as pets, where they are a potential hazard. In the United States it was estab-lished in 1957 there were 100,000 monkeys, 10,000 skunks and 6000 turtles kept as pets. The guinea pig, white rat and mouse, the rabbit, parrot, parakeet, lovebird and other psittacine birds all are common inhabitants of the home, sharing intimate contact with its occupants. In fact there is scarcely a wild animal or bird that is not from time to time captured and kept as a pet. The hazards consist not only of the animal diseases which may be conveyed to man, but also some-times human diseases that are acquired by animals and birds and passed back to man.

TABLE 84

REVIEW OF DISEASES WHICH ANIMALS TRANSMIT TO MAN, WITH THE ANIMAL HOSTS

Disease	Etiologic Agent	Common Animal Host	Usual Method of Human Infection
Acanthocheilonemiasis	*Acanthocheilinema streptocera*	Monkey Chimpanzee	Mosquito bite
Actinomycosis	*Actinomyces bovis* *A. israeli* *A. bandetti*	Cow, horse, hog, many domestic and wild animals	Method uncertain

TABLE 84—(*cont'd*)

Disease	Etiologic Agent	Common Animal Host	Usual Method of Human Infection
Adiaspiromycosis	*Emmonsia parva* *E. crescens*	Rabbit, beaver, muskrat, water-rat, vole, squirrel, mouse, mink, skunk, weasel, pine marten	Contact
Amebiasis, (amebic dysentery)	*Entamoeba histolytica*	Dog, cat, monkey, rat	Contaminated food and drinking water
Amebiasis, porcine	*Entamoeba polecki*	Hog	Contaminated food and water
Amphistomiasis (see Gastrodiscoides infection)			
Ancylostomiasis (dog hookworm)	*Ancylostoma ceylonicum*	Dog, cat, wild carnivores	Through broken skin
Anthrax	*Bacillus anthracis*	Cow, horse, sheep, goat, hog, dog, cat, hen, wild animals and birds	Contact; hair and hide; biting insects; contaminated food
Antibiotics in animal products (see Chemicals)			
Anthelmintics in animal products (see Chemicals)			
Ascariasis, porcine	*Ascaris lumbricoides* var. *suum*	Hog	Contaminated food and water
Aspergillosis	*Aspergillus fumigatus* and other members of species	Young poultry, horse, cow, lamb, cat, hog	Inhalation of spores, probably
B virus infection (see Herpes virus simiae infection)			
Balantidiasis	*Balantidium coli*	Monkey, dog	Food and drinking water contaminated with animal feces
Beef tapeworm infection (see Taeniasis, bovine)			
Bertiella infection	*Bertiella studeri*	Monkey	Swallowing infected mite
Bilharziasis (see Schistosomiasis)			
Blastomycosis (North American)	*Blastomyces dermatitidis*	Dog, horse	Inhalation, trauma
Bot (see ox bot, also oestrus ovis conjunctivitis)			
Botulism	*Clostridium botulinum* and *Cl. parabotulinum*	Birds, hog, cow, other animals	Home-canned foods
Boutonneuse fever	*Rickettsia conori*	Dog	Tick bite
Brazilian typhus	*Rickettsia rickettsi*	Dog	Tick bite
Brucellosis	*Brucella abortus* *Br. melitensis* *Br. suis*	Cow, sheep, goat, hog, horse, mule, dog, cat, deer, buffalo, European hare, jackrabbit, hen, turkey	Through milk, and by contact (abrasions and inhalation)
Brugia infection	*Brugia malayi*	Cat, wild felines	*Anopheles* or *Mansonia* mosquito bite

TABLE 84—*(cont'd)*

Disease	Etiologic Agent	Common Animal Host	Usual Method of Human Infection
California encephalitis	Virus	Horse, cow, rabbit, ground squirrel probably	Mosquito bite
Canicola fever (see Leptospirosis)			
Cat scratch disease	Virus	Cat	Cat scratch or bite; puncture wounds
Cattle bot (see Ox bot)			
Central European encephalitis	Virus	Sheep, goat, wild rodents	Tick bite
Chemicals in animal products	Sulfonamides Antibiotics Anthelmintics Insecticides, Others	Cow, sheep, goat, hog, hen	By ingesting milk or meat
Chickenpox (varicella)	Virus	Chimpanzee, orangutan, gorilla	Contact
Chigger mite dermatitis	*Trombicula irritans*	Wild birds and rodents, other animals	Contact
Chigoe dermatitis (jigger flea)	*Tunga penetrans*	Dog, hog, other animals	Contact with soil contaminated by infested animal
Clonorchiasis	*Clonorchis sinensis*	Cat, dog, hog, wild animals	Eating raw fish
Coccidioidomycosis	*Coccidioides immitis*	Dog, cow, hog, horse, sheep, monkey, rodents, other animals	Inhalation and through wounds
Colombian spotted fever	*Rickettsia rickettsi*	Dog	Tick bite
Colorado Tick fever	Virus	Porcupine, ground squirrel, pine squirrel, chipmunk, field mice	Tick bite
Common cold	Virus	Chimpanzee	Contact
Contagious ecthyma of sheep and goats	Virus	Sheep, goats	Contact; through skin abrasions
Cowpox	Virus	Cow	Skin abrasions and vaccination
Creeping eruption (see Larva migrans, also ox bot)			
Crimean hemorrhagic fever	Virus	Hares	Tick bite
Cryptococcosis	*Cryptococcus neoformans*	Cow, horse, hog, goat, other animals and birds	Method uncertain, possibly inhalation or through milk
Cutaneous streptothricosis	*Dermatophilus congolensis*	Cow, goat, dog, horse, deer, eland	Contact
Cysticercosis (see Taeniasis, bovine and porcine)			
Diphasic meningoencephalitis	Virus	Sheep, goats, wild rodents and birds	Tick bite
Diphtheria	*Corynebacterium diphtheriae*	Cow, dog, cat, hen	Through milk and by contact

TABLE 84—(*cont'd*)

Disease	Etiologic Agent	Common Animal Host	Usual Method of Human Infection
Diphyllobothriasis	*Diphyllobothrium latum*	Dog, cat, bear, fish eating mammals	Eating raw fish
Dirofilariasis (see Larva migrans, filarial)			
Dog hookworm (see Ancylostomiasis)			
Dog mite dermatitis	*Demodex folliculorum*	Dog, cat, other animals	Contact
Dog tapeworm infection	*Dipylidium caninum*	Dog, cat	Swallowing infected fleas
Dracontiasis	*Dracunculus medinensis*	Dog, fur bearing animals	From drinking water
Duck tapeworm infection	*Drepanidotaenia lanceolata*	Duck	Contaminated water and food
Dwarf tapeworm infection	*Hymolepis nana*	Rat, mouse	From contaminated food
Eastern encephalitis	Virus	Small wild birds, duck, turkey, pheasant	Mosquito bite
Echinochasmus infection	*Echinochasmus perfoliatus*	Dog	Eating fresh water fish
Echinococcosis (Hydatid disease)	*Echinococcus granulosus*	Dog, cow, sheep, hog, wolf, dingo, camel, moose, caribou, reindeer, and rodents	Contaminated food and water; swallowing parasite eggs from dog feces
Echinococcosis	*Echinococcus multilocularis*	Fox, wild mice	By mouth
Echinostomiasis	*Echinostoma ilocanum*	Cat, dog, hog, rat	From eating infected snail
Echinostomiasis	*Echinostoma revolutum*	Duck, goose, hen	From mollusks
Encephalomyocarditis	Virus	Cotton rat, squirrels, mongoose, monkey, baboon, chimpanzee	Method in doubt
Endemic relapsing fevers	*Borrelia* genus of spirochetes	Wild rodents, birds	Tick bite
Epizootic lymphangitis	*Histoplasma farciminosum*	Horse, mule, donkey	Contact
Equine infectious anemia	Virus	Horse, mule, donkey	Fly bite, contact
Espundia (see Leishmaniasis)			
Fascioliasis	*Fasciola hepatica F. giganticum*	Sheep, cow, other herbivorous animals	Raw plant foods
Fasciolopsiasis	*Fasciolopsis buski*	Hog, dog	Raw aquatic plants
Favus (see Ringworm)			
Fish tapeworm infection (see Diphyllobothriasis)			
Foot-and-mouth disease	Virus	Cow, other cloven-footed animals	Contact
Fowl mite dermatitis	*Dermanyssus gallinae*	Hen	Contact
Gas gangrene	*Clostridium perfringens* and others	Cow, sheep, goat, hog, dog, cat, and intestines of other animals	Through broken skin

TABLE 84—(*cont'd*)

Disease	Etiologic Agent	Common Animal Host	Usual Method of Human Infection
Gastrodiscoides infection	*Gastrodiscoides hominis*	Hog	Contaminated food and drinking water
Giardiasis	*Giardia lamblia*	Chinchilla	Contaminated food or water
Glanders	*Actinobacillus mallei*	Horse, mule, donkey	Contact
Gnathostomiasis	*Gnathostoma hispidum*	Hog	Eating infected fish
Gnathostomiasis	*Gnathostoma spinigerum*	Dog, cat, other animals	Eating infected fish
Gongylonemiasis	*Gongylonema pulchrum*	Cow, hog, bear, monkey, hedgehog	Drinking contaminated water; eating infected cockroaches
Haplomycosis (see Adiaspiromycosis)			
Haverhill fever (see rat-bite fever)			
Hemorrhagic septicemia	*Pasteurella multocida*	Horse, cow, sheep, goat, hog, dog, cat, rat, poultry, others	Animal bite; contact; ingestion; obscure methods
Herpes-virus simiae infection	Virus	Monkey	Monkey bite or abrasions contaminated with monkey saliva
Heterophyiasis	*Heterophyes* sp.	Dog, cat, birds	Eating fresh water fish
Histoplasmosis	*Histoplasma capsulatum*	Dog, cat, cow, horse, rat, mouse, hen, bat, other wild animals	Inhalation of dust; sometimes ingestion
Hydatidosis (see Echinococcosis)			
Hypoderma bovis infection (see Ox bot)			
Ilheus encephalitis	Virus	Monkey, marmoset, marsupials	Mosquito bite
Influenza	Virus	Hog, hose, sheep, duck, suspected	Contact
Insecticides in animal products (see Chemicals)			
Japanese B encephalitis	Virus	Marsh birds, hog	Mosquito bite
Jungle yellow fever	Virus	Monkey, marsupials, jungle rodents	Mosquito bite
Kala-azar (see Leishmaniasis)			
Kenya typhus fever	*Rickettsia conori*	Dog	Tick bite
Korean hemorrhagic fever	Unknown	Insectivores and small rodents suspected	Chigger suspected
Kyasanur forest disease	Virus	Monkey	Tick bite
Larva migrans, bovine	*Bunostomum phlebotomum*	Cow	Through unbroken skin
Larva migrans, cutaneous	*Ancylostoma braziliense Uncinaria stenocephala*	Dog, cat, fox	Through unbroken skin

TABLE 84—*(cont'd)*

Disease	Etiologic Agent	Common Animal Host	Usual Method of Human Infection
Larva migrans, filarial	*Dirofilaria conjunctivae*	Dog, cat, fox, wolf	Mosquito bite
	D. immutis and other filaria of domestic animals	Dog, cat	Mosquito bite
Larva migrans, visceral	*Toxicara canis*	Dog, cat, domestic animals	Swallowing dog and cat round-worm eggs
Leishmaniasis, cutaneous Oriental sore (old world)	*Leishmania tropica*	Dog, other canines, wild rodents	Sandfly bite
Espundia (new world)	*L. braziliensis*	Dog, other canines, wild rodents	Sandfly bite
Leishmaniasis, visceral (Kala-azar)	*Leishmania donovani*	Dog, other canines, wild rodents	Sandfly bite
Leptospirosis	*Leptospira* spp.	Dog, cat, cow, hog, horse, sheep, goat, deer, bat, many wild animals	Contact, ingestion, immersion, exposure
Listeriosis	*Listeria monocytogenes*	Cow, sheep, hen, goat, pig, horse, rat, many animals and birds	Method uncertain
Loaiasis	*Loa loa*	Chimpanzee	Fly bite
Louping ill	Virus	Sheep, goat, cow, wild rodents and passerine birds	Tick bite and through milk
Lymphocytic chorio-meningitis	Virus	Mouse, dog, monkey, guinea pig, cotton rat, fox, chinchilla, hog, monkey	Food and dust
Malaria, quartan and simian	*Plasmodium malariae* and simium types	Monkey and higher apes	Anopheles mosquito bite
Mange mite dermatitis	*Sarcoptes* species	Horse, cow, sheep	Contact
Measles (rubeola)	Virus	Monkey, dog	Contact
Melioidosis	*Pseudomonas pseudomollei*	Rodents, cat, dog, sheep, goat, horse, rabbit	Mosquito bite, flea bite
Metagonimiasis	*Metagonimus* species	Birds, fish-eating mammals	Eating raw fish
Metastrongyliasis	*Metastrongylus elongatus*	Hog, sheep, cow	By mouth
Milk sickness	Trematol and other chemicals	Cow	Milk
Milkers nodules	Virus	Cow	Contact
Mite typhus (see Tsutsugamushi disease)			
Mumps	Virus	Monkey, dog, cat	Contact
Murine typhus fever	*Rickettsia mooseri*	Rats, many wild rodents, rabbit, chimpanzee, monkey	Flea bite
Murray Valley encephalitis	Virus	Many land and swamp birds, domestic fowl, opossum, fox, others	Mosquito bite
Nemotodiasis (see Larva migrans, visceral)			
Newcastle disease	Virus	Hen, turkey, all avian species	Contact

TABLE 84—(*cont'd*)

Disease	Etiologic Agent	Common Animal Host	Usual Method of Human Infection
Nocardiosis	*Nocardia asteroides N. brasiliensis*	Cow, goat, dog, cat, horse, hog, wild animals	Contact
Oesophagostomum infection	*Oesophagostomum* sp.	Monkey	Infective larvae by mouth
Oestrus ovis conjunctivitis (sheep bot)	*Oestrus ovis*	Sheep, goat, game animals	Fly maggots deposited on skin
Omsk hemorrhagic fever	Virus	Wild rodents	Tick bite
Opisthorchiasis	*Opisthorchis felineus O. viverini O. sinensis*	Dog, cat, other animals	Eating raw fresh water fish
Oriental lung fluke disease (see Paragonomiasis)			
Oriental sore (see Leishmaniasis cutaneous)			
Ornithosis	Virus	Psitticine birds, hen, pigeon, duck	Contact
Ostertagia infection	*Ostertagia* sp.	Cow, sheep, goat, other herbiverous animals	Food and water
Ox bot	*Hypoderma bovis* or *H. lineatum*	Cow, goat, horse, deer, game animals	Fly maggots deposited on skin
Paragonomiasis	*Paragonimus kellicoti*	Fur bearing animals	Eating raw crayfish
Paragonimiasis (Oriental lung fluke disease)	*Pargonimus westermani*	Dog, cat, hog, wild carnivores	Eating raw crayfish and crabs
Pasteurellosis (Pasteurella multocida infection—see Hemorrhagic septicemia)			
Pork tapeworm infection (see Taeniasis, porcine)			
Powassan encephalitis	Virus	Wild animal host suspected	Tick bite
Plague	*Pasteurella pestis*	Brown rat, black rat, roof rat and 227 other species of rodents and lagomorpha, monkeys, other animals	Flea bite and inhalation
Pseudocowpox (see Milkers nodules)			
Pseudotuberculosis	*Pasteurella pseudotuberculosis*	Sheep, hog, cat, monkey, fox, mink, many wild animals and birds	Method uncertain
Psittacosis (see Ornothosis)			
Q fever	*Coxiella burneti*	Cow, sheep, goat, bandicoot, other bush animals and wild birds	Tick bite; air borne; infection; milk
Rabies	Virus	Dog, wolf, coyote, skunk, fox, bat, all warm-blooded animals	Animal bites and abrasions
Radioactive materials in animal products	Various radioactive materials	Cow, sheep, goat, hog, hen	By ingesting milk or meat

TABLE 84—(cont'd)

Disease	Etiologic Agent	Common Animal Host	Usual Method of Human Infection
Rat-bite fever, Haverhill fever	*Streptobacillus moniliformis*	Rat, cow, weasel, squirrel	Rat bite, milk
Sodoku	*Spirillum minus*	Rat, mouse, cat, others	Rat bite
Rat mite dermatitis	*Bdellonyssus bacoti*	Rat	Contact
Rat tapeworm infection	*Hymolepis diminuta*	Rat, mouse	Swallowing infected insects
Relapsing fever, endemic (see Endemic relapsing fever)			
Rhinosporidiosis	*Rhinosporidium seeberi*	Cow, horse, mule	Method uncertain
Rickettsialpox	*Rickettsia akari*	Horse, mouse, wild rodents	Mite bite
Rift Valley fever	Virus	Sheep, cow, probably wild and forest rodents	Mosquito bite; contact
Ringworm, body (Tinea corporis)	Various *Microsporum* and *Trichophyton*	Many wild and domestic animals	Contact
Ringworm, scalp (Tinea capitis)	*Microsporium canis* *Trichophyton menta grophytes*, var. *grann-ulare* and other *Microsporum* and *Trichophyton*	Dog, cat, horse, monkey, many animals	Contact
Rocky Mountain spotted fever	*Rickettsia rickettsi*	Squirrel, rat, mouse, wood-chuck, cottontail rabbit, other wild animals and rodents	Tick bite or crushing tick on skin
Russian spring-summer encephalitis	Virus	Wild rodents	Tick bite
Salivary gland virus infection	Virus	Monkey, rat, mouse, others	Contact
Salmonellosis	*Salmonella* group of bacteria	Cow, sheep, hog, horse, dog, cat, rat, skunk, monkey, poultry, other birds	Infected meat, food contaminated by rat droppings
Sarcocystiasis	*Sarcocystis* sp.	Cow, sheep, horse, hog, rabbit, other mammals	Contaminated food and water
Scarlet fever (see Strepto-coccal infection)			
Schistosomiasis, bovine	*Schistosoma bovis*	Cow, sheep	Through the skin
Schistosomiasis, Bilharziasis	*Schistosoma japonicum*	Dog, cat, rat, cow, horse, deer, other animals	Through the skin
	Schistosoma haemato-bium	Monkey	Through the skin
	Schistosoma mansoni	Monkey	Through the skin
Scrub typhus (see Tsutsugamushi disease)			
Sealers finger (see Swine erysipelas)			
Sheep bot (see Oestrus ovis conjunctivitis)			
Sheep wireworm infection	*Haemonchus contortus*	Sheep, cow, goat	Drinking water

TABLE 84—*(cont'd)*

Disease	Etiologic Agent	Common Animal Host	Usual Method of Human Infection
Sodoku (see Rat-bite fever)			
South African tick fever	*Rickettsia pijperi*	Dog	Tick bite
Sporotrichosis	*Sporotrichum schenckii*	Rat, horse, mule, dog, other animals	Through broken skin, (animal bite or other injury)
Spotted fever (see Rocky Mountain spotted fever)			
St. Louis encephalitis	Virus	Wild birds, domestic hen	Mosquito bite
Staphylococcal infections	*Staphylococcus aureus*	Cow, hog	Ingestion of milk, contact
Streptococcal infection, hemolytic			
A. Scarlet fever	*Streptococcus pyogenes*	Cow, dog	Milk and contact
B. Streptococcal sore throat	*Str. epidemicus (str. pyogenes)*	Cow	Ingestion of milk
Streptothricosis, cutaneous	*Dermatophilus congolensis*	Goat, horse, eland, deer, cow, dog	Contact
Strongylodiasis	*Strongyloides stercoralis*	Dog, chimpanzee	Through the skin
Sulfonamides in animal products (see Chemicals)			
Swine erysipelas	*Erysipelothrix insidiosa*	Hog, sheep, rat, mouse, turkey, pigeon, young chickens	Through skin abrasions
Swineherds disease (see Leptospirosis)			
Syngamosis	*Syngamus laryngeus*	Cow, goat	By mouth
Taeniasis, bovine	*Taenia saginata*	Cow	Insufficiently cooked beef
Taeniasis, porcine	*Taenia solium*	Hog	Insufficiently cooked pork
Ternidens infection	*Ternidens deminutus*	Monkey	By mouth
Tetanus	*Clostridium tetani*	Horse, cow, rabbit, guinea pig, others	Through skin abrasions
Thelaziasis	*Thelazia californiensis*	Dog, cat	Method uncertain
Thelaziasis	*Thelazia callipaeda*	Dog	Method uncertain
Toxoplasmosis	*Toxoplasma* sp.	Rodents, birds, cow, hog, sheep, goat, dog, cat, mink	Method uncertain
Trichinosis	*Trichinella spiralis*	Hog, bear, walrus, dog, cat, rat	Insufficiently cooked pork and other flesh
Trichostrongylosis	*Trichostrongylus* sp.	Cow, sheep, goat, other herbivorous animals	Food and water
Trypanosomiasis, African	*Trypanosoma gambiense* and *Tr. rhodesiense*	Cow, sheep, horse, hog, antelope	By tsetse fly bite
Trypanosomiasis, American (Chagas' disease)	*Trypanosoma cruzi*	Dog, cat, hog, monkey, bat, opossum, armadillo, squirrel, other rodents	Fecal material of triatomid bug

TABLE 84—*(cont'd)*

Disease	Etiologic Agent		Usual Method of Human Infection
Tsutsugamushi disease (Scrub typhus, mite typhus)	*Rickettsia tsutsugamushi*	Field rats and mice, vole, swamp birds, parrot, monkey, bush hen	Mite bite
Tuberculosis, avian	*Mycobacterium avium*	Hen, hog, wild birds in captivity	Ingestion, inhalation, (human infection rare)
Tuberculosis, bovine	*Mycobacterium bovis*	Cow, hog, dog, goat, cat, horse	Ingestion of milk or meat, contact
Tuberculosis, human	*Mycobacterium tuberculosis*	Monkey, hog, dog	Ingestion of contaminated pork, contact
Tularemia	*Pasteurella tulareusis*	Rabbit, sheep, dog, cat, horse, cow, many wild animals and birds	Handling; ingestion; insect bite
Tumor virus infection	Virus	Monkey	Probably by bite of arthropod
Typhus fever (see Murine typhus fever)			
Vesicular stomatitis	Virus	Cow, horse, hog, deer, raccoon, bobcat, skunk	Contact and possibly insect bites
Vibriosis	*Vibrio fetus*	Cow, sheep	Contact, other methods uncertain
Warble fly (see ox bot and oestrus ovis conjunctivitis)			
Weil's disease (see Leptospirosis)			
West Nile fever	Virus	Wild birds	Mosquito bite
Western encephalitis	Virus	Wild birds, hen, horse, deer, squirrels	Mosquito bite
Venezuelan encephalitis	Virus	Horse, wild animal host suspected	Mosquito bite
Yellow fever (see Jungle yellow fever)			

INDEX

H